Psychotropic Drugs

EXPERIMENTAL AND CLINICAL PSYCHIATRY

Volume 1: HANDBOOK OF BIOLOGICAL PSYCHIATRY, *edited by Herman M. van Praag, Malcolm H. Lader, Ole J. Rafaelsen, and Edward J. Sachar*

Part I: Disciplines Relevant to Biological Psychiatry
Part II: Brain Mechanisms and Abnormal Behavior—Psychophysiology
Part III: Brain Mechanisms and Abnormal Behavior—Genetics and Neuroendocrinology

(in preparation)

Part IV: Brain Mechanisms and Abnormal Behavior—Chemistry
Part V: Drug Treatment in Psychiatry
Part VI: Practical Application of Psychotropic Drugs and Other Biological Treatments

Volume 2: A PSYCHODYNAMIC APPROACH TO ADOLESCENT PSYCHIATRY: THE MOUNT SINAI EXPERIENCE, *edited by Don R. Heacock*

Volume 3: PSYCHIATRIC CONSULTATION IN THE GENERAL HOSPITAL, *Lewis S. Glickman*

Volume 4: PSYCHOTROPIC DRUGS: PLASMA CONCENTRATION AND CLINICAL RESPONSE, *edited by Graham D. Burrows and Trevor R. Norman*

(other volumes in preparation)

Psychotropic Drugs

Plasma Concentration and Clinical Response

Edited by

GRAHAM D. BURROWS
TREVOR R. NORMAN
Department of Psychiatry
University of Melbourne
Parkville, Victoria, Australia

MARCEL DEKKER, INC. New York and Basel

Library of Congress Cataloging in Publication Data

Main entry under title:

Psychotropic drugs.

(Experimental and clinical psychiatry ; v. 4)
Includes bibliographical references and indexes.
1. Psychotropic drugs--Physiological effect.
2. Blood plasma--Effect of drugs on. I. Burrows,
Graham D. II. Norman, Trevor R., [date]
III. Series. [DNLM: 1. Psychotropic drugs--Blood.
2. Psychotropic drugs--Pharmacodynamics. W1 EX465
v. 4 / QV 77 P9754]
RM315.P8 615'.788 80-25685
ISBN 0-8247-1009-6

MARCEL DEKKER, INC.
270 Madison Avenue, New York, New York 10016

Current printing (last digit):
10 9 8 7 6 5 4 3 2 1

PRINTED IN THE UNITED STATES OF AMERICA

Foreword

This book makes a significant contribution to the field of plasma levels of psychotropic drugs and response.

The use of plasma levels to monitor treatment with anticonvulsants, cardiac glycosides, and some antirheumatic drugs is now routine in clinical medicine. In psychiatric practice lithium is the only drug in which regular plasma level estimations are obligatory.

With most psychotropic drugs there are considerable problems: firstly, in the actual assay of the active metabolite(s) and secondly, in planning studies that will provide data from which to come to conclusions about the relationships between plasma levels and therapeutic results. The authors of the chapters in this book review problems in their field as they exist today. It is a changing subject and it will be of interest to reread this book 10 years from now to see in what way progress has been made. As they are, almost any page from any of the papers could be the basis of continuing research.

I believe the book will be of special value to pharmacologists and psychiatrists in training and those in research. It should help each group understand the very real problems that are present in this field of study.

The editors are to be congratulated in achieving a book with chapters written by experts from different countries, providing an overview of this complex area in 1980.

Brian Davies
University of Melbourne
Parkville, Victoria, Australia

Preface

The advent of the psychotropic drugs in the 1950s revolutionized the treatment of psychiatric disorders, particularly in mania, depression, schizophrenia, and anxiety states. The understanding of the etiology of these disorders, while still mainly limited, has been facilitated by the use of pharmacological agents. Recently, attention has focused on the more efficient prescribing of psychotropic drugs, and a subdiscipline of psychiatry, clinical neuropsychopharmacology, has developed. Of paramount importance has been the issue of the relationship between plasma concentration and clinical effect. Many contradictory studies have now been reported in the literature, with no emergence of a consensus. This book is an attempt to present all the evidence relating to plasma level clinical effects of psychotropic drugs, and so provide a basis for further discussion. With this in mind, the book has arisen from people actively involved in the field and well known for their contributions to clinical psychopharmacology.

As editors we thank each of the contributors for his or her participation. We wish also to express our appreciation to Ms. Angela Lane and Mrs. Gertrude Rubinstein for secretarial and editorial assistance.

Graham D. Burrows
Trevor R. Norman

Contributors

William J. Annitto Second Annex Community Unit, Fair Oaks Hospital, Summit, New Jersey, and New Jersey Medical School, Newark, New Jersey, United States

Graham D. Burrows Department of Psychiatry, University of Melbourne, Parkville, Victoria, Australia

John L. Crammer Institute of Psychiatry, University of London, London, England

Stephen H. Curry* Department of Pharmacology and Therapeutics, The London Hospital Medical College, London, England

Mervyn J. Eadie Department of Medicine, University of Queensland, Brisbane, Queensland, Australia

Larry Evans Department of Psychiatry, University of Queensland, Brisbane, Queensland, Australia

Ann Fulton Department of Psychiatry, University of Melbourne, Parkville, Victoria, Australia

Samuel Gershon Department of Psychiatry, School of Medicine, New York University Medical Center, New York, New York, United States

Lars F. Gram† Western Psychiatric Institute and Clinic, University of Pittsburgh, Pittsburgh, Pennsylvania, United States

Present Affiliation

*College of Pharmacy, University of Florida, Gainesville, Florida, United States

†Department of Clinical Pharmacology, Institute of Pharmacology, Odense University, Odense, Denmark

Veronika E. Grimm* Department of Psychiatry, Karolinska Hospital, Stockholm, Sweden

Leo E. Hollister Psychopharmacology Research, Veterans Administration Hospital, and Department of Psychiatry and Pharmacology, Stanford University School of Medicine, Palo Alto, California, United States

William J. Lang Department of Pharmacology, University of Melbourne, Parkville, Victoria, Australia

Jan Lundström Astra Läkemedel AB, Research and Development Laboratories, Södertälje, Sweden

Kay P. Maguire Department of Psychiatry, University of Melbourne, Parkville, Victoria, Australia

George Moore Astra Pharmaceuticals Pty. Ltd., Medical Department, Sydney, New South Wales, Australia

Trevor R. Norman Department of Psychiatry, University of Melbourne, Parkville, Victoria, Australia

Sven-Ove Ögren Astra Läkemedel AB, Research and Development Laboratories, Södertälje, Sweden

George Sakalis Department of Psychiatry, New York University Medical Center, New York, New York, United States

Bruce A. Scoggins Howard Florey Institute of Experimental Physiology and Medicine, University of Melbourne, Parkville, Victoria, Australia

Göran Sedvall Department of Psychiatry, Karolinska Hospital, Stockholm, Sweden

Louis Traficante† Department of Psychiatry, New York University Medical Center, New York, New York, United States

Denis N. Wade Department of Clinical Pharmacology, University of New South Wales, and Department of Clinical Pharmacology, St. Vincent's Hospital, Sydney, New South Wales, Australia

Jeremy M. E. Wurm Department of Psychiatry, University of Melbourne, Parkville, Victoria, Australia

Present Affiliation

*The Hebrew University of Jerusalem and The Weizmann Institute of Science, Rehovot, Israel

†Department of Biobehavioral Sciences, Boston University Medical Center, Boston Massachusetts, United States

Contents

1

Pharmacological Basis of Mechanism of Action of Psychotropic Drugs

William J. Lang / *Department of Pharmacology, University of Melbourne, Parkville, Victoria, Australia*

I. INTRODUCTION

Substances that act primarily on the central nervous system (CNS) to modify behavior number among them many drugs of considerable significance. Man seems always to have been aware of the fact that substances of plant and animal origin can induce desirable or undesirable behavioral effects, and special significance has been attached to a variety of such preparations in primitive cultural or religious ceremonies throughout recorded history. Indeed, man's ingenuity has hardly been more evident than in his unlimited capacity to ferment alcohol successfully from whatever food source was available. The social use of the tranquilizing or the stimulant effects of alcoholic and caffeinated beverages is worldwide, and in both cases it far outweighs the valid therapeutic uses of these substances. Since the 1950s, the use of psychotropic drugs has increased to such an extent, both in psychiatric and general medical practice, that the drugs account for more than 20% of all prescriptions written. Despite the unquestioned benefit of such drugs, their use is not without problems. In addition to the difficulties associated with their inherent side effects and abuse liability, there is now concern also about their possible overuse. Perhaps greater understanding of the pharmacological basis of the actions of psychotropic drugs can lessen these shortcomings.

Classification of drugs acting on the CNS is not completely satisfactory. The most acceptable approach has been to subdivide psychotropic drugs on the basis of their principal clinical use. However, apart from the difficulties associated with their overlapping clinical effects, this approach is also complicated by confusion in terminology used to describe psychotropic drugs. Another approach has been to subdivide the drugs on the basis of their chemical structures; combining both of these approaches is advantageous. As experimental findings are accumulated, the other possibility, namely, classifying the compounds on the pharmacological basis of their mechanisms of action, may be approaching.

For many reasons, drugs acting within the CNS, however, cannot as yet be adequately classified in terms of their mechanisms of action. Undoubtedly the complexity of organization in the brain is such as to limit the understanding of neuronal integration and response. The technical difficulties are only slowly being overcome in elaborating drug effects on neurons. Relating drug actions on neuronal function to behavior will involve an even slower step.

Generally, various authorities [1] have subdivided drugs acting in the CNS into three broad groups. *General (nonselective) CNS depressants,* including anesthetic agents, the aliphatic alcohols, the barbiturates, and other related sedative hypnotic drugs, are claimed to share the ability to depress excitable tissue at all levels. *General (nonselective) CNS stimulants,* including analeptics and convulsants, are believed to excite the CNS either by blocking inhibition or by direct neuronal excitation. *Drugs that selectively modify CNS function,* the third group, are the most important in this text. These agents include the psychotropic drugs, as well as anticonvulsants, analgesics, and drugs used in treating Parkinson's disease. Interestingly, increasing evidence suggests that many of these drugs with selective action modify neurohumoral transmission in various regions of the CNS.

Psychotropic drugs have been introduced into clinical use in various ways. Reserpine, present in rauwolfia plant extracts, was used in primitive Hindu medicine for a variety of diseases, including insanity, before its introduction into Western medicine. At about the same time chlorpromazine was included by Laborit in his "lytic cocktail" which combined pethidine, promethazine, and chlorpromazine as a treatment in manic patients. Laborit had sought a compound with more central effects than the antihistamine promethazine and subsequently predicted that the new agent would be used in psychiatry. Indeed, because chlorpromazine affected mental alertness and induced a condition related to akinesia, Laborit proposed the name *neuroleptic* for this class of drugs. The third type of chemical substances with neuroleptic properties, butyrophenone derivatives, came by way of a program of synthesizing compounds with morphinelike properties. Janssen later expressed surprise that from the point of view of its chemical structure, haloperidol, apparently unrelated to the then known major tranquilizers and derived from norpethidine, should exhibit chlorpromazinelike activity. The first monoamine oxidase inhibitor-antidepressant, iproniazid, was originally used in the treatment of tuberculosis. Surprisingly, the first reported use of iproniazid in psychiatry was of its evaluation by Jackson Smith [2] as a tranquilizer. The first tricyclic antidepressant, imipramine, initially introduced as an antihistaminic, was clinically tested following a request to see whether it could be used as a sedative. It is clear that all these important psychotropic drugs found their way into clinical use, and their efficacies were established, without any understanding of their mechanisms of action being established.

Nonetheless, by whatever way the psychotropic drugs came into psychiatric use, there can be no doubt their clinical usefulness has had dramatic impact on basic concepts and the treatment of mental illness. In addition, tremendous energy and resource have gone into attempts to study the mechanisms of action of these drugs. The consequences have had far-reaching implications for pharmacology in various attempts to improve the original drugs and lessen their side effects and to elaborate on the role of various putative neurotransmitter substances in the CNS. For psychiatry, the studies on the mechanisms of action of psychotropic drugs have given impetus to and insight into understanding or hypothesizing on the etiology of mental illness.

II. NEUROHUMORAL TRANSMITTERS IN THE CENTRAL NERVOUS SYSTEM

Attempts to explain the mechanisms of action of most psychotropic drugs are usually concerned with the ways the drugs may modify neurohumoral transmission in the CNS. Some of the suggested mechanisms include mimicking, releasing, or prolonging the effects of neurotransmitters, or conversely depleting, preventing the synthesis or release, or antagonizing the action of neurotransmitters. The roles of putative central transmitters are therefore of considerable significance.

Several chemical compounds are currently considered to be likely candidates for a transmitter role; these include acetylcholine (AC), certain amino acids such as γ-aminobutyric acid (GABA), glycine, and glutamate, as well as the monoamines, norepinephrine (NE), dopamine (DA), and serotonin (5-HT). Not one of these substances, however, meets all the rigid criteria formulated to characterize neurotransmitters. Other substances such as histamine, prostaglandins, substance P, other amino acids, and various trace amines have also been proposed as transmitters, but the evidence for their role is not as compelling.

The largest mass of literature relating psychoactive drugs and central neurotransmitters concerns the monoamines, as do the various theories on the neurochemical bases of mental illness. This emphasis has in part arisen because no doubt the concepts of synaptic transmission in the CNS have been heavily biased by findings about peripheral neurons. Furthermore, psychoactive drugs as a group modify many autonomic functions. Recently, other putative transmitters are assuming greater importance in understanding the mechanisms of action of these drugs.

A. Catecholamines

The presence of catecholamines in nerves was first demonstrated by von Euler [3]. Brain tissue contains three catecholamines, NE, DA, and epinephrine, the last of which occurs in the lowest amount. A certain amount of DA occurs in all adrenergic nerves as a precursor to NE, but there are neurons in which the synthesis stops at the DA stage. NE and DA are considered now to have independent roles as neurotransmitters in the CNS.

B. Norepinephrine

Vogt [4] described the uneven distribution of NE in the dog brain, and subsequently using histochemical fluorescence techniques Ungerstedt [5] was able to map NE-containing pathways in the rat brain. An association of nerve endings containing large granular vesicles, with regional brain levels of NE [6], suggested storage sites within brain neurons. The enzymatic steps described for the synthesis of NE have been shown in the brain. In the periphery, the enzymes monoamine oxidase (MAO), located both intra- and extraneuronally, and catechol-O-methyltransferase (COMT), located primarily outside the neuron, are responsible for the metabolism of NE. These enzymes also occur in the CNS [7].

Most of the NE released from sympathetic adrenergic nerves has its action terminated, however, by active reuptake back into the nerve. This is considered to account for 80% of the released catecholamine. Glowinski and associates [8] showed that radioactively labeled NE was also taken up by the brain.

A variety of approaches have been used to determine the likely functions of NE. Application by microiontophoresis to single cells may cause either excitation or inhibition of firing [9,10]. However, the view has been expressed [11] that the excitatory responses of nerve cells to injected NE may be an artifact. In the intact cat, when NE was injected into the cerebral ventricles to bypass the blood-brain barrier, it caused a stuporous state [12]. Intravenous injections of NE into newly hatched chickens which have a deficient blood-brain barrier produced sleep [13]. Despite these findings, Fuxe and associates [14] concluded that increased NE receptor activity in the cerebral cortex probably results in alertness and increased drive. They also concluded that activation of NE receptors in the CNS results in aggression and increased locomotor activity, and that noradrenergic neurons participate in the control of somatic and autonomic reflex activity as well as in the control of some hormonal release. In addition, noradrenergic neurons along with dopaminergic ones are claimed to be involved in conditioned processes [14] and the reward system [15].

C. Dopamine

Dopamine (DA) is the immediate precursor in the biosynthesis of NE, and its presence [16] and distribution [17,18] in the brain have been known for many years. DA is the principal catecholamine in three neuronal systems, the nigroneostriatal, the mesolimbic, and the tuberoinfundibular [14]. The enzymes responsible for the synthesis and degradation of DA in the brain are the same as those concerned with NE. The uptake system in dopaminergic neurons in the CNS is similar to that for NE, but it is known to be differently affected by drugs [19].

Iontophoretic application of DA suppresses the rapid discharge elicited by AC on some cells in the caudate nucleus [20], and there is good evidence that this DA action mimics the response to stimulation of the substantia nigra [21, 22]. In the mammalian brain 80% of the total DA and its metabolic end product homovanillic acid (HVA) is found within the basal ganglia complex [23]. Neurophysiological findings and the pathological evidence of a severe loss of DA in the striatum of patients with Parkinson's disease have led to the view that these dopaminergic neurons are of great importance in normal movements and posture. Increased DA receptor activity in the neostriatum is generally accepted as leading to stereotyped behavior in animals; similar behavior in patients with schizophrenia has led to the assumption that an abnormally increased activity in the nigrostriatal DA neurons could at least partly be responsible for the psychotic state [14]. Less is known about the role of the DA neurons in the limbic system, but their importance in mental function has been deduced from the action of various classes of neuroleptic drugs in antagonizing DA effects. The tuberoinfundibular DA neurons are believed to be related to various endocrine systems.

D. Serotonin

Since serotonin (5-HT) was detected in the CNS by Amin and associates [24] the pathways of serotonergic nerves have been mapped [14]. Cell bodies of neurons containing 5-HT are localized mainly in the raphe complex of the reticular formation, and these as well as those in the ventromedial reticular tegmentum give rise to large numbers of ascending axons running in the middle third of the tegmentum. Descending pathways containing 5-HT go to the spinal cord, and in addition other neurons innervate the lower brainstem. The enzymes tryptophan-5-hydroxylase and aromatic L-amino acid decarboxylase responsible for the synthesis of 5-HT, and MAO which metabolizes it to 5-hydroxyindoleacetic acid

(5-HIAA), have been demonstrated in the CNS. Like the catecholamines, 5-HT also has its postsynaptic actions terminated by reuptake into the presynaptic terminal. However, again the structure/activity relationships of drugs affecting reuptake [19] suggest that there may be differences in the various uptake processes.

Several functions have been proposed for 5-HT-containing neuronal systems. Direct application of 5-HT onto single neurons by iontophoretic techniques has usually caused depressant effects, but some excitant actions have been shown [10]. When Feldberg and Myers [25] injected 5-HT into the cerebral ventricles of cats they found it raised body temperature and suggested a role in temperature regulation. Myers and Beleslin [26] observed that the amount of 5-HT collected from the anterior preoptic area of monkeys increased above resting levels when the animals were exposed to a cold environment. Destruction of cell bodies in the raphe nucleus of the cat and a subsequent loss of 5-HT from nerve terminals disrupted sleep patterns [27], and evidence suggests a functional relation in sleep control. Also, 5-HT pathways have been implicated in sexual behavior, neuroendocrine function, and autonomic and somatic reflex activity [14]. Abnormal levels of 5-HT and its metabolite have been related to mental deficiency and the pathogenesis of parkinsonism. It is claimed that there is evidence for both a positive and negative relationship of 5-HT to brain reward behavior [15].

E. Acetylcholine

The presence of acetylcholine (AC) and of the two enzymes responsible respectively for its synthesis and degradation and their distribution is well documented [28]. Using techniques of differential centrifugation and hypoosmotic shock it has been shown that AC occurs in particles in nerve endings, choline acetylase in the soluble cytoplasm fraction of nerve endings, and cholinesterase in the microsomal fraction suggestive of postsynaptic localization [10]. Because fluorescence techniques are not appropriate for AC, histological staining for the presence of cholinesterase has been used to map various cholinergic pathways in the CNS.

Iontophoretic application of AC onto Renshaw cells and pharmacological analysis of the action [29] provides a classic example for studying the nature of transmission of central neurons. Whereas in the spinal cord AC produces only excitation of neuronal activity, in other parts of the CNS and brain both excitatory and inhibitory effects have been observed. Furthermore, the action is exerted on both muscarinic-type and nicotinic-type cholinoceptive sites. Cholinergic transmission also seems to occur in the cerebral cortex and most subcortical brain regions. The release of AC from the CNS has been shown to vary depending on the behavioral state of the animal [30].

The possible functional roles of central cholinergic systems have been studied in various ways, and together the findings support an association between cholinergic mechanisms and behavior. The major functional roles of AC in the CNS have been discussed at length by De Feudis [31]. Cholinergic elements appear to be involved in reticulocortical pathways responsible for arousal, and in addition cholinergic systems seem to play a role in motor reflexes and postural mechanisms through the spinal pathways and the extrapyramidal tracts. Feldberg and Sherwood [32] showed that intraventricular injections of AC and anticholinesterases in animals produce a "catatoniclike" state, and earlier Sherwood [33] had interrupted catatonic stupor in some schizophrenic patients with intraventricular injections of a preparation of "true" cholinesterase. Studies since then have indicated that central cholinergic mechanisms may be involved in emotion, learning, and memory.

F. Histamine

Although the presence of histamine in mammalian brain was first demonstrated by Kwiatkowski [34] in 1943, its role as a central transmitter has been seriously entertained only recently (for reviews, see Refs. 35-38). Regional differences in brain concentration occur, and the amine appears to be contained in both mast cells and neurons. Studies indicate it is localized in the subcellular fraction containing nerve terminals. Radioactively labeled histamine does not cross the blood-brain barrier, and it has been concluded therefore that it must be synthesized within the brain [36]. The amino acid precursor is histidine, and although in some tissues conversion is known to involve nonspecific aromatic amino acid decarboxylase, White [39] expressed the view that there was a specific histidine decarboxylase in brain. The distribution of the converting enzyme in brain roughly parallels that of histamine. The only demonstrated metabolic route for endogenous histamine in brain tissue is through methylation by the highly specific enzyme histamine-N-methyltransferase, and the product is then a substrate for MAO. By the method of producing selective lesions and following the loss of histamine in specific regions, a pathway from the hypothalamus to the cerebral cortex [40] and another to the hippocampus have been described [37]. A histamine-sensitive adenylate cyclase system has been found in the hippocampus.

Iontophoretic application of histamine onto individual brain neurons produces both excitation and depression, but the classification of their receptors into histamine H_1 or H_2 types remains to be confirmed [38]. Intraventricular injection of histamine into the cerebral ventricles of animals causes hypothermia, emesis, and an increase in water intake. No positive statements can be made about the actions of histamine on complex behavior, but it has been proposed that histamine abnormalities may be involved in schizophrenia and parkinsonism.

G. γ-Aminobutyric Acid

The CNS contains high concentrations of free amino acids, several of which are thought to play a transmitter role. In mammals, γ-aminobutyric acid (GABA) has been detected in the brain and to a lesser extent in the spinal cord, but virtually not at all in peripheral tissues. The regional distribution in the monkey brain was found to vary over a 10-fold range [41]. GABA is synthesized in the brain from glutamate, and the enzyme responsible for catalyzing the reaction, glutamic decarboxylase (GAD), is located exclusively in the CNS. The enzyme requires pyridoxal phosphate as a coenzyme. GABA loss from nerve terminals can be produced by the destruction of cell bodies of specific nerves. It has been shown by Otsuka and Miyata [42] that cerebellar ablation causes a marked decrease of GABA from normally high levels in isolated Deiters cells; experimental evidence of this sort indicates that Purkinje cell axons terminate with dorsal Deiters cells and that this is a GABAergic pathway.

GABA is transaminated by GABA-α-ketoglutamate transaminase, an enzyme found chiefly in the gray matter of the CNS, and like GAD it requires pyridoxal phosphate as a coenzyme. The product of this reaction is glutamic acid and succinic semialdehyde which ultimately enters the tricarboxylic acid cycle.

There is general consensus that there is a GABA uptake mechanism in the brain with a high degree of structural specificity. Autoradiographic studies have shown GABA is taken up mainly by nerve terminals and glial cells [43], and active uptake appears to be the mechanism responsible for terminating the proposed transmitter action of GABA. However, because uptake inhibitors have not yet been shown to have any direct influence on GABA-mediated synaptic inhibition, a word of caution has been expressed by Johnston [44]. His view is that at the present time there is thus no direct evidence that GABA uptake terminates the action of synaptically released GABA.

Microiontophoretic application of GABA has a depressant effect on single nerve cells in the cerebral cortex, medulla, spinal cord, and various other sites of the CNS (for review, see Ref. 45). The specificity of this effect in the brain was demonstrated with the alkaloid bicuculline, which suppresses the inhibitory effect of GABA but not that of the other important inhibitory amino acid, glycine [46]. Administration of GABA into the cerebral ventricles of cats produced only slight behavioral consequences. Electroencephalograms changed to sleep patterns, conditioned avoidance latency increased, and body activity diminished [47]. However, in some cases the effects produced were no different from those in saline controls.

GABA fulfills many of the criteria one would expect of an inhibitory neurotransmitter in the brain. It has been suggested that altered GABA functions may be related to various forms of convulsions, movement disorders, sleep, and wakefulness. A defect in the GABA system may underlie schizophrenia [48].

H. Other Possible Central Transmitters

The substances previously discussed, the biogenic amines and the amino acid GABA, are obviously not the only candidates for neurotransmitter roles in the

CNS. However, they have been selected for discussion because they more commonly have been implicated in attempts to explain the mechanisms of action of many psychotropic drugs. In the future it is possible that other putative transmitters will become fashionable in theories on the mechanisms of action of these drugs. Such substances include several other amino acids, including glycine and glutamate, various peptides including substance P, several prostaglandins, and some trace amines.

The other well-studied inhibitory amino acid in the CNS besides GABA is glycine. Four times as high a concentration of glycine occurs in the spinal cord as in the cerebral cortex; this sort of uneven distribution led Aprison and Werman [49] to suggest glycine was a spinal cord neurotransmitter. The action of intracellularly applied glycine on single neurons and its selective inhibition by strychnine have been part of the evidence suggestive of glycine being probably the major inhibitory transmitter in the cord and brainstem (for review, see Ref. 50). Studies with glutamate have indicated this amino acid may be the principal excitatory amino acid transmitter in the CNS, but the findings have been hindered so far by lack of specific antagonists of its action. Other amino acids have also been shown to have characteristics suggestive of their being excitatory or inhibitory transmitters.

The role of peptides as neurotransmitters is more controversial, but there is an extensive literature on substance P and the endorphins. The occurrence and regional distribution of substance P in the brain [51] and its action when applied intracellularly to central neurons [52] suggest a transmitter role. A very interesting relationship with the central monoaminergic system was shown by Carlsson and associates [53], and a possible implication in the pathogenesis of depression and schizophrenia has been suggested. Polypeptides with opiate properties have been isolated from the brain, and the first to be defined were methionine- and leucine enkephalin [54]. The pentapeptide enkephalins compete with opiates for receptor sites in brain homogenates and produce transient analgesia when injected into the cerebral ventricles of animals. These and similar peptides have since become collectively known as the endorphins. Of the endorphins which have been described to date the enkephalin pentapeptides appear to be the prime candidates for a neurotransmitter role (for review, see Ref. 55). Since some enkephalins and stereospecific receptors occur in areas not implicated in nociception, a general role has been proposed also for endorphins in more complex mood and behavior. There have been already several reports implicating disorders in brain endorphins in mental illness.

The concepts of central transmission have been biased by results found with peripheral neurotransmission processes and the role of similar compounds in the CNS. However, first the amino acid transmitters and more recently the peptides and fatty acids have added new dimensions. The role of trace amines and other alternative transmitters in the CNS have recently been highlighted (for commentary, see Ref. 56). New analytical methods have made it possible to identify an increasing number of aromatic amines in the CNS, and there is increasing evidence of their synthesis and storage in, and release from, nerve terminals. The biogenic amines appear to be associated with a small percentage of nerve terminals relative to the amino acid transmitters [57], and yet they have been afforded greater importance in relation to the psychotropic drugs. Although the postsynaptic functions of the trace amines is still obscure, the future may find a place for them in understanding psychiatric disorders and the action of drugs used in their treatment.

III. NEUROLEPTICS

Neuroleptic agents can be subdivided into several chemically different types, phenothiazines and thioxanthenes, butyrophenones and diphenylbutylpiperidines, and the rauwolfia alkaloids. Chemical differences endow these compounds with pharmacological properties which determine their use in special circumstances or particular patients. Pharmacological differences provide insight into their side effects. Pharmacological similarities, particularly with regard to the way dopaminergic systems are altered, albeit by different means, have helped understand their basis of action. The proposed mechanism of action of neuroleptic drugs has provided some clues to the etiology of mental illness.

A. Chemistry

1. Phenothiazines and Thioxanthenes

The phenothiazine nucleus is a three-ring structure in which two benzene rings designated a and c are linked by a sulfur and a nitrogen atom (see Table 1). Phenothiazine itself has no significant central effect but has been used as an anthelmintic and urinary antiseptic. Substitution on the phenothiazine nucleus alters its pharmacological properties, the first derivative with reported CNS effects being methylene blue. The antihistamine promethazine first directed attention to a significant sedative action of some phenothiazines and in turn resulted in the study of chlorpromazine and other neuroleptic drugs. Variations of the most frequently used phenothiazines include compounds with substituents at position 2, the most common being Cl, CF_3, and SCH_3, and within the side chain at position 10. On the basis of substituents of the side chain attached to the N atom, neuroleptic phenothiazines can be divided into three groups, the aliphatic type like chlorpromazine, the piperidine type like thioridazine, and the piperazine type like trifluoperazine. Neuroleptic-type phenothiazines have a 3-carbon bridge between the N atom of the ring and that of the side chain. In contrast, phenothiazines commonly used in treating Parkinson's disease or aller-

Table 1 Structures of Selected Phenothiazines

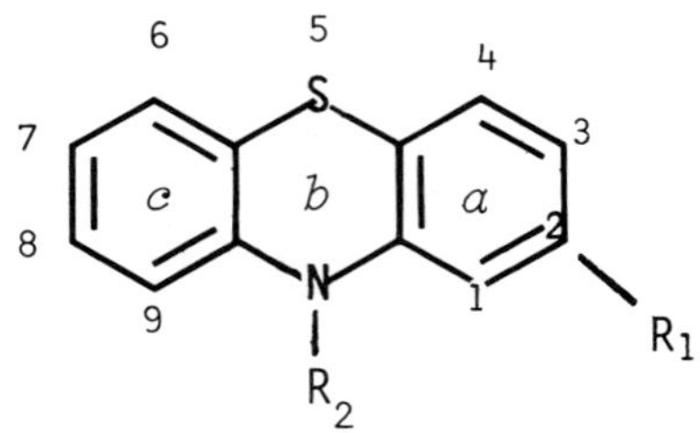

Phenothiazine nucleus

Drug	R_1	R_2	Classification
Chlorpromazine	$-Cl$	$-CH_2-CH_2-CH_3$	Aliphatic-type Neuroleptic
Thioridazine	$-SCH_3$	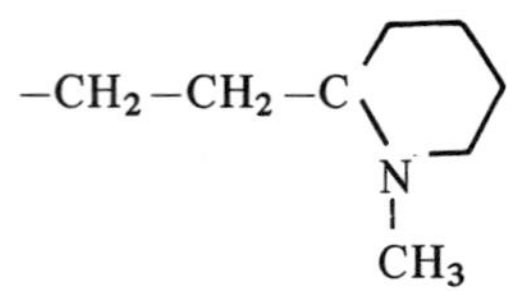	Piperidine-type Neuroleptic
Trifluoperazine	$-CF_3$	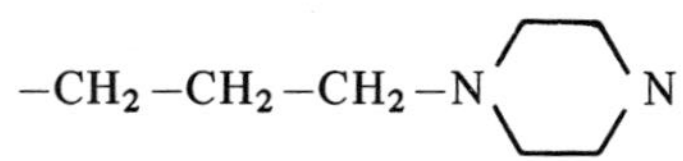	Piperazine-type Neuroleptic
Fluphenazine	$-CF_3$	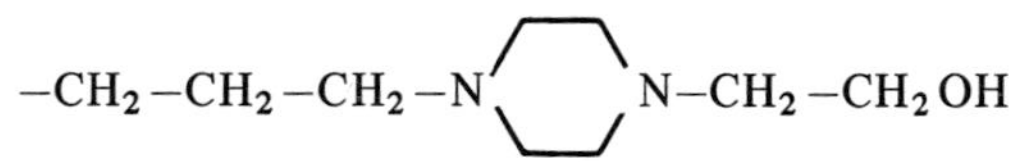	Piperazine-type Neuroleptic
Ethopropazine		$-CH_2-CH(CH_3)-N(CH_2-CH_3)_2$	Antiparkinsonian Drug
Promethazine		$-CH_2-CH(CH_3)-N(CH_3)_2$	Antihistamine

gies, like ethopropazine and promethazine respectively, usually have a 2-carbon bridge. These differences are shown in Table 1.

Conformational similarities between chlorpromazine and DA were described by Horn and Snyder [58] and claimed to support the DA concept of antipsychotic activity. Using Dreiding models these authors demonstrated that DA in its solid-state conformation could be superimposed upon a portion of the known X-ray structure of chlorpromazine. The structure/activity relationships proposed explain the importance of the substituent in ring a, the 3-carbon side chain bearing the amino group, and a hetero atom between rings a and c.

If the N atom in the phenothiazine ring is replaced by a C atom with a double bond to the side chain, the compound is a thioxanthene derivative. Chlorprothixene is an example of a thioxanthene neuroleptic and like chlorpromazine has a Cl atom substituent at position 2 and the same dimethylaminopropyl side chain except for the double bond at position 10. Comparisons can be drawn also between the major thioxanthenes and their phenothiazine analogues.

2. *Butyrophenones and Diphenylbutylpiperidines*

The butyrophenones were developed in a systematic attempt to produce pethidinelike substances, and therefore are chemically quite unrelated to the phenothiazines. Literally hundreds of butyrophenones were synthesized by Janssen and his colleagues, but only haloperidol has had extensive clinical use. An interesting similarity can be seen in the structures of haloperidol and the inhibitory amino acid neurotransmitter GABA (see Fig. 1). Replacement of the carbonyl in the propylene chain of the butyrophenone structure by a fluorophenyl resulted in a chemically new group of drugs, referred to as diphenylbutylpiperidines; pimozide is the best-studied neuroleptic drug in this chemical class, and its structure also is shown in Fig. 1.

3. *Rauwolfia Alkaloids*

Almost simultaneously with the use of phenothiazines in the treatment of psychosis in the 1950s came the introduction of the rauwolfia alkaloid reserpine. Reserpine is still used as an antihypertensive drug but nowadays rarely as a psychotropic agent because it has been shown to be less effective than phenothiazine derivatives in many well-controlled clinical trials. As well, reserpine poses a serious problem in that it may precipitate severe mental depression. Reserpine is only one of the several alkaloids found in *Rauwolfia serpentina* (Benth), and has a complex indole-containing structure (see Fig. 2). Although of diminished clinical importance, reserpine is still of considerable significance in understanding the mechanism of action of psychotropic drugs.

4. *Dibenzodiazepines*

The only member of this interesting class of drugs to be discussed is clozapine. Although this compound has undergone only limited clinical trial, it is reported

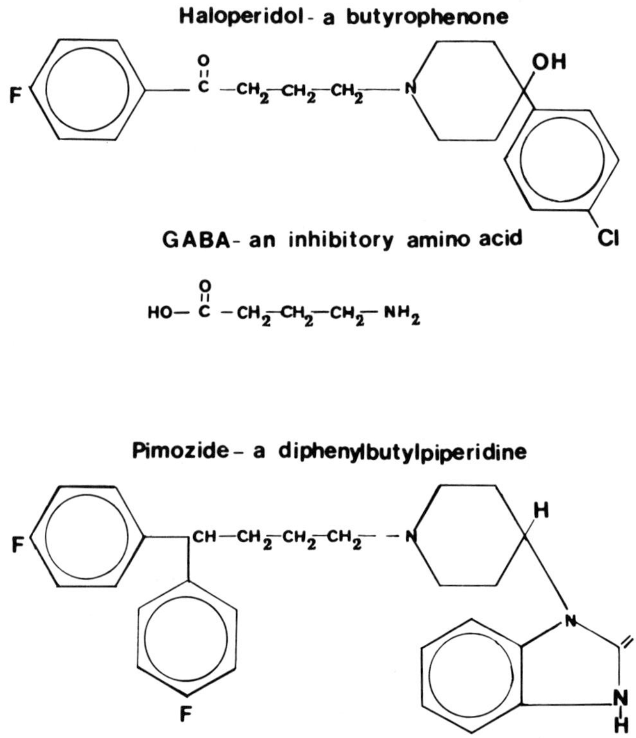

Figure 1 Chemical structures of haloperidol, pimozide, and GABA.

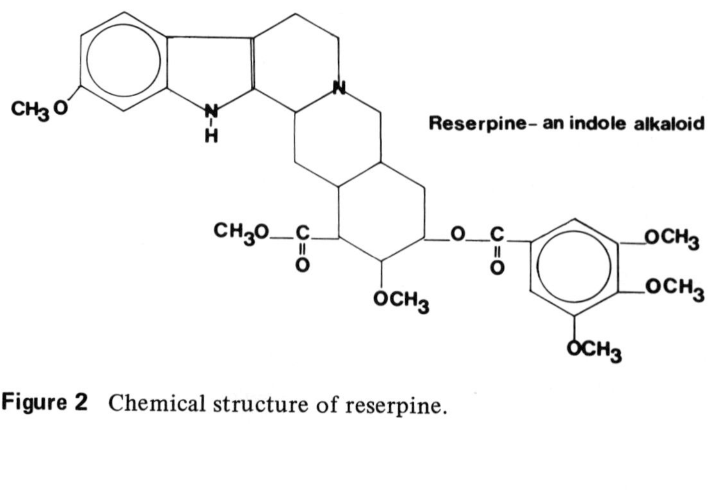

Figure 2 Chemical structure of reserpine.

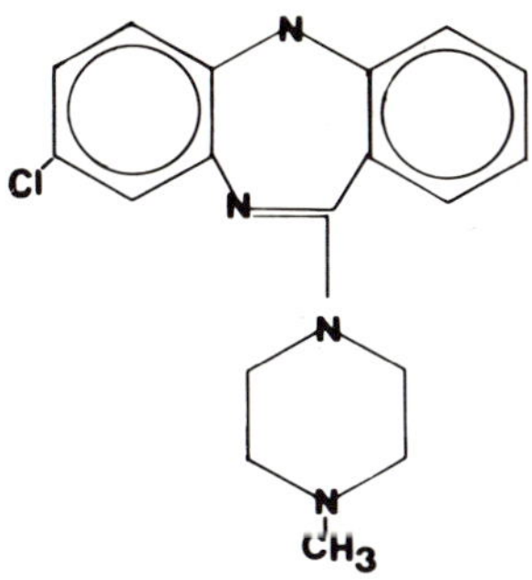

Clozapine - a dibenzodiazepine

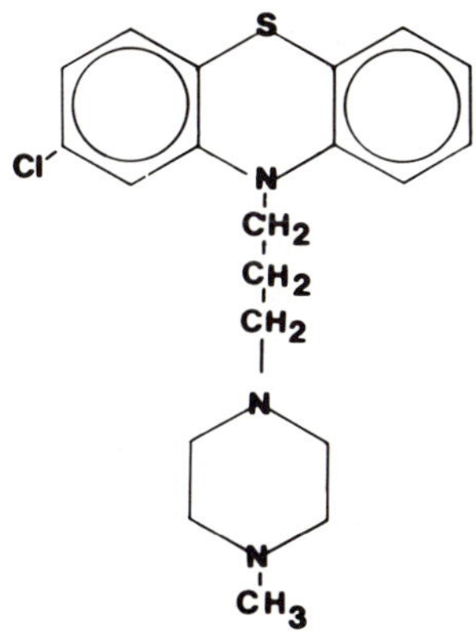

Prochlorperazine - a piperazine-type phenothiazine

Figure 3 Chemical structures of clozapine and prochlorperazine.

to have antipsychotic action and is claimed to be unique in that few extrapyramidal side effects occur during its use [59]. Like the phenothiazines, clozapine is a potent antagonist of the ability of DA to activate adenylate cyclase, and it has a superficial similarity in chemical structure to the piperazine-type phenothiazine prochlorperazine (see Fig. 3).

B. Relationship of Neuroleptics to Dopamine in the Central Nervous System

Very persuasive evidence can be presented to implicate DA in the mechanism of action of neuroleptic drugs, both with regard to their ability to alleviate psychoses and more particularly to cause motor disturbances through disturbance of the extrapyramidal system. All of the clinically useful neuroleptics have been shown to interfere with dopaminergic mechanisms, and this common feature among a variety of other pharmacological actions provides the best correlation with their efficacy. As well, the amphetamines which can cause a psychoticlike state resembling paranoid schizophrenia [60] are believed to activate DA mechanisms in the CNS; the neuroleptics antagonize amphetamine-induced behavior in animals and are effective in the treatment of amphetamine psychosis in man. The extrapyramidal side effects common to the various chemical classes of neuroleptics resemble in many ways the symptoms of naturally occurring Parkinson's disease. The role of DA in the basal ganglia and the therapeutic implications of its loss from the caudate nucleus and putamen in parkinsonism, as well as the clinical use of levodopa to replenish DA in alleviating the condition, are well established (for review, see Ref. 61). Of course, there are other factors involved in Parkinson's disease that are also important even though DA changes appear to be critical.

The fundamental pharmacological paper on chlorpromazine of Courvoisier and associates [62] demonstrated the many actions of this drug. Since then phenothiazine derivatives have been shown to antagonize certain of the responses produced by catecholamines, 5-HT, AC, and histamine in a variety of pharmacological preparations. The potencies, however, of the various phenothiazines are often found to differ in specific actions. As a consequence of chlorpromazine being a more potent α-adrenoreceptor antagonist than trifluoperazine, it therefore causes more hypotension; on the other hand, promethazine is a more potent antagonist of histamine- and acetylcholine-induced contracture of guinea pig ileum than is chlorpromazine and is preferred in the treatment of allergies even though unfortunately it suffers from having atropinelike side effects. Phenothiazines also exert a host of biochemical effects, including inhibition of oxidative phosphorylation and inhibition of adenosine triphosphatase (for review, see Ref. 63), which may bear on their clinical use.

Matthysse [64] correlated the clinical usefulness of various phenothiazine, butyrophenone, and diphenylbutylpiperidine compounds as antipsychotics, with their effects on DA turnover and their so-called nonspecific properties. Matthyse concluded that the nonspecific properties, such as their actions of inhibiting oxidative phosphorylation, stabilizing membranes, and donating electrons, are common to many phenothiazines, including promethazine, ethopropazine, and thiethylperazine, which do not have antipsychotic efficacy in addition to the various neuroleptic phenothiazines. In contrast, only the neuroleptic phenothiazines enhance DA turnover in the brain. It is also known that the neuroleptic phenothiazines increase the turnover of brain NE, but since promethazine does as well, Matthysse also called this a nonspecific phenothiazine effect. Further support for the Matthysse argument was claimed with the finding that pimozide augments DA turnover without affecting the metabolism of NE [65].

All classes of neuroleptics except reserpine block the DA receptor, and this action is thought to be responsible for increasing the turnover of DA in the brain. Reserpine, however, has long been known to deplete biogenic amines, and this effect also extends to brain DA. The end result, therefore, whether by postsynaptic receptor blockade or presynaptic depletion, is that DA nerve transmission in the CNS is diminished by all neuroleptic drugs. The conformational similarity of chlorpromazine and DA also supports this concept of action [58]. In addition, Horn and Snyder [58] claimed that if molecular models were constructed, it could be shown that butyrophenones could assume a conformation resembling part of the phenothiazine ring.

The limbic system and the corpus striatum contain adenylate cyclase that is specifically activated by DA. Activation of this enzyme is antagonized by neuroleptic drugs, and this DA-sensitive adenylate cyclase has been postulated to represent the immediate receptor molecule ultimately responsible for the physiological effects of DA.

General consensus is that if the DA systems underlie the action of neuroleptics, then the one in the limbic area is concerned more with behavioral and emotional effects and that in the corpus striatum has to do with motor responses. However, according to Hornykiewicz [66] there is evidence from animal experiments that both of these systems and a third one arising in the hypothalamus and terminating in the external layer of the median eminence may all have relevance to the behavioral disturbances of psychotic patients.

If it be assumed that neuroleptics bring about clinical improvement by interfering with DA transmission in the limbic area and extrapyramidal side effects result from a similar action in the basal ganglia, there still remains a question. How can behavioral improvement with the neuroleptics be dissociated from drug-induced parkinsonism? There appear to be some possible answers, one discussed at length by Snyder and associates [67] being that the drugs exert a varying degree of central cholinergic blockade which reduces the extent of their extrapyramidal side effects. Another possibility is that the DA receptor, the DA-sensitive adenylate cyclase system, is differently affected in different regions of the brain.

Because it was thought that peripheral anticholinergic action may not correspond precisely with that in the brain, Snyder and colleagues [67] used the binding of 3-quinuclidinyl benzilate (QNB), an antagonist of muscarinic cholinergic receptors, to membrane preparations from the CNS as a technique to determine central anticholinergic potency. The binding of highly radioactive QNB represents an almost exclusive interaction with muscarinic cholinergic receptors, and the potency of antagonism by several neuroleptics was experimentally determined. In this way it was found that clozapine, a neuroleptic almost devoid of extrapyramidal side effects, has similar potency to anticholinergic antiparkinsonian drugs such as benztropine and trihexyphenidyl. Thioridazine displayed the second greatest affinity and was claimed to rank next with regard to freedom from these side effects, and chlorpromazine with moderate side effects had somewhat less affinity for the sites. Fluphenazine and trifluoperazine, piperazine-type phenothiazine derivatives with considerably more extrapyramidal side effects than chlorpromazine, were even less effective in binding to the muscarinic receptors. Finally, haloperidol with as high or higher an incidence of extrapyramidal effects as the piperazine phenothiazines had very little affinity for the muscarinic receptor. The presumed different balance of cholinergic and dopaminergic blockade in the corpus striatum therefore was thought to account for the differences in side effects of the neuroleptics. The relative muscarinic receptor blocking action of the antipsychotics has been confirmed using other assay systems [68,69]. One drug, however, that does not fit into this explanation is pimozide. This neuroleptic was shown by Laduron and Leysen [69] not to possess antimuscarinic properties although it produces a low incidence of extrapyramidal side effects. It was suggested by Laduron and Leysen [69] that pimozide may be retained at aspecific sites of binding and only slowly be dissociated. If so, this could modulate the free drug concentration in the vicinity of DA receptors in such a way that these receptors are only slowly occupied, allowing an easier adaptation after postsynaptic blockade.

The ability of neuroleptics to inhibit the activation by DA of adenylate cyclase has been compared in two central areas, the limbic and caudate [70]. The inhibitory effects were not found to be different in the two sites and could not account for their different tendencies to produce extrapyramidal effects. However, Anden and Stock [71] reported that compared to haloperidol, clozapine, which produces significantly less extrapyramidal effects, caused greater DA turnover in the limbic system than in the corpus striatum.

C. Relationship of Butyrophenones to γ-Aminobutyric Acid Mechanisms

It was shown earlier that haloperidol, a typical butyrophenone, has a structural similarity to GABA (Fig. 1), and when neuroleptic action was initially demonstrated, Janssen [72] suggested that the butyrophenones may act by mimicking GABA and blocking the excitatory action of glutamic acid, particularly in the extrapyramidal system. Although these drugs, like most other neuroleptics, are usually interpreted as acting through DA receptor antagonism, there are experimental findings that suggest they may affect GABA neurons.

The butyrophenone droperidol, used in the technique of neuroleptanalgesia, has a synergistic action with GABA when applied microelectrophoretically onto Purkinje cells in the cat cerebellum, and its inhibitory effect on cell firing also is antagonized by bicuculline [73]. An affinity for the GABA receptor is also suggested by the finding that haloperidol can displace bicuculline bound to membrane preparations from rat cerebellum [74].

Inhibition by haloperidol of the electrically stimulated release of GABA from preloaded slices of rat corpus striatum [75] is an effect that may relate to the extrapyramidal symptoms associated with this drug. Inhibition of GABA uptake into slices of rat cerebral cortex [76] produced by haloperidol is not inconsistent with a possible effect on behavior.

Kim and Hassler [77] have shown that haloperidol causes a decrease in GABA levels in the striatum and substantia nigra of rats. A stimulant effect on DA turnover has also been shown. Although this latter effect is usually thought to result from DA receptor antagonism, Kim and Hassler [77] blocked the increased turnover with aminooxyacetic acid. Aminooxyacetic acid is one of the most widely used agents for increasing the levels of GABA in the brain, and its action suggests that the effect of haloperidol described may be mediated by GABA. Unfortunately, doubts have been raised about the specificity of aminooxyacetic acid [44].

It seems fitting to leave the last word on the relationship of haloperidol and GABA to a Janssen. Cool and Janssen [78] injected haloperidol and GABA into cannulae implanted in the neostriatum of cats and found the compounds produced identical effects. The GABA antagonist picrotoxin counteracted both compounds.

D. Pharmacological Basis of Side Effects of Neuroleptics

The side effects of neuroleptics can be considered in two categories, the more serious hypersensitivity reactions, particularly blood dyscrasias, but also jaundice and dermatological reactions [79] and the bothersome autonomic, extrapyramidal system and endocrine effects which by and large may be considered as extensions of the inherent pharmacological actions of the drugs.

Extrapyramidal side effects can fairly convincingly be attributed to antagonism or depletion of DA in the basal ganglia. A reasonable correlation has been shown between severity of these side effects and a lack of anticholinergic activity (see earlier discussion). Neuroleptics exert a variety of actions on the autonomic nervous system. In part these effects originate in the CNS, but peripheral actions can readily be demonstrated. Reserpine depletes amines from neurons both in the brain and the sympathetic adrenergic system; an antihypertensive effect results along with sedation. The phenothiazines also modify autonomic function. Both α-adrenoreceptor antagonism and inhibition of the reuptake of NE occurs; these actions vary with different phenothiazine derivatives and are also influenced by the duration of administration of the drugs. Phenothiazines of the aliphatic type like chlorpromazine produce greater hypotensive effects than those of the piperazine type like trifluoperazine [79], and this general difference is apparently related to potency of α-adrenoreceptor antagonism. However, tolerance develops to the cardiovascular effects with continued treatment of the phenothiazines. Butyrophenone derivatives resemble the piperazine-type phenothiazines in having minimal effect on the autonomic nervous system. Some phenothiazines are reported to block both the nicotinic and muscarinic actions of AC, but in clinical use parasympathetic effects only occur with large doses. A correlation can be seen between severity of parasympathetic side effects and effects on blood pressure of the neuroleptic drugs. Clinical findings suggest that autonomic side effects appear to be less frequent with the more potent piperazine derivatives like trifluoperazine and fluphenazine [80], and this also seems true of the butyrophenones. A recent study of Fjalland and colleagues [68] compared the muscarinic receptor affinity of a wide range of psychotropic drugs. Among the more potent antagonists of AC were clozapine, thioridazine, and chlorprothixene, while fluphenazine and perphenazine were among the weakest. The endocrine effects of phenothiazines are due primarily to actions on the brain, mainly in the hypothalamus [81]. Disturbance of temperature regulation produced by neuroleptics may be related to alteration in biogenic amine mechanisms in the hypothalamus also.

IV. ANTIDEPRESSANTS

The main groups of clinically useful antidepressants can be subdivided into several groups—MAO inhibitors of the hydrazide and nonhydrazide type; the tricyclic antidepressants, of which the principal types are dibenzazepine and dibenzocycloheptadine derivatives; as well as dibenzoxepine, N-substituted cycloalkylindole, and tetracyclic piperazine compounds.

A. Chemistry

1. MAO Inhibitors

Following the findings that the hydrazide derivative iproniazid had clinical antidepressant effects and was an inhibitor of MAO, a series of related compounds were used in psychiatry. Because hydrazines are hepatotoxic, however, their clinical applications were limited. Compounds structurally related to the amphetamines have proven to be useful MAO inhibitors, including the hydrazine phenelzine and the nonhydrazine tranylcypromine, which is produced by cyclization of the side chain of amphetamine (see Fig. 4).

2. Tricyclic Antidepressants

The tricyclics, like the phenothiazines, are three-ring structures (see Table 2). The structure of the dibenzazepines, like imipramine, consists of two benzene rings linked by a nitrogen atom and an ethylene grouping. Imipramine has the same dimethylaminopropyl side chain attached to the N atom as has chlorpromazine. The demethylated derivative of imipramine, desipramine (the secondary amine), is both a metabolite of imipramine and an antidepressant in its own right.

Amitriptyline has a carbon atom substituted for the nitrogen in the central ring structure of imipramine and therefore is a dibenzocycloheptadine. The side chain is attached to a double bond in an analogous way to the conversion of a phenothiazine to a thioxanthene. Nortriptyline is a secondary amine, the demethylated derivative of amitriptyline and a metabolite, and likewise is a useful antidepressant.

Other tricyclic antidepressants include doxepin, which is related to amitriptyline except that an oxygen atom is substituted for one of the methylene groups in the center ring. Iprindole is a N-substituted cycloalkylindole. Mian-

Table 2 Chemical Structures of Typical Tricyclic Antidepressants

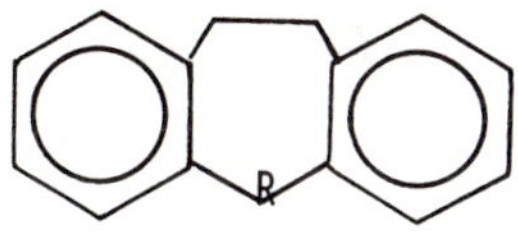

Tricyclic antidepressant nucleus

Drug	R	Classification
Imipramine	$N-CH_2-CH_2-CH_2N(CH_3)_2$	Dibenzazepine; Tertiary Amine
Desipramine	$N-CH_2-CH_2-CH_2-NHCH_3$	Dibenzazepine; Secondary Amine
Amitriptyline	$C=CH-CH_2-CH_2-N(CH_3)_3$	Dibenzocycloheptadine; Tertiary Amine
Nortriptyline	$C=CH-CH_2-CH_2-NHCH_3$	Dibenzocycloheptadine; Secondary Amine

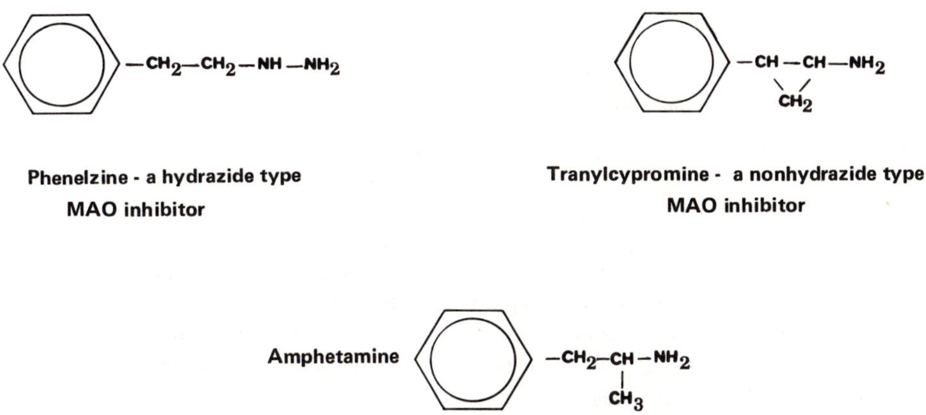

Figure 4 Chemical structures of MAO inhibitors and amphetamine.

serin is a tetracyclic piperazine. Structures of these antidepressants are shown in Fig. 5.

The structure/activity relationships of antidepressants have been discussed by Wilhelm [82] and compared with those of the phenothiazines and thioxanthenes. All have a tricyclic primary framework, and the difference in these primary skeletons is claimed to contribute to the pharmacological differences seen

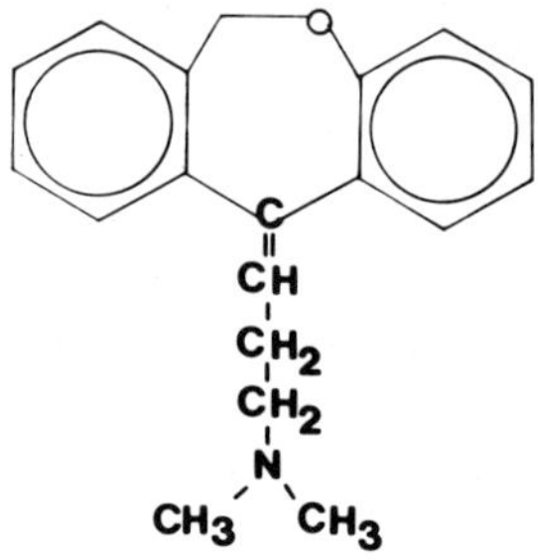

Doxepin - a dibenzoxepine

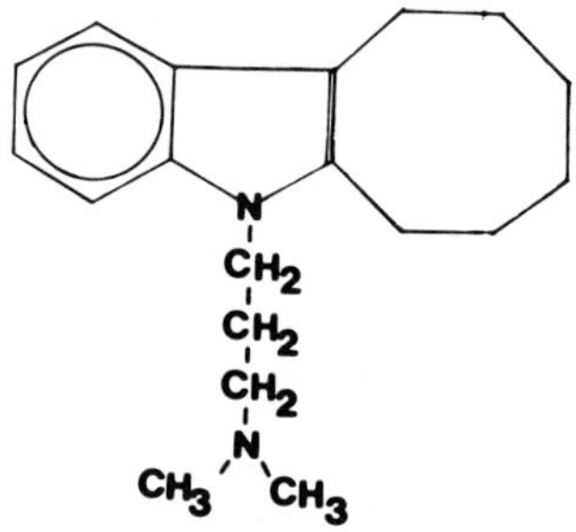

Iprindole - a N-substituted cycloakyl indole

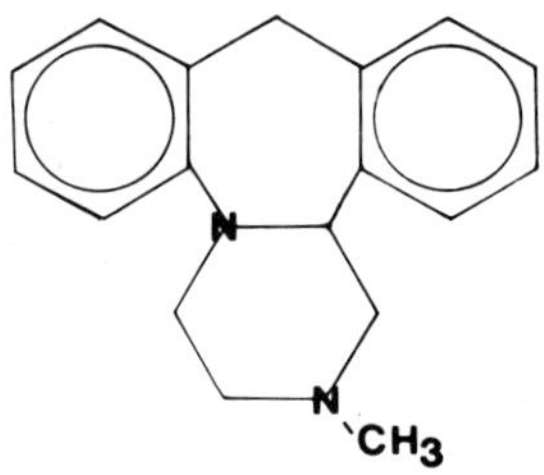

Mianserin - a tetracyclic piperazine

Figure 5 Chemical structures of atypical tricyclic antidepressants.

with these compounds. The effect exerted by the side chain on the clinical activity of all these compounds is apparently to modulate the main action produced by the primary skeleton. Nonbranching, 3-membered carbon chains are deemed preferable for the purest type action, and shortening or adding a branch to the side chain enhances sedative properties. Other properties conferred by the substituents such as basicity and solubility contribute mainly to the ability of antidepressant drugs getting to their site of action. Wilhelm [82] suggested that the constellation type C adopted by the neuroleptics influences DA, whereas the constellation type D of the antidepressants influences NE more.

B. Inhibition of MAO

The clinically used MAO inhibitors produce irreversible inactivation of MAO by forming stable complexes with the enzyme. The synthesis of biogenic amines is not inhibited, and the MAO inhibitors ultimately produce increased levels of NE, DA, and 5-HT in the brain and various peripheral tissues. The drugs do not affect diamine oxidase and therefore do not significantly affect histamine. Type-B MAO is claimed to be relatively more inhibited by tranylcypromine and pargyline, but this finding is controversial [83]. It is interesting, however, that many tricyclics inhibit type B of the enzyme in vitro [83], although generally these compounds are not considered MAO inhibitors.

There are two aspects of the pharmacological actions of MAO inhibitors that are controversial. The first is that it is difficult to differentiate between the significance of the various biogenic amines in the antidepressant action, if indeed they contribute singly. The second relates to the central effects compared to the peripheral cardiovascular actions of these drugs. The MAO inhibitor pargyline is an antihypertensive agent, and the generally accepted view of its action is that it leads to the formation of "false transmitters" in sympathetic nerves. The "false transmitter" is then thought to be released instead of, or with, NE, and the vasoconstrictor effect of sympathetic nerves is thereby reduced because the "false transmitter" is less active than NE. This proposed action creates a dilemma in that one proposal for the antidepressant effect of MAO inhibitors is that NE levels in the brain are increased and so too is noradrenergic transmission.

Earlier attempts to relate catecholamine metabolism to the mechanism of action of antidepressants were embraced in the so-called catecholamine hypothesis of affective disease [84,85]. Subsequently the "indoleamine hypothesis" of Lapin and Oxenkrug [86] and the "permissive hypothesis" of Wilson and Prange [87] extended the explanation to incorporate a role for 5-HT in antidepressant action. Certainly the inhibition of MAO in the brain can increase the levels of 5-HT, and it has been reported that there is a significant lowering of 5-HT in the brains of depressive suicides [88,89].

C. Inhibition of Neuronal Uptake of Norepinephrine

Sigg [90] demonstrated that imipramine potentiated peripheral effects of NE and proposed that increased noradrenergic effects in the CNS might explain antidepressant action. Glowinski and Axelrod [91] reported the inhibition of uptake of tritiated NE in the intact rat brain by imipramine and structurally related compounds. It has earlier been pointed out that the reuptake of NE by neurons is the principal mechanism of terminating its action after release from the nerve terminal. Blocking the uptake prolongs the duration of transmitter in the synaptic cleft and thereby potentiates the transmission process. The tricyclic antidepressants also, therefore, have been proposed to overcome depression by increasing central noradrenergic activity.

Several findings complicate such a simple interpretation of the actions of tricyclics. First, in some clinical studies it has been claimed that some phenothiazines have comparable antidepressant effects to the tricyclics, and yet they are much weaker inhibitors of NE uptake. In addition, iprindole, a newer drug with antidepressant effects, does not significantly inhibit the neuronal uptake of the catecholamine [92]. On the other hand, desipramine is the most active uptake inhibitor of the typical tricyclics and yet is somewhat less useful clinically than imipramine and amitriptyline. Finally, it has been shown that lithium enhances rather than inhibits the uptake of NE into brain synaptosomes [93]. Whereas this has been argued as an explanation for its antimanic effect, recent studies have shown lithium also exerts an antidepressant effect [94].

D. Inhibition of Neuronal Uptake of Serotonin

Sigg and colleagues [95] found that imipramine, amitriptyline, and their demethylated derivatives also potentiate some peripheral actions of 5-HT in addition to those of NE. However, some 5-HT actions were antagonized also, especially by large doses of the tricyclics. It was subsequently shown that tricyclic antidepressants inhibit the uptake of 5-HT into central neurons [96-98]. The tertiary amine compounds among the tricyclics are more potent in this regard than are their secondary amine derivatives.

As is the case with noradrenergic neurons, the reuptake of 5-HT into nerve terminals is an important mechanism in terminating neurotransmitter activity. It also could be anticipated that 5-HT transmission in the CNS would be increased by inhibiting reuptake into the neuron, thereby prolonging the presence of transmitter in the synaptic gap.

E. Effects of Antidepressant Compounds on Acetylcholine Receptors

Peripheral antimuscarinic effects were first reported with imipramine by Domenjoz and Theobald [99], and it is recognized that imipramine and amitriptyline are more powerful anticholinergic drugs in therapeutic doses than are the neuroleptic phenothiazines. It has been suggested that a central atropinelike action might in part contribute to the antidepressant effect of tricyclics; however, there is little convincing evidence of this. On the other hand, some of the side effects of tricyclic antidepressants can be attributed to blockade of muscarinic receptors. Dry mouth, blurred vision, hesitancy in micturition, and impotence fit into this category. Tachycardia and palpitations may in part be explained by muscarinic blockade, but inhibition of reuptake of NE released from sympathetic nerve endings in the heart also contributes to this effect. The side effect of sweating is difficult to reconcile with an atropinelike action, and it has been claimed that this could be due to a central effect of the tricyclics increasing sympathetic output [100]. The MAO inhibitors are not thought to exert atropinelike action.

F. Effects of Antidepressant Drugs on Histamine

Despite the fact that imipramine was originally introduced as an antihistamine, little attempt has been made to relate its mechanism of action as an antidepressant to effects on histamine. Although histamine is generally accepted as being involved in allergic manifestations, its physiological role is not well established. Interest in histamine H_1 and H_2 receptors and increasing evidence that histamine may be a neurotransmitter in the mammalian CNS [38] had directed attention recently to brain histamine receptors being possible sites of action for antidepressant drugs [101].

Hegstrand and co-workers [102] described a histamine-sensitive adenylate cyclase present in homogenates of guinea pig and human hippocampus and neocortex which has pharmacological properties similar to those of the histamine H_2 receptor. The histamine H_2 antagonist metiamide prevented activation of this adenylate cyclase by histamine, but α- and β-adrenoreceptor or muscarinic antagonists failed to do so. In addition, the enzyme was observed to be present in subcellular fractions of brain rich in synaptic membranes, suggesting a relationship with a physiological transmitter role in the CNS.

Because iprindole and mianserin did not conform to the pattern of the classical tricyclic antidepressant drugs in their effect on neuronal uptake of biogenic amines and therefore weakened the argument favoring such a mechanism being the basis of their action, Kanof and Greengard [101] studied the effects of various antidepressants on activation of brain adenylate cyclase by histamine. Antidepressant drugs of the dibenzazepine class (imipramine and derivatives), the dibenzocycloheptadine class (amitriptyline and derivatives), and iprindole and mianserin were found to be competitive inhibitors of histamine-sensitive adenylate cyclase activity. Of particular interest was the potent inhibition produced by the "atypical" antidepressants, mianserin and iprindole. Some other psychotropic drugs including phenothiazines were investigated, and it was claimed that while some phenothiazines with reported antidepressant properties also inhibited activation of the enzyme, not all neuroleptics did.

Kanof and Greengard [101] concluded that the inhibition constants of the antidepressant drugs obtained in vitro were sufficiently low to be consistent with possible in vivo effects. This was based on determinations from recent clinical studies of plasma levels of antidepressants and the assumption that steady-state ratios of brain/plasma concentrations of tricyclic antidepressants are similar in the rat to those in man during therapy with these drugs. The other interesting consequence of these studies is the possibility that new antidepressant drugs may be derived from such an approach. In the past, the use of screening procedures based on models such as reserpine antagonism or modification, able to select known active tricyclic or MAO inhibitors, has restricted available antidepressant drugs to compounds of similar classes. The introduction of new chemical types able to modify histamine mechanisms may have far-reaching implications in the treatment of depression.

G. Pharmacological Effects Related to Duration of Administration

One shortcoming in attempts to relate pharmacological actions of the antidepressants to their mechanism of action in the clinical treatment of depression revolves around a difference in duration of administration. Most pharmacological data are derived from experiments in which effects were studied immediately or soon after acute drug administration. In contrast, clinical use of antidepressants is long term, and of even greater significance is the well-established observation that improvement is not immediate but rather slow in onset.

During long-term administration of chlorpromazine in dogs [103] and humans [104] it was observed that pharmacological responses were modified. In particular, whereas initially chlorpromazine decreased pressor responses to NE because of α-adrenoreceptor antagonism, after continued administration chlorpromazine potentiated the cardiovascular response. This change suggested that after long-term administration chlorpromazine was having an imipraminelike effect and, indeed, there is some clinical evidence suggestive of an antidepressant effect of chlorpromazine [105] and thioridazine [106].

Altered pharmacological effects of tricyclic antidepressants have also been reported following their chronic administration. Long-term treatment with tricyclics decreased the levels of NE [107], whereas acute administration did not [108]. Prolonged treatment with imipramine also decreased the levels of 5-HT and its metabolite 5-HIAA in rat brain [109].

A recent commentary by Sulser and associates [83] is pertinent to a consideration of altered pharmacological actions after long-term administration with the antidepressants. This group has studied the effect of various antidepressant treatments on the sensitivity of the NE-cyclic AMP generating system of the limbic forebrain. This system was chosen because it displays a number of characteristics compatible with those of a central NE receptor and because the function of the limbic forebrain is related to emotion and sensory mechanisms. A single dose of desipramine and iprindole or short-term administration with tricyclic antidepressants was found not to alter the basal level of cyclic nucleotides or the response to NE. However, administration of the same drugs for 3-6 weeks markedly reduced the sensitivity of the noradrenergic receptor-coupled adenylate cyclase system [110]. This delayed subsensitivity following long-term administration of antidepressants has been verified. With MAO inhibitors a decrease in the reactivity of the noradrenergic receptor-coupled adenylate cyclase system also occurred after chronic administration. On the basis of the effect of long-term treatment, Sulser and associates [83] were tempted to speculate that the drugs bring about a desensitization of enhanced noradrenergic receptor functions in depression. This speculation dramatically revises the catecholamine hypothesis of affective disease, or, indeed, reverses the earlier implication. Thus the increased amounts of NE produced by blocking reuptake or metabolism with the antidepressant drugs is seen as causing decreased sensitivity to the neurotransmitter rather than replenishing a deficiency of neurotransmitter. The concept shifts the possible underlying cause of depression from an abnormality in presynaptic function to one of abnormal postsynaptic receptor sensitivity.

V. ANTIMANIC DRUGS: LITHIUM

Lithium is one of the alkali metals like sodium and potassium, and salts of lithium have been used in medicine for a variety of reasons for many years. Although lithium bromide was thought to be the most sedative of bromides when it was used as an antiepileptic agent, it was not until Cade [111] claimed a specific antimanic action that significant interest was taken in its use, in psychiatry. Even then, because of its toxic nature when improperly used and the unfortunate deaths resulting from the use of lithium salts as sodium replacement in hypertensive patients, lithium only slowly attained its current status in therapy.

Currently established therapeutic uses of lithium are in mania and in prophylaxis against recurrent manic-depressive disorder, although it finds other applications [112]. Considerable information has been derived from pharmacological studies with lithium, but there are several problems in relating its basic actions to therapeutic effects. These include the general observation that when administered to animals lithium does not produce much change in activity except in quite toxic doses. Also, in healthy human volunteers there are no significant effects on mood and only subtle mental changes. The other problem is that traditional amine hypotheses relating to mood disorders have it that mania is associated with an excess and depression with a deficiency of amine transmitters in the CNS. Whereas the evidence that lithium decreases the availability of NE at central receptor sites could explain its efficacy in mania [113], lithium also prevents the recurrence of depression. The hypotheses should therefore include a stabilizing action of lithium on the metabolic process underlying mood changes in either direction [112].

As a biologically important electrolyte lithium in many respects resembles sodium, potassium, magnesium, and calcium. Lithium administration causes a decrease of brain magnesium [114,115]. In man there is an increase in plasma magnesium, and it has been suggested that an early rise during lithium treatment predicts a good response in the treatment of depression [116]. There is a decrease in urinary calcium excretion in man [117,118]. It has long been known that lithium can substitute for sodium in extracellular fluid, and it can substitute for sodium in the process of depolarization. Lithium is not as easily removed from cells by cationic transport systems. Impairment of general electrophysiological neuronal processes by lithium, however, might be too general a process to account for the rather specific effects observed on mood.

A variety of effects on biogenic amines have been attributed to lithium both in vivo and in vitro [112]. These include stimulation of NE turnover and both stimulation or inhibition of 5-HT turnover. Other effects include alteration of catecholamine metabolism, inhibition of stimulus-induced release, and both stimulation or inhibition of amine reuptake. Colburn and associates [93] reported that lithium facilitated the uptake of NE into brain synaptosomes, and Pomeroy and Rand [119] suggested a similar action on noradrenergic neurons. These effects are consistent with a decrease in NE available in the synaptic cleft perhaps inhibiting normal transmission in central noradrenergic pathways.

Singer and Rotenberg [120] have suggested two mechanisms of action for lithium. The first is alteration of the neurophysiological process by lithium entering neuronal processes with sodium and modifying ion transport. Changes in the electroencephalograms of patients on lithium have been noted. The second mechanism relates to suppression by lithium of hormone-activated adenylate cyclase in the CNS as has been shown to occur in thyroid and kidney. Argument for this second mechanism was based on the knowledge that neurotransmitters in part activate adenylate cyclase to produce cyclic AMP and that urinary cyclic AMP levels seem to be high in manic patients. Schou [112] stated that, although the idea that lithium might produce a general lowering of all hormone responses mediated via cyclic AMP is attractive, the assumption is not supported by experimental testing. Lithium in fact enhances glucagon-stimulated excretion of cyclic AMP [121].

Lithium affects carbohydrate metabolism at several stages and may therefore in turn affect neuronal transmission. The relevance of this, if any, to lithium therapy is not clear.

VI. ANTIANXIETY AGENTS

Many classes of drugs are used to alleviate anxiety symptoms. Traditional treatment was with barbiturate derivatives or other sedative agents until the introduction of antianxiety agents such as meprobamate and the benzodiazepine derivatives. Before the advent of benzodiazepines, the effectiveness of antianxiety agents left a lot to be desired when evaluated in reliably controlled clinical trials. For instance, the drug benactyzine was widely used as an antianxiety agent following the thorough studies of Jacobsen [122,123] in which it was shown to reduce stress-induced or conflict behavior in animals. However, controlled clinical studies [124,125] proved it to be no better than placebo, and benactyzine no longer has clinical usage. Even meprobamate, despite its extensive use, was shown in a survey of psychiatric literature to be less active than placebo in a majority of well-controlled clinical studies (see references in Ref. 126).

Other drugs are used in anxiety states, including sedatives like amobarbital and the antihistamines diphenhydramine and promethazine, some of the antidepressants in certain circumstances, and the β-adrenoreceptor antagonists. The latter group include propranolol and satolol, but although useful in reducing autonomic symptoms associated with anxiety, there is no strong evidence that these two drugs have significant effect on psychological symptoms including worry, tension, and fear [127].

Benzodiazepines have been reliably demonstrated to be effective antianxiety agents and are now the most extensively used drugs in this class because of their minimal sedative effect, large safety factor, and reduced liability to produce dependency problems. Only the mechanism of action of the benzodiazepines will be discussed.

A. Chemistry of Benzodiazepines

The early promise of chlordiazepoxide and diazepam led to an extensive investigation of the chemical and pharmacological properties of derivatives belonging to the class of 1,4-benzodiazepines. Many of these are available for clinical use, and the structures of some of the more common ones are shown in Fig. 6. Only compounds bearing a substituent in position 7 are highly active, the most common substituent being a Cl or a NO_2 group in the clinically used drugs. Some active derivatives also have a halogen atom substituted at the ortho position of ring C, and activity is also associated with a methyl group at position 1 [128]. The metabolism of the benzodiazepines shows considerable variation in different species, and many metabolites have been characterized. A striking characteristic of many benzodiazepines is their biotransformation to active metabolites [129]. In fact, one of the metabolites of diazepam is oxazepam, which itself is used as an antianxiety agent. The formation of pharmacologically active metabolites means that most benzodiazepine derivatives have a long biological half-life. One notable exception is nitrazepam, which is used as an hypnotic rather than an antianxiety agent, and in this case it is the parent compound rather than its metabolites which accounts for the pharmacological activity [130].

The benzodiazepine derivatives have effects in common with barbiturates —for instance, sedative and anticonvulsant actions—but electrophysiological studies suggest their major action in the CNS is exerted on the hippocampus in contrast to that of the barbiturates on the brainstem reticular formation.

B. Action on Monoamines

Because of the effects of established tranquilizers on the metabolism and action of monoamines, interest early was directed in this area. Benzodiazepines de-

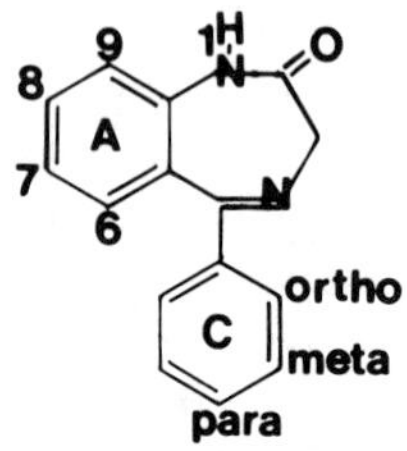

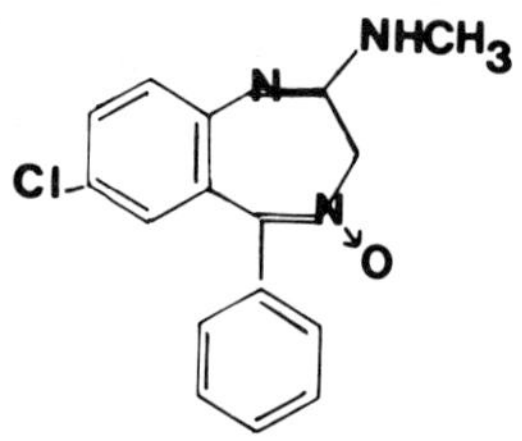

Chlordiazepoxide

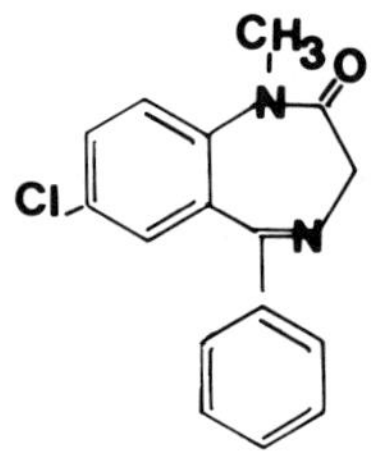

Diazepam

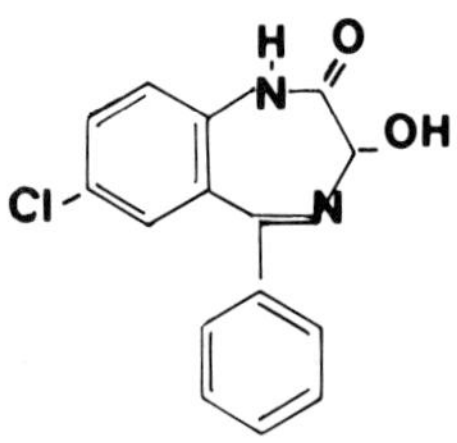

Oxazepam

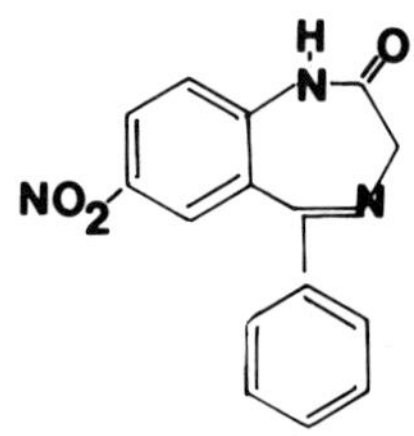

Nitrazepam

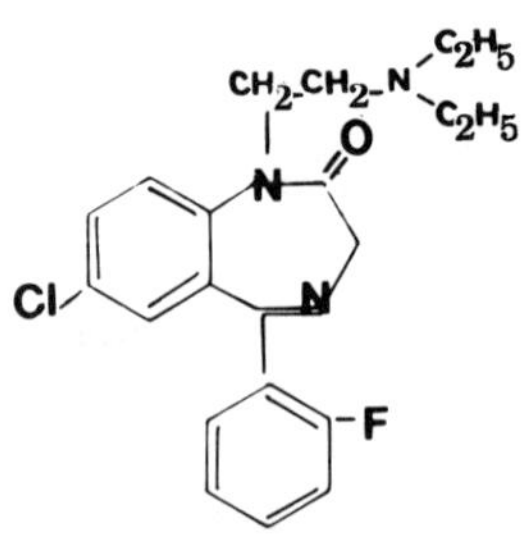

Flurazepam

Figure 6 Chemical structures of benzodiazepine derivatives.

crease NE turnover in the thalamus-hypothalamus-midbrain, cortex, and cerebellum regions of the brain, and DA turnover in the corpus striatum; in addition, at least some benzodiazepine derivatives are weak inhibitors of NE uptake into hypothalamic synaptosomes and DA uptake into striatal synaptosomes [131]. Lidbrink and associates [132] concluded that benzodiazepines probably cause reduction of NE and 5-HT turnover in the cortical areas and of DA turnover in the forebrain, and suggested that this was due to an inhibition of transmitter release. Meprobamate and barbiturates exhibit similar actions on monoamine neurons.

Schallek and associates [133] suggested that the general sedative properties of the benzodiazepines may be related to modification of catecholaminergic and serotonergic neurons. General depressant properties, however, do not account for their other properties, including specific antianxiety effects. The consequences of changes in DA turnover are not clear, but extrapyramidal side effects are not commonly associated with benzodiazepines, as is the case with the neuroleptics.

C. Effects on Acetylcholine

The benzodiazepines are considered to have very weak, if any, effects on the peripheral autonomic nervous system, and although Leeuwin and associates [134] reported an antagonist effect of several benzodiazepines against AC-induced contractions of guinea pig ileum, on a molar basis, the doses used were very high. Benzodiazepines have also been shown to antagonize the depolarizing effect of carbachol on nicotinic receptors in the rat superior cervical ganglion [135]. Again the molar concentrations required were of a high order. It seems unlikely these effects would be produced during therapeutic use of the drugs.

Diazepam has been shown to increase whole brain levels of AC but not to affect choline levels or choline acetylase and cholinesterase activities [136]. These findings suggest that diazepam blocks the release of AC from central neurons. The effect occurred in the hemisphere and diencephalon but not in cerebellum and mesencephalon, and Consolo and associates [136] related it to the anticonvulsant effect of diazepam. Inhibition of the release of AC may be the basis of the advice that diazepam should not be used in patients with glaucoma [79].

D. Benzodiazepines and Central Glycine Receptors

Strychnine is regarded as a potent glycine antagonist, and by measuring the binding of radioactively labeled strychnine to synaptic membrane preparations, it has been possible to label glycine receptors in the brainstem and spinal cord [137]. It was claimed that the receptor labeling was reliable because the regional distribution of strychnine binding could be correlated with the synaptic features of glycine biochemistry and neurophysiology. The rather specific ability of benzodiazepine derivatives to displace bound strychnine from such preparations led Snyder and Enna [138] to postulate a role of central glycine receptors in the antianxiety, anticonvulsant, and muscle relaxant properties of these drugs. Benzodiazepines were thus considered to act by mimicking the inhibitory amino acid transmitter glycine.

Various groups using microelectrophoretic techniques failed to provide support for such a mechanism of action. In studies on single medullary neurons in the rat, Dray and Straughan [139] found that while flurazepam depressed firing rate in a similar manner to glycine, this effect was not blocked by strychnine. In experiments on interneurons in the cat spinal cord, chlordiazepoxide neither depressed firing as did glycine nor altered the interaction of strychnine with glycine [140]. In mice, diazepam in doses that had little or no influence on convulsions or death produced by strychnine provided some degree of protection against these effects produced by bicuculline [140].

Johnston [44] has argued that the in vitro binding studies can be interpreted as indicating that the benzodiazepines bind to strychnine rather than the glycine binding site. This view is based on the affinity of the benzodiazepines for the strychnine binding site being several orders of magnitude lower than that of strychnine.

E. Benzodiazepine Actions Involving γ-Aminobutyric Acid Mechanisms

One of the most telling arguments against the explanation of the action of benzodiazepines being mediated primarily by way of altering glycine effects is the relative potency of benzodiazepine derivatives in preventing convulsions induced by different stimulants. Thus, although benzodiazepines modify strychnine-produced convulsions in animals only in high doses, much better protection is afforded against the convulsant effects of the GABA antagonists bicuculline [140] and picrotoxin [141], or of leptazol [142]. At the same time, these findings support the many studies which relate benzodiazepine actions to central mechanisms involving both the presynaptic and postsynaptic inhibitory actions of GABA.

Experiments carried out by Suria and Costa [143] on the bullfrog sympathetic ganglion have provided evidence for the involvement of GABA in the actions of diazepam on presynaptic nerve terminals. Posttetanic potentiation (PTP) of synaptic potentials can be generated in the curare-treated ganglion [144, 145] and are thought to reflect neurophysiological events that occur presynaptically. PTP has been described also in other neural tissues where it is claimed it may contribute to the spread of seizure discharge [146], and modification of the phenomenon has been used to explain the mechanisms of some antiepileptic drugs such as diphenylhydantoin [147].

Suria and Costa [143] used PTP of synaptic potentials in bullfrog sympathetic ganglia to study various drugs, including benzodiazepines. It was found that diazepam inhibited PTP probably because it can depolarize the preganglionic nerve terminals. As a result of this depolarization, the release of AC was thought to be reduced, and this was believed to be mediated initially through a release of GABA. Depolarization of nerve terminals of cholinergic fibers in the ganglia of bullfrog by diazepam failed to occur if GABA formation was inhibited [148].

A postsynaptic relationship was suggested in studies in which flurazepam and GABA were applied iontophoretically to single cells in the rat medulla [139]. It was shown that flurazepam, like GABA, depressed neuronal firing rates and that in both cases iontophoretically applied bicuculline blocked the responses; at the same time bicuculline did not affect the depressant action of glycine. Another benzodiazepine, clonazepam, in experiments in which it was ad ministered systemically, reversed the block of GABA responses produced by iontophoretic bicuculline on central neurons [135].

Some discrepancies with these results were found in similar experiments by Curtis and associates [149]. Intravenous diazepam was not observed to influence the sensitivity of neurons in the cat to either GABA or glycine applied electrophoretically. Diazepam did not modify either bicuculline or strychnine effects on the inhibitory actions of either amino acid. These authors concluded that their findings suggested benzodiazepines neither mimicked nor antagonized these two inhibitory amino acids on spinal and cerebellar neurons in cats anesthetized with pentobarbital. Straughan [135] suggested that the conflicting findings may be accounted for by differences in anesthesia. In support of this possibility he described experiments in which small doses of barbiturates reversed the blocking action of bicuculline.

There is other support for the view that benzodiazepines potentiate GABA-mediated postsynaptic inhibition. Diazepam enhanced synaptic inhibition of Purkinje cell firing [149] and GABA inhibition in the cat cuneate nucleus [150]. Diazepam inhibited the spontaneous activity of single sensory motor neurons in the rabbit and potentiated the action of microiontophoretically applied GABA [151].

The apparent GABA-like action of benzodiazepines cannot be explained on the basis of inhibition of reuptake of the amino acid by nerve terminals. Chlordiazepoxide, diazepam, and flurazepam did not affect the uptake of GABA in cat and rat cerebellum [149], and although diazepam did reduce the uptake of tritiated GABA by slices of rat cerebral cortex [152], the concentration required was far in excess of that likely to be achieved in therapy.

The most puzzling experimental findings in relating the proposed action of benzodiazepine derivatives to facilitation of GABA transmission or activating GABA receptors are those of Steiner and Felix [153]. Their experiments have shown that iontophoretically applied chlordiazepoxide in fact blocked the effect of exogenous GABA and of GABA-mediated cerebellar Purkinje cells in the rat and the cat.

F. Involvement of γ-Aminobutyric Acid in the Action of Benzodiazepines on Other Transmitters in the Central Nervous System

The findings of Suria and Costa [143] of a possible relationship of GABA in the decreased release of AC by benzodiazepines may be extended to embrace other possible central transmitters. Costa [148] suggested that the evidence relating the action of diazepam being mediated by GABA established a unified concept to explain the reported effect of diazepam in slowing down the turnover rate of catecholamines and 5-HT, as well as AC.

Fuxe and associates [154] investigated the effect of the benzodiazepine reduction of NE and DA turnover with quantitative microspectrofluorimetry. They proposed a possible involvement of GABA mechanisms in this reduction. Diazepam was found to reduce DA turnover in the caudate nucleus, olfactory tubercle, accumbens nucleus, and limbic cortex. A hypothermic action was ruled out as the cause and so too was DA receptor blockade. However, because bicuculline counteracted the effect of benzodiazepines on DA turnover, and because certain GABAergic drugs such as p-chlorphenyl-GABA, aminooxyacetic acid, and γ-hydroxybutyrolactone reduce DA turnover and counteract neuroleptic-induced increase in DA turnover in the limbic system, Fuxe and associates [154] concluded that GABA mechanisms were implicated. It was an interesting finding that the turnover of DA was not affected in the neostriatum since this appears to be in keeping with the lack of extrapyramidal effects of benzodiazepines.

Because recent findings had indicated the existence of inhibitory epinephrine (E) innervation of the locus ceruleus, and because the benzodiazepine reduction of cortical NE turnover was previously thought to be due to a reduction of nervous impulses in parts of the cerulocortical NE pathway, Fuxe and associates [154] thought the effect of benzodiazepines may be due to an E receptor stimulating action. Some support for this is the similarity of effects of diazepam and clonidine, an α-adrenoreceptor agonist, and an interaction between diazepam and piperoxane, an α-adrenoreceptor antagonist. The GABA antagonist picrotoxin was claimed to block some of the effects of diazepam thought to be mediated by activation of this E receptor.

Additional evidence for the speculated relationship of diazepam, GABA, and E receptor activity in anxiety is provided by findings in different studies with yohimbine. Yohimbine causes an anxietylike state in man [155] and has been found to block E receptors [156]. Yohimbine increases the turnover of NE in the brain, and this effect is slowed down by diazepam [154]. The behavioral and cardiovascular responses to yohimbine in the conscious dog also are markedly reduced by the benzodiazepine chlordiazepoxide [126], and this is at least consistent with the speculated relationship.

G. Benzodiazepine Receptor in the Central Nervous System

The presence of benzodiazepine receptors in the CNS has recently been reported independently by Möhler and Okada [157] and Squires and Braestrup [158]. The receptors originally were identified by high-affinity tritiated diazepam binding in rat brain, and it was found that barbiturates and meprobamate did not bind with the sites. Möhler and Okada [157] described a variation in density of binding sites in different regions with the highest occurring in cerebral cortex followed by hypothalamus, cerebellum, midbrain, and hippocampus. Less was found in striatum and medulla-pons, and relatively small levels in the spinal cord. A similarity of the rank order of density of receptors was claimed with that of the GABA receptor [74]. Although this supports the relevance of GABA mechanisms in the action of benzodiazepines, the two receptors are not identical with regard to binding characteristics. The failure of benzodiazepines to block tritiated GABA binding to brain membrane [138] and the inability of GABA, its agonist muscimol, or its antagonists picrotoxin and bicuculline to displace tritiated diazepam suggests that benzodiazepines do not bind to GABA receptors. It is possible that benzodiazepine effects may be indirect ones, for instance by facilitating the release of GABA.

Subcellular distribution findings suggest that 60% of the tritiated diazepam binding sites occur in the synaptosomal fraction [157]. This may mean that the more important site of action of the drugs is a presynaptic one. The binding is stereospecific, and the pharmacological potency of benzodiazepines correlates with their affinity for the receptor. Benzodiazepine receptors have also been identified in human brain corresponding to those of rat brain in affinity, stereospecificity, and regional distribution [157].

These interesting and detailed findings offer promise of rapid advance in further elaborating the mechanism of action of benzodiazepine derivatives.

REFERENCES

1. D. N. Franz, Drugs acting on the central nervous system. In *The Pharmacological Basis of Therapeutics* (L. S. Goodman and A. Gilman, eds.). New York, Macmillan, 1975.
2. N. Kline, Monoamine oxidase inhibitors: An unfinished picaresque tale. In *Discoveries in Biological Psychiatry* (F. J. Ayd and B. Blackwell, eds.). Philadelphia, Lippincott, 1970.

3. U. S. von Euler, A specific sympathomimetic ergone in adrenergic nerve fibres (sympathin) and its relations to adrenaline and noradrenaline. *Acta Physiol. Scand. 12:*73-97, 1946.
4. M. Vogt, The concentration of sympathin in different parts of the central nervous system under normal conditions and after administration of drugs. *J. Physiol.* (London) *123:*451-481, 1954.
5. U. Ungerstedt, Stereotaxic mapping of the monoamine pathways in the rat brain. *Acta Physiol. Scand., Suppl. 367:*1-48, 1971.
6. F. E. Bloom and G. K. Aghajanian, An electron microscopic analysis of large granular synaptic vesicles of the brain in relation to monoamine content. *J. Pharmacol. Exp. Ther. 159:*261-273, 1968.
7. J. Musacchio, Enzymes involved in the biosynthesis and degradation of catecholamines. In *Handbook of Psychopharmacology,* vol. 3: *Biochemistry of Biogenic Amines* (L. L. Iversen, S. D. Iversen, and S. H. Snyder, eds.). New York, Plenum Press, 1975.
8. J. Glowinski, I. J. Kopin, and J. Axelrod, Metabolism of (^{3}H) norepinephrine in the rat brain. *J. Neurochem. 12:*25-30, 1965.
9. P. B. Bradley and J. H. Wolstencraft, Excitation and inhibition of brainstem neurones by noradrenaline and acetylcholine. *Nature 196:*840, 873 1962.
10. P. B. Bradley, The pharmacology of synapses in the central nervous system. In *Recent Advances in Pharmacology* (J. M. Robson and R. S. Stacey, eds.). London, Churchill, 1968.
11. T. W. Stone, Are noradrenaline excitations artefacts? *Nature 234:*145-146, 1971.
12. W. Feldberg and S. L. Sherwood, Injections of drugs into the lateral ventricle of the cat. *J. Physiol.* (London) *123:*148-167, 1954.
13. W. G. Dewhurst and E. Marley, Action of sympathomimetic and allied amines on the central nervous system of the chicken. *Brit. J. Pharmacol. 25:*705-727, 1965.
14. K. Fuxe, T. Hökfelt, and U. Ungerstedt, Morphological and functional aspects of central monoamine neurons. *Int. Rev. Neurobiol. 13:*93-126 1970.
15. J. Olds, *Drives and Reinforcement. Behavioral Studies of Hypothalamic Functions.* New York, Raven Press, 1977.
16. A. Carlsson, M. Lindqvist, T. Magnusson, and B. Waldeck, On the presence of 3-hydroxytyramine in brain. *Science 127:*471, 1957.
17. U. S. von Euler, Distribution and metabolism of catechol hormones in tissues and axones. *Rec. Progr. Horm. Res. 14:*483-507 1959.
18. A. Carlsson, The occurrence, distribution, and physiological role of catecholamines in the nervous system. *Pharmacol. Rev. 1:*490-493, 1959.
19. S. D. Iversen and L. L. Iversen, *Behavioral Pharmacology.* New York, Oxford University Press, 1975.
20. F. E. Bloom, E. Costa, and G. C. Salmoiraghi, Anesthesia and the responsiveness of individual neurons of the caudate nucleus of the cat to acetyl-

choline, norepinephrine, and dopamine administered by microelectrophoresis. *J. Pharmacol. Exp. Ther. 150:*244-252, 1965.
21. D. H. York, Possible dopaminergic pathway from substantia nigra to putamen. *Brain Res. 20:*233-249, 1970.
22. J. A. Gonzalez-Vegas, Actions of papaverine and bulbocapnine on synaptic transmission in the nigro-striatal pathway in the rat. *J. Physiol.* (London) *226:*102P, 1972.
23. O. Hornykiewicz, Dopamine (3-hydroxytyramine) and brain function. *Pharmacol. Rev. 18:*925-964, 1966.
24. A. H. Amin, T. B. B. Crawford, and J. H. Gaddum, The distribution of substance P and 5-hydroxytryptamine in the central nervous system of the dog. *J. Physiol.* (London) *126:*596-618, 1954.
25. W. Feldberg and R. D. Myers, Changes in temperature produced by microinjections of amines into the anterior hypothalamus of cats. *J. Physiol.* (London) *177:*239-245, 1965.
26. R. D. Myers and D. B. Beleslin, Changes in serotonin release in hypothalamus during cooling or warming of the monkey. *Amer. J. Physiol. 220:* 1746-1754, 1971.
27. M. Jouvet, Biogenic amines and the states of sleep. *Science 163:*32-41, 1969.
28. W. Feldberg and M. Vogt, Acetylcholine synthesis in different regions of the central nervous system. *J. Physiol.* (London) *107:*372-381, 1948.
29. D. R. Curtis and R. M. Eccles, The excitation of Renshaw cells by pharmacological agents applied electrophoretically. *J. Physiol.* (London) *141:*435-445, 1958.
30. J. F. Mitchell, The spontaneous and evoked release of acetylcholine from the cerebral cortex. *J. Physiol.* (London) *165:*98-116, 1963.
31. F. V. De Feudis, *Central Cholinergic Systems and Behaviour.* London, Academic Press, 1974.
32. W. Feldberg and S. L. Sherwood, Injections of drugs into the lateral ventricle of the cat. *J. Physiol.* (London) *123:*148-167, 1954.
33. S. L. Sherwood, Intraventricular medication in catatonic stupor. *Brain 75:* 68-75, 1952.
34. H. Kwiatkowski, Histamine in nervous tissue. *J. Physiol.* (London) *102:*32-41, 1943.
35. K. M. Taylor, Brain histamine. In *Handbook of Psychopharmacology,* vol. 3. *Biochemistry of Biogenic Amines* (L. L. Iverson, D. S. Iverson, and S. H. Snyder, eds.). New York, Plenum Press, 1975.
36. C. Calcutt, The role of histamine in the brain. *Gen. Pharmacol. 7:*15-25, 1976.
37. J.-C. Schwartz, G. Barbin, M. Garbarg, H. Pollard, C. Rose, and M. Verdiere, Neurochemical evidence for histamine acting as a transmitter in mammalian brain. *Advan. Biochem. Psychopharmacol. 15:*111-126, 1976.
38. J.-C. Schwartz, Histaminergic mechanisms in brain. *An. Rev. Pharmacol. 17:*325-339, 1977.

39. T. White, Biosynthesis, metabolism, and function of histamine in the nervous system. *Fed. Proc. 23:*1103-1106, 1964.
40. M. Garbarg, G. Barbin, J. Feger, and J.-C. Schwartz, Histaminergic pathways in rat brain evidenced by lesions in the medial forebrain bundle. *Science 186:*833-835, 1974.
41. S. Fahn and L. J. Côté, Regional distribution of γ-aminobutyric acid (GABA) in brain of the Rhesus monkey. *J. Neurochem. 15:*209-213, 1968.
42. N. Otsuka and Y. Miyata, Application of enzymatic cycling to the measurement of gamma-aminobutyric acid in single neurons of the mammalian central nervous system. *Advan. Biochem. Psychopharmacol. 6:*61-74, 1972.
43. L. Iversen and J. S. Kelly, Uptake and metabolism of γ-aminobutyric acid by neurones and glial cells. *Biochem. Pharmacol. 24:*933-938, 1975.
44. G. A. R. Johnston, Neuropharmacology of amino acid inhibitory transmitters. *An. Rev. Pharmacol. 18:*269-289, 1978.
45. F. V. De Feudis, Amino acids as central neurotransmitters. *An. Rev. Pharmacol. 15:*105-130, 1975.
46. D. R. Curtis, A. W. Duggan, D. Felix, G. A. R. Johnston, and H. McLennan, Antagonism between bicuculline and GABA in the cat brain. *Brain Res. 33:*57-73, 1971.
47. E. R. John, K. F. Killam, B. M. Wenzel, and R. D. Tschirgi, Effects of intraventricular injections of gamma-aminobutyric acid on performance of conditioned responses in cats. In *Inhibition in the Nervous System and Gamma-aminobutyric Acid* (E. Roberts, ed.). New York, Pergamon Press, 1960.
48. E. Roberts, An hypothesis that there is a defect in the GABA system in schizophrenia. *Neurosci. Res. Program Bull. 10:*468-482, 1972.
49. M. H. Aprison and R. Werman, Distribution of glycine in cat spinal cord and roots. *Life Sci. 4:*2075-2083, 1965.
50. N. Davidson, *Neurotransmitter Amino Acids.* London, Academic Press, 1976.
51. E. A. Mroz, M. J. Brownstein, and S. E. Leeman, Distribution of immunoassayable substance P in the rat brain: Evidence for the existence of substance P-containing tracts. In *Substance P* (U. S. von Euler and B. Pernow, eds.). New York, Raven Press, 1977.
52. K. Krnjević, Effects of substance P on central neurons in cats. In *Substance P* (U. S. von Euler and B. Pernow, eds.). New York, Raven Press, 1977.
53. A. Carlsson, T. Magnusson, G. H. Fisher, D. Chang, and K. Folkers, Effect of synthetic substance P on central monoaminergic mechanisms. In *Substance P* (U. S. von Euler and B. Pernow, eds.). New York, Raven Press, 1977.
54. J. Hughes, Isolation of an endogenous compound from the brain with pharmacological properties similar to morphine. *Brain Res. 88:*295-308, 1975.
55. R. C. A. Frederickson, Enkephalin pentapeptides: A review of current evidence for a physiological role in vertebrate neurotransmission. *Life Sci. 21:*23-42, 1977.

56. R. J. Baldassarini and J. E. Fischer, Trace amines and alternative neurotransmitters in the central nervous system. *Biochem. Pharmacol. 27:*621-626, 1978.
57. S. H. Snyder, W. J. Logan, J. P. Bennett, and A. Arregui, Amino acids as central nervous transmitters: Biochemical studies. In *Neurosciences Research,* vol. 5 (S. Ehrenpreis and I. J. Kopin, eds.). New York, Academic Press, 1973.
58. A. S. Horn and S. H. Snyder, Chlorpromazine and dopamine: Conformational similarities that correlate with the antischizophrenic activity of phenothiazine drugs. *Proc. Nat. Acad. Sci. U.S. 68:*2325-2328, 1971.
59. D. De Maio, Clozapine: A novel major tranquilizer. *Arzneimittel–Forsch. 22:*919-923, 1972.
60. D. S. Bell, The experimental reproduction of amphetamine psychoses. *Arch. Gen. Psychiat. 29:*34-40, 1973.
61. O. Hornykiewicz, Dopamine in the basal ganglia: Its role and therapeutic implications (including the clinical use of L-DOPA). *Brit. Med. Bull. 29:* 172-178, 1973.
62. S. Courvoisier, J. Fournel, R. Ducrot, M. Kolsky, and P. Koetschet, Properties pharmacodynamiques du chlorhydrate de chloro-^{3}(dimethylamine-$^{3'}$propyl)-^{10}phenothiazine (4560 RP). *Arch. Int. Pharmacodyn. 92:*305-361, 1953.
63. E. F. Domino, R. D. Hudson, and G. Zografi, Substituted phenothiazines: Pharmacology and chemical structure. In *Drugs Affecting the Central Nervous System* (F. Burger, ed.). London, Edward Arnold, 1968.
64. S. Matthysse, Antipsychotic drug actions: A clue to the neuropathology of schizophrenia? *Fed. Proc. 32:*200-205, 1973.
65. H. Nybäck, J. Schubert, and G. Sedvall, Effect of apomorphine and pimozide on synthesis and turnover of labelled catecholamines in mouse brain. *J. Pharm. Pharmacol. 22:*622-624, 1970.
66. O. Hornykiewicz, Psychopharmacological implications of dopamine and dopamine antagonists: A critical evaluation of current evidence. *An. Rev. Pharmacol. 17:*545-559, 1977.
67. S. H. Snyder, S. P. Banerjee, H. I. Yamamura, and D. Greenberg, Drugs, neurotransmitters, and schizophrenia. *Science 184:*1243-1253, 1974.
68. B. Fjalland, A. V. Christensen, and.J. Hytell, Peripheral and central muscarinic receptor affinity of psychotropic drugs. *Naunyn-Schmiedebergs Arch. Pharmakol. Exp. Pathol. 301:*5-9, 1977.
69. P. M. Laduron and J. E. Leysen, Is the low incidence of extrapyramidal side-effects of antipsychotics associated with antimuscarinic properties? *J. Pharm. Pharmacol. 30:*120-122, 1978.
70. Y. C. Clement-Cormier, J. W. Kebabian, G. L. Petzold, and P. Greengard, Dopamine-sensitive adenylate cyclase in mammalian brain: A possible site of action of antipsychotic drugs. *Proc. Nat. Acad. Sci. U.S. 71:*1113-1117, 1974.
71. N.-E. Anden and G. Stock, Effect of clozapine on the turnover of dopamine

in the corpus striatum and in the limbic system. *J. Pharm. Pharmacol. 25:* 346-348, 1973.
72. P. A. J. Janssen, The pharmacology of haloperidol. *Int. J. Neuropsychiat. 3:*S10-S18, 1967.
73. S. Maruyama and T. Kawasaki, Synergism between γ-aminobutyric acid and butyrophenones administered microelectrophoretically in the Purkinje cells of the cat cerebellum. *Japn. J. Pharmacol. 25:*209-213, 1975.
74. H. Möhler and T. Okada, GABA receptor binding with ^{3}H(+)-bicuculline methiodide in rat CNS. *Nature 267:*65-67, 1977.
75. K. Dismukes and A. H. Mulder, Effects of neuroleptics on release of ^{3}H-dopamine from slices of rat corpus striatum. *Naunyn-Schmiedebergs Arch. Pharmakol. Exp. Pathol. 297:*23-29, 1977.
76. L. L. Iversen and G. A. R. Johnston, GABA uptake in rat central nervous system: Comparison of uptake in slices and homogenates and the effects of some inhibitors. *J. Neurochem. 18:*1939-1950, 1971.
77. J.-S. Kim and R. Hassler, Effects of acute haloperidol on the gamma-aminobutyric acid system in rat striatum and substantia nigra. *Brain Res. 88:*150-153, 1975.
78. A. R. Cool and H.-J. Janssen, γ-Aminobutyric acid: The essential mediator of behaviour triggered by neostriatally applied apomorphine and haloperidol. *J. Pharm. Pharmacol. 28:*70-74, 1976.
79. M. E. Jarvik, Drugs used in the treatment of psychiatric disorders. In *The Pharmacological Basis of Therapeutics* (L. S. Goodman and A. Gilman, ed.). New York, Macmillan, 1965.
80. E. F. Domino, Psychosedative drugs, I: Substituted phenothiazines, reserpine, and derivatives. In *Drill's Pharmacology in Medicine* (J. R. Di Palma, ed.). New York, McGraw-Hill, 1965.
81. D. de Wied, Chlorpromazine and endocrine function. *Pharmacol. Rev. 19:* 251-288, 1967.
82. M. Wilhelm, The chemistry of polycyclic psycho-active drugs: Serendipity or systematic investigation? In *Depressive Illness: Diagnosis, Assessment, Treatment* (P. Kieholz, ed.). Bern, Hans Huber, 1972.
83. F. Sulser, J. Vetulani, and P. L. Mobley, Mode of action of antidepressant drugs. *Biochem. Pharmacol. 27:*257-261, 1978.
84. J. J. Schildkraut, The catecholamine hypothesis of affective disorders: A review of supporting evidence. *Amer. J. Psychiat. 122:*509-522, 1965.
85. W. E. Bunney and J. M. Davis, Norepinephrine in depressive reactions. *Arch. Gen. Psychiat. 13:*483-494, 1965.
86. I. P. Lapin and G. F. Oxenkrug, Intensification of the central serotonergic processes as a possible determinant of the thymoleptic effect. *Lancet 1:* 132-136, 1969.
87. I. C. Wilson and A. J. Prange, Tryptophan in mania: Theory of affective disorders. *Psychopharmacologia, Suppl. 26:*76, 1972.
88. D. M. Shaw, F. E. Camps, and E. C. Eccleston, 5-Hydroxytryptamine in the hind-brain of depressive suicides. *Brit. J. Psychiat. 113:*1407-1411, 1967.

89. C. M. B. Pare, D. P. H. Yeung, K. Price, and R. S. Stacey, 5-Hydroxytryptamine, noradrenaline, and dopamine in brainstem, hypothalamus, and caudate nucleus of controls and of patients committing suicide by coal-gas poisoning. *Lancet 2:*133–135, 1969.
90. E. B. Sigg, Pharmacological studies with Tofranil. *Can. Psychiatr. Ass. J., Suppl. 4:*75–85, 1959.
91. J. Glowinski and J. Axelrod, Inhibition of uptake of tritiated noradrenaline in the intact rat brain by imipramine and structurally related compounds. *Nature 204:*1318–1319, 1964.
92. W. E. Fann, J. M. Davis, D. S. Janowsky, J. S. Kaufmann, J. D. Griffith, and J. A. Oates, Effect of iprindole on amine uptake in man. *Arch. Gen. Psychiat. 26:*158–162, 1972.
93. R. W. Colburn, F. K. Goodwin, W. E. Bunney, and J. M. Davis, Effect of lithium on the uptake of noradrenaline by synaptosomes. *Nature 215:* 1395–1397, 1967.
94. F. K. Goodwin, D. L. Murphy, D. L. Dunner, and W. E. Bunney, Lithium response in unipolar versus bipolar depression, *Amer. J. Psychiat. 129:*44–47, 1972.
95. E. B. Sigg, L. Soffer, and L. Gyermek, Influences of imipramine and related psychoactive agents on the effect of 5-hydroxytryptamine and catecholamines on the cat nictitating membrane. *J. Pharmacol. Exp. Ther. 142:*13–20, 1963.
96. A. Carlsson, K. Fuxe, and U. Ungerstedt, The effect of imipramine on central 5-hydroxytryptamine neurons. *J. Pharm. Pharmacol. 20:*150–151, 1968.
97. K. Fuxe and U. Ungerstedt, Histochemical studies on the effect of (+)-amphetamine, drugs of the imipramine group, and tryptamine on central catecholamine and 5-hydroxytryptamine neurons after intraventricular injections of catecholamines and 5-hydroxytryptamine. *Eur. J. Pharmacol. 4:*135–144, 1968.
98. P. Lidbrink, G. Jonsson, and K. Fuxe, The effect of imipramine-like drugs and antihistamine drugs on uptake mechanisms in the central noradrenaline and 5-hydroxytryptamine neurons. *Neuropharmacol. 10:*521–536, 1971.
99. R. Domenjoz and W. Theobald, Zur pharmakologie des Tofranil® (N-[3-Dimethylaminopropyl]-iminodibenzyl-hydrochloride). *Arch. Int. Pharmacodyn. 120:*450–489, 1959.
100. E. B. Sigg, Autonomic side-effects induced by psychotherapeutic agents. In *Psychopharmacology: A Review of Progress, 1957-1967.* (D. H. Efron, J. O. Cole, J. Levine, and J. R. Wittenborn, eds.). Public Health Service Publication No. 1836. Washington, D.C., U.S. Government Printing Office, 1968.
101. P. D. Kanof and P. Greengard, Brain histamine receptors as targets for antidepressant drugs. *Nature 272:*329–333, 1978.
102. L. R. Hegstrand, P. D. Kanof, and P. Greengard, Histamine-sensitive adenylate cyclase in mammalian brain. *Nature 260:*163–165, 1976.
103. W. J. Lang, M. L. Brown, S. Gershon, I. Sletten, and B. Korol, Effects of chronic chlorpromazine administration upon the blood pressure response

to autonomic drugs in conscious dogs. *Arch. Int. Pharmacodyn. 162:* 330-344, 1966.

104. I. W. Sletten, W. J. Lang, M. L. Brown, S. R. Ballou, and S. Gershon, Chronic chlorpromazine administration: Some pharmacological and psychological effects in man. *Clin. Pharmacol. Ther. 6:*575-586, 1965.

105. M. Fink, M. Pollack, D. F. Klein, A. G. Blumberg, I. Belmont, E. Karp, J. C. Kramer, and A. Willner, Comparative studies of chlorpromazine and imipramine, I: Drug discriminating patterns. In *Neuropsychopharmacology* (P. B. Bradley, F. Flügel, and P. H. Hoch, eds.). Amsterdam, Elsevier, 1964.

106. J. E. Overall, L. E. Hollister, F. Meyer, I. Kimbell, and J. Shelton, Imipramine and thioridazine in depressed and schizophrenic patients: Are there specific antidepressant drugs? *JAMA 189:*605-608, 1964.

107. J. J. Schildkraut, A. Winokur, P. R. Draskoczy, and J. H. Henzle, Changes in norepinephrine turnover in rat brain during chronic administration of imipramine and protriptyline: A possible explanation for the delay in onset of antidepressant effects. *Amer. J. Psychiat. 127:*1032-1039, 1971.

108. F. Sulser, M. H. Bickel, and B. B. Brodie, The action of desmethylimipramine in counteracting sedation and cholinergic effects of reserpine-like drugs. *J. Pharmacol. Exp. Ther. 144:*321-330, 1964.

109. H. S. Alpers and H. E. Himwich, The effect of chronic imipramine administration on rat brain levels of serotonin, 5-hydroxyindoleacetic acid, norepinephrine, and dopamine. *J. Pharmacol. Exp. Ther. 180:*531-538, 1972.

110. J. Vetulani, R. J. Stawirz, J. V. Dingell, and F. Sulser, A possible common mechanism of action of antidepressant treatments: Reduction in the sensitivity of the noradrenergic cyclic AMP generating system in the rat limbic forebrain. *Naunyn-Schmiedebergs Arch. Pharmakol. Exp. Pathol. 293:* 109-114, 1976.

111. J. F. J. Cade, Lithium salts in the treatment of psychotic excitement. *Med. J. Aust. 2:*349-352, 1949.

112. M. Schou, Pharmacology and toxicology of lithium. *An. Rev. Pharmacol. 16:*231-243, 1976.

113. M. J. Rand and M. W. McCulloch, Modes of action of antidepressants. In *Handbook of Studies on Depression* (G. Burrows, ed.). Amsterdam, Excerpta Medica, 1977.

114. N. J. Birch and F. A. Jenner, The distribution of lithium and its effects on the distribution and excretion of other ions in the rat. *Brit. J. Pharmacol. 47:*586-594, 1973.

115. P. A. Bond, B. A. Brooks, and A. Judd, The distribution of lithium, sodium, and magnesium in rat brain and plasma after various periods of administration of lithium in the diet. *Brit. J. Pharmacol. 53:*235-239, 1975.

116. J. S. Carman, R. M. Post, T. A. Teplitz, and F. K. Goodwin, Divalent cations in predicting antidepressant response to lithium. *Lancet 2:*1454, 1974.

117. J. Crammer, Lithium, calcium, and mental illness. *Lancet 1:*215-216, 1975.
118. N. Bjørum, I. Hornum, E. T. Mellerup, P. K. Plenge, and O. J. Rafaelsen, Lithium, calcium, and phosphate. *Lancet 1:*1243, 1975.
119. A. Pomeroy and M. J. Rand, Facilitation of noradrenaline uptake by lithium. *Aust. N.Z. Psychiat. 5:*280-285, 1971.
120. I. Singer and D. Rotenberg, Mechanisms of lithium action. *N. Engl. J. Med. 289:*254-260, 1973.
121. O. V. Olesen, J. Jensen, and K. Thomsen, Effect of lithium on glucagon-stimulated cyclic AMP excretion in rats. *Acta Pharmacol. Toxicol. 35:* 403-411, 1974.
122. E. Jacobsen and Y. Skaarup, Experimental induction of conflict-behaviour in cats: The effect of some anticholinergic compounds. *Acta Pharmacol. Toxicol. 11:*125-134, 1955.
123. E. Jacobsen and E. Sonne, The effect of benzilic acid diethylaminoester, HCl (Benactyzine) on stress-induced behaviour in the rat. *Acta Pharmacol. Toxicol. 11:*135-147, 1955.
124. A. Coady and E. C. O. Jewesbury, A clinical trial of benactyzine hydrochloride ("Suavitil") as a physical relaxant. *Brit. Med. J. 1:*485-487, 1956.
125. H. Scott Forbes and B. V. Earle, Benactyzine in psychoneurosis. *Brit. Med. J. 1:*226, 1977.
126. W. J. Lang and S. Gershon, Effects of psychoactive drugs on yohimbine-induced responses in conscious dogs: A proposed screening procedure for anti-anxiety agents. *Arch. Int. Pharmacodyn. 142,* 457-472, 1963.
127. M. Lader, Antianxiety drugs: Clinical pharmacology and therapeutic use. *Drugs 12:*362-373, 1976.
128. L. H. Sternbach, Chemistry of 1,4-benzodiazepines and some aspects of the structure-activity relationship. In *The Benzodiazepines* (S. Garattini, E. Mussini, and L. O. Randall, eds.). New York, Raven Press, 1973.
129. M. A. Schwartz, Pathways of metabolism of the benzodiazepines. In *The Benzodiazepines* (S. Garattini, E. Mussini, and L. O. Randall, eds.). New York, Raven Press, 1973.
130. L. O. Randall and B. Kappell, Pharmacological activity of some benzodiazepines and their metabolites. In *The Benzodiazepines* (S. Garattini, E. Mussini, and L. O. Randall, eds.). New York, Raven Press, 1973.
131. K. M. Taylor and R. Laverty, The interaction of chlordiazepoxide, diazepam, and nitrazepam with catecholamines and histamine in regions of the rat brain. In *The Benzodiazepines* (S. Garattini, E. Mussini, and L. O. Randall, eds.). New York, Raven Press, 1973.
132. P. Lidbrink, H. Corrodi, K. Fuxe, and L. Olson, The effects of benzodiazepines, meprobamate, and barbiturates on central monoamine neurons. In *The Benzodiazepines* (S. Garattini, E. Mussini, and L. O. Randall, eds.). New York, Raven Press, 1973.
133. W. Schallek, W. Schlosser, and L. O. Randall, Recent developments in the

pharmacology of the benzodiazepines. *Advan. Pharmacol. Chemother. 10:*119-183, 1972.
134. R. S. Leeuwin, R. N. Djojodibroto, and E. Th. Groenwoud, The effects of three benzodiazepines and of meprobamate on the actions of smooth muscle stimulants on the guinea-pig ileum. *Arch. Int. Pharmacodyn. 217:* 18-21, 1975.
135. D. W. Straughan, Current views on the mechanism of action of the benzodiazepines. *Arch. Pharmacol. Toxicol. 3:*3-22, 1977.
136. S. Consolo, H. Ladinsky, G. Peri, and S. Garattini, Effect of diazepam on mouse whole brain and brain area acetylcholine and choline levels. *Eur. J. Pharmacol. 27:*266-268, 1974.
137. A. B. Young and S. H. Snyder, Strychnine binding associated with glycine receptors of the central nervous system. *Proc. Nat. Acad. Sci. U.S. 70:* 2832-2836, 1973.
138. S. H. Snyder and S. J. Enna, The role of central glycine receptors in the pharmacologic actions of benzodiazepines. *Advan. Biochem. Psychopharmacol. 14:*81-91, 1975.
139. A. Dray and D. W. Straughan, Benzodiazepines: GABA and glycine receptors on single neurones in the rat medulla. *J. Pharm. Pharmacol. 28:* 314-315, 1976.
140. D. R. Curtis, C. J. A. Game, and D. Lodge, Benzodiazepines and central glycine receptors. *Brit. J. Pharmacol. 56:*307-311, 1976.
141. E. Costa, A. Guidotti, and C. C. Mao, Evidence for involvement of GABA in the action of benzodiazepines: Studies on rat cerebellum. *Advan. Biochem. Psychopharmacol. 14:*113-130, 1975.
142. G. Zbinden and L. O. Randall, Pharmacology of benzodiazepines: Laboratory and clinical correlations. In *Advances in Pharmacology* (S. Garattini and P. A. Shore, eds.). New York, Academic Press, 1967.
143. A. Suria and E. Costa, Evidence for GABA involvement in the action of diazepam on presynaptic nerve terminals in bullfrog sympathetic ganglia. *Advan. Biochem. Psychopharmacol. 14:*103-112, 1975.
144. B. Libet, S. Chichibu, and T. Tosaka, Slow synaptic responses and excitability in sympathetic ganglia of the bullfrog. *J. Neurophysiol. 31:*383-395, 1968.
145. R. M. Eccles and B. Libet, Origin and blockade of synaptic responses of curarized sympathetic ganglia. *J. Physiol.* (London) *157:*484-503, 1961.
146. D. W. Esplin, Effects of diphenylhydantoin on synaptic transmission in cat spinal cord and stellate ganglion. *J. Pharmacol. Exp. Ther. 120:*301-323, 1957.
147. D. M. Woodbury and D. W. Esplin, Neuropharmacology and neurochemistry of anticonvulsant drugs. *Proc. Ass. Res. Nerv. Ment. Dis. 37:*24-56, 1959.
148. E. Costa, New concepts on the mechanisms of action of benzodiazepines. *Life Sci. 17:*167-185, 1975.
149. D. R. Curtis, D. Lodge, G. A. R. Johnston, and S. J. Brand, Central actions of benzodiazepines. *Brain Res. 118:*344-347, 1976.

150. P. Polc and W. Haefely, Effects of two benzodiazepines, phenobarbitone, and baclofen on synaptic transmission in the cat cuneate nucleus. *Nauyn-Schmiedebergs Arch. Pharmakol. Exp. Pathol. 294:*121-131, 1976.

151. V. V. Zakusov, R. U. Ostrovskaya, S. N. Kozhechkin, V. V. Markovich, E. M. Molodavkin, and T. A. Voronina, Further evidence for GABA-energic mechanisms in the actions of benzodiazepines. *Arch. Int. Pharmacodyn. 229:*313-326, 1977.

152. M. Harris, J. M. Hopkins, and M. J. Neal, Effect of centrally acting drugs on the uptake of γ-aminobutyric acid (GABA) by slices of rat cerebral cortex. *Brit. J. Pharmacol. 47:*229-239, 1973.

153. F. A. Steiner and D. Felix, Antagonistic effects of GABA and benzodiazepines on vestibular and cerebellar neurones. *Nature 260:*346-347, 1976.

154. K. Fuxe, L. F. Agnati, P. Bolme, T. Hökfelt, P. Lidbrink, A. Ljungdahl, M. de la Mora, and S. O. Ögren, The possible involvement of GABA mechanisms in the actions of benzodiazepines on central catecholamine neurons. *Advan. Biochem. Psychopharmacol. 14:*45-61, 1975.

155. G. Holmberg and S. Gershon, Autonomic and psychic effects of yohimbine hydrochloride. *Psychopharmacologia 2:*93-106, 1961.

156. P. Bolme, H. Corrodi, K. Fuxe, T. Hökfelt, P. Lidbrink, and M. Goldstein, Possible involvement of central adrenaline neurons in vasomotor and respiratory control: Studies with clonidine and its interactions with piperoxane and yohimbine. *Eur. J. Pharmacol. 28:*89-94, 1974.

157. H. Möhler and T. Okada, Benzodiazepine receptor: Demonstration in the central nervous system. *Science 198:*844-851, 1977.

158. R. F. Squires and C. Braestrup, Benzodiazepine receptors in rat brain. *Nature 266:*732-734, 1977.

2

Methods for the Measurement of Psychotropic Drugs
Antidepressants

Bruce A. Scoggins / *Howard Florey Institute of Experimental Physiology and Medicine, University of Melbourne, Parkville, Victoria, Australia*

Kay P. Maguire / *Department of Psychiatry, University of Melbourne, Parkville, Victoria, Australia*

I. TRICYCLIC ANTIDEPRESSANTS

A variety of methods for the measurement of tricyclic antidepressant drugs have been described since 1960. An outline of the chemical structure of the tricyclics and related drugs is shown in Fig. 1. Common to the majority of methods is the need for extraction of the drug from the biological medium prior to analysis (Sec. I.A). This usually involves extraction of an alkaline medium with an organic solvent. The extract is then assayed by spectrofluorimetry (Sec. I.B), isotope-derivative dilution analysis (Sec. I.C), gas-liquid chromatography (Sec. I.D), high performance liquid chromatography (Sec. I.F) or radioimmunoassay (Sec. I.G), to name the most commonly used techniques. Although most of the methods referred to apply to blood plasma, the majority of these could be used for whole blood, tissue, urine, or cerebrospinal fluid (CSF) with slight modification of the extraction procedure.

The first studies requiring the measurement of tricyclic antidepressants were concerned with the metabolism, distribution, and excretion of the drugs. The assay was usually by spectrophotometry or simple chemical analyses, some of which involved separation of parent drug from its metabolites by chromatography (IMI* [1-3], AT [4-7], NT [8], and DMI [9]). None of these assays were sensitive enough for plasma level analysis. Fluorimetric techniques were developed which had adequate sensitivity but were usually nonspecific due to metabolite interference (IMI [10], DMI [11], IMI and DMI [12]).

More suitable assays were developed in 1967, first by Moody and colleagues [13] who described a more advanced fluorimetric procedure for IMI and DMI, and second by Hammer and Brodie [14] who developed an isotope-derivative assay for NT or DMI. A further advance came in 1970-71 with the first suitable gas-liquid chromatography (GLC) techniques (AT [15], AT and NT [16], NT [17], and DMI [18]).

Since then, the majority of published methods have utilized GLC, initially with the more conventional detectors, flame ionization or electron capture, but more recently with either nitrogen-specific detection or mass fragmentography. Other contemporary methods investigated include thin-layer chromatography-densitometry (TLC-D), high-pressure liquid chromatography (HPLC), and radioimmunoassay (RIA).

In this review, the approaches used since 1967 will be discussed with emphasis on specificity, sensitivity, accuracy, precision (reproducibility), expense,

*Abbreviations: AT = amitriptyline; BUT = butriptyline; CMI = clomipramine; DMI = desipramine; DCMI = desmethylclomipramine; DDOX = desmethyl-doxepin; DNT = desmethyl-nortriptyline; DOX = doxepin; IMI = imipramine; MAP = maprotiline; MIAN = mianserin; NBUT = norbutriptyline; NT = nortriptyline; NOMI = nomifensine; NZIM = norzimelidine; PT = protriptyline; TRI = trimipramine; ZIM = zimelidine.

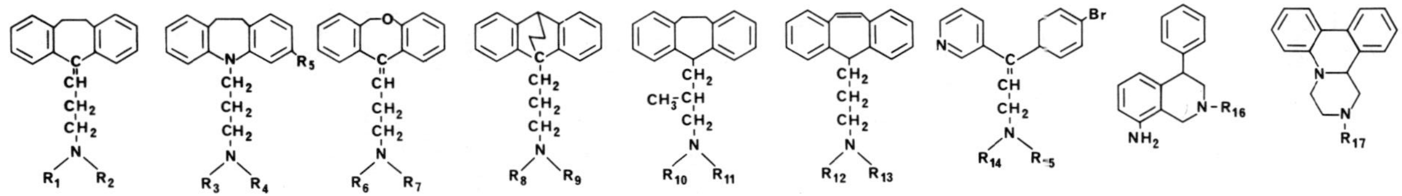

COMPOUND		R_1	R_2	R_3	R_4	R_5	R_6	R_7	R_8	R_9	R_{10}	R_{11}	R_{12}	R_{13}	R_{14}	R_{15}	R_{16}	R_{17}
AMITRIPTYLINE	AT	CH_3	CH_3	-	-	-	-	-	-	-	-	-	-	-	-	-	-	-
NORTRIPTYLINE	NT	H	CH_3	-	-	-	-	-	-	-	-	-	-	-	-	-	-	-
IMIPRAMINE	IMI	-	-	CH_3	CH_3	-	-	-	-	-	-	-	-	-	-	-	-	-
DESIPRAMINE	DMI	-	-	H	CH_3	-	-	-	-	-	-	-	-	-	-	-	-	-
CHLOMIPRAMINE	CMI	-	-	CH_3	CH_3	Cl	-	-	-	-	-	-	-	-	-	-	-	-
DESMETHYLCHLOMIPRAMINE	DCMI	-	-	H	CH_3	Cl	-	-	-	-	-	-	-	-	-	-	-	-
DOXEPIN	DOX	-	-	-	-	-	CH_3	CH_3	-	-	-	-	-	-	-	-	-	-
DES METHYLDOXEPIN	D DOX	-	-	-	-	-	H	CH_3	-	-	-	-	-	-	-	-	-	-
MAPROTILINE	MAP	-	-	-	-	-	-	-	H	CH_3	-	-	-	-	-	-	-	-
BUTRIPTYLINE	BUT	-	-	-	-	-	-	-	-	-	CH_3	CH_3	-	-	-	-	-	-
NORBUTRIPTYLINE	NBUT	-	-	-	-	-	-	-	-	-	H	CH_3	-	-	-	-	-	-
PROTRIPTYLINE	PT	-	-	-	-	-	-	-	-	-	-	-	H	CH_3	-	-	-	-
ZIMELIDINE	ZIM	-	-	-	-	-	-	-	-	-	-	-	-	-	CH_3	CH_3	-	-
NORZIMELIDINE	NZIM	-	-	-	-	-	-	-	-	-	-	-	-	-	H	CH_3	-	-
NOMIFENSINE	NOMI	-	-	-	-	-	-	-	-	-	-	-	-	-	-	-	CH_3	-
MIANSERIN	MIAN	-	-	-	-	-	-	-	-	-	-	-	-	-	-	-	-	CH_3

Figure 1 Structures of tricyclic antidepressants.

convenience and ease of sample processing. A procedure will be considered as specific if drug metabolites do not interfere and only drugs which have been shown not to interfere with the assay procedure are administered concomitantly. The sensitivity required for the routine analysis of plasma levels of the majority of tricyclic drugs is approximately 5-10 ng/ml. The assay should be capable of a precision of approximately ±5-10% over the total concentration range required, and a rapid assay is defined as one in which an answer can be given within 24 hours of receipt of the sample. In addition, reference will be made to the relevant clinical or pharmacokinetic studies in which particular techniques have been utilized.

A. Extraction of Plasma Samples

The tricyclic drugs are lipophilic strong bases; thus at high pH (approximately 10), the free base can be extracted from the aqueous phase into an organic solvent such as n-heptane, diethylether, or petroleum ether, while at pH < 3, the base can be reextracted into the aqueous phase. A comprehensive evaluation of the partition of IMI and its metabolites between aqueous solutions of varying pH and organic solvents has been described by Weder and Bickel [19]. A similar partition pattern is observed for the other tricyclics [20,21].

Plasma extraction procedures generally involve either one or three steps, depending on the method of analysis to follow. For isotope-derivative techniques utilizing TLC, mass fragmentography, or HPLC, a single alkaline extraction into an organic solvent is carried out. For techniques such as GLC with flame ionization detection, extensive cleanup of the sample is required; thus a threestep procedure is necessary. This involves an initial extraction into solvent, a back-extraction into acid, followed by a further extraction into solvent. These extraction procedures are reproducible, and yields are $> 90\%$ for a single extraction. This drops to 60-80% for the three-step procedure. The yield is dependent on the biological medium being extracted; for example, plasma extractions result in a lower yield than extractions from aqueous solutions. Thus if standards are to be used for quantitation, they must be prepared by mixing the drug to be analyzed with the appropriate biological material. The use of internal standards for correction of losses will be dealt with later on.

Either silanization of glassware or addition of isoamyl alcohol to the solvent can be used to reduce adsorption to glassware. Isoamyl alcohol also helps prevent emulsion formation during extraction. For all techniques, it has been found essential to use either analytical-grade solvents which have been redistilled or nanograde-quality solvents to obtain minimal nonspecific blanks.

Storage of samples in 0.1 mol/liter HCl (1:5, acid:plasma) at -20°C or at -4°C has been common practice, although acidification may not be essential. Plasma samples were found to be stable for several weeks at room temperature and for at least 2 years when frozen [22].

The only novel approach to plasma extraction procedures to be published is that of Hartvig and colleagues [23,24]. Plasma samples were applied to a cellulose column and AT was eluted at pH 5 into heptane, the NT was eluted with dichloromethane butanol (4:1). Others [25] have reported that solid phase extraction using either Celite 545 or XAD-2 columns are unsatisfactory. Of particular interest has been the development of techniques which allow separation of secondary and tertiary amines during extraction. This has been achieved by two methods. In the first selective extraction of AT and NT was achieved by varying the pH of the plasma [26]. The other approach formed a derivative of the secondary amine (DMI) and once again used pH changes to produce selective extraction [27].

B. Spectrophotofluorimetry

Initially, fluorimetric measurements involved a one-step extraction followed by acidification of the solvent extract and fluorimetric analysis of the acid phase [28]. This technique was nonspecific since metabolites could interfere. An improved method [13] was developed in 1967 which involved a three-step extraction after which the extract was split into two portions. One extract was acetylated, then both parts acidified and their fluorescence determined. This gave estimates of IMI and IMI-like substances, with DMI being determined by difference. The only metabolite shown to interfere was didesmethylimipramine; hence total specificity was not achieved. The sensitivity of the method was approximately 30 ng/ml. This technique, with minor modifications, has been widely used probably due to its low cost and simplicity. Clinical studies have been carried out by Walter ([29], IMI), Zeidenberg et al. ([30], IMI and DMI) and Glassman et al. ([31], IMI and DMI). Whyte et al. [32] and Moody et al. [33] studied PT plasma levels based on the method of Moody [28] while Olivier-Martin et al. [34] used the early method of Dingell et al. [12] for DMI. A more sensitive assay capable of measuring 5 ng/ml of AT has recently been described [35]. This method is based on the reaction of AT with α-bromomethylacridine to form a quaternary product which on photolysis yields fluorescence in a stoichiometric fashion.

C. Isotope Derivative Dilution Analysis

In this procedure, the compound to be determined is made to react quantitatively with a radioactive reagent of known specific activity. The radioactive product is then separated and purified. The amount of activity in the pure product indicates the amount of radioactive reagent it contains; thus from the stoichiometry of the reaction, the amount of compound present can be calculated.

In 1967, Hammer and Brodie [14] described an isotope derivative dilution procedure for the measurement of the secondary amine tricyclics DMI and NT.

The method involved a one-step extraction followed by formation of a derivative using [^{3}H] acetic anhydride. The labeled acetyl derivative was extracted into heptane and assayed by liquid scintillation spectrometry. The sensitivity of the method of 5 ng/ml and hence became extensively used not only by the Swedish workers [36-38] but also by others [39-46] with slight modification.

The major drawback to the method was its lack of specificity. Any secondary or primary amine could undergo the chemical reaction involved, thus the hydroxylated and demethylated metabolites of the drugs could interfere. Incorporation of a chromatographic separation step would overcome this problem and was carried out by Zuleski et al. ([47], NT), Riess, ([20], MAP), Maguire et al. ([22], NT), Carnis et al. ([21], DCMI), and Jones and Luscombe ([48], CMI).

The latter four methods also incorporated a second isotope to correct for procedural losses. Synthesis of high-specific-activity ^{14}C-labeled tricyclic drugs has allowed the development of these double-isotope derivative dilution assays (DIDDA). The technique is sensitive, specific, precise, rapid and relatively inexpensive if one has access to a liquid scintillation spectrometer. It has been used in a variety of studies [49-51]. An interlaboratory comparison of NT standards and plasma samples assayed by both GLC and double-isotope dilution has validated the specificity of this methodological approach [52]. Similarly, close agreement has been found when the same samples were assayed by radioimmunoassay [53].

This methodological approach is suitable for measurement of any of the secondary amine tricyclic drugs. An isotope derivative assay for tertiary amines using [^{14}C] methyliodide was described by Harris et al. [54] for IMI. More recently, Carnis et al. [21] converted CMI to its carbamate with trichloroethylchloroformate, which on hydrolysis gave DCMI. Since many steps were involved, yields of the labeled derivative were low (4-6%) thus making the procedure unsuitable for routine use. "In vitro" demethylation of AT by rat liver homogenates prior to acetylation has been attempted but also gave poor yields [55].

Both methods described by Reiss [20] and that by Carnis et al. [21] use low specific activity ^{14}C-tracer and relatively low-specific-activity [^{3}H] acetic anhydride. When consideration is given to the very large mass of ^{14}C-tracer added to each sample, it is surprising that the sensitivity of their assays are as low as stated. Also, neither of these two methods takes full advantage of the principle of isotope dilution in which the known specific activity of the derivative reagent is used to determine mass [22,56]. Comparison of unknown samples with a calibration curve determined with each run is both unnecessary and time consuming. The specificity of the double isotope assays is very good if chromatography after derivative formation is carried out. Incorporation of salicyclic aldehyde to block primary amines such as desmethyl NT from acetylation as used by Gram and Fredrickson-Overφ [39] in their modification of the original Hammer and Brodie [14] assay appears to be unnecessary for NT [22].

D. Gas-Liquid Chromatography

Gas-liquid chromatography (GLC) has been the most widely used approach for the measurement of the tricyclic drugs. Initial studies involved flame ionization detection (FID) or electron capture detection (ECD); however, the development of the alkali flame ionization detection (AFID), which is selective to nitrogen, and the coupling of gas chromatography-mass fragmentography (GC-MF) have led to these becoming the most widespread methods currently in use for the complete range of tricyclic drugs.

1. Flame Ionization Detection

Weder and Bickel [19] used flame ionization detection (FID) to quantitate IMI and seven of its metabolites after selective extraction of the various compounds. This study showed the separation capability of GLC but was not sensitive enough for therapeutic analyses. The first practical method was that described by Braithwaite and his colleagues [15,16] for determining AT and NT. The technique involved a single extraction step, derivatization of NT, and quantitation by comparison with nonextracted standards, with the internal standard being added just prior to the GLC analysis.

Hucker and Stauffer [57] developed a more acceptable method of analysis of AT and NT. Reproducibility was improved by addition of the internal standard to the plasma samples prior to extraction, and nonspecific interference was eliminated by use of a three-step extraction procedure. The GLC column packing chosen was OV-17, a more stable and simpler packing than that used by Braithwaite and colleagues. It also had greater separative power; hence no derivatization of NT was necessary. (Derivatization is usually carried out to improve separation or to reduce peak tailing and irreversible absorption to the column.) The function of the internal standard is to compensate for errors introduced by factors which are otherwise difficult to control, such as variations in extraction or derivative formation, thus the internal standard should be added to the original biological sample.

FID methods published since 1974 have fallen into two categories, the first being concerned with forensic measurement of the tricyclics and thus not been concerned with sensitivity [58,59] or specificity in that estimations of parent drug and metabolites were sufficient [60,61]. The second category includes those measuring therapeutic levels and involves methods based on that of Hucker and Stauffer [57] with minor modifications according to the drug to be analyzed. Published methods include O'Brien and Hinsvark ([62], DOX), Corona and Bonferoni ([63], AT and NT), Norman et al. ([64], BUT), Bruderlein et al. ([65], BUT), and Nyberg and Martensson ([66], AT, NT, IMI, DMI, CMI, DCMI, and PT). An outline of the major publications using this technique appears in Table 1.

These techniques are quite acceptable in terms of specificity, accuracy,

Table 1 Summary of GC-FID and GC-ECD Methods for the Measurement of Antidepressant Plasma Levels

Reference	Drugs	Plasma volume (ml)	Extraction and solvent[a]	Derivative formed[b]	Detector	Sensitivity (ng/ml)	Precision (%)	Assessment of Specificity[c]	Application
[16]	AT, NT	5	1-Step; Pet. Spirit	TFA	FID	20	7 (AT) 5 (NT)	R_T data for metabolites and other drugs	Steady-state plasma levels from 12 patients; single and multiple doses in 2 volunteers
[57]	AT, NT	3-5	3-Step; Heptane–IAA, Ether	–	FID	20	8.2 (AT) 9.4 (NT)	R_T data for metabolites	Steady-state levels in 3 patients
[62]	DOX, DDOX	5	3-Step; n-Hexane	–	FID	10	11 (DOX)	–	Steady-state levels in 7 patients
[63]	AT, NT	5	3-Step; n-Heptane	TFA	FID	–	–	R_T data for other drugs	Steady-state levels
[66]	AT, NT, IMI, DMI, CMI, DCMI, PT	4	3-Step; Hexane-IAA	–	FID	–	7-13	–	Steady-state levels in 3 patients
[64]	BUT	4	3-Step; n-Hexane	–	FID	10	–	R_T for other tricyclics	Steady-state levels in 3 patients
[18]	DMI	4	1-Step; Benzene	TFA	ECD	1	3-7	–	Single doses in 2 patients

[71]	NT and metabolites	4	3-Step; n-Hexane	HFBA	ECD	10	3–6	No endogenous interference	Single doses in 4 patients
[72]	MAP	1	3-Step; n-Heptane-iso-propanol	HFBA	ECD	10	3–10	Comparison with DIDDA	12 patient samples
[73]	NOMI	2	3-Step; Diethyl ethyl	HFBA	ECD	1	–	Benzodiazepines and barbiturates didn't interfere	Single oral dose in 3 volunteers
[24]	AT, NT	0.5	Cellulose Column	TEC	ECD	1	5.5 (AT) 7.5 (NT)	No metabolite interference	Single oral doses in patients

[a]IAA = isoamyl alcohol.
[b]TFA = trifluoroacetate; HFBA = heptafluorobutyrate; TEC = trichloroethylchloroformate.
[c]R_T = retention time.

and precision but are time-consuming. The limit of sensitivity is 10-20 ng/ml, which is adequate for routine monitoring of most of the tricyclic drugs but is not sufficiently low enough for pharmacokinetic studies after single doses. Recent papers emphasize the need for thoroughly clean glassware and very pure solvents to eliminate interfering chromatographic peaks.

The method of Braithwaite and Widdop [16] has been used in clinical studies on AT and NT [67-69] while that of Norman et al. [64] has been used to measure BUT levels [70].

2. *Electron Capture Detection*

To utilize this type of GLC detector, the tricyclic must be derivatized to a compound which gives a high response on the ECD. The secondary amine tricyclics can be easily converted to their trifluoroacetyl or hepta fluorobutyryl derivatives which can be detected in pg amounts. Methods have been described by Ervik et al. ([18], DMI), Walle and Ehrsson ([17], NT), Borgå and Garle ([71], NT and metabolites), Geiger et al. ([72], MAP), and Vereczkey et al. ([73], NOMI). These methods basically involve a three-step extraction, derivatization and quantitation by ECD. They all have acceptable specificity, precision, accuracy and sensitivity is approximately 1-10 ng/ml. Their major disadvantage is that they are only applicable to the secondary amine tricyclic drugs. The method of Borgå and Garle [71] has been used by Kragh-Sorensen et al. [74-76] and Montgomery et al. [77].

Hartvig and colleagues [23,24] have developed methods of converting AT to an ECD-sensitive compound. Their method involved a column extraction which separated AT from its metabolites, followed by either oxidation to anthraquinone, or conversion using trichloroethylchloroformate to a carbamate. The latter conversion could also be applied to NT; hence by prior separation on the column, AT and NT could be determined. The sensitivity was 1 ng/ml and was free from metabolite interference. The column extraction seemed quicker than the conventional three-step technique; thus this method appears to have great potential. It has also been applied to the measurement of IMI and DMI, DMI and DCMI [24]. A summary of a number of methods using this method appears on Table 1.

3. *Alkali Flame Ionization Detection*

Modification of the conventional FID by Karmen and Guiffrida [78] has led to a detector selective to compounds containing nitrogen [79,80]. The AFID or nitrogen detector has an increased sensitivity to the tricyclic compounds compared to that of an FID. This has led to the development of assay techniques based on those previously described for the FID, which allow reliable estimation of levels as low as 5 ng/ml using only 2-3-ml plasma samples. More recently a method has been described with a sensitivity of 1-2 ng/ml for IMI [81].

The majority of published methods utilize a three-step extraction, but others [82-84] find that only a single extraction is necessary. Similarly, some investigators find that derivatization of secondary amines is necessary (Jorgensen [83], AT and NT, Bailey and Jatlow [85], IMI and DMI, Gupta et al. [86], AT and metabolites, Bailey et al. [87], NOMI, and Connor et al. [88], AT and NT), whereas others do not (Gifford et al. [82], IMI; Cooper et al. [89], IMI and DMI; Bailey and Jatlow [90], AT and NT; Vasiliades and Bush [91], AT and NT; Hucker and Stauffer [92], AT and NT).

Several improvements in general technique (apart from the increased sensitivity of the detector) have been described in these recent studies. Cooper et al. [89] and Hucker and Stauffer [92] have reduced the volume of solvent used for the last extraction to 50 μliter. This avoids the concentration of solvent impurities during the evaporation step which is required when larger volumes are used, and may also avoid losses during concentration and reconstitution of samples. Gupta et al. [86] and Connor et al. [88] have incorporated two internal standards, a tertiary and a secondary amine compound, into their techniques. The secondary amine undergoes derivatization along with the drug that is being measured, thus allowing for correction of losses during this step.

Open glass capillary columns were used by Bailey et al. [87] and Rosseel et al. [93], which have greater separative capabilities than the conventional packed column. Bailey and colleagues [87] as well as Witts and Turner [84] have automated the GLC analysis by use of injector systems.

The basic extraction and AFID analysis can be used for all the tricyclic drugs with appropriate choice of internal standards and chromatographic conditions. This prompted Gifford [94] to suggest that extraction and detection coefficients for each drug should be established; then quantitation of any of the drugs could be made using a single standard curve and the appropriate "correction factor." Witts and Turner [84] evaluated this approach and concluded that it was not feasible. Thus separate standard curves must be extracted for each particular drug. Recently Dawling and Braithwaite [95] have published a simplified procedure which gives details of retention times for a wide range of antidepressants. A summary of published methods using this procedure appears in Table 2.

As this approach is a recent development, few clinical applications have been published. The method of Gifford et al. [82] has been used to study DMI, BUT, and NT [96,97] while that of Jorgensen [83] has been used by Jorgensen and Staehr [98].

4. Gas Chromatography-Mass Fragmentography

Gas chromatography-mass fragmentography (GC-MF) involves the use of a mass spectrometer as an ion-specific detector for the gas chromatographic effluent. Simultaneous and continuous monitoring of mass-spectral ions representing typical fragments of the compounds to be measured gives a gas chromatogram in which compounds can be identified by their retention times and by the presence

Table 2 Summary of GC-AFID Methods for the Measurement of Antidepressant Plasma Levels

Reference	Drugs	Plasma volume (ml)	Extraction and solvent[a]	Derivative formed[b]	Sensitivity (ng/ml)	Precision (%)	Assessment of specificity[c]	Application
[89]	IMI, DMI	1-3	3-Step; n-Heptane-IAA	–	3-5	5.2 (IMI) 8.1 (DMI)	R_T data for metabolites	Single doses for 20 volunteers
[83]	AT, NT	2	1-Step; Hexane	Acetate	5 AT 15 NT	7.6	R_T data for metabolites and benzodiazepines	Single doses in 2 volunteers; steady-state levels in 9 patients
[82]	IMI	4	1-Step; n-Heptane	–	1-10	3-10	–	See Ref. 84
[86]	AT, NT MAP	1-3	2-Step; Pentane	Acetate	10 AT, MAP 20 NT	11 Inter 12-20 Intra	–	Steady-state levels in patients
[91]	AT, NT	2	3-Step; n-Heptane-isobutanol	–	1	4.1 Inter 12.8 Intra	–	7 overdoses
[85]	AT, NT	3	3-Step; Hexane-IAA	–	5	4.6 Inter 8.6 Intra	R_T for 47 drugs	25 overdoses; 9 patients

[90]	IMI, DMI	3	3-Step; Hexane-IAA	TFA	5	6 Inter 5 Intra	R_T data for 46 drugs	8 patients on therapeutic doses
[92]	AT, NT	2	3-Step; Hexane	-	5	3.3-18.5	–	Steady-state levels in patients
[87]	NOMI	2	3-Step; Diethylether	HFBA	2	5-10	No endogenous interference; confirmed by GC-MF	Single doses in 2 volunteers; steady-state levels in 9 volunteers
[183]	NOMI	1	1-Step; Ether	–	10	–	Compared with HPLC and RIA	Single doses in 3 volunteers
[95]	AT, NT	1	3-Step; n-Hexane	–	10	<5	No interference from endogenous compounds or other drugs	Steady-state levels in 103 patients
[93]	DOX; DDOX, cis, trans Isomers	1	1-Step; n-Hexane	TFA	2	3-8	Confirmed by GC-MF	Steady-state levels in 2 patients

[a]IAA = isoamyl alcohol.
[b]TFA = trifluoroacetate; HFBA = heptafluorobutyrate.
[c]R_T = retention time.

and relative intensities of the characteristic fragments. This combination of the separative powers of GLC and the selectivity of MF has produced one of the most powerful analytical techniques available.

GC-MF was initially used to qualitatively study NT metabolism [99,100]. Borgå et al. [101] developed the first quantitative GC-MF technique for NT and DNT, while Frigerio and colleagues developed assays for IMI, DMI, DOX and DDOX [102-104]. These techniques required 1-3-ml plasma samples and could detect down to a few ng/ml.

The use of stable isotope-labeled compounds as internal standards was first introduced by Gaffney et al. [105]. Hence deuterium-labeled analogues of the drug to be analyzed were used by Borgå et al. ([106], NT), Biggs et al. [107], Dubois et al. ([108], CMI, DCMI and IMI), Alfredsson et al. ([109], CMI, DCMI) and Garland ([110], AT and NT). The deuterium analogue provides an ideal internal standard as its extraction performance, adsorption to glass surfaces and chromatographic behavior should be identical to that of the nonlabeled drug. In addition, it can be detected separately by the mass spectrometer.

The method of Biggs et al. [107] allows for the measurement of AT, NT, IMI, DMI, DOX, DDOX, or PT. Fifteen samples can be analyzed per hour after a single-step extraction and derivatization of the secondary amine tricyclics. This procedure has been used to measure plasma levels of AT, NT, and PT [107, 111-117]. While the majority of methods use electron ionization, a procedure using chemical ionization has been developed for a wide range of tricyclics (DOX, DDOX, AT, NT, DMI, IMI, PT) [118]. A summary of the major methods using this approach appears on Table 3.

The major disadvantage of this technique is the highly sophisticated equipment. Computer systems interfaced to the mass spectrometer allow for accurate control of the ion detector leading to high sensitivity and selectivity but also to high cost. For this reason, this technique, although highly desirable, is likely to be available to only a few in the near future.

Borgå et al. [106] have compared the sensitivity of GC-MF with their GC-ECD method for NT and found GC-MF to be 10 times more sensitive. GC-MF is approximately 10 and 20 times more sensitive than AFID and FID, respectively. This sensitivity enables reliable measurement of plasma levels after single oral doses of 25 mg CMI [108] and 50 mg AT [110].

A further application of the technique of GC-MF is the screening of plasma from overdose patients. Because of its selectivity, identification of unknown drugs can be readily carried out. GC-MF is also a useful technique for characterizing drug metabolites.

E. Thin-Layer Chromatography-Densitometry

Nagy and Treiber [119] described a simple procedure for the measurement of IMI and DMI based on TLC. Following a one-step extraction, TLC in one dimen-

Table 3 Summary of GC-MF Methods for the Measurement of Antidepressant Plasma Levels

Reference	Drugs	Plasma volume (ml)	Extraction and solvent	Derivative formed[a]	EI/CI[b]	Sensitivity (ng/ml)	Precision (%)	Application
[101,106]	NT, DNT, 10-OH-NT	2-3	3-Step; n-Hexane	HFBA	EI	<5	3-6	Patient samples (19, 68)
[104]	IMI, DMI	1	1-Step; n-Hexane	Acetate	EI	10	–	Steady-state levels and single doses
[108]	CMI, DCMI, IMI	1	3-Step; n-Heptane	PFP	EI	2	4	Single doses in 6 volunteers
[107]	AT, NT, IMI, DMI, DOX, DDOX, PT	4	3-Step; Pet. Ether	TFA	EI	10	–	Steady-state and overdose levels
[184]	IMI, DMI	2	1-Step; n-Hexane	TFAI	CI	–	–	Steady-state levels in 8 patients
[109]	CMI, DCMI	2	3-Step; n-Heptane	PFP	EI	2-5	6 (CMI) 4 (DCMI)	Single doses and steady-state levels
[145]	MIAN	1-2	n-Hexane followed by HPLC	–	EI	1	6-7	Steady-state levels and single doses
[185]	AT, NT, IMI, DMI, DOX, DDOX, PT	2	1-Step; n-Hexane	TFA	CI	5	4-12	Patient samples
[110]	AT, NT	1	2-Step; n-Hexane	TFA	CI	1	–	Steady-state levels and single doses
[118]	AT, NT, IMI, DMI, DOX, DDOX	2	3-Step; Heptane-isobutanol	HFBA	CI	1	5	Steady-state levels

[a] HFBA = heptafluorobutyrate; PFP = pentafluoropropyl; TFA = trifluoroacetate; TFAI = trifluoroacetylimidazole.
[b] EI = electron ionization; CI = chemical ionization.

sion was performed to separate IMI and its metabolites. After allowing the drugs to react with nitrous gases to give an intense yellow, densitometric measurement was carried out. The sensitivity of the technique was 5 ng/ml using 5 ml plasma samples, and has been used by Gram and Christiansen [120] ; and Gram et al. [121,122].

A similar technique for the measurement of AT and NT was developed by Faber et al. [123]. Breyer and Villumsen [124] used TLC to separate either AT or IMI and their demethylated metabolites followed by quantitation by reflectance photometry in ultraviolet light. These techniques have acceptable specificity and reproducibility, and detection limits of 5-10 ng/ml.

High-performance thin-layer chromatography has been used by Fenimore et al. [125] for AT, NT, IMI, and DMI. Better resolution and sensitivity was achieved compared to the conventional TLC plates. Detection of concentrations as low as 5 ng/ml from 1-ml plasma samples were possible. A similar assay with even greater sensitivity (0.5 ng/ml) has been described by Haefelfinger [126] for AT and NT.

F. High-Performance Liquid Chromatography

The application of high-speed ion pair partition and liquid-solid adsorption chromatography to the separation of tricyclic drugs was first described by Knox and Jurand [127] in 1975. In the four years following that 1975 article there was extensive development of this analytical approach for the quantitative determination of the majority of tricyclic drugs in plasma (Mellstrom and Eksborg [128], CMI and DCMI; Persson and Lagerström [129], IMI and DMI; Lagerström, et al. [130], CMI; Mellstrom and Tybring, [131], CMI and DCMI; Brodie et al. [132], AT and NT; Van Den Berg et al. [133], IMI, AT, CMI; Kraak and Bijster, [134], AT and metabolites; Watson and Stewart, [135], AT and NT; Moyes and Moyes, [136], CMI; Uihlein and Hajdu, [137], NOMI; Emanuelsson and Moore [138], ZIM and NZIM; Westenberg et al. [139], CMI, DCMI; Proelss et al. [25], DOX, DMI, NT, IMI, AT; Vandemark et al. [140], AT, NT, IMI, DMI). The technique has also been applied to assays of tablet formulations [141,142] and urine [143]. Others have used HPLC for sample purification prior to GLC [136], or mass fragmentography [144-146].

Detailed evaluation of a number of aspects of the chromatographic technique to improve resolution of individual drugs from each other and from their metabolites has also been described [147-149].

A summary of the major features of 12 different methodological approaches which are suitable for and which have been used to measure a wide variety of antidepressants in plasma are shown in Table 4. These methods are basically all very similar. All require solvent extraction of basic plasma followed by either ion pair partition, adsorption or reversed phase liquid chromatography using a number of different types of column packing and elution solvents. With the exception of those used in conjunction with a mass spectrometer, a UV detector is used.

With few exceptions the sensitivity of the methods are similar to those using GLC. However, HPLC does have the advantage of greater carrying capacity and also that the sample is not destroyed as occurs in GLC. The methods are also very rapid, with 10-20 minutes usually the time for a single estimation.

At the present time it is not possible to generalize as to whether adsorption, ion pair partition, or reverse-phase chromatography is the most suitable for this class of compounds. All give similar sensitivities if the UV detector wavelength is similar. This latter point is important if elution solvents interfere with the primary absorbance of the drug. However, for routine clinical applications reversed phase HPLC may have advantages over adsorption silica columns because of marked improvement in column efficiency.

A number of studies have examined in detail the role of individual components of the elution solvent profile. Of these those by Kraak and Bijster [134] and Johansson et al. [149] are of particular interest. Separation of tertiary from secondary amines is dependant on pH for resolution in samples containing both amines (e.g., AT and NT) [25].

If a UV detector is used, an internal standard of a similar drug or a derivative is most often used to correct for procedural losses. It is important to realize that if an isotopic internal standard is used, as is often done if mass fragmentography is to be carried out, isotopic effects may be observed on the column with separation of the deuterated form from the unlabeled drug [144,145].

Overall the majority of methods describing the use of HPLC require further evaluation as to their sensitivity, specificity, accuracy and precision and their suitability for measurement of patient plasma samples. One important aspect of specificity—interference from structurally related psychotropic drugs—has recently been assessed in detail [25]. Comparison of results from HPLC with those of other techniques using the same plasma samples is also important [131].

The technique will probably gain in popularity and if used in conjunction with mass fragmentography will be a powerful and useful procedure for measuring plasma levels of drugs and their metabolites.

G. Radioimmunoassay

Although radioimmunoassay has been widely used for measurement of many drugs, peptides, proteins, and steroid hormones, it is only recently that this approach has been used for psychotropic drugs. The first brief report was in 1974 by Sathananthan et al. [150] who described a method for IMI. Since that time eight other methods have been described. A summary of the published procedures used to measure tricyclic drugs in plasma appears in Table 5. A screening method for tricyclics using this approach has also been reported [151].

Table 4 Summary of HPLC Methods for Measurement of Antidepressant Plasma Levels

Reference	Drugs	Plasma volume (ml)	Internal standard[a]	Extraction solvent	Type of HPLC (column)	UV (nM)	Sensitivity (ng/ml)	Precision (%)	Application
[128]	CMI, DCMI	2	TRI	Ether	Ion Pair Partition (Diachrom 37–44 μm)	255	?	4.3 (CMI) 6.3 (DCMI)	Single doses in 3 patients
[132]	AT, NT	4	AT derivative	Ether	Reversed Phase (Partisil-10 ODS)	254	5	4.7 (AT) 4.5 (NT)	No patient studies
[144,145]	MIAN	1	[^{2}H]	n-Hexane	Adsorption (μ-Porasil)	280	–	–	Clean up prior to MS
[138]	ZIM, NZIM	1	GI	Ether	Adsorption (Partisil 5)	258	25	7 (ZIM)	Single patient after 42-d ZIM
[134]	AT and metabolites	1	–	n-Hexane	Reversed Phase (C8 and Nucleosil 10)	–	0.3	7 (AT)	Single patient after 14-d AT
[131]	CMI, DCMI	1	TRI	n-Hexane	Ion Pair Partition (Partisil-10)	254	–	7.3 (CMI)	Compared with GLC on 34 patients
[137]	NOMI and metabolites	2	CMN	Ether	Adsorption (Mercko-sorb S1100)	242	30	3.5 (NOM)	Compared with MF and 1 patient single dose

[135]	AT, NT	2	DMI	Dichloro-methane	Adsorption (Micropak)	240	10	10	No patient studies
[139]	CMI, DCMI	1-4	IMI	n-Hexane	Adsorption (Lichro-sorb Si 60)	250	2 CMI 10 DCMI		Single-dose study in 2 patients
[146]	IMI	4	[^{2}H]	n-Hexane	Adsorption (Lichro-sorb Si 60)	250	0.4	8	Cleanup prior to MF bioavailability in 8 patients
[140]	AT, NT, IMI, DMI	2	PT	n-Hexane	Adsorption (Silica B/5)	211	10	5-6 Intra 6-8 Inter	No patient studies
[25]	AT, NT, DMI, IMI, DOX	2	βNA	n-Hexane	Ion Pair Partition (μ-Bondapak)	254	2	2-3 Intra 2-7 Inter	No patient studies

[a] [^{2}H] = deuterium-labeled; GI = geometrical isomers; CMN = 3-chloro-4-methoxy NOMI; βNA = β-napthylamine.

Table 5 Summary of Radioimmunoassay Methods for Measurement of Antidepressant Plasma Levels

Reference	Drugs	Plasma volume	Extraction solvent	Tracer (SA)	Sensitivity	Precision (%)	Assessment of specificity[a]	Application
[182]	DMI	μl	Pet. Ether	$[^3H]$ DMI (20 Ci/mmol)	200 pg/ml	?	X-react.: IMI and metabolites	Rat Brain–Plasma
[152]	NT	0.1 ml	None	$[^{14}C]$ NT (20 mCi/mmol)	200 ng/ml	?	X-react.: Various tricyclics	None
[26]	AT, NT	0.5 ml	n-Heptane	$[^3H]$ AT (28 Ci/mmol)	2 ng/ml	<9 Intra	Compared with GC-MF; X-react.: Various tricyclics and metabolites	Steady-state and single dose
[156]	NOMI	0.1 ml	None	$[^3H]$ NOMI (2 Ci/mmol)	300 pg/ml	6-7 Inter	Compared with HPLC; X-react.: metabolites	Single doses
[155]	CMI	0.1 ml	Pet. Ether	$[^3H]$ CMI (39 Ci/mmol)	200 pg/ml	6-7 Intra 12 Inter	Compared with DIDDA; X-react.: Various tricyclics and metabolites	Single doses
[53]	NT, IMI	0.1 ml	None	$[^3H]$ IMI (30 Ci/mmol)	1-2 ng/ml	6 Intra-NT 11 Inter-NT	Compared with DIDDA; X-react.: Various tricyclics and metabolites	Steady-state 150 mg/day
[158]	AT, NT	0.05 ml	None	$[^3H]$ AT (2 Ci/mmol)	2 ng/ml	?	Compared with GLC; X-react.: Various tricyclics, metabolites, and drugs	Single doses
[27]	IMI, DMI	0.1 ml	n-Heptane	$[^3H]$ IMI (5 Ci/mmol)	10 ng/ml	3 Intra-DMI 10 Inter-DMI	Compared with GLC; X-react.: Various tricyclics and metabolites	Steady-state 150-300 mg/day IMI

[a]X-react. = cross-reactivity.

Antisera have been prepared by injection of a variety of tricyclic drugs, coupled to bovine serum albumin (BSA), into rabbits or sheep. In the main, derivatization of the parent tricyclic drug has involved modification of the side chain to form either N-4-bromobutyl NT [152], N-4-succinyl NT [26,27], or N-3-carboxypropionyl NT or DMI and N-2-carboxyethyl NT or DMI [153]. Coupling through the ring structure using 10/11-hydroxy-CMI to prepare 10/11-hemisuccinate-CMI has been described by Read et al. [154] and Read and Riad-Fahmy [155]. N-(8-NOMI)succinamic acid was formed as a derivative by Heptner et al. [156]. Complete details of the chemistry of some of these reactions were described by Hubbard et al. [153].

The extent of incorporation of the hapten into the BSA has been variable [27,152,153,155] and although many of the hapten-carrier protein complexes have been less than ideal [157] satisfactory antisera have been produced.

The majority of antisera show substantial cross-reactivity between the secondary and tertiary structures as well as to other tricyclic drugs with similar ring structures [53]. Major changes in the tricyclic nucleus, as in a change from a seven membered to a six membered ring, decreased binding. Those with only two rings showed no cross-reactivity. This would be expected if coupling was carried out on the side chain. There is, however, substantial evidence based on Scatchard plot analysis of the Aherne et al. [152] antisera to show that the side chain structure is also an important antigenic determinant [53].

The majority of antisera also show little or no cross-reactivity to the 2- or 10-hydroxy metabolites [27,53,153], or to other common psychotropic drugs [53].

The described radioimmunoassays are sensitive ($<$2 ng/ml) and enable rapid analysis of small volumes of plasma ($\leqslant$0.5 ml). One antiserum [152] described by Maguire et al. [53] and Robinson et al. [158] can be used as a direct assay without extraction. This is also true for the NOMI radioimmunoassay [156]. Where extraction is required either petroleum ether or n-heptane has been used.

The precision of the various radioimmunoassays are adequate for routine clinical plasma measurements. The specificity of the methods using the Aherne et al. [152] NT antiserum have been rigorously checked by duplicate assay of plasma samples by both double iostope derivative dilution analysis [53] and by gas liquid chromatography [159,160] and shown to be in close agreement with the more rigorous methods. Similar comparisons using GLC have been carried out for IMI and DMI [27] and for AT and NT [26]. The major problem of specificity has been the cross reactivity of the tertiary amines for antisera raised against a secondary amine. Further, for many of the antisera the cross-reactivity of the secondary and tertiary amines are not identical [152], and it is thus not possible to accurately measure either total AT plus NT or AT alone in patients receiving the tertiary amines [158]. Lucek and Dixon [26] described a method of selective extraction of AT and NT based on changes in the pH of the plasma to avoid this problem. A novel approach has been described by Brunswick et al. [27] and enables the separation of IMI from DMI during extraction. In this procedure succinyl-DMI is formed in the heptane extract of plasma. After acidification IMI partitions into the acid layer while the succinyl DMI remains in the basic layer.

One of the major problems limiting the development of radioimmunoassay has been the unavailability of high-specific-activity tritiated tracer. As shown by Aherne et al. [152] ^{14}C-labeled antigens are unsuitable, having inadequate sensitivity for plasma measurements. More recently high-specific activity [^{3}H] IMI (30 Ci/mmol) and [^{3}H] CMI (39 Ci/mmol) have been available from the Radiochemical Centre, Amersham. Lower-specific activity [^{3}H] IMI (4-6 Ci/mmol) have been prepared by catalytic exchange labeling. Improved exchange labeling using activated palladium as a catalyst has enabled the synthesis of high specific activity DMI (44 Ci/mmol) and IMI (15 Ci/mmol); however, this approach does not appear suitable for NT or AT [161].

Although ^{125}I-labeled antigens have not been described for plasma measurements clearly their use would offer many advantages. Problems related to radioiodination of drugs have been discussed by Robinson et al. [162]. A procedure for the iodination of MAP following introduction of a tyrosine residue has been described by Riess (personal communication).

Recently a nonisotopic double-antibody enzyme immunoassay has been described for NT [163]. The antiserum used is that described by Aherne et al. [152] and in the assay DNT coupled to β-D-galactosidase is used as the label. Unlabeled antigen (NT) competes with the enzyme labeled antigen for the antiserum. A second antibody is used to separate antibody bound from free antigen. Enzyme activity is then measured on the bound fraction in the precipitate. The assay has similar sensitivity (1 ng/ml), specificity and precision to the previously described RIA using this antiserum and tritiated antigen as a label [53,158].

Although at the present time radioimmunoassays for this class of psychotropic drugs are not widely used, this will change with the increasing availability of suitable antisera. However it is important to realize that the specificity and other characteristics of all antisera are different, and each new assay must be rigorously checked against a more definitive method. This is of particular importance if commercial kit assays are to be used for clinical studies.

H. Summary

Contemporary analytical techniques for the measurement of plasma levels of tricyclic antidepressant drugs are reviewed. Table 6 presents in a simplified form a comparison of some of the practical aspects of each of the different types of method. The methods of choice for routine plasma measurements are GLC, double isotope derivative dilution, HPLC, and immunoassay. The highly specific

Table 6 Summary of Evaluation of Procedures Used to Measure Antidepressant Plasma Levels

Method	Sensitivity (ng/ml)	Accuracy and precision	Specificity	Convenience	Cost		Drugs assayed
					Materials	Equipment	
Spectrophotometry	>100	Poor	Poor	++	++	+	Not suitable for plasma assay
Fluorimetry	5-30	Poor	Poor	++	++	+	IMI, DMI, AT, NT
Quantitative TLC	5	Adequate	Adequate	++	++	+	AT, NT, IMI, DMI
Double-isotope Derivative dilution	2-5	Excellent	Very good	+++	++++	+++	NT, DMI, MAP, DCMI
GLC-FID	10-20	Adequate	Adequate	++	+++	++	AT, NT, DOX, IMI, DMI, CMI, DCMI, BUT
GLC-ECD	1-10	Good	Adequate	++	+++	++	AT, NT, MAP, DMI, NOMI
GLC-AFID	1-10	Good	Adequate	++	+++	++	AT, NT, IMI, DMI, MAP, NOMI, DOX
GLC-MS	1	Excellent	Excellent	+++	+++	+++++	AT, NT, DOX, IMI, DMI, PT, CMI, DCMI, MIAN
HPLC-UV	2-10	Good	Adequate	++++	+++	+++	AT, NT, CMI, DCMI, IMI, DMI, ZIM, NZIM, NOMI
HPLC-MS	0.5	Excellent	Excellent	+++	+++	+++++	IMI, MIAN
Radioimmunoassay	0.1-2	Good	Adequate	+++++	+	+++	AT, NT, IMI, CMI, DMI, NOMI

technique of GC-MF has an important role in definitive studies involved with the characterization of metabolites and drug pharmacokinetics. The high cost of the instrumentation will prevent this technique becoming widely used for routine analysis. The technique with the most potential is immunoassay since these are simple, inexpensive and rapid methods which could be automated. The development of further antisera specific for either bicyclic, tricyclic or tetracyclic drugs along with the recently developed enzyme immunoassays [163] will undoubtedly lead to immunoassay being the method of choice in the future for routine analysis.

II. MONOAMINE OXIDASE INHIBITORS

A variety of methods have been described for the measurement of concentrations of the monoamine oxidase inhibitors in biological media. These include spectrophotometric [164], fluorimetric [165], enzymatic [166], thin-layer chromatographic [167], and gas-chromatographic techniques [168]. Plasma concentrations of phenelzine were in the 1-10 μg/ml range [164]; hence any of the above techniques would be suitable. However, it appears to be more appropriate to monitor plasma or platelet monoamine oxidase activity. A relationship between inhibition of the enzyme activity and response to therapy has been demonstrated [169].

III. LITHIUM

The role of lithium in mania is well established [170] and it has been used for the treatment of recurrent affective illnesses [171]. The workers in the latter reference have established a therapeutic range of 0.6-2.0 meq/liter. At levels above this, toxic symptoms may be observed hence it is essential to monitor plasma concentrations.

Recently, it has been suggested that erythrocyte levels or erythrocyte/plasma ratios may be related to therapeutic response [172,173]. Both plasma and erythrocyte levels can be measured by virtually the same procedure involving either atomic emission or atomic absorption spectrometry.

A. Atomic Emission Spectrometry or Flame Photometry

Flame photometry is based on the fact that a metal salt will emit a characteristic radiation, and the intensity of the emitted light correlates directly with the concentration of the metal ion. The sample solution is sprayed into a flame, the radiation emitted is isolated and measured, and then it is compared to that obtained from solutions of known concentrations. Techniques for the measurement of lithium ion have been described by Fournis and Chazot [174], Brown and Legg [175], Sideman [176], and Coombs [177].

B. Atomic Absorption Spectrophotometry

This technique is based on the fact that metal ions absorb light at characteristic wavelengths. A solution of the metal ion is sprayed into a flame such that 99% of the atoms are at their ground state. Light of the appropriate wavelength directed at the sample is absorbed as the atoms are excited to a higher transition state. The amount absorbed is directly related to the concentration of the metal in the sample. Published methods using this technique include Amidsen [178], Brown and Legg [175], Frazer et al. [179], Pybus and Bowers [180], and Levy and Katz [181].

Atomic absorption is the more commonly used technique; however, both it and atomic emission are quite acceptable. They are rapid, requiring only sample dilution prior to analysis and the sensitivity required routinely is well above the lower limits of both techniques.

REFERENCES

1. T. Berti and M. Ferrari, Metabolism and estimation of imipramine. *Arch. Ital. Sci. Farmacol. 10:*2-8, 1960.
2. B. Hermann and R. Pulver, The metabolism of Tofranil. *Arch. Int. Pharmacodyn. 126:*454-469, 1960.
3. M. H. Bickel and H. J. Weder, The total fate of a drug: kinetics of distribution, excretion, and formation of 14 metabolites in rats treated with imipramine. *Arch. Int. Pharmacodyn. 173:*433-463, 1968.
4. H. B. Hucker and C. C. Porter, Studies on the metabolism of amitriptyline. *Fed. Proc. 20:*172, 1961.
5. H. B. Hucker, Metabolism of amitriptyline. *Pharmacologist 4:*171, 1962.
6. J. E. Wallace and E. V. Dahl, The determination of amitriptyline by ultraviolet spectrophotometry. *J. Forensic Sci. 12:*484-496, 1967.
7. G. L. Corona and M. R. Facino, Identification and evaluation of amitriptyline and its basic metabolites in rabbit's urine. *Biochem. Pharmacol. 17:*2045-2050, 1968.
8. M. E. Amundson and J. A. Manthey, Excretion of nortriptyline hydrochloride in man. *J. Pharm. Sci. 55:*277-280, 1966.
9. J. L. Crammer and B. Scott, The excretion of desmethylimipramine and its metabolites in depressive patients. *Excerpta Medica Foundation, I.C.S. 150:*1942-1944, 1968.
10. G. C. Haydu, A. Dhrymiotis, and G. P. Quinn, Plasma imipramine level in syndromes of depression. *Am. J. Psychiat. 119:*574-575, 1962.
11. C. M. Yates, A. Todrick, and A. C. Tait, Aspects of the clinical chemistry of desmethylimipramine in man. *J. Pharm. Pharmacol. 15:*432-438, 1963.

12. J. V. Dingell, F. Sulser, and J. R. Gillette, Species differences in the metabolism of imipramine and desmethylimipramine. *J. Pharmacol. Exp. Ther. 143:*14-22, 1964.
13. J. P. Moody, A. C. Tait, and A. Todrick, Plasma levels of imipramine and desmethylimipramine during therapy. *Brit. J. Psychiat. 113:*183-193, 1967.
14. W. H. Hammer and B. B. Brodie, Application of isotope derivative technique to assay of secondary amines: Estimation of desipramine by acetylation with ^{3}H-acetic anhydride. *J. Pharmacol. Exp. Ther. 157:*503-508, 1967.
15. R. A. Braithwaite and J. A. Whatley, Specific gas chromatographic determination of amitriptyline in human urine following therapeutic doses. *J. Chromatogr. 49:*303-307, 1970.
16. R. A. Braithwaite and B. Widdop, A specific gas-chromatographic method for the measurement of steady-state plasma levels of amitriptyline and nortriptyline in patients. *Clin. Chim. Acta 35:*461-472, 1971.
17. T. Walle and H. Ehrsson, Quantitative gas chromatographic determination of picogram levels of amino and alcoholic compounds by electron-capture detection. *Acta Pharm. Suec. 8:*27-38, 1971.
18. M. Ervik, T. Walle, and H. Ehrsson, Quantitative gas chromatographic determination of nanogram levels of desipramine in serum. *Acta Pharm. Suec. 7:*625-634, 1970.
19. H. J. Weder and M. H. Bickel, Separation and identification of imipramine and its metabolites from biological samples by gas-liquid chromatography. *J. Chromatogr. 37:*181-189, 1968.
20. W. Riess, The double radio-iostope derivative technique for the assay of drugs in biological material. I: The measurement of maprotiline. *Anal. Chim. Acta 68:*363-376, 1974.
21. G. Carnis, J. Godbillon, and J. P. Metayer, Determination of clomipramine in plasma or urine by the double-radioisotope derivative technique. *Clin. Chem. 22:*817-823, 1976.
22. K. P. Maguire, G. D. Burrows, J. P. Coghlan, and B. A. Scoggins, Rapid radioisotopic procedure for the determination of nortriptyline in plasma. *Clin. Chem. 22:*761-764, 1976.
23. P. Hartvig, S. Strandberg, and B. Naslund, Determination of plasma amitriptyline by electron-capture gas chromatography after oxidation to anthraquinone. *J. Chromatogr. 118:*65-74, 1976.
24. P. Hartvig and B. Naslund, Simultaneous determination of plasma amitriptyline and nortriptyline as trichloroethyl carbamates by electron-capture gas chromatography. *J. Chromatogr. 133:*367-371, 1977.
25. H. F. Proelss, H. J. Lohmann, and D. G. Miles, High performance liquid chromatographic simultaneous determination of commonly used tricyclic antidepressants. *Clin. Chem. 24:*1948-1953, 1978.
26. R. Lucek and R. Dixon, Specific radioimmunoassay for amitriptyline and nortriptyline in plasma. *Res. Comm. in Chem. Path. Pharmacol. 18:*125-136, 1977.

27. D. J. Brunswick, B. Needelman, and J. Mendels, Radioimmunoassay of imipramine and desmethylimipramine. *Life Sci. 22:*137-146, 1978.
28. J. P. Moody, S. F. Whyte, and G. J. Naylor, A simple method for the determination of protriptyline in plasma. *Clin. Chim. Acta. 43:*355-359, 1973.
29. C. J. S. Walter, Drug plasma levels and clinical effect. *Proc. Roy. Soc. Mec. 64:*4-12, 1971.
30. P. Zeidenberg, J. M. Perel, M. Kanzler, R. N. Wharton, and S. Malitz, Clinical and metabolic studies with imipramine in man. *Amer. J. Psychiat. 127:*1321-1326, 1971.
31. A. H. Glassman, J. M. Perel, M. Shostak, S. J. Kantor, and J. L. Fleiss, Clinical implications of imipramine in plasma levels for depressive illness. *Arch. Gen. Psychiat. 34:*197-204, 1977.
32. S. F. Whyte, A. J. Macdonald, G. J. Naylor, and J. P. Moody, Plasma concentrations of protriptyline and clinical effects in depressed women. *Brit. J. Psychiat. 128:*384-390, 1976.
33. J. P. Moody, S. F. Whyte, A. J. Macdonald, and G. J. Naylor, Pharmacokinetic aspects of protriptyline plasma levels. *Eur. J. Clin. Pharmacol. 11:* 51-56, 1977.
34. R. Olivier-Martin, D. Marzin, E. Buschsenschutz, P. Pichot, and J. Boissier, Plasma levels of imipramine and desmethylimipramine and antidepressant effect during controlled therapy. *Psychopharmacologia 41:*187-195, 1975.
35. P. N. Kaul, L. R. Whitfield, and M. L. Clark, Quantitative determination of amitriptyline in blood. *J. Pharm. Sci. 67:*60-62, 1978.
36. W. Hammer and F. Sjöqvist, Plasma levels of monomethylated tricyclic antidepressants during treatment with imipramine-like compounds. *Life Sciences 6:*1895-1903, 1967.
37. B. Alexanderson, D. A. Price-Evans, and F. Sjöqvist, Steady-state plasma levels of nortriptyline in twins: Influence of genetic factors and drug therapy. *Brit. Med. J. 4:*764-768, 1969.
38. M. Åsberg, B. Cronholm, F. Sjöqvist, and D. Tuck, Relationship between plasma level and therapeutic effect of nortriptyline. *Brit. Med. J. 3:* 331-334, 1971.
39. L. F. Gram and K. Fredricson-Overφ, Drug interaction: Inhibitory effect of neuroleptics on metabolism of tricyclic antidepressants in man. *Brit. Med. J. 1:*463-465, 1972.
40. K. Fredricson-Overφ, L. F. Gram, and V. Hansen, Kinetics of nortriptyline in man according to a two compartment model. *Eur. J. Clin. Pharmacol. 8:*343-347, 1975.
41. K. Fredricson-Overφ, L. F. Gram, and V. Hansen, Interaction of perphenazine with the kinetics of nortriptyline. *Acta Pharmacol. Toxicol. 40:*97-105, 1977.
42. G. D. Burrows, B. Davies, and B. A. Scoggins, Plasma concentration of nortriptyline and clinical response in depressive illness. *Lancet 2:*619-623, 1972.

43. G. D. Burrows, B. A. Scoggins, L. R. Turecek, and B. Davies, Plasma nortriptyline and clinical response. *Clin. Pharmacol. Ther. 16:*639-644, 1974.
44. G. D. Burrows, L. R. Turecek, B. Davies, R. Mowbray, and B. A. Scoggins, A sequential trial comparing two plasma levels of nortriptyline. *Aust. N.Z. J. Psychiat. 8:*21-23, 1974.
45. A. Jori, D. Bernardi, G. Muscettola, and S. Garattini, Brain levels of imipramine and desipramine after combined treatment with these drugs in rats. *Eur. J. Pharmacol. 15:*85-90, 1971.
46. E. Riva, P. D. Hrdina, and P. L. Morselli, Measurement of desipramine in brain tissue by a radioisotope derivative technique. *J. Pharm. Pharmacol. 27:*797-799, 1975.
47. F. R. Zuleski, A. Loh, and F. J. Di Carlo, Assay of human plasma for nortriptyline by radioacetylation and thin-layer chromatography. *J. Chromatogr. 132:*45-49, 1977.
48. R. B. Jones and D. K. Luscombe, Single dose studies with clomipramine in normal subjects. *Postgrad. Med. J., Suppl. 3, 52:*62-67, 1976.
49. B. A. Scoggins, J. P. Coghlan, K. P. Maguire, G. D. Burrows, and B. Davies, The measurement of plasma levels of tricyclic antidepressant drugs. *Aust. N. Z. J. Psychiat. 10:*7-12, 1976.
50. G. D. Burrows, K. P. Maguire, B. A. Scoggins, J. Stevenson, and B. Davies, Plasma nortriptyline and clinical response: A study using changing plasma levels. *Psychol. Med. 7:*87-91, 1977.
51. G. D. Burrows, J. Vohra, P. Dumovic, K. P. Maguire, B. A. Scoggins, and B. Davies, Tricyclic antidepressants and cardiac conduction. *Progr. in Neuro-Psychopharmacol. 1:*329-334, 1977.
52. G. D. Burrows, B. Davies, K. P. Maguire, T. R. Norman, B. A. Scoggins, R. P. Hullin, and J. Burch, Interlaboratory comparison of nortriptyline levels. *Biochem. Med. 20:*125-127, 1978.
53. K. P. Maguire, G. D. Burrows, T. R. Norman, and B. A. Scoggins, A radioimmunoassay for nortriptyline (and other tricyclic antidepressants) in plasma. *Clin. Chem. 24:*549-554, 1978.
54. S. R. Harris, L. E. Gaudette, D. H. Efron, and A. A. Manian, A method for the measurement of plasma imipramine and desmethylimipramine concentrations. *Life Sciences 9:*781-788, 1970.
55. K. P. Maguire, Measurement of plasma nortriptyline. M.Sc. thesis, University of Melbourne, 1975.
56. J. P. Coghlan and B. A. Scoggins, Measurement of aldosterone in peripheral blood of man and sheep. *J. Clin. Endocrinol. Metab. 27:*1470-1486, 1967.
57. H. B. Hucker and S. Stauffer, GLC method for quantitative determination of amitriptyline in human plasma. *J. Pharm. Sci. 63:*296-297, 1974.
58. G. Norheim, The simultaneous determination of amitriptyline and nortriptyline in post mortem blood and urine using gas liquid chromatography. *J. Chromatogr. 88:*403-406, 1974.
59. M. Sheehan and P. Haythorn, Combined thin-layer and gas-liquid chromatographic identification of tricyclic antidepressants in urine. *J. Chromatogr. 132:*237-247, 1977.

60. P. C. N. Eichholtz, Determination of therapeutic levels of amitriptyline in serum by gas-liquid chromatography. *J. Chromatogr. 3:*456-458, 1975.
61. H. E. Hamilton, J. E. Wallace, and K. Blum, Spectrophotometric and gas-liquid chromatographic determination of amitriptyline. *Anal. Chem. 47:* 1139-1143, 1975.
62. J. E. O'Brien and O. N. Hinsvark, GLC determination of doxepin plasma levels. *J. Pharm. Sci. 65:*1068-1069, 1976.
63. G. L. Corona and B. Bonferoni, Simultaneous determination of therapeutic levels of amitriptyline and nortriptyline in plasma by gas-liquid chromatography. *J. Chromatogr. 124:*401-404, 1976.
64. T. R. Norman, K. P. Maguire, and G. D. Burrows, Determination of therapeutic levels of butriptyline in plasma by gas-liquid chromatography. *J. Chromatogr. 134:*524-528, 1977.
65. H. Bruderlein, M. Kraml, and D. Dvornik, A gas-liquid chromatographic method for the determination of butriptyline in serum. *Clin. Biochem. 10:* 3-7, 1977.
66. G. Nyberg and E. Martensson, Quantitative analysis of tricyclic antidepressants in serum from psychiatric patients. *J. Chromatogr. 143:*491-497, 1977.
67. R. A. Braithwaite, R. Goulding, G. Theano, J. Bailey, and A. Coppen, Plasma concentration of amitriptyline and clinical response. *Lancet 1:* 1297-1300, 1972.
68. R. A. Braithwaite, B. R. S. Nakra, and R. Gaind, Steady-state plasma concentrations during single and multiple dosage schedules of amitriptyline. *Psychol. Med. 4:*338-341, 1974.
69. W. H. Lyle, P. W. Brooks, D. F. Early, W. P. Leggett, G. Silverman, G. E. Strang, R. A. Braithwaite, J. M. Cuthill, R. Goulding, I. B. Pearson, and R. P. Snaith, Plasma concentration of nortriptyline as a guide to treatment. *Postgrad. Med. J. 50:*282-287, 1974.
70. G. D. Burrows, T. R. Norman, K. P. Maguire, G. Rubinstein, B. A. Scoggins, and B. Davies, A new antidepressant butriptyline: Plasma levels and clinical response. *Med. J. Aust. 2:*604-606, 1977.
71. O. Borgå and M. Garle, A gas chromatographic method for the quantitative determination of nortriptyline and some of its metabolites in human plasma and urine. *J. Chromatogr. 68:*77-88, 1972.
72. U. P. Geiger, T. G. Rajagopalan, and W. Riess, Quantitative assay of maprotiline in biological fluids by gas-liquid chromatography. *J. Chromatogr. 114:*167-173, 1975.
73. L. Vereczkey, G. Bianchetti, V. Rovei, and A. Frigerio, Gas chromatographic method for the determination of nomifensine in human plasma. *J. Chromatogr. 116:*451-456, 1976.
74. P. Kragh-Sorensen, M. Åsberg, and C. Eggert-Hansen, Plasma nortriptyline levels in endogenous depression. *Lancet 1:*113-115, 1973.
75. P. Kragh-Sorensen, C. Eggert-Hansen, N. E. Larsen, J. Naestoft, and E. F. Hvidberg, Long-term treatment of endogenous depression with nortriptyline with control of plasma levels. *Psychol. Med. 4:*174-180, 1974.

76. P. Kragh-Sorensen, C. E. Hansen, P. C. Baastrup, and E. F. Hvidberg, Self-inhibiting action of nortriptyline's antidepressive effect at high plasma levels. *Psychopharmacologia 45:*305-312, 1976.
77. S. A. Montgomery, R. A. Braithwaite, and J. L. Crammer, Routine nortriptyline levels in treatment of depression. *Brit. Med. J. 2:*166-167, 1977.
78. A. Karmen and L. Guiffrida, Enhancement of the response of the hydrogen flame ionization detector to compounds containing halogens and phosphorus. *Nature 201:*1204-1205, 1964.
79. B. Kolb and J. Bischoff, A new design of a thermionic nitrogen and phosphorus detector for GC. *J. Chromatogr. Sci. 12:*625-629, 1974.
80. M. J. Hartigan, J. E. Purcell, M. Novotny, M. L. McConnell, and M. L. Lee, Analytical performance of a novel nitrogen-sensitive detector and its applications with glass open tubular columns. *J. Chromatogr. 99:*339-348, 1974.
81. M. Bertrand, C. Dupuis, M. Gagnon, and R. Dugal, Nanogram-range determination of plasma imipramine by gas-liquid chromatography using a selective nitrogen/phosphorus detector. *Clin. Biochem. 11:*117-120, 1978.
82. L. A. Gifford, P. Turner, and C. M. B. Pare, Sensitive method for the routine determination of tricyclic antidepressants in plasma using a specific nitrogen detector. *J. Chromatogr. 105:*107-113, 1975.
83. A. Jorgensen, A gas chromatographic method for the determination of amitriptyline and nortriptyline in human serum. *Acta Pharmacol. Toxicol. 36:*79-90, 1975.
84. D. J. Witts and P. Turner, A single comprehensive gas chromatographic assay for tricyclic and tetracyclic antidepressant drugs and their major metabolites in plasma. *Brit. J. Clin. Pharmacol. 4:*249-252, 1977.
85. D. N. Bailey and P. I. Jatlow, Gas-chromatographic analysis for therapeutic concentrations of imipramine and desipramine in plasma, with use of a nitrogen detector. *Clin. Chem. 22:*1697-1701, 1976.
86. R. N. Gupta, G. Molnar, R. E. Hill, and M. L. Gupta, Estimation of amitriptyline and its metabolites in serum and urine by GLC using nitrogen-specific detection. *Clin. Biochem. 9:*247-251, 1976.
87. E. Bailey, M. Fenoughty, and L. Richardson, Automated high resolution gas chromatographic analysis of psychotropic drugs in biological fluids using open tubular glass capillary columns, 1. Determination of nomifensine in human plasma. *J. Chromatogr. 131:*347-355, 1977.
88. J. N. Connor, G. F. Johnson, and H. M. Solomon, Quantitation of amitriptyline and nortriptyline in human serum. *J. Chromatogr. 143:*415-421, 1977.
89. T. B. Cooper, D. Allen, and G. M. Simpson, A sensitive GLC method for the determination of imipramine and desmethylimipramine using a nitrogen detector. *Psychopharmacol. Comm. 1:*445-454, 1975.
90. D. N. Bailey and P. I. Jatlow, Gas-chromatographic analysis for therapeutic concentrations of amitriptyline and nortriptyline in plasma, with use of a nitrogen detector. *Clin. Chem. 22:*777-781, 1976.
91. J. Vasiliades and K. C. Bush, Gas liquid chromatographic determination of

therapeutic and toxic levels of amitriptyline in human serum with a nitrogen-sensitive detector. *Anal. Chem. 48:*1708-1711, 1976.
92. H. B. Hucker and S. C. Stauffer, Rapid, sensitive gas-liquid chromatographic method for determination of amitriptyline and nortriptyline in plasma using a nitrogen-sensitive detector. *J. Chromatogr. 138:*437-442, 1977.
93. M. T. Rosseel, M. G. Bogaert, and M. Claeys, Quantitative GLC determination of cis- and trans-isomers of doxepin and desmethyldoxepin. *J. Pharm. Sci. 67:*802-805, 1978.
94. L. A. Gifford, Progress towards a comprehensive plasma assay for the tricyclic and tetracyclic antidepressants. *Postgrad. Med. J., Suppl. 3, 52:*69-71, 1976.
95. S. Dawling and R. A. Braithwaite, Simplified method for monitoring tricyclic antidepressant therapy using gas-liquid chromatography with nitrogen detection. *J. Chromatogr. 146:*449-456, 1978.
96. R. S. B. Ehsanullah, K. Ghose, M. J. Kirby, and D. J. Witts, Some clinical pharmacological studies with tandamine hydrochloride, a potential antidepressive agent. *Brit. J. Clin. Pharmacol. 3:*950P, 1976.
97. K. Ghose, G. J. Huston, M. J. Kirby, D. J. Witts, and P. Turner, Some clinical pharmacological studies with butriptyline, an antidepressive drug. *Brit. J. Clin. Pharmacol. 4:*91-93, 1977.
98. A. Jorgensen and P. Staehr, On the biological half-life of amitriptyline. *J. Pharm. Pharmacol. 28:*62-64, 1976.
99. C. G. Hammar, B. Alexanderson, B. Holmstedt, and F. Sjöqvist, Gas chromatography-mass spectrometry of nortriptyline in body fluids of man. *Clin. Pharmacol. Ther. 12:*496-505, 1971.
100. D. R. Knapp, T. E. Gaffney, R. E. McMahon, and G. Kiplinger, Studies of human urinary and biliary metabolites of nortriptyline with staple isotope labelling. *J. Pharmacol. Exp. Ther. 180:*784-790, 1972.
101. O. Borgå, L. Palmer, A. Linnarsson, and B. Holmstedt, Quantitative determination of nortriptyline and desmethylnortriptyline in human plasma by combined gas chromatography-mass spectrometry. *Anal. Letts. 4:*837-849, 1971.
102. A. Frigerio, G. Belvedere, F. DeNadai, R. Fanelli, C. Pantarotto, E. Riva, and P. L. Morselli, A method for the determination of imipramine in human plasma by gas-liquid chromatography-mass fragmentography. *J. Chromatogr. 74:*201-208, 1972.
103. A. Frigerio, C. Pantarotto, R. Franco, R. Gomeni, and P. L. Morselli, Quantitative determination of doxepin and desmethyldoxepin in rat plasma by means of gas-liquid chromatography-mass fragmentography. *J. Chromatogr. 130:*354-360, 1977.
104. G. Belvedere, L. Burti, A. Frigerio, and C. Pantarotto, Gas chromatographic-mass fragmentographic determination of "steady-state" plasma levels of imipramine and desipramine in chronically treated patients. *J. Chromatogr. 111:*313-321, 1975.
105. T. E. Gaffney, C. G. Hammar, B. Holmstedt, and R. E. McMahon, Ion

specific detection of internal standards labelled with stable isotopes. *Anal. Chem. 43:*307-310, 1971.

106. O. Borgå, L. Palmer, F. Sjöqvist, and B. Holmstedt, Mass fragmentography used in quantitative analysis of drugs and endogenous compounds in biological fluids. In *Pharmacology and the Future of Man,* Proc. 5th Int. Congr. Pharmacology, Karger-Basel, vol. 3:56-68, 1973.

107. J. T. Biggs, W. H. Holland, S. Chang, P. P. Hipps, and W. R. Sherman, Electron beam ionization mass fragmentographic analysis of tricyclic antidepressants in human plasma. *J. Pharm. Sci. 65:*261-268, 1976.

108. J. P. Dubois, W. King, W. Theobald, and B. Wirz, Measurement of clomipramine, N-desmethylclomipramine, imipramine, and dehydroimipramine in biological fluids by selective ion monitoring, and pharmacokinetics of clomipramine. *Clin. Chem. 22:*892-897, 1976.

109. G. Alfredsson, F. A. Wiesel, B. Fyro, and G. Sedvall, Mass fragmentographic analysis of clomipramine and its mono-demethylated metabolite in human plasma. *Psychopharmacology 52:*25-30, 1977.

110. W. A. Garland, Quantitative determination of amitriptyline and its principal metabolite, nortriptyline, by GLC-chemical ionization mass spectrometry. *J. Pharm. Sci. 66:*77-81, 1977.

111. J. T. Biggs, W. H. Holland, and W. R. Sherman, Steady-state protriptyline levels in an outpatient population. *Amer. J. Psychiat. 132:*960-962, 1975.

112. V. E. Ziegler, P. J. Clayton, and J. T. Biggs, A comparison study of amitriptyline and nortriptyline with plasma levels. *Arch. Gen. Psychiat. 34:* 607-612, 1977.

113. V. E. Ziegler, P. J. Clayton, J. R. Taylor, B. T. Co, and J. T. Biggs, Nortriptyline plasma levels and therapeutic response. *Clin. Pharmacol. Ther. 20:*458-463, 1976.

114. V. E. Ziegler, B. T. Co, J. R. Taylor, P. J. Clayton, and J. T. Biggs, Amitriptyline plasma levels and therapeutic response. *Clin. Pharmacol. Ther. 19:*795-801, 1976.

115. V. E. Ziegler, T. A. Fuller, and J. T. Biggs, Nortriptyline and 10-hydroxynortriptyline plasma concentrations. *J. Pharm. Pharmacol. 28:*849-850, 1976.

116. V. E. Ziegler, J. W. Knesevich, L. T. Wylie, and J. T. Biggs, Sampling time, dosage schedule, and nortriptyline plasma levels. *Arch. Gen. Psychiat. 34:*613-615, 1977.

117. V. E. Zeigler, D. A. Meyer, S. H. Rosen, J. W. Knesevich, and J. T. Biggs, Amitriptyline dosage schedule, sampling time and tricyclic plasma levels. *Brit. J. Psychiat. 131:*168-171, 1977.

118. R. G. Jenkins and R. O. Friedel, Analysis of tricyclic antidepressants in human plasma by GLC-Chemical ionization mass spectrometry with selected ion-monitoring. *J. Pharm. Sci. 67:*17-23, 1978.

119. A. Nagy and L. Treiber, Quantitative determination of imipramine and desipramine in human blood plasma by direct densitometry of thin-layer chromatograms. *J. Pharm. Pharmacol. 25:*599-603, 1973.

120. L. F. Gram and J. Christiansen, First-pass metabolism of imipramine in

man. *Clin. Pharmacol. Ther. 17:*555-563, 1975.
121. L. F. Gram, N. Reisby, I. Ibsen, A. Nagy, S. J. Dencker, P. Bech, G. O. Petersen, and J. Christiansen, Plasma levels and antidepressive effect of imipramine. *Clin. Pharmacol. Ther. 19:*318-324, 1976.
122. L. F. Gram, P. B. Andreasen, K. Fredrickson-Overø, and J. Christiansen, Comparison of single dose kinetics of imipramine, nortriptyline, and antipyrine in man. *Psychopharmacology 50:*21-27, 1976.
123. D. B. Faber, C. Mulder, and W. A. Man in 'T Veld, A thin-layer method for the determination of amitriptyline and nortriptyline in plasma. *J. Chromatogr. 100:*55-61, 1974.
124. U. Breyer and K. Villumsen, Measurement of plasma levels of tricyclic psychoactive drugs and their metabolites by UV reflectance photometry of thin layer chromatograms. *Europ. J. Clin. Pharmacol. 9:*457-465, 1976.
125. D. C. Fenimore, C. J. Meyer, C. M. Davis, F. Hsu, and A. Zlatkis, High-performance thin-layer chromatographic determination of psychopharmacologic agents in blood serum. *J. Chromatogr. 142:*399-409, 1977.
126. P. Haefelfinger, Determination of amitriptyline and nortriptyline in human plasma by quantitative thin-layer chromatography. *J. Chromatogr. 145:*445-451, 1978.
127. J. H. Knox and J. Jurand, Separation of tricyclic psychosedative drugs by high-speed ion-pair partition and liquid-solid adsorption chromatography. *J. Chromatogr. 103:*311-326, 1975.
128. B. Mellstrom and S. Eksborg, Determination of chlorimipramine and desmethylchlorimipramine in human plasma by ion-pair partition chromatography. *J. Chromatogr. 116:*475-479, 1976.
129. B. A. Persson and P. O. Lagerström, Ion-pair partition chromatography in the analysis of drugs and biogenic substances in plasma and urine. *J. Chromatogr. 122:*305-316, 1976.
130. P. O. Lagerström, I. Carlsson, and B. A. Persson, Determination of chloroimipramine and its demethyl-metabolite in plasma by ion-pair partition chromatography. *Acta Pharm. Suecica 13:*157-166, 1976.
131. B. Mellstrom and G. Tybring, Ion-pair liquid chromatography of steady-state plasma levels of chlorimipramine and demethylchlorimipramine. *J. Chromatogr. 143:*597-605, 1977.
132. R. R. Brodie, L. F. Chasseaud, and D. R. Hawkins, Separation and measurement of tricyclic antidepressant drugs in plasma by high-performance liquid chromatography. *J. Chromatogr. 143:*535-539, 1977.
133. J. H. M. Van Den Berg, J. J. M. deRuwe, R. S. Deelder, and T. A. Plomp, Column liquid chromatography of tricyclic antidepressants. *J. Chromatogr. 138:*431-436, 1977.
134. J. C. Kraak and P. Bijster, Determination of amitriptyline and some of its metabolites in blood by high-pressure liquid chromatography. *J. Chromatogr. 143:*499-512, 1977.
135. I. D. Watson and M. J. Stewart, Quantitative determination of amitriptyline and nortriptyline in plasma by high-performance liquid chromatography. *J. Chromatogr. 132:*155-159, 1977.
136. R. B. Moyes and I. C. A. Moyes, Measurement of plasma antidepressant

levels by high-performance liquid chromatography. *Postgrad. Med. J. Suppl. (4)53:*117-123, 1977.

137. M. Uihlein and P. Hajdu, High performance liquid chromatography in research of pharmacokinetics and metabolism. *Arzneim.-Forsch. 27:*98-102, 1977.

138. R. Emanuelsson and R. G. Moore, Quantitation of zimelidine and norzimelidine in plasma by HPLC. *J. Chromatogr. 146:*113-119, 1977.

139. H. G. M. Westenberg, B. F. H. Drenth, R. A. deZeeuw, H. DeCuyper, H. M. van Praag, and J. Korf, Determination of clomipramine and desmethylclomipramine in plasma by means of liquid chromatography. *J. Chromatogr. 142:*725-733, 1977.

140. F. L. Vandemark, R. F. Adams, and G. J. Schmidt, Liquid-chromatographic procedure for tricyclic drugs and their metabolites in plasma. *Clin. Chem. 24:*87-91, 1978.

141. J. R. Salmon and P. R. Wood, Determination of nortriptyline in sugar coated tablets by high performance liquid-chromatography. *Analyst 101:* 611-615, 1976.

142. A. G. Butterfield and R. W. Sears, High performance liquid chromatographic determination of perphenazine and amitriptyline hydrochloride in two-component tablet formulations. *J. Pharm. Sci. 66:*1117-1119, 1977.

143. I. D. Watson and M. J. Stewart, Assay of tricyclic structured drugs and their metabolites in urine by high-performance liquid chromatography. *J. Chromatogr. 134:*182-186, 1977.

144. J. J. deRidder, P. C. J. M. Koppens, and H. J. M. vanHal, The use of high performance liquid chromatography for sample clean-up in mass fragmentographic assays. *J. Chromatogr. 143:*281-287, 1977.

145. J. J. deRidder, P. C. J. M. Koppen, and H. J. M. vanHal, Mass-fragmentographic assay of nanogram amounts of the antidepressant drug Mianserin Hydrochloride (org GB 94) in human plasma. *J. Chromatogr. 143:*289-297, 1977.

146. H. d'A, Heck, N. W. Flynn, S. E. Buttrill, R. L. Dyer, and M. Anbar, DeTermination of imipramine in plasma by high pressure liquid chromatography and field ionization mass spectrometry: Increased sensitivity in comparison with gas chromatography mass spectrometry. *Biomed. Mass Spectrometry 5:*250-257, 1978.

147. I. D. Watson and M. J. Stewart, Separation and quantitative determination of tricyclic antidepressants by high-performance liquid chromatography. *J. Chromatogr. 110:*389-392, 1975.

148. M. R. Detaevernier, L. Dryon, and D. L. Massart, The separation of some tricyclic antidepressants by high-performance liquid chromatography. *J. Chromatogr. 128:*204-207, 1976.

149. I. M. Johansson, K. G. Wahlund, and G. Schill, Reversed-phase ion-pair chromatography of drugs and related organic compounds. *J. Chromatogr. 149:*281-296, 1978.

150. G. L. Sathananthan, S. Gershon, S. Spector, and M. Almeida, Correlation of plasma and cerebrospinal fluid levels of imipramine. *Clin. Pharmacol. Ther. 15:*218, 1974.

151. B. Kaul, B. Quame, and B. Davidow, Screening for tricyclic antidepressant drugs in biological specimens by radioimmunoassay. *J. Anal. Toxicol. 1:*236-243, 1977.
152. G. W. Aherne, E. M. Piall, and V. Marks, The radioimmunoassay of tricyclic antidepressants. *Brit. J. Clin. Pharmacol. 3:*561-565, 1976.
153. J. W. Hubbard, K. K. Midha, J. K. Cooper, and C. Charette, Radioimmunoassay for psychotropic drugs, II: Synthesis and properties of haptens for tricyclic antidepressants. *J. Pharm. Sci. 67:*1571-1577, 1978.
154. G. F. Read, D. Riad-Fahmy, and R. F. Walker, A specific radio-immunoassay procedure for plasma clomipramine. *Postgrad. Med. J. Suppl. (4)53:* 110-116, 1977.
155. G. F. Read and D. Riad-Fahmy, Determination of a tricyclic antidepressant, clomipramine (Anafranil), in plasma by a specific radioimmunoassay procedure. *Clin. Chem. 24:*36-40, 1978.
156. W. Heptner, M. J. Badian, S. Baudner, O. E. Christ, H. M. Fraser, W. Rupp, K. E. Weimer, and H. Wissmann, Determination of nomifensine by a sensitive radioimmunoassay. *Brit. J. Clin. Pharmacol. 4:*123-127, 1977.
157. J. D. Robinson, B. A. Morris, E. M. Piall, G. W. Aherne, and V. Marks. The use of rats in the screening of drug-protein conjugates for immunoactivity. In *Radioimmunoassay in Clinical Biochemistry* (C. A. Pasternak, ed.). London, Heyden & Son, 1975, pp. 101-111.
158. J. D. Robinson, D. Risby, G. Riley, and G. W. Aherne, A radioimmunoassay for the determination of combined amitriptyline and nortriptyline concentrations in microliter samples of plasma. *J. Pharmacol. Exp. Ther. 205:*499-502, 1978.
159. G. W. Aherne, V. Marks, G. Mould, and G. Stout, Radioimmunoassay for nortriptyline and amitriptyline. *Lancet 1:*1214, 1977.
160. J. D. Robinson, R. A. Braithwaite, and S. Dawling, Measurement of plasma nortriptyline concentrations: Radioimmunoassay and gas chromatography compared. *Clin. Chem. 24:*2023-2025, 1978.
161. O. Buchman and I. Pri-Bar, High specific acitvity labelling of some tricyclic antidepressants. *J. Labelled Compounds and Radiopharmaceuticals 14:*263-269, 1978.
162. J. D. Robinson, G. W. Aherne, J. D. Teale, B. A. Morris, and V. Marks, Problems encountered in the use of radioiodination tags in radioimmunoassays for drugs. In *Radioimmunoassay in Clinical Biochemistry* (C. A. Pasternak, ed.), London, Heyden & Son, 1975, pp. 113-123.
163. M. N. Al-Bassam, M. J. O. O'Sullivan, E. Gnemmi, J. W. Bridges, and V. Marks, Double-antibody enzyme immunoassay for nortriptyline. *Clin. Chem. 24:*1590-1594, 1978.
164. D. A. P. Evans, K. A. Manley, and U. A. McKusick, Genetic control of isoniazid metabolism in man. *Brit. Med. J. 2:*485-491, 1960.
165. P. Turner, J. H. Young, and E. F. Scowen, Fluorimetric determination of tranylcypromine in urine. *J. Pharm. Pharmacol. 18:*550-551, 1966.
166. J. A. Fuentes, M. A. Oleshansky, and N. H. Neff, A sensitive enzymatic assay for dextro- or levo-tranylcypramine in brain. *Biochem. Pharmacol. 24:*1971-1973, 1975.
167. R. M. deSagher, A. P. deLeenheer, and A. E. Claeys, Thin-layer chromatog-

graphy of hydrazidic monoamine oxidase inhibitor drugs. *J. Chromatogr. 106:*357-362, 1975.
168. R. M. deSagher, A. P. deLeenheer, and A. E. Claeys, Identification and quantitative GLC determination of Iproniazid in human urine. *J. Pharm. Sci. 65:*878-882, 1976.
169. A. Nies, D. S. Robinson, K. R. Lamborn, C. L. Ravaris, and J. O. Ives, The efficacy of the MAO inhibitor phenelzine: Dose effects and prediction of response. *IX Cong Collegium Internationale Neuropsychopharmacologicum Symposium No. 11,* Paris, 1976.
170. J. F. J. Cade, Lithium salts in the treatment of psychotic excitement. *Med. J. Aust. 36:*349-352, 1949.
171. P. C. Baastrup and M. Schou, Lithium as a prophylactic agent. *Arch. Gen. Psychiat. 55:*162-172, 1967.
172. J. Mendels and A. Frazer, Intracellular lithium concentration and clinical response towards a membrane theory of depression. *J. Psychiat. Res. 10:* 9-18, 1973.
173. J. Mendels and A. Frazer, Alterations in cell membrane activity in depression. *Amer. J. Psychiat. 131:*1240-1246, 1974.
174. Y. Fournis and G. Chazot, Determination du lithium dans les milieux biologiques. *Pathol. et Biol. 19:*787-795, 1971.
175. P. B. Brown and E. F. Legg, The estimation of lithium in serum. *Ann. Clin. Biochem. 7:*13-18, 1970.
176. L. Sideman, Revision of flame photometric Li determination. *Clin. Chem. 16:*618-619, 1970.
177. H. I. Coombs, The estimation of lithium in serum. *Brit. J. Psychiat. 118:* 225-226, 1971.
178. A. Amidsen, Serum lithium determinations for clinical use. *Scand. J. Clin. Lab. Invest. 20:*104-108, 1967.
179. A. Frazer, S. K.Secunda, and J. Mendels, A method for the determination of sodium, potassium, magnesium, and lithium concentrations in erythrocytes. *Clin. Chim. Acta 36:*499-509, 1972.
180. J. Pybus and G. N. Bowers, Jr., Measurement of serum lithium by atomic absorption spectroscopy. *Clin. Chem. 16:*139-143, 1970.
181. A. L. Levy and E. M. Katz, Comparison of serum lithium determinations by flame photometry and atomic absorption spectrophotometry. *Clin. Chem. 16:*840-842, 1970.
182. S. Spector, N. L. Spector, and M. P. Almeida, Radioimmunoassay for desmethylimipramine. *Psychopharmacol. Comm. 1:*421-429, 1975.
183. J. Chamberlain and H. M. Hill, A simple gas chromatographic method for the determination of nomifensine in plasma and a comparison of the method with other available techniques. *Brit. J. Clin. Pharmacol. 4* (Suppl.): 117-121, 1977.
184. M. Claeys, G. Muscettola, and S. P. Markey, Simultaneous measurement of imipramine and desipramine by selected ion recording with deuterated internal standards. *Biomed. Mass Spectrometry 3:*110-116, 1976.
185. J. M. Wilson, L. J. Williamson, and V. A. Raisys, Simultaneous measurement of secondary and tertiary tricyclic antidepressants by ac/MS chemical ionization mass fragmentography. *Clin. Chem. 23:* 1012-1017, 1977.

3

Methods for the Measurement of Psychotropic Drugs
Antipsychotics and Antianxiety Agents

Trevor R. Norman and Graham D. Burrows /
Department of Psychiatry,
University of Melbourne, Parkville, Victoria, Australia

ANTIPSYCHOTICS

The antipsychotic drugs are broadly defined as those drugs effective in the treatment of schizophrenia. Antipsychotics are usually of three chemical classes: phenothiazines, thioxanthenes, and butyrophenones. Further subdivisions of these drugs exist, based on chemical structural relationships. Some miscellaneous agents, belonging to the dibenzoxazepine and indole chemical classes, are also effective antipsychotic agents (see Fig. 1).

The introduction of chlorpromazine (CPZ) into psychiatric practice brought about a revolution in the treatment of schizophrenia. Clinically, chlorpromazine alone was not the complete answer. Problems of side effects and toxicity soon became obvious. The concept of the measurement of plasma levels to identify therapeutic levels, toxic concentrations, and problems of side effects became possible with the introduction of sensitive, specific analytical techniques. These methods have been reviewed [1,2], but recent advances in methodology have largely superseded the techniques described.

I. PHENOTHIAZINES

A. Extraction from Biological Specimens

Essentially the same methods for extraction of tricyclic antidepressants from biological specimens can be used for the phenothiazines. A detailed scheme for the extraction of chlorpromazine and metabolites from urine has been developed at the National Institute of Mental Health [3]. This involves extraction of drug and metabolites with an organic solvent from the alkalinized ($pH > 10$) urine sample. Back-extraction into acid, followed by a further extraction into solvent after alkalinization and hydrolysis of the conjugates then follows. The sample is then ready for quantitation. This method leads to the extraction of the metab-

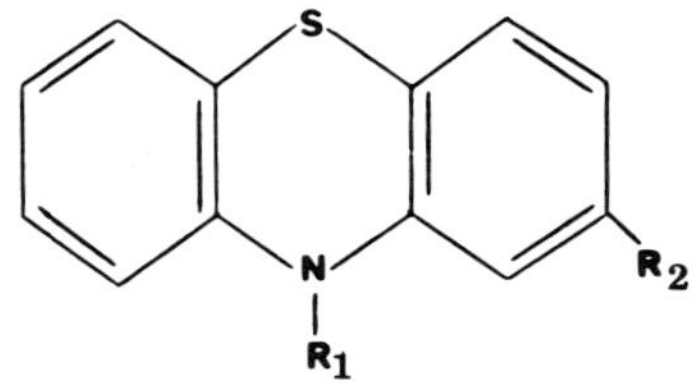

DRUG	R_1	R_2
CHLORPROMAZINE	$-(CH_2)_3-N(CH_3)_2$	$-Cl$
TRIFLUPROMAZINE	$-(CH_2)_3-N(CH_3)_2$	$-CF_3$
THIORIDAZINE	$-(CH_2)_2-$ (N-CH_3)	$-SCH_3$
PERPHENAZINE	$-(CH_2)_3-N\quad N-(CH_2)_2-OH$	$-Cl$
PROCHLORPERAZINE	$-(CH_2)_3-N\quad N-CH_3$	$-Cl$
FLUPHENAZINE	$-(CH_2)_3-N\quad N-(CH_2)_2-OH$	$-CF_3$
ACETOPHENAZINE	$-(CH_2)_3-N\quad N-(CH_2)_2-OH$	$-COCH_3$
TRIFLUOPERAZINE	$-(CH_2)_3-N\quad N-CH_3$	$-CF_3$

THIOXANTHENES

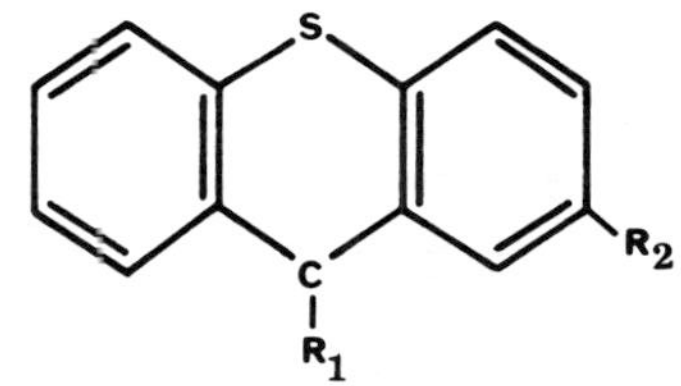

DRUG	R_1	R_2
CHLORPROTHIXENE	$=CH-(CH_2)_2-N(CH_3)_2$	$-Cl$
THIOTHIXENE	$=CH(CH_2)_2-N\quad N-CH_3$	$-SO_2N(CH_3)_2$

BUTYROPHENONES

HALOPERIDOL

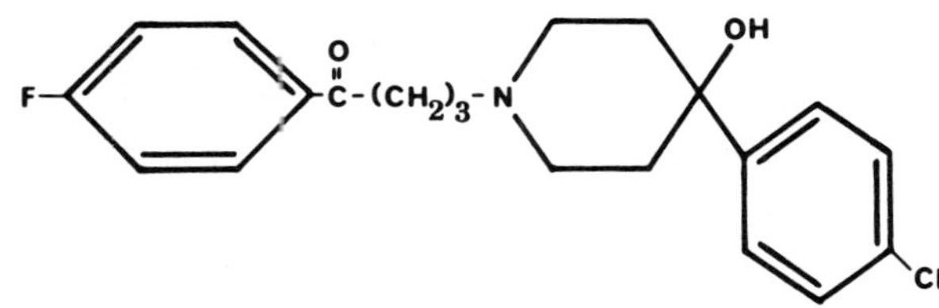

Figure 1 Structures of some antipsychotic drugs.

olites of the drug, and nonseparative analytical techniques (e.g., spectrophotometry) would give a total chlorpromazine concentration.

A detailed scheme for the extraction of drugs from toxicological specimens has been given by Goldbaum and Dominguez [4]. The principles outlined are readily applicable to phenothiazine analysis. Tompsett [2] has outlined extraction procedures for phenothiazines and their sulfoxides in serum, soft tissues, and urine. Other metabolites are not specifically separated by the techniques employed, and under the conditions used some metabolites may be destroyed or converted back to the parent drug.

To overcome the difficulty of separation of drug and metabolites Whelpton and Curry [5] developed a method of separation of fluphenazine and its metabolites based on pH-dependent partition ratios. The method was originally used by Brodie et al. [6] for drug analysis. A solution of an ionizable solute, shaken with an immiscible organic phase, is distributed between the two phases. By careful adjustment of the pH of the aqueous phase the amount of solute extracted into one phase or the other can be regulated. This approach provided a good separation of fluphenazine, fluphenazine sulfoxide, and 7-hydroxyfluphenazine from plasma, urine, and feces.

A simplified version of the first extraction technique has been applied to the extraction of phenothiazines from plasma before quantitation. For use in quantitative studies, the extraction method must be reproducible. This can be ensured by use of an internal standard, carried through the entire extraction process. Storage of samples of the phenothiazines may present some difficulties. Frozen fluphenazine plasma samples have been found to decompose after two months in the dark and to decompose on excessive exposure to light [7].

The introduction of XAD resins and large-pore kieselguhr granular columns may provide a simple, reproducible, and fast extraction procedure for biological samples. However, the use of such columns is developmental at this time, but if shown to be successful they will doubtless be of great utility.

B. Spectrophotometric Analysis

Spectrophotometry can readily be used for the determination of most drugs in biological specimens. Perhaps the most widely used technique is based on the ability of the drug to absorb light in the ultraviolet or visible regions of the spectrum. Most drugs do not possess absorption in the visible region, but they can be reacted with a variety of reagents to produce a colored species. This is the technique of colorimetry.

Brodie and Udenfriend [8] described the determination of amine compounds, after their extraction from biological samples, from the color formed with methyl orange. However, this method has not been widely applied to phenothiazine determination, and it is doubtful that the specificity and sensitivity are sufficient for use in plasma level determinations. In a series of papers, Forrest and co-workers [9-18] described rapid tests for the identification of phenothiazines in the urine. After separation of the drug by ion exchange chromatography, a colored derivative could be formed by reaction with ferric ion and sulfuric acid or potassium dichromate and mineral acids or the FPN reagent (ferric ion, perchloric, and nitric acids), or nitrite ion in sulfuric acid. The nature and intensity of the color was related to the patient's dose. Such reagents may be useful in the detection of overdoses of phenothiazines, but were not applied to the determination of plasma concentrations. Slight modifications by other workers have failed to improve the sensitivity [19-22]. Reaction of the phenothiazines with palladium chloride leads to the formation of a blue complex, but this reaction has not been applied to plasma level studies [23]. A method for the determination of a mixture of secondary and tertiary amines in urine depends on the ability of the secondary amine to form a dithiocarbamate with carbon disulfide. The reaction of this dithiocarbamate with copper ion to form a yellow complex allows quantitation of the secondary amine. The tertiary amine can be quantitated by differential extraction [24]. The sensitivity of the method is of the order of 10-20 μg/ml of each drug, not sufficient to allow for routine plasma level determination.

Colorimetry has major disadvantages for the routine determination of drug concentrations. The sensitivity of the method is usually not adequate; specificity is often poor; the complex responsible for the color is sometimes unstable. Under these conditions quantitative analysis is difficult to achieve. These reactions are at best a qualitative test for the presence of phenothiazine and phenothiazine-like drugs.

Direct measurement of the extracted drug by ultraviolet (UV) spectrophotometry or extraction, oxidation, and measurement of the oxidized species constitute alternative methods of drug quantitation. Oxidation with cobalt (III) oxide and measurement of the resultant species has been used for a range of phenothiazines in blood, serum, and urine [25]. A sensitivity of a few μg/ml was found. Direct measurement of methotrimeprazine in brain [26] and chlorpromazine in plasma extracts [27] from their UV absorbances have similar levels of sensitivity. These methods lack specificity, which may be increased by the inclusion of a chromatography step [3], and sensitivity for routine use in monitoring patient plasma samples.

The first useful fluorimetric determination of the phenothiazines chlorpromazine, thioridazine, and trifluoperazine in biological fluids involved extraction and oxidation with hydrogen peroxide, then measurement of fluorescence [28]. Such a method is a total phenothiazine assay. However, it was applied to urine, blood, and tissue samples with a sensitivity of about 50 ng/ml. It is most useful for urine samples where the levels of drug are higher. No data on the precision and accuracy of the assay were recorded, but extraction and oxidation conditions and recoveries were extensively investigated. Pacha [29] described fluorimetric determination of thioridazine and mesoridazine after oxidation with potassium permanganate. A sensitivity of 0.05 μg/ml of plasma was recorded, with a linear spectrophotometer response up to 10 μg. The method was used to study the pharmacokinetics of thioridazine in volunteers. Chlorpromazine and 11 of its metabolites were determined after thin-layer chromatography (TLC) and reaction with dansylchloride, by fluorimetry [30-33]. A sensitivity of 10 ng/ml was claimed for samples extracted from plasma or urine. Simpson et al. [34] determined butaperazine levels in whole blood by spectrofluorimetry after extraction into an organic solvent. Recovery of the drug was greater than 96%, and the coefficient of variation at 150 ng/ml was 2.4% (n = 20). Specificity was evaluated using TLC. The sulfoxide did not significantly interfere in the determination of patient samples. Butaperazine concentrations in blood were determined after a three-step extraction [35]. Sensitivity was 20 ng/ml with a linear fluorimeter response over the 0-400-ng/ml range. Specificity was checked using thin-layer chromatography. The method was subsequently used by Davis and coworkers in clinical [36] and pharmacokinetic studies [37]. A less sensitive method was used for the determination of urinary levels of thioridazine, trifluoperazine, and their sulfoxides in urine [38]. Fluorescence was measured after oxidation with potassium permanganate. A sensitive, precise assay for chlorpromazine and its sulfoxide was based on the reaction of the amine base with 9-bromomethylacridine to form a fluorescent derivative [33]. As little as 15-20 ng of chlorpromazine can be determined with a precision (coefficient of variation) of 3%.

Fluorimetry offers a sensitive method for determination of the phenothiazines in biological fluids. Specificity can be adequately achieved if a chromatography or differential extraction step is included. For routine measurement, fluorimetry offers no particular advantages over other methods of analysis.

C. Radioimmunoassay

Radioimmunoassay (RIA) is potentially the most useful technique, because of its technical simplicity, for the measurement of the phenothiazines and indeed all drugs. However, the production of antisera specific to the drug to be measured is a crucial factor in the RIA technique. Phenothiazine immunogenicity has been extensively studied in rabbits and guinea pigs [39,40]. Both perphenazine and nor_2-chlorpromazine, when individually covalently bonded to a carrier molecule (bovine serum albumin, BSA), elicited hapten-specific antibody synthesis [39]. Both antisera were investigated for the determination of chlorpromazine concentrations. The nor_2-chlorpromazine-BSA antiserum was more thoroughly investigated with respect to its cross-reactivity toward other phenothiazines and chlorpromazine metabolites. Promazine and triflupromazine were both weakly bound, as was 7-hydroxychlorpromazine and chlorpromazine sulfoxide. However, nor_2-chlorpromazine and mono- and didesmethylchlorpromazine had cross-reactivities similar to those of chlorpromazine itself. The antiserum is not specific, but would be useful where total chlorpromazine and metabolite levels are required. The assay had good sensitivity (25 ng using a 30-mCi/mmol-specific-activity [^{14}C] chlorpromazine tracer). Use of a higher-specific-activity ^{3}H-labeled tracer would improve sensitivity. The method was not applied to the measurement of patient plasma samples, and the lack of specificity of the antiserum is problematic where such a large number of metabolites may be responsible for the therapeutic effect of the drug.

Following this work, a more specific antiserum against chlorpromazine (CPZ) was developed [41]. The sensitivity of the assay was improved by using 3.0-Ci/mmol [^{3}H] chlorpromazine as tracer. As little as 10 pg could be assayed, with none of the major metabolites (CPZ sulfoxide, nor_1- and nor_2-chlorpromazine) binding significantly to the antibody in the 10-2,000-pg range. However, 7- and 8-hydroxychlorpromazine and promazine were significantly bound to the antibody in this range. Brain and plasma levels of chlorpromazine were determined in rats after intravenous infusion of 10 mg/kg. Prior extraction of the sample was not necessary. The method has not been applied to the measurement of patient samples, nor was the precision of the assay evaluated.

A radioimmunoassay for fluphenazine in plasma which does not require extraction has been developed [42]. The antiserum was raised in sheep against bovine serum albumin coupled to 7-carboxyflupenthixol by the carbodiimide reaction. A sensitivity of 50 pg/ml using a 200-μl sample of plasma was found for the assay. The intraassay precision over the range 20-500 pg was 6-10% (coefficient of variation). At higher concentrations, 1 and 2 ng, the precision was 20 and 15%, respectively, suggesting that samples at this concentration should be diluted. The hydroxy metabolites of fluphenazine showed significant cross-reactivity with the antiserum, as did perphenazine and trifluoperazine. Other antipsychotics, benzodiazepines, and tricyclic antidepressants exhibited negligible cross-reactivity. The method was applied to patient samples, and the preliminary data indicate this is a useful method for routine application.

The development of specific antibodies to the phenothiazines and the availability of high-specific-activity tritium-labeled drugs make the development of radioimmunoassay feasible. The RIA technique is rapid and simple, usually does not require prior extraction of plasma sample, and is sensitive and precise. For routine monitoring of phenothiazine plasma levels it is the ideal technique. Specificity of the antibodies developed so far is problematic, but further research should ensure that this is overcome.

D. Isotope Derivative Dilution Analysis

The principles of radioisotopic assays have been described in detail [43]. Two types of assay can be distinguished: single-isotope derivative and double-isotope derivative. Both are technically demanding and more readily applied to primary or secondary amine drugs. The double-isotope derivative dilution analysis is the better of the two methods since the second isotope acts as an internal recovery marker and there is no need to construct standard curves [44].

Isotope assays have not been fully exploited for the measurement of antipsychotic plasma levels. In a series of papers, Efron and associates have described a radioassay of chlorpromazine [45-47]. The method is designed to measure unmetabolized chlorpromazine and some metabolites after extraction from plasma. Chlorpromazine, nor_1-CPZ, and nor_2-CPZ are extracted from alkalinized (pH 8.5) plasma into heptane, then extracted into acid, and finally back-extracted into heptane-isoamyl alcohol. The sulfoxides (chlorpromazine sulfoxide [CPZSO], nor_1-CPZSO, and nor_2-CPZSO) can be extracted from the residual plasma with ethyl acetate, then into acid and back-extracted into ethyl acetate. Both extracts are acetylated with [^{3}H]acetic anhydride and quaternized with [^{14}C]methyliodide. The secondary and primary amines (nor_1-CPZ, nor_2-CPZ, nor_1-CPZSO, and nor_2-CPZSO) react with the acetic anhydride. The tertiary amines (CPZ and CPZSO) react with the methyliodide. The acetylated and quaternized compounds in each tube are separated by extraction into butanol or heptane-isoamyl alcohol. The respective fractions are then counted in a scintillation spectrometer, and unknown samples can be calculated from a standard curve. When applied to the measurement of human plasma samples, the sensitivity was 10-15 ng/ml of CPZ. A greater sensitivity could be achieved if higher-specific-activity tracers were used. The use of solvent extraction steps after derivatization could be replaced by thin-layer chromatographic separation of the derivatives. A better recovery may be obtained in this step, while specificity would be improved.

This method has general applicability to the amine-type drugs but has not been pursued for compounds other than chlorpromazine. The complexities of phenothiazine metabolism make the development of an assay for the parent drug and metabolites difficult. Use of high-specific-activity ^{3}H-labeled chlorpromazine and ^{14}C-labeled metabolites would allow the more specific, sensitive, and accurate double-isotope technique to be developed for this drug. As a rapid, routine assay for the phenothiazines, isotope dilution techniques are not yet practical.

E. Thin-Layer Chromatographic Analysis

Some of the earliest methods for the determination of phenothiazines relied on the use of thin-layer chromatography (TLC) plates and spray reagents. These methods were mainly used for the detection of phenothiazines and phenothiazinelike substances in urine or plasma [16,48-56] or for the study of phenothiazine metabolism [57-59]. Such methods are useful in the rapid identification of phenothiazine overdose but have not been applied to plasma level measurement. Zingales in a series of papers [60-62] has systematically investigated the behavior of psychotropic drugs on thin-layer plates in several solvent systems following extraction from urine or blood. The method is not sensitive enough to be applicable to plasma level measurements.

Arons et al. [63] used a spectrophotometric method to determine chlorpromazine levels in urine after separation by TLC. This method has not been applied to any plasma level studies of chlorpromazine. Kaul and associates [30, 32,33,119] have reported two sensitive methods for chlorpromazine determination based on quaternization of the tertiary amine with dansylchloride or 9-bromoethylacridine, followed by separation on thin-layer plates and spectrofluorimetry. Both techniques are capable of measuring down to 10 ng/ml of chlorpromazine with ±5% quoted for the precision of the duplicates. The dansylation technique also allows the determination of 11 chlorpromazine metabolites. Turano and associates [64,65] used direct-scanning densitometry after two-dimensional TLC for the determination of chlorpromazine and metabolites in blood, plasma, erythrocytes, and urine. A detection limit of about 0.1 μg was claimed for the method, but no evaluation in terms of accuracy and precision was carried out.

Chan et al. [66] have described a TLC-spectrodensitometry procedure for chlorpromazine metabolism, and this method has been used in some clinical studies [67]. Kapadia et al. [68] determined butaperazine by a combination of TLC and ultraviolet spectrophotometry. However, this method was not applied to plasma samples. Breyer and Villumsen [69] determined perazine plasma levels following TLC and ultraviolet reflectance photometry of the plates. Good separation of perazine and its metabolites, desmethylperazine and perazine sulfoxide, was achieved. Calibration curves were linear over the range 0-400 ng/ml with recoveries of 80-90% for perazine, desmethylperazine, perazine sulfoxide, and perazine N-oxide. Duplicate assays varied about 5%. This assay method could be applied to other phenothiazines, since Breyer and Villumsen have demonstrated its utility for the measurement of tricyclic antidepressants, in addition to perazine.

The utilization of thin-layer chromatography, combined with spectrofluorimetry, direct-scanning densitometry, or ultraviolet reflectance spectrometry, in clinical studies is a possibility, since adequate sensitivity has been demonstrated. The problem of separation and quantitation of metabolites is most difficult, correct choice of the solvent system being crucial. For laboratories without access to more sophisticated equipment, TLC is an efficient, reliable technique.

F. Gas-Liquid Chromatographic Analysis

Gas-liquid chromatography (GLC), as in other forms of chromatographic analysis, is a separative technique, the degree of separation achieved being dependent on the choice of stationary phase. Methyl and phenyl silicone phases (e.g., OV-1, OV-17) have been successfully used for quantitative determination of antipsychotic drugs. Choice of detector in gas chromatography is not as critical as stationary phase, but the N-P specific detector (i.e., alkali flame ionization detector, AFID) can be more sensitive than either conventional flame ionization or electron capture. Mass fragmentography offers a further refinement of detection, and methods using this technique are discussed in Sec. I.H. GLC provides a sensitive, specific, and precise method of analysis for phenothiazines in biological fluids at levels normally observed on therapeutic doses. In psychiatric practice blood plasma or serum has been the usual biological fluid studied. The extraction procedures described in Sec. I.A can be applied to the serum sample to recover the drugs. Extensive cleanup of the samples is required for gas chromatography, especially where flame ionization detection (FID) is used. For electron capture detection (ECD) and AFID, rigorous cleanup of samples may not be essential, but is advisable to avoid possible contamination by endogenous substances. Table 1 lists the GLC methods in terms of the specificity (minimum detectable amount), precision (coefficient of variation at a given concentration), and evaluation (recovery, linearity of standard curves) for a number of the commonly prescribed phenothiazines. Most of the methods described have adequate sensitivity and precision for routine monitoring programs. However, some published methods of analysis, although demonstrating adequate sensitivity and precision for plasma or serum standards, have not been applied to clinical studies or samples from patients. Table 1 indicates if a method has been applied clinically and so is a suitable routine method. The stationary phase of choice in published papers is 3% OV-17. However, SE-30 and OV-1 have been used successfully, while other stationary phases have not been fully exploited. Whelpton and Curry [70] used OV-255 and demonstrated good separation of chlorpromazine, diazepam, and N-desmethyldiazepam, two potential interfering substances with CPZ analysis, as diazepam is often administered concomitantly.

The extensive metabolism of the phenothiazines presents some problems for the analyst. Not all metabolites are separated by the one extraction process, and some metabolites are changed back to the parent drug during the extraction steps. This second problem is most important for studies which attempt to relate plasma concentrations to clinical effect. Any evaluation of analytical methods for phenothiazine determination should take this possibility into account. Curry [71] has reviewed these principles for chlorpromazine analysis. Despite the long list of GLC methods for the phenothiazines, Curry's method [72] remains the most often used in clinical studies of chlorpromazine and is readily adaptable to the other phenothiazines [7,73].

Table 1 Gas Chromatographic Analysis of Phenothiazines

Biological specimen	Stationary phase	Precision, specificity, and evaluation	Detector	Comments	Reference
		Chlorpromazine			
None	3% SE-30	–	FID	Conversion of CPZSO to CPZ for identification	[75]
Blood	3% Versamid 1.5% Versilube	Not used for quantitation	ECD	Applied to patient samples for identification	[76]
Blood	3% SE-33		Ni^{63} ECD	Preliminary report of *Anal. Chem.* paper [72]	[77]
Plasma	3% OV-17	Specificity ensured by extraction of blanks; sensitivity 10 ng/ml; CV = 6% at 200 ng/ml (n = 7)	Ni^{63} ECD	Applied to patient plasma CPZ; DMCPZ, CPZSO also determined	[72]
Plasma, Urine, Feces	3% OV-17	Duplicates agree to within ±5%	ECD	Application of Curry's [72] method to clinical trial	[74]
Nonhuman liver	3% OV-25	No evaluation of the method	FID	CPZ and its major metabolites studied	[78]
Plasma	3% OV-17	Linear standard curve in range 0–10 ng/ml; no precision studies	Ni^{63} ECD	2,4-Dichloropromazine used as internal standard	[79]
Brain	2.8% SE-30	No evaluation	ECD	Used GLC as proof that 7- and 8-OH-CPZ lodged in rat and monkey brain	[80]
Plasma	3% OV-17	No evaluation; modifications suggested by Flint et al. [79] included in method	Ni^{63} ECD	Application to inpatient samples of Curry's [72] method	[81]
Serum	3% OV-17	95% recovery of CPZ in extractions; linear standard curve 0–250 ng/ml; sensitivity of 400 pg/ml	Ni^{63} ECD	Modification of Curry's [72] method using trifluoperidol as internal standard; no application to patient samples	[82]

(continued)

Table 1 (continued)

Biological specimen	Stationary phase	Precision, specificity, and evaluation	Detector	Comments	Reference
		Chlorpromazine (continued)			
Serum	–	–	AFID	Note on artifacts in sera if glassware is not thoroughly cleaned	[83]
Plasma	4% XE-60	Specific assay; linear standard curve 0-500 ng/ml; 87% recovery of CPZ; no internal standard	Ni^{63} ECD	Applied to inpatient samples (n = 8) on a weekly basis	[84]
Plasma	–	85% recovery of CPZ; no internal standard	–	Slight modification of Curry's [72] method; application to patient samples	[85]
Blood	3% OV-17	Recovery CPZ 60-70%; reassessment of 1968 paper	Ni^{63} ECD	Benzodiazepines interfere with the analysis	[86]
Plasma	OV-225	No evaluation	–	Separation of CPZ, diazepam, and N-desmethyldiazepam	[70]
Plasma	3% OV-17	Conditions used as for CPZ analysis	Ni^{63} ECD	7-OH-CPZ determined as silylated derivative	[87]
Plasma, Urine	–	–	–	CPZNO and CPZSO determined	[88]
Plasma	3% OV-17	Review of GLC principles	ECD	No application to patient samples	[71]
Blood	3% OV-17	Investigation of a possible problem arising in CPZ analysis	Ni^{63} ECD	Dedimethyl CPZ determination; reaction of nor_1- and nor_2-CPZ with aldehydes and ketones to form GC stable imines	[95]

		Fluphenazine			
Urine	2% SE-30	Recovery FLU exceeded 100%; FLU-SO recovery 98%; sensitivity and precision not recorded	FID	Trimethylsilyl derivatives of drug used	[89]
Urine	3% OV-17	Minimum detectable amount 2 ng/ml	FID AFID	Comparison of FID and AFID; drugs determined as acetyl or TMS derivatives	[90]
Plasma	3% OV-17	Sensitivity 3 ng/ml; 80% recovery of FLU; r = 0.99 for standards; no precision studies	Ni^{63} ECD	Applied to patient samples; TMS derivatives formed	[7]
Plasma	3% SE-30	CV evaluated over the range 0.5-17 ng/ml was 31-8%; 1 ng/ml sensitivity	AFID	Applied to patient samples; Perphenazine internal standard; TMS derivatives formed	[91]
		Thioridazine			
Plasma	3% OV-17	Recovery 90-100%; sensitivity 0.2 μg/ml (FID); 0.05 μg/ml (argon); specificity assessed with blanks; no precision studies	FID Argon FID	Applied to patient samples	[73]
Serum	3% OV-17	Recovery 75%; linear response in range 0-0.5 μg/ml; CV = 6%, n = 20 at 1.03 μg/ml; CV = 9%, n = 15 at 0.29 μg/ml	FID	Applied to both inpatients and volunteers	[92]
Plasma	3% XE-60	Linear standard curves over 0-2 μg/ml; accuracy and recovery evaluated at 0.5 and 1.0 μg/ml	FID	Thioridazine, sulforidazine, mesoridazine and perazine evaluated; applied to patient samples	[93]
Plasma	3% OV-17	Recovery 40-80% for thioridazine and metabolites; sensitivity 50 ng/ml; CV = 8%	FID	Applied to patient samples	[94]

(continued)

Table 1 (continued)

Biological specimen	Stationary phase	Precision, specificity, and evaluation	Detector	Comments	Reference
		Thioridazine (continued)			
Blood Urine	3% OV-17	93% recovery; CV = 0.53%, n = 6; duplicates agree to within 15%	FID	Applied to patient samples; TFA derivatives used	[96]
		Perphenazine			
Blood	3% SE-52	Linear calibration over 0–40 ng/ml; specificity established; accuracy ±7%	ECD	Hepta fluorobutyrate ester prepared; limited application to patient samples	[97]
Blood	3% SE-32	Recovery 90-100%; detection limit 0.2 ng/ml	Ni^{63} ECD	Application to patient samples	[98]
Plasma	1% OV-17	Linear calibration 1-5 ng/ml; CV at 1 and 5 ng/ml of 5% and 2%; recovery 100%	ECD	Application to patient plasma; TMS derivatives formed; PPZ and PPZ-SO determined	[99]
		Methotrimeprazine			
Urine	5% OV-1 2% FFAP	Recovery 80-90%; trifluoperazine as internal standard; no precision studies	FID	Application to patient samples; acetate derivative formed	[100]
Plasma	3% OV-17	Sensitivity 2-3ng/ml; CV of 8-15% for concentrations between 10 and 100 ng/ml	FID	Applied to patient samples; sulfoxide metabolite also determined	[101]

		Promazine and Trifluoperazine			
Blood	3% OV-1	No details of precision or recovery	ECD	Bromination of compounds before chromatography	[102]
		Phenothiazines			
None	Various	No precision studies	FID	Information on the separation of drugs on various stationary phases	[103]
Urine	5% OV-1	Calibration data for perazine, trifluoperazine, prothipendyl, propericiazine	FID	Identification and quantitation in urine of patients receiving therapeutic doses	[104]

G. High-Performance Liquid Chromatographic Analysis

The principles and terminology of high-performance liquid chromatography (HPLC) have been described by Dixon et al. [105] and Knox [106]. As with GLC, HPLC is a separative and specific technique, but the quality of the separation depends both on the choice of the stationary and mobile phases. Detector selection is also of importance; however, the fixed- or variable-wavelength "UV detectors" appear to be satisfactory in drug analyses.

Relatively little application of the HPLC technique has been made for the determination of phenothiazines. Muusze and Huber [107] evaluated a number of liquid-liquid systems for the separation of thioridazine and its metabolites. A 254-nm-wavelength ultraviolet photometer was used as a detector. The method was not applied to patient samples. Further development using a fluorimetric detector allowed the method to be applied to plasma samples [108]. Rodgers [109] used HPLC for the separation and analysis of a range of phenothiazines in several pharmaceutical preparations. The method was not used to determine patient plasma samples. Ion pair partition chromatography has been compared with adsorption chromatography for a series of phenothiazines, adsorption chromatography being more selective [110]. The paper demonstrated the feasibility of HPLC for phenothiazine determination. Analyses of patient samples were not carried out.

A coulometric detector for HPLC, with a detection limit in the picogram range, has been described [111]. This detector was used by Tjaden et al. [112] for the determination of perphenazine and fluphenazine in plasma. The plasma was extracted into an organic phase, cleaned up by two back-extractions, and injected onto a column. Separation of the drug from internal standard was achieved using a reversed-phase system. A limited application of the method to patient plasma samples was made. The limit of detection of the method was less than 1 ng/ml, with a standard deviation of 7 and 16% at 8 ng/ml for perphenazine and fluphenazine, respectively. Metabolites of the drugs were not determined. Fluphenazine, perphenazine, trifluoperazine, chlorpromazine, and thioridazine were determined in serum on silica columns using methanol as the mobile phase [113]. A limit of detection of 0.1 mg/liter was claimed for the technique, but no other details were given.

Other methods for phenothiazine determination, based on HPLC, have been described [114,115] but have not been applied to plasma level measurement. HPLC is outpacing GLC as the method of choice for antidepressant determination in biological fluids and should in the future prove to be an efficient means of phenothiazine analysis.

H. Mass Fragmentographic Analysis

Gas chromatography-mass spectrometry combines the separative power of the gas chromatograph with the resolution of the mass spectrometer. The mass spectrometer can be operated in two modes, either as a monitor of the total number of ions eluting from the gas chromatograph with time (total ion chromatogram, TIC) or focusing on particular ions characteristic of the compound of interest (mass fragmentography). The latter mode is the most valuable technique for quantitation of drugs, while the former is valuable in drug metabolism studies. Hammar and co-workers [116] first introduced mass fragmentography and applied it to chlorpromazine determination. Since that time the technique has been applied to the determination of a range of psychotropic drugs.

A limit of detection of around 1 picogram of chlorpromazine was claimed for mass fragmentography [116]. No evaluation of the precision and accuracy of the method was carried out in this study. However, the paper did demonstrate the feasibility of the technique for routine analysis. Alfredsson et al. [117] have quantitated chlorpromazine and its metabolites nor_1-chlorpromazine and 7-hydroxychlorpromazine in plasma, cerebrospinal fluid (CSF), and tissues. Trideuterated derivatives of the compounds to be measured were used as the internal standards. Samples were extracted and chromatographed on 3% SP-2100. Chlorpromazine was determined from the ratio of the m/e values at 323 and 318. The settings for nor_1-CPZ and 7-OH-CPZ were m/e 405/400 and 406/409 respectively. Detection limits for the compounds were about 1 ng/ml in plasma and 0.2 ng/ml in CSF. The relative standard deviation was between 3 and 14% at 25 ng/ml of CPZ and nor_1-CPZ and 10% at 10 ng/ml of 7-OH-CPZ. Good linearity was achieved for each compound over the range of 0-150 ng/ml. Application of the method to plasma samples was made. This method is suitable for routine analysis of chlorpromazine levels.

Mass fragmentography has not been extensively applied to the study of the phenothiazines. Perhaps because of the complexity of their metabolism many workers have been daunted by the prospect of quantitation of the metabolites. Not all metabolites are biologically active, and the possibility of separation and quantitation of all active metabolites in a single assay makes mass fragmentography an important area of development for phenothiazine determination.

I. Interlaboratory Comparison of Assays

Most of the assay methods described for the phenothiazines have been applied to patient samples. However, in a sense, these methods are unproven since they have not been applied in other laboratories. The method of Curry [72] has proven to be the most widely applied for the determination of chlorpromazine and is adaptable to the determination of other phenothiazines. An attempt to establish quality control in chlorpromazine determination was carried out by Turner et al. [118].

Samples of calf plasma were spiked with high and low concentrations of chlorpromazine, chlorpromazine sulfoxide, nor_1-chlorpromazine, and nor_2-chlorpromazine and these were lyophilized and sent to seven different analysts.

Three analytical techniques were employed: gas chromatography, combined TLC fluorescence, and TLC. The results of the study established good agreement among all methods and the spiked value for high and low chlorpromazine concentration. However, simple TLC methods gave consistently low values compared to the spike concentration and GLC or fluorescence methods. Metabolite values gave poorer results, especially in the high spiked concentrations. Curry's method gave a CPZSO concentration about twice that of the true spike concentration. There is no obvious explanation for this result. Only one method, that of Kaul (fluorescence) [119] gave values consistent with the spike concentration for both high and low concentrations. It should be noted that in the high-spike nor_1-chlorpromazine all other methods, except for Kaul, gave a consistent value of about 90 ng/ml. This may be the result of sample decomposition.

The results of the multilaboratory comparison, while they do not give perfect agreement, illustrate the comparability of results for chlorpromazine analysis. The study points up the need for standardized methods of analysis and the availability of guaranteed quality control standards for psychotropic drugs. When such standards are available, only then can full credence be given to plasma level-clinical effect relationships. For the present, however, the method of choice for phenothiazine determination is GLC with an electron capture detector.

II. OTHER ANTIPSYCHOTIC DRUGS

A. Butyrophenones

The butyrophenones are a group of drugs chemically distinct from the phenothiazines but equally as effective in the treatment of schizophrenia. Haloperidol is the best-known member of this class and the most extensively investigated. Other butyrophenones are either without antipsychotic activity or have not been as thoroughly investigated.

Metabolism of haloperidol occurs by oxidative dealkylation in the liver, forming fluorocarbonic acids [120]. Subsequently this metabolic pathway has been confirmed in man [121]. Haloperidol has no active metabolites, and analytical methods are required which are specific only for the parent drug. Methods based on colorimetry or TLC, while they are suitable for examining dosage forms of the drug, are not suitable for determination of blood levels of the drug following administration of the therapeutic doses [122,123]. Methods based on gas chromatography or radioimmunoassay have adequate sensitivity and specificity for routine plasma level determinations.

Zingales [124] reported a gas chromatographic method for haloperidol using an electron capture detector and 2% OV-1 as the stationary phase. The drug was extracted from plasma or urine into an organic solvent, back-extracted in acid, and then extracted into an organic phase before injection onto the column. Haloperidol recovery by this method was greater than 85% in the range 5-50 ng/ml. A linear detector response was obtained in the 5-500-ng range. Tricyclic antidepressants, 1-4-benzodiazepines, and phenothiazines except for chlorpromazine did not interfere with the determination. The method was used to determine patient samples, but no precision studies were carried out.

A method based on electron capture detection using OV-17 as a stationary phase was described and applied to seven butyrophenones including haloperidol, trifluperidol, and penfluridol [125]. An extraction method similar to that described by Zingales [124] was evaluated and used in the quantitation of haloperidol and trifluperidol, using 2-N-benzylamino-5-chlorobenzophenone as an internal standard. Linear calibration curves were obtained in the range 1-10 ng for haloperidol and 0.5-5 ng for trifluperidol. Recoveries for both drugs were between 70 and 90% from blood and tissues. The method proved satisfactory for animal studies, but when applied to patient studies the sensitivity was only 20 ng/ml. No haloperidol was detected in the plasma of 10 patients receiving 4 mg orally or in 3 patients receiving 4 mg intramuscularly. For patients receiving higher oral doses (up to 9 mg/day) for extended periods of time the method had adequate sensitivity.

A gas chromatographic method for the determination of haloperidol suitable for both pharmacokinetic studies and routine monitoring has also been described [126]. Haloperidol was extracted from alkalinized plasma into heptane, then back-extracted into sulfuric acid. A final extraction into heptane ensured a chromatographically clean extract. A Ni^{63} electron capture detector (ECD) was used for the analysis and either 0.3% Versamid or 0.6% OV-17 were suitable stationary phases. Quantitation was achieved using chloro-substituted haloperidol (HAC) as the internal standard. Recovery of haloperidol was 71% and remained constant in the 0.5-20-ng/ml range. A linear standard curve was found for this concentration range. Precision of the assay was assessed with standards, the coefficient of variation lying between 2 and 6% in the concentration range 2-10 ng/ml. Duplicate analyses of patient samples in the range 0.5-9.5 ng/ml did not vary more than ±8%. Of several drugs assessed, only thioridazine and dibenzepin gave interferences with the determinations. The method is precise and specific and is readily applicable to routine monitoring. It has sufficient sensitivity to be applicable to pharmacokinetic studies. Haloperidol, droperidol, and penfluridol have also been determined gas chromatographically after Hofmann degradation of the drug [127].

Radioimmunoassay has also been used for haloperidol determination [128]. An antibody was raised in rabbits against a haloperidol-hydrazone-BSA conjugate. Cross-reactivity of the antiserum to haloperidol metabolites and other antipsychotic drugs, including chlorpromazine, thioridazine, and droperidol, showed the antibody to be specific for the drug. The sensitivity of the assay was 0.01 ng.

Triplicate measurements on six patient samples within the concentration range 6-245 ng/ml gave an intra- and interassay variability of around 7%. This assay is specific and has sufficient sensitivity to be used in clinical studies. It has an added advantage in that patient samples do not need to be extracted from plasma or serum. As with other radioimmunoassays, the production of the antiserum is the critical factor in assay development.

Butyrophenone analysis is most easily accomplished using specific radioimmunoassays, but for laboratories without access to liquid scintillation counters, the electron capture gas chromatograph provides an equally specific and precise assay.

B. Thioxanthenes

Derivatives of thioxanthene are effective antipsychotic agents but are not as widely used as either the phenothiazines or butyrophenones. Fewer analytical techniques have been reported for this group than for some others. Early gas chromatographic systems for toxicological identification of drugs included chlorprothixene and thiothixene among the compounds studied [103,129]. This work was not used for quantitation of biological samples.

An ultraviolet spectrophotometric method for the determination of chlorprothixene has been described [130]. The absorbance of the drug is measured after extraction and oxidation with alkaline potassium permanganate. Metabolites as well as the parent compound are determined in this nonspecific assay. The method has been applied to urinary determinations of total chlorprothixene in man after single 50-mg oral doses. The sensitivity of this method and of an earlier fluorimetric procedure [131] make them unsuitable for routine plasma level monitoring. The inclusion of a thin-layer chromatography step gave good specificity to a chlorprothixene assay [132]. The metabolites chlorprothixene sulfoxide, N-monodemethylchlorprothixene, and N-monodemethylchlorprothixene sulfoxide were determined separately from chlorprothixene from their ultraviolet absorbances at 230 nm. Only autopsy samples were assessed, and the sensitivity of the method did not allow blood levels to be determined.

A modification of Pacha's [29] method for the fluorimetric estimation of phenothiazines has been described for thioxanthene estimations [133]. After extraction of the drug and metabolites into heptane from alkalinized plasma, they are back-extracted into sulfuric acid. A further extraction into pH-5.5 acetate buffer was performed and the compounds oxidized with potassium permanganate. The fluorescence of the oxidized drug was determined at 440 nm after excitation at 310 nm. Recovery of the drug varied from 70 to 100% and the sensitivity was 3 ng/ml for extracted plasma. Linear fluorescence was observed up to 500 ng/ml. Only the N-demethyl metabolite interfered with the determination. No precision studies were carried out, but the method was applied to single-dose studies in volunteers and to clinical studies on inpatients [134]. The same method can be used for the determination of chlorprothixene, clopenthixol, and flupenthixol by a change of excitation and fluorescence wavelengths and modification of the pH [133].

A mass fragmentographic analysis of thiothixene was used to evaluate the pharmacokinetics of this drug in man [135]. An internal standard (trideuterothiothixene) was added to the plasma samples prior to extraction with dicthyl ether after alkalinization. The organic phase was evaporated and reconstituted in methanolic acetic acid and 50 μl aliquots injected into the GC-MS. The stationary phase was 1% Pentasil TM-350. Ions at m/e 113 and 116 from thiothixene and trideuterothiothixene were used to accomplish the quantitation. The sensitivity of the assay was 1 ng/ml and the accuracy of the method was 93 ± 8% of added values in the concentration range 1-30 ng/ml. No precision studies were carried out.

Thiothixene has also been determined by high-performance liquid chromatography [136]. Liquid-solid chromatography was used with Corasil II as the stationary phase and a mixture of ethanolamine, water, and methanol as the mobile phase. Quantitation was achieved by comparison of the peak area of thiothixene to that of the internal standard N-1-naphthylethylenediamine. This method has not been applied to patient samples, but the high recoveries (95%) and the excellent precision (3%) suggest that it is a feasible proposition.

A sensitive radioimmunoassay has been developed for the determination of flupenthixol concentrations in human plasma [137]. Antibodies for the assay were raised in sheep against ovalbumin coupled to 7-carboxyflupenthixol by the carbodiimide reaction. The sensitivity of the assay, with [^{3}H] flupenthixol as tracer, was 2 ng/ml in a 100-μl plasma sample. The intraassay coefficient of variation was 7%, and the interassay coefficient of variation was 10%. Recovery was greater than 90%. The antiserum showed no cross-reactivity with tricyclic drugs, and the major metabolites of flupenthixol (sulfoxide and Lu 5-051) showed low interferences. Plasma concentrations after single oral and multiple intramuscular injections were measured with the assay. This assay allows for rapid, sensitive, and precise determination of flupenthixol in human plasma, without the necessity of extraction of the samples.

Specific, sensitive, and precise thioxanthene assay is best carried out using mass fragmentography. The development of specific antibodies to the thioxanthenes and their metabolites will allow radioimmunoassay to play a bigger role.

ANTIANXIETY AGENTS

A diverse group of substances have been used as specific antianxiety agents, including benzodiazepines, propanediols, antihistamines, barbiturates, and occasionally tricyclic antidepressants. Meprobamate was one of the first popular agents used in the treatment of anxiety. With the advent of the benzodiazepines, meprobamate has been replaced as a treatment modality. The benzodiazepines with relatively short biological half-lives and a wide therapeutic index are the most widely prescribed of the antianxiety agents. Because of their widespread usage in clinical practice and the large literature concerning their measurement, the emphasis in this section will be placed on the benzodiazepines, and a brief mention made of some of the other agents. The methodology for the determination of the benzodiazepines has been extensively reviewed [138-140].

III. BENZODIAZEPINES

The structural relationships between the various benzodiazepines are outlined in Fig. 2. Most of the benzodiazepines undergo extensive metabolism in humans, giving rise to a number of metabolites, which are themselves pharmacologically active. Quantitation becomes not only a matter of the measurement of the parent drug but also of the measurement of active metabolites. Techniques possessing high specificity are required both for the determination of clinical pharmacokinetics and studies relating plasma levels and clinical response. The first step in the determination of any drug is its extraction from the biological matrix (most often blood plasma, but sometimes cerebrospinal fluid or whole blood) in which it occurs. Such methods are described in the next section.

A. Extraction from Biological Specimens

Several methods have been used for the extraction of benzodiazepines prior to determination. The pH of the extraction medium is important in influencing the behavior of the benzodiazepines, which all have an acidic pK_1. Generally it has been found that at a pH between 8 and 10 the benzodiazepines are readily extracted from biological media into an organic solvent [141-144]. Most organic solvents would appear to be suitable, but diethyl ether, dichloroethane, ethyl acetate, and n-heptane have been the preferred solvents. Further extraction from the organic phase into acid and then back-extraction into the organic phase may be required, particularly if the sample is to be used for gas chromatography. Often this method does not extract all the metabolites.

Extraction of drugs using XAD-2 resins has been described [145-148] and evaluated for certain psychotropic drugs [149]. Drugs can be extracted from blood, serum, and urine samples after the pH of the medium has been adjusted to between 7 and 8. The drugs are adsorbed onto the column by hydrophobic bonding and dipole-dipole interactions and can be desorbed by washing with an organic solvent. An additional extraction step may be necessary, as some en-

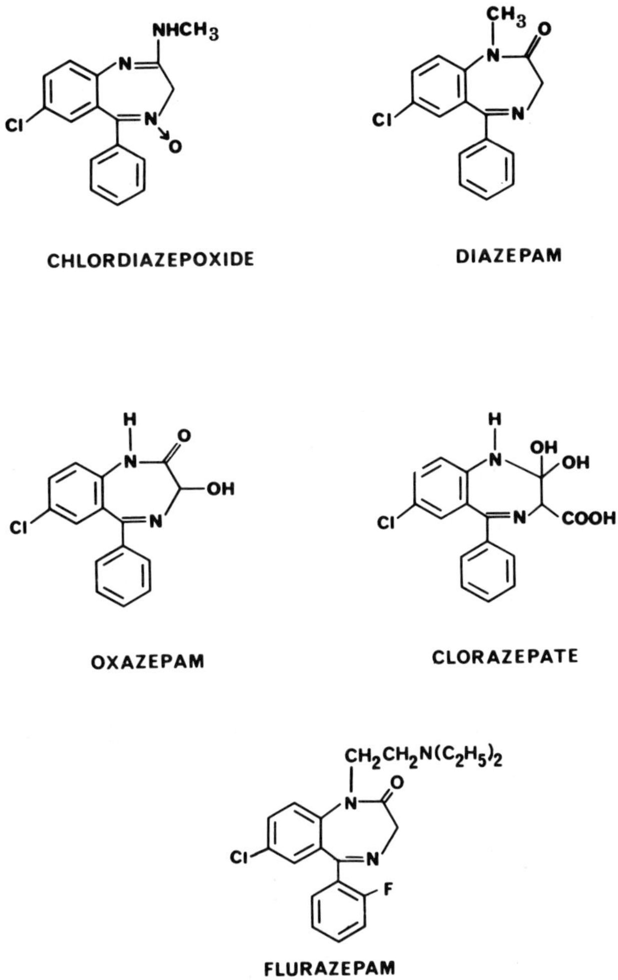

Figure 2 Structures of some benzodiazepines.

dogenous components of the matrix can be eluted from the column as well. Extraction of benzodiazepines from urine using this method has been described [150]. Charcoal and ion-exchange resins have had limited application to the isolation of drugs from biological media [151,152]. Column chromatography as an extraction procedure provides a rapid means of sample cleanup prior to the determination of drugs. Quantitation requires that the technique gives reproducible recoveries. This may not always be achieved.

A third technique for drug extraction is a combination of solvent extraction and salting out. Basic drugs can be extracted into alcohol from urine saturated with potassium carbonate [153]. Greater than 90% recovery of diazepam and chlordiazepoxide at concentrations of 100 μg/ml and 200 μg/ml respectively were obtained. Similar procedures using ammonium carbonate-ethyl acetate were developed for plasma samples [154]. A high recovery of diazepam was achieved. Methylene chloride, benzene, chloroform, and isopropanol were also evaluated, but the recoveries were generally lower. This technique provides a rapid and quantitative method of recovery.

B. Spectrophotometric Analysis

Three separate techniques of analysis based on the absorption of light by a drug can be distinguished: ultraviolet spectrometry, colorimetry, and fluorimetry. The molar absorption coefficients of the benzodiazepines are all of the order of 10^4 liters/mol-cm [155]. Plasma chlordiazepoxide levels were measured after extraction of the drug into chloroform and then back-extraction in hydrochloric acid. Quantitation was achieved from the absorbance of the drug at 247 nm. A recovery of 84% was achieved with a sensitivity of 2.0 μg/ml. The precision, expressed as the coefficient of variation, at 17 μg/ml was 3% [156]. Similar methods for nitrazepam [157] and chlordiazepoxide [158] determination, with comparable sensitivity and precision, have been reported for blood and urine. Oxazepam was an interfering substance in these determinations. Ultraviolet spectrometry is not a useful method for the routine measurement of benzodiazepines in plasma samples. Such a technique is nonspecific, providing a total drug analysis. This specificity problem is further compounded by the use of an acid back-extraction technique, which probably results in hydrolysis of parent drug and metabolite to their respective benzophenones.

Colorimetric procedures for benzodiazepine measurement have been based on the Bratton-Marshall reaction [159]. After extraction, the drug is hydrolyzed to an aromatic amine, diazotized and coupled to N-(1-naphthyl)ethylenediamine. The resultant colored dye is read at 550 nm. This method has been used to measure chlordiazepoxide concentrations in plasma [160,161]. A similar technique has been used for the determination of chlordiazepoxide, nitrazepam, and oxazepam in urine [162] and for chlordiazepoxide and medazepam in blood [163]. Evaluation of the precision and recovery of the method has been carried out for blood samples [164]. Beer's law was obeyed up to 40 μg/ml of chlordiazepoxide, and the extraction method used gave 100% recovery. The precision at 10 μg/ml was 7% based on 40 determinations. The method was applicable to oxazepam determination. Of the drugs tested only sulfanilamide and procainamide gave interferences. Barbiturates and phenothiazines did not interfere. Recent colorimetric procedures have been based on the oxidation-reduction reaction of diazepam, chlordiazepoxide, and nitrazepam with metal complexes, notably hexathiocyanato chromium (III) [165-167]. These colorimetric assays are nonspecific and lack the sensitivity required for routine plasma level determinations. They do provide a rapid means of identification in cases of overdose.

Assays based on fluorimetry provide the most sensitive optical methods for the determination of benzodiazepines. Under optimum conditions the sensitivity of this method is suitable for routine use in clinical applications. One of the earliest methods for chlordiazepoxide determination was based on its extraction from plasma and acid hydrolysis to the lactam [168]. The procedure is specific for the drug with a sensitivity of 0.25 μg/ml. Recovery from plasma was 73%. An excitation wavelength of 380 nm was used, and the fluorescence was measured at 480 nm. The method was applied to three patients who received a single oral dose of 30 mg of chlordiazepoxide. Precision studies were not carried out. Slight modification of the procedure allows for N-desmethylchlordiazepoxide determination as well [169]. Flurazepam and its metabolites were determined in blood and urine after extraction and hydrolysis to their respective benzophenones [170]. The hydrolysis product was further reacted with dimethyl formamide in potassium carbonate to give the 9-acridanone and the fluorescence intensity measured. A 50-70% recovery was obtained, with a sensitivity of 5-10 ng/ml claimed. Nitrazepam and its two metabolites, 7-amino- and 7-acetamidonitrazepam, were determined in human plasma with a sensitivity of 0.01 μg/ml [171]. Recovery of 80% or more for all three compounds was achieved and the fluorescence determined at 480 nm. Precision of the assay was 6% at 0.2 μg/ml. Conversion to the 9-acridanone has been used as a screening method for the detection of diazepam, chlordiazepoxide, oxazepam, clorazepate, and their major metabolites in blood or urine [172]. The method can be adapted for therapeutic levels. A modification of the fluorescence technique involves conjugation of the acid hydrolysis product of chlordiazepoxide to fluorescamine [173]. Application to clinical samples has not been extensive. The fluorescence technique has been widely applied for the determination of chlordiazepoxide, but has not found as wide an application for the other benzodiazepines.

Spectrophotometric analysis generally lacks the sensitivity of other analytical techniques, and specificity is also problematic. Many of the methods described for the benzodiazepines involve hydrolysis of the samples to a common benzophenone intermediate, and so provide a total benzodiazepine concentration. The inclusion of a chromatography step can provide greater specificity and sensitivity may also be improved.

C. Thin-Layer Chromatographic Analysis

Thin-layer chromatography (TLC) can be applied to quantitative problems in two forms. Once the chromatogram is developed individual spots can be located under ultraviolet light or with spray reagents, eluted, and quantitated with any suitable technique. Usually optical methods are employed, but GLC, GC-MS, or RIA may also be suitable. Alternatively, direct-scanning spectrodensitometry can be used. This technique has advantages over elution since recovery is likely to be higher and sensitivity is better.

TLC has found its greatest application in the separation and identification of the metabolites of the benzodiazepines. In combination with infrared, nuclear magnetic resonance, and mass spectroscopy, TLC can provide unequivocal identification of drug substances. The metabolism of several benzodiazepines has been studied in this manner [150,174-176]. TLC in combination with spray reagents has been used for the detection of impurities in pharmaceutical preparations of benzodiazepines [177] and for rapid detection in overdoses [178-184]. None of these methods has adequate sensitivity to be applied to routine plasma level measurement.

Medazepam was determined using combined TLC-spectrophotofluorimetry [185]. The minimum detectable level in plasma was 0.01-0.02 μg. Fluorescence was determined at 490 nm, after excitation at 360-370 nm. Application to patient samples was not assessed. Flurazepam and its metabolites were determined by direct-scanning spectrofluorodensitometry after hydrolysis and cyclization to their 9-acridanones [186]. Fluorescence was measured at 457 nm and a detection limit of 0.5-1.0 ng/ml based on a 4-ml plasma sample determined. The method was applied to patient samples, and its sensitivity and reproducibility make it suitable for use in routine measurement. A similar method has been used for the determination of flunitrazepam and its main metabolites in plasma [187]. Five solvent systems were evaluated for the separation of the parent compound and its three metabolites, and all proved adequate. After reduction with stannous chloride the compounds were reacted with fluorescamine to produce a fluorescent derivative. Linearity was achieved in the range 1-20 ng with a sensitivity of 1-2 ng/ml. Samples from two patients were determined by this method. Diazepam and its metabolites were determined after two-dimensional TLC and measurement of the diffuse reflectance of the chromatogram at 230 nm [188,189]. Recoveries for diazepam, N-desmethyldiazepam, 3-hydroxydiazepam, and oxazepam were greater than 90%. The coefficients of variation at 0.8 μg/ml of diazepam and 0.5 μg/ml of each of the metabolites was about 5-6%. The precision and sensitivity of the method are adequate for clinical studies. It has been applied to patients receiving diazepam for "status epilepticus." A sensitive method for the determination of chlordiazepoxide, diazepam, and the major metabolites in blood and serum based on spectrodensitometry has been described [190]. The method has been applied to patient samples, and the results showed good agreement with a radioimmunoassay. Chlordiazepoxide and its metabolites, demoxepam and N-desmethylchlordiazepoxide, were determined by fluorescence TLC-densitometry after extraction from serum with ether [191]. Adequate sensitivity for routine use was achieved. The same method was employed to measure diazepam and N-desmethyldiazepam levels in serum standards, but not patient samples [192]. The methods described have adequate sensitivity and precision for routine application, but have so far not been applied widely. A comprehensive review of TLC solvent systems and detection methods is presented elsewhere [140].

D. High-Performance Liquid Chromatographic Analysis

As with the phenothiazines, the relatively new technique of high-performance liquid chromatography (HPLC) has not been extensively applied to the determination of benzodiazepines. Liquid-solid chromatography was used to separate diazepam, its metabolites, and several other benzodiazepines [193]. A sensitivity of about 2 μg per compound was achieved, not sufficient for routine application. Ketazolam, an oxazolobenzodiazepine, was determined by HPLC with a sensitivity limit of 30 ng [194]. This compound is immediately pyrolyzed to diazepam at the temperature required for gas chromatography. HPLC represents the only practical method of analysis for ketazolam. Triflubazam and its metabolites were measured in blood and urine using adsorption chromatography on silica gel [195]. The detection limit was 50 ng/ml, and application to clinical samples was made. Bugge [196] employed a porous silica (Partisil) for the separation of diazepam and N-desmethyldiazepam after their extraction from blood. Recoveries of the drugs from standards were greater than 90%. A sensitivity of 100 ng/ml was determined for a 1-ml blood sample, greater sensitivity being possible with a larger sample. Nitrazepam [197] and flunitrazepam [198] have also been determined in urine or blood by HPLC. Unchanged benzodiazepines and their metabolites have been analyzed in tissue samples following enzymic digestion with subtilisin [199]. After filtering, the enzymic digests were extracted with diethyl ether, the ether evaporated, and the residues dissolved in ethanol and microliter amounts injected onto the column. Sensitivities of the order of 10 ng/g of liver were obtained. The method was applied to forensic samples. A well-evaluated method for the determination of diazepam, oxazepam, and N-desmethyldiazepam showed adequate sensitivity for routine application [200]. Prazepam was added as an internal standard, and the interassay precision (coefficient of variation) was 3-10%. A reversed-phase system using acetonitrile-sodium acetate buffer as the mobile phase was employed. A similar reversed-phase system, using methanol-water as the mobile phase, was used for diazepam, N-desmethyldiazepam determination [201]. The limit of detection for diazepam was 4 ng/ml and for N-desmethyldiazepam was 2 ng/ml. The method has been applied to pharmacokinetic and steady-state data in patients receiving therapy with diazepam.

Although not extensively applied to benzodiazepine analysis, HPLC is well suited to the problem. It offers the advantage of less tedious extraction procedures and can be carried out at ambient temperatures, an important consideration for this class of compound, since thermal rearrangement can produce misleading analyses.

E. Gas-Liquid Chromatographic Analysis

The most widely used method of benzodiazepine analysis is gas-liquid chromatography (GLC). Conservatively, over 100 methods for the benzodiazepines have been published. Not all of these methods are applicable to blood or plasma samples, and those that are have not always been evaluated for routine use. Gas chromatographic methods and their associated problems have been reviewed [138,202]. The benzodiazepines have been determined, after extraction, as the unchanged drugs, as derivatives, or as their benzophenones after acid hydrolysis. Some of the GLC methods used are summarized in Table 2 with their respective precision and reproducibility.

Electron capture detectors have found a wide application for benzodiazepine analysis, as has the flame ionization detector. The nitrogen-phosphorus detector has not been as widely used as the other two. A variety of stationary phases have been used, with apparently little to choose between 3% OV-17, 2% XE-60, 3% OV-25, 3% OV-225, and 2% Carbowax. All of these phases give an adequate separation of the drugs and their metabolites within a reasonable on-column analysis time.

GLC techniques which are based on the acid hydrolysis to the corresponding benzophenone can lead to a total benzodiazepine analysis, as some drugs and their major metabolites give rise to the same product. Chlordiazepoxide and desmethylchlordiazepoxide are both hydrolyzed to 2-amino-5-chlorobenzophenone; diazepam and 3-hydroxydiazepam are hydrolyzed to 2-methylamino-5-chlorobenzophenone [138]. A complication in the analysis of some benzodiazepines is that they are thermally unstable, and at the temperatures required for gas chromatography they may be decomposed on the column. Oxazepam is readily dehydrated on the column to form 6-chloro-4-phenylquinazoline-2-carboxaldehyde [203]; 3-hydroxydiazepam gave smaller-than-expected retention times in some systems, suggesting a partial decomposition [138]. N-oxide derivatives may also be decomposed on GLC columns [203]. Despite these problems, GLC remains the analytical mainstay for benzodiazepines. It is sensitive, specific, reliable, and readily applied to most biological fluids. Its major disadvantage is the time taken for an analysis to be performed. For clinical research studies this may not be as important as sensitivity and precision.

F. Mass Fragmentographic Analysis

There have been few applications of the combined gas chromatography-mass spectrometry technique to benzodiazepine quantitation. Mostly GC-MS has been used to establish metabolic profiles of the benzodiazepines, for the identification

Table 2 Gas Chromatographic Analysis of Some Benzodiazepines

Drug(s)	Stationary phase	Precision, sensitivity, and evaluation	Detector	Remarks	Reference
Diazepam	3% OV-17	Linear standard curve over 0-1 μg/ml for diazepam and N-desmethyldiazepam; no other evaluation	Ni^{63} ECD	Method applied to pharmacokinetic study of diazepam in 7 patients; both drugs determined without prior hydrolysis	[204]
Diazepam	3% OV-225	Linear standard curves 0-1 μg/ml for oxazepam; N-desmethyldiazepam and 3-OH-diazepam; diazepam gave nonlinear responses; sensitivity 0.02 μg/ml for each component	Ni^{63} ECD	Method not used for clinical samples; can be used for plasma or urine (2-ml samples); prazepam used as internal standard; simple extraction into ethylbenzoate and determination without hydrolysis	[205]
Diazepam	3% E-350	Recovery 90% for diazepam, oxazepam, N-desmethyldiazepam and hydroxydiazepam; duplicate determinations from patients gave SD of 8% diazepam, 10% for desmethyldiazepam; linear standards 0-1.2 μg/ml	Ni^{63} ECD	Method used in determining the bioavailability of two forms of diazepam in humans and rats; simple extraction into benzene before GC analysis. Chlordiazepoxide used as internal standard	[206]
Diazepam, Deskalkylflurazepam	3% OV-17	Quantitative recovery of diazepam, desmethyldiazepam, N-desalkylflurazepam; between- and within-run precision evaluated at 100, 250, and 500 ng/ml for diazepam (CV = 1-3%, n = 16) and for desmethyldiazepam (CV = 3-5%, n = 16)	ECD	Extraction from serum into toluene-heptane-isoamyl alcohol from a pH 9 phosphate buffer; medazepam used as internal standard; method applied to clinical samples but results not reported; no interferences from other psychotropic drugs found	[207]

(continued)

Table 2 (continued)

Drug(s)	Stationary phase	Precision, sensitivity, and evaluation	Detector	Remarks	Reference
Diazepam	3% OV-225	Quantitative recovery of diazepam (95%) and internal standard (prazepam: 98%); CV at 100 ng/ml was 6.5%; linear standard curve over the range 0-1 μg/ml; sensitivity of 2.5 ng/ml of diazepam	Ni^{63} ECD	A microsample (100 μl) of serum extracted into 5 ml of diethyl ether; ether separated and evaporated, reconstituted in 100 μl of ethanol and 2 μl aliquots injected onto column; no metabolites determined; no application to clinical samples	[208]
Diazepam	3% SE-30	Linear standard curve up to 4 μg/ml; recovery of drugs was quantitative; sensitivity 0.1 μg/ml	FID	Not applied to patient samples; suitable for toxicological analyses; O-aminobenzophenone used as internal standard; diazepam and N-desmethyldiazepam determined after acid hydrolysis to benzophenones	[209]
N-desmethyldiazepam	1% Poly–A–103	Sensitivity is 1 ng/ml; recovery greater than 70%; other benzodiazepines do not interfere with the analysis	Ni^{63} ECD	Three-stage extraction procedure used; N-desmethyltetrazepam as internal standard; applied in a study of chlorazepate pharmacokinetics	[210]
Diazepam, Desmethyldiazepam	3% OV-7	Quantitative recovery of drugs; specificity of assay checked; no precision studies; no sensitivity data for the assay	Ni^{63} ECD	Single extraction into n-butyl acetate; prazepam used as the internal standard; applied to clinical samples	[211]
Diazepam, Desmethyldiazepam	3% OV-17	Quantitative recovery; sensitivity 5 ng/ml and 10 ng/ml for diazepam and nordiazepam, respectively; no precision studies	Ni^{63} ECD	Single extraction into benzene; methylnitrazepam used as the internal standard; applied to chronic and single oral doses	[212]

Desmethyl-diazepam	–	Quantitative recovery of drug and internal standard; sensitivity 5 ng/ml; CV = 5% at 25 ng/ml (n = 72)	Ni^{63} ECD	Single extraction into benzene-isoamyl alcohol; diazepam as internal standard; used for a study of clorazepate pharmacokinetics	[213]
Desmethyl-diazepam	3% OV-17	Recovery 82% over 10-20 ng/ml; sensitivity 10 ng/ml; no precision studies; good agreement with an RIA	Ni^{63} ECD	Desmethyldiazepam identified in the plasma of patients receiving chlordiazepoxide; applied to patient samples	[214]
Nitrazepam	3% OV-17	Quantitative recovery of drug and internal standard (92%); SD = 5% over range 10-100 ng/ml; sensitivity 1 ng/ml	Ni^{63} ECD	Single extraction step; SCOT columns employed; applied to bioavailability and pharmacokinetic studies; clonazepam used as internal standard	[215]
Nitrazepam	3% OV-17	Recovery 95%; linear calibration in range 0-0.2 μg/ml; sensitivity 0.1 ng/ml; no evaluation	Ni^{63} ECD	Extraction from plasma into ether followed by two-step cleanup and acid hydrolysis of drug and clonazepam internal standard; applied to patient samples	[216]
Nitrazepam	3% OV-17	Quantitative recovery; sensitivity 5 ng/ml; SD between determinations on different days 13%	Ni^{63} ECD	Extraction from serum into benzene followed by acid hydrolysis and reextraction into benzene; desmethyldiazepam used as internal standard; used for clinical samples	[217]
Nitrazepam	–	Recovery 96%; linear calibration in range 0-200 ng/ml; precision assessed by comparison of detector response at 25 ng/ml	Ni^{63} ECD	Clonazepam, methylbromazepam, and methylnitrazepam used as internal standards; two extraction techniques—without and with hydrolysis—compared; no statistical differences observed; applied to patient samples	[218]

(continued)

Table 2 (continued)

Drug(s)	Stationary phase	Precision, sensitivity, and evaluarion	Detector	Remarks	Reference
Bromazepam	3% OV-225	Sensitivity 5 ng/ml; no precision studies; linear calibration over range 0-100 ng/ml; 3% OV-17 gave inadequate separation of hydrolysis products	Ni^{63} ECD	Extraction from plasma into ether followed by hydrolysis and cleanup; methylbromazepam used as internal standard; not applied to clinical samples	[219]
Bromazepam	3% OV-17	Recovery 85%; sensitivity 5-10 ng/ml; no other evaluation	Ni^{63} ECD	Single extraction into ether after protein precipitation; methylbromazepam used as internal standard; applied to patient samples; 3-OH metabolite not detectable in blood of chronically treated patients	[220]
Chlordiazepoxide	2% OV-17	Sensitivity 0.5 ng/ml; recovery 90% over range 0.03-10 μg/ml	ECD	Single extraction from plasma into heptane; no internal standard used; applied to patient samples; other psychotropic drugs do not interfere with the method	[221]
Oxazepam	3% OV-225	Sensitivity 1 ng/ml; recovery 98%; method cross-validated with different GC method; no precision studies	Ni^{63} ECD	Drug extracted into an organic solvent and alkylated; lorazepam used as internal standard; method specific for oxazepam; applied to pharmacokinetic analysis	[222]
Oxazepam	2% XE-60	Sensitivity of 20 ng/ml; recovery of 50-60%; no precision studies	Ni^{63} ECD	Extraction of the drug from plasma into ether followed by hydrolysis and cleanup; no internal standard; possible specificity problem if more than one benzodiazepine administered; applied to patient samples	[223]

Medazepam, Diazepam, Nitrazepam	1% OV-17	Recovery of drugs 75%; interassay precision CV = 5% at 500 ng/ml for medazepam, CV = 6% at 200 ng/ml for diazepam, CV = 9% at 400 ng/ml for nitrazepam	FID	Medazepam and diazepam analyzed intact after extraction using nitrazepam TMS derivative as internal standard; medazepam could be used as internal standard for determining the other two drugs; applied to therapeutic and overdose situations	[224]
Medazepam	3% OV-225	Linear calibration over range 0.005-2.0 μg/ml; no other evaluation	Ni^{63} ECD	Three-step extraction without hydrolysis; prazepam used as internal standard; applied to plasma samples	[225]
Medazepam	3% OV-225	No evaluation of the method	Electrolytic Conductivity	Single extraction into ether; no clinical samples; medazepam, desmethylmedazepam, diazepam, and desmethyldiazepam all determined intact	[226]
Medazepam, Diazepam	3% OV-17	Sensitivity 20 ng/ml	Electrolytic Conductivity	Three-step extraction; medazepam, desmethylmedazepam, diazepam, desmethyl diazepam all determined; detailed evaluation of detector characteristics	[227]
Medazepam, Diazepam	3% OV-17	Sensitivity 40-50 ng for 1-ml plasma; recovery medazepam 97%, diazepam 86%, desmethyldiazepam 94%; no precision studies	Ni^{63} ECD	Three-step extraction procedure; no suitable internal standard because of the complex metabolism; diazepam and desmethyldiazepam the major metabolites in blood; applied to patient samples	[144]
Flurazepam	3% QF-1	Sensitivity 5-10 ng/ml; no other evaluation	Ni^{63} ECD	Drug extracted from plasma into ether, then purified by extraction into acid and back-extraction into ether; diazepam used as internal standard; applied to patient samples	[228]

(continued)

Table 2 (continued)

Drug(s)	Stationary phase	Precision, sensitivity, and evaluation	Detector	Remarks	Reference
Clorazepate, Desmethyl-diazepam	3% OV-17	Sensitivity for clorazepate and desmethyldiazepam 4 ng/ml; recovery of clorazepate 60%, of desmethyldiazepam 95%	Ni^{63} ECD	Single extraction into benzene-methylene chloride; griseofulvin used as the internal standard; applied to patient samples	[229]
Clorazepate	3% Poly-A-103	Linear calibration over range 0–1 μg/ml; sensitivity 0.01 μg/ml; CV = 4% at 0.15 μg/ml (n = 8)	Ni^{63} ECD	Extraction and hydrolysis followed by cleanup; diazepam used as internal standard; used in a study in dogs; clorazepate determined by subtraction of the immediately determined desmethyldiazepam level from those obtained after overnight hydrolysis of plasma; method not specific if oxazepam present	[230]
Flunitrazepam, Desmethyl-flunitrazepam	3% OV-225	Sensitivity 0.5 ng/ml; linear calibration in range 0–15 ng/ml; no evaluation	Ni^{63} ECD	Extraction from plasma into ether followed by hydrolysis and cleanup; methylclonazepam used as internal standard; applied to patient pharmacokinetics	[231]
Flunitrazepam, Desmethyl-flunitrazepam	8% SE-30	Recovery flunitrazepam 99%, desmethylflunitrazepam 99%; sensitivity 1 ng/ml; no evaluation	Ni^{63} ECD	Single extraction from serum into benzene; lorazepam or flurazepam used as internal standard; applied to patient samples	[232]
Lorazepam	3% OV-17	Linear calibration 0-125 ng/ml; 10-15% SD for duplicates; sensitivity 20 ng/ml	Ni^{63} ECD	Single extraction from plasma into benzene; flurazepam used as internal standard; applied to clinical samples	[233]

Lorazepam	3% OV-1	Recovery 86%; sensitivity 0.01 μg/ml; linear calibration 0.01–0.8 μg/ml; no precision studies	H^3Sc ECD	Plasma extracted twice with ethylacetate; extracts combined, evaporated, and reconstituted in toluene; applied to overdose and therapeutic levels; griseofulvin internal standard	[234]
Pinazepam	3% OV-17	Linear calibration 5–40 ng/ml; recovery; pinazepam 77%; desmethyldiazepam, oxazepam, hydroxypinazepam, 90%; CV = 5% at 5 ng/ml for pinazepam, CV = 3–4% at 25 ng/ml for metabolites	Ni^{63} ECD	Pinazepam and metabolites determined intact; lorazepam used as internal standard; measured in patient plasma, urine, and milk	[235]
Benzodiazepines	3% OV-17	Recovery 85% for drugs and metabolites; sensitivity 1–10 ng/ml diazepam, bromazepam, clonazepam, flunitrazepam, and metabolites; no other evaluation	Ni^{63} ECD	Three-step extraction with or without hydrolysis; extraction procedure modified for 1-ml samples. applied to patient samples; specific for parent drug and metabolite if drug is administered alone	[236]
Benzodiazepines	3% OV-1	Recovery of several benzodiazepines from rat blood determined as 90% diazepam, 100% desmethyldiazepam, 65% N-methyloxazepam, 63% oxazepam, 87% nitrazepam; no evaluation	FID	Single extraction step into organic phase; drugs determined intact; 2-N-benzylamino-5-chlorobenzophenone used as internal standard; no application to patient samples	[237]
Benzodiazepines	2% OV-17	Linear standard curve 0.2–2.0 μg/ml, CV = 5–20% at 1 μg/ml for oxazepam, diazepam, nordiazepam, chlordiazepoxide, flurazepam, desalkylflurazepam; recoveries quantitative	FID	Three-step extraction; prazepam internal standard; useful for toxicological purposes	[238]

of the drugs after overdose, and for investigations of the thermal stability of the compounds.

Forgione et al. [239] were the first to establish the utility of the GC-MS method for identification of a mixture of benzodiazepines. Using 3% OV-17 as a stationary phase, good separation of oxazepam, diazepam, N-desmethyldiazepam, N-methyloxazepam, and nitrazepam were achieved. Under similar conditions, with a similar stationary phase (1.5% OV-1), oxydiazepam and oxazepam were found to be thermally unstable [240]. In quantitative analysis this may not be important, but for qualitative studies it may lead to an incorrect identification.

The most extensive use of GC-MS has been in the study of benzodiazepine metabolism. Oxazepam and lorazepam glucuronides were positively identified by their mass spectra after extraction from urine [241]. An extensive investigation of flurazepam metabolites has been carried out using GC-MS [242]. Separation of the metabolites was achieved on a 3% OV-17 stationary phase after extraction from urine. Application to forensic analysis was described.

Oxazepam and lorazepam glucuronides were determined as their methyl- and trimethylsilyl esters in urine [243]. An internal standard was used with a linear calibration over the range from 50 ng/ml to 1 μg/ml. The specificity of the method was established using blank samples. The method was applied to both animal and human studies, but so far has not been widely applied to clinical studies. In a study of the determination of pinazepam and its metabolites in serum, mass spectrometry was used to establish the identity of the peaks eluting from the gas chromatograph [244]. Multiple ion detection (MID) was used to study blood and urine concentrations of benzodiazepine esters in pharmacokinetic studies [245]. In particular, pivoxazepam, the pivalic ester of oxazepam, was determined using both MID and Ni^{63} ECD and a 3% OV-17 stationary phase to accomplish the separation. MID was 10 times as sensitive as ECD, and at 5-10 ng/ml of pivoxazepam the confidence limit was ±10%.

Mass fragmentographic analysis of the benzodiazepines has not been applied to quantitative studies in clinical trials or in a routine monitoring capacity. The increased sensitivity of this form of analysis compared with the others described is probably unnecessary in most clinical situations. Gas chromatography with conventional EC detectors has proven more than adequate for routine monitoring. Mass fragmentography may be required for accurate quantitation of the levels achieved during pharmacokinetic studies.

G. Radioimmunoassay

The potential of radioimmunoassay (RIA) for benzodiazepine quantitation has been recognized. Two reports have focused on diazepam and chlordiazepoxide determination. Peskar and Spector [246] described the production of two antibodies against diazepam analogues. One formed by diazo coupling of 5-3-(4-aminophenylazo)-4-hydroxyphenyl-7-chloro-1,3-dihydro-1-methyl-2,H-1,4-benzodiazepine-2-one to bovine serum albumin and immunization of rabbits was specific for diazepam, with only oxydiazepam showing a slight cross-reaction. The second antiserum, raised against a slightly different benzodiazepine, showed almost equal affinity for diazepam and N-desmethyldiazepam. Use of both antisera would give parent drug and metabolite levels. The sensitivity of the assay was 1 ng/ml of blood. Neither drug nor metabolite were determined directly, but were extracted from blood with diethylether. The assay was used to measure blood samples taken from two volunteers after intravenous and oral administration of 10 mg of diazepam, and the results compared with a Ni^{63} ECD gas chromatographic method. Good agreement was found between the two assays. The specificity of the assay was assessed, and neither antibody gave a cross-reaction with oxazepam, medazepam, N-desmethylmedazepam, chlordiazepoxide, or demoxepam.

Gelbke et al. [247] used the RIA developed by Peskar and Spector in a screening program for the identification of diazepam. The assay was more thoroughly evaluated and also compared with a gas chromatographic method. The sensitivity of the assay was 5 ng/ml with a precision (coefficient of variation) between 5 and 12% in the range 10-160 ng/ml. Intraassay precision was 12% at 25 ng/ml and 8% at 69 ng/ml. Only 3-hydroxydiazepam (temazepam) exhibited any significant cross-reaction with the antiserum. A comparison of 219 samples by GC and RIA gave a good correlation between the two methods (correlation coefficient 0.98; slope 1.06). The RIA provides a rapid, specific, and sensitive assay for diazepam.

Chlordiazepoxide has also been determined by RIA [248]. In this case the antiserum was raised by immunization of rabbits against an immunogen produced by diazo coupling of 7-chloro-5-(4-hydrazinocarbonylmethoxyphenyl)-2-methylamino-3H-1,4-benzodiazepine-4-oxide to bovine serum albumin. The antiserum is specific for chlordiazepoxide, no cross-reaction occurring with N-desmethylchlordiazepoxide, demoxepam, N-desmethyldiazepam, diazepam, and clonazepam. A sensitivity of 20 ng/ml was assessed for a 0.1-ml plasma sample. Greater sensitivity could be achieved with a larger sample. An advantage of this assay is that prior extraction of plasma samples is not required. Precision of the assay, expressed as the coefficient of variation, was 4% over the range 20-1000 ng/ml, and triplicate assays agreed to within ±0.07 μg/ml over the range 0.22-1.35 μg/ml. The method was applied to single- and chronic-dose studies, and the results compared with those obtained by spectrofluorimetry. The results were subjected to a linear regression analysis, and the intercept and slope were not significantly different from 0 and 1 at the 0.05 level.

Radioimmunoassay, while proving itself to be sensitive, precise, and specific and offering the advantage of a rapid determination of diazepam or chlordiazepoxide levels, has not been fully exploited in clinical studies. The production of a specific antiserum is a difficult and time-consuming task, but once achieved offers significant advantages over other analytical techniques.

H. Polarographic Analysis

The polarographic behavior of several benzodiazepines has been used as a means of analysis. Although the direct-current polarographic reduction waves have been extensively used for the assay of formulations, there are fewer applications to quantitation at therapeutic levels.

Oelschlager and colleagues [249,250] made an extensive study of the polarographic behavior of oxazepam and medazepam. Both drugs were reduced at a dropping mercury electrode in a single wave, wave height being linearly related to concentration, but also dependent on the pH. Sensitivity of the method was not sufficient for application to therapeutic levels.

Diazepam was determined in plasma by cathode-ray polarography after extraction from alkalinized plasma with petroleum spirit [251]. The organic phase was evaporated and the residues dissolved in hydrochloric acid. Sodium tetraborate was added as the supporting electrolyte and the drug quantitated from the peak height at -1.22 V versus the standard calomel electrode. Recovery of diazepam was 90% but with nordiazepam was about 20%. A sensitivity of 0.02 μg/ml was claimed for the method, with a linear calibration in the range 0-5 μg/ml. The method was applied to patient samples, but no precision studies were carried out.

Cyclic voltammetry and chronopotentiometry were used to determine nitrazepam in untreated serum [252]. Wave height was proportional to drug concentration in the range 2-50 μg/ml at $E_{1/2}$ = -0.51 V versus Ag/AgCl electrode. No application was made to patient samples, and the method does not have adequate sensitivity for routine use at therapeutic dosages.

Differential pulse polarography was used for diazepam determination in serum [253]. Serum samples were saturated with potassium chloride and extracted into benzene. The benzene was evaporated and the residue dissolved in sulfuric acid and the polarogram determined. Peak height at -0.6 V versus Ag/AgCl electrode was proportional to diazepam concentration in the range 0.05-1.0 μg/ml. The sensitivity was 0.01 μg/ml, and an error of 0.5-7.0% was found for diazepam samples in the range 0.05-2.3 μg/ml. As other benzodiazepines reduce at different half-wave potentials, specificity of the method was ensured. Determination of traces of chlordiazepoxide, other 1,4-benzodiazepines, and their metabolites has also been carried out using differential-pulse polarography [254,255]. Using this technique, a method suitable for toxicological quantitation of benzodiazepines in blood and plasma has been described [256]. The sensitivity of the method is 0.25-0.5 μg/ml. It serves as a screening procedure to determine total benzodiazepine concentration before more specific methods are applied.

A list of polarographic reduction potentials in various supporting electrolytes has been published [140]. The polarographic methods of analysis have not been fully exploited, but at this time they do not appear to have adequate sensitivity for routine determination of therapeutic levels of benzodiazepines.

IV. OVERVIEW

Modern developments in analytical techniques have made it possible to measure accurately and precisely the range of psychotropic drugs. Some of these methods have sufficient sensitivity to be applicable to the determination of plasma, blood, or CSF levels of these agents. Mass fragmentography is the most specific and sensitive method of drug analysis available, but its costs are almost prohibitive. Radioimmunoassay offers sensitivity and precision with a reduction in specificity. For routine monitoring of samples RIA is an ideal technique because direct analysis on plasma samples can be carried out. Gas-liquid chromatography with a nitrogen-specific detector also offers a specific and precise analytical technique, but the sensitivity may not be adequate in some determinations (e.g., for fluphenazine determinations after intramuscular injections). Other techniques lack general applicability, do not have adequate sensitivity, or their specificity is poor. The choice of analytical technique will most often depend on the techniques available within the laboratory conducting the study. All techniques need to be thoroughly investigated and analytical variables delineated before they are applied in clinical studies.

REFERENCES

1. G. Cimbura, Review of methods of analysis for phenothiazine drugs. *J. Chromatogr. Sci. 10:*287-293, 1972.
2. S. L. Tompsett, The phenothiazines. In *Progress In Chemical Toxicology,* vol. 5 (A. Stolman, ed.). New York, Academic Press, 1974, pp. 151-185.
3. A. A. Manian, J. Levine, D. Johnson, C. A. Rodriguez, and E. Usdin, Assay of chlorpromazine and some of its metabolites in urine samples. *Psychopharmacol. Bull. 6:*44-56, 1970.
4. L. R. Goldbaum and A. M. Dominguez, A system for the toxicological analysis of drugs in biological specimens. In *Progress In Chemical Toxicology,* vol. 5 (A. Stolman, ed.). New York, Academic Press, 1974, pp. 101-149.
5. R. Whelpton and S. H. Curry, Solvent extraction as applied to fluphenazine and its metabolites. In *Assay of Drugs and Other Trace Compounds*

In Biological Fluids (E. Reid, ed.). London, Longmans, 1975, pp. 115-120.

6. B. B. Brodie, S. Udenfriend, J. E. Baer, W. Dill, T. Chenkin, G. Downing, J. V. Taggert, and E. S. Josephson, The estimation of basic organic compounds in biological materials, I-VI. *J. Biol. Chem. 168:*299-344, 1947.
7. L. Rivera-Calimlim and A. Siracusa, Plasma assay of fluphenazine. *Commun. Psychopharmacol. 1:*233-242, 1977.
8. B. B. Brodie and S. Udenfriend, The estimation of basic orgainc compounds and a technique for the appraisal of specificity. *J. Biol. Chem. 158:*705, 1945.
9. F. M. Forrest and I. S. Forrest, A simple test for the detection of chlorpromazine in urine. *Amer. J. Psychiat. 113:*931-932, 1957.
10. F. M. Forrest, I. S. Forrest, and A. S. Mason, A rapid urinary test for chlorpromazine, promazine, and pacatal: A supplementary report. *Amer. J Psychiat. 114:*931-932, 1958.
11. I. S. Forrest and F. M. Forrest, Urine colour test for the detection of phenothiazine compounds. *Clin. Chem. 6:*362, 1960.
12. I. S. Forrest, F. M. Forrest, and A. S. Mason, A rapid urine colour test for thioridazine. *Amer. J. Psychiat. 116:*928-929, 1960.
13. F. M. Forrest, I. S. Forrest, and A. S. Mason, Review of rapid urine tests for phenothiazine and related drugs. *Amer. J. Psychiat. 118:*300-307, 1961.
14. I. S. Forrest, M. B. Wechsler, and J. Sperco, A comprehensive method for the determination of urinary chlorpromazine and its oxidative metabolites. *Amer. J. Psychiat. 120:*44, 1963.
15. I. S. Forrest, S. L. Kanter, J. E. Sperco, and M. Wechsler, A comprehensive determination of thioridazine and its metabolites in urine. *Amer. J. Psychiat. 121:*1049, 1965.
16. I. S. Forrest, A. G. Bolt, and M. T. Serra, Applejack concentration of urinary phenothiazine metabolites. *Proc. West. Pharmacol. Soc. 9:*24, 1966.
17. A. G. Bolt and I. S. Forrest, Assay of chlorpromazine glucuronides in human urine. *J. Pharm. Sci. 56:*1533, 1967.
18. A. G. Bolt, I. S. Forrest, and M. T. Serra, Quantitative studies of urinary excretion of chlorpromazine metabolites in chronically-dosed psychiatric patients. *J. Pharm. Sci. 55:*1205, 1966.
19. B. Gotheif and A. G. Karczmar, Quantitative colorimetric method and extraction procedure for determination of chlorpromazine in animal tissues. *Int. J. Neuropharmacol. 2:*95, 1963.
20. C. A. Hitzel, Method for the estimation of phenothiazine derivatives in urine and blood. *Clin. Chem. 7:*130, 1961.
21. P. Haux and S. Natelson, A practical method for the assay of phenothiaaines in biologic fluids. *Amer. J. Clin. Pathol. 53:*77, 1970.
22. J. E. March, D. Donato, P. Turano, and W. S. Turner, Interpatient variation and significance of plasma levels of chlorpromazine in psychotic patients. *J. Med.* (Basel) *3:*146, 1972.

23. L. Cavatorta, Assay of promazine and its separation from chlorpromazine and promethazine. *J. Pharm. Pharmacol. 11:*49, 1959.
24. B. M. Phillips, P. J. Kraus, and M. E. Stratmeyer, Spectrophotometric determination of a mixture of secondary and tertiary amines in urine. *J. Pharm. Sci. 54:*803, 1965.
25. J. E. Wallace and J. D. Biggs, Determination of phenothiazine compounds in biologic specimens by UV spectrophotometry. *J. Pharm. Sci. 60:*1346, 1971.
26. A. H. Afifi and E. L. Way, Estimation of methotrimeprazine in brain and correlation of brain levels with pharmacologic activity. *J. Pharm. Sci. 56:*720, 1967.
27. N. Salzman and B. B. Brodie, Physiological disposition and fate of chlorpromazine and a method for its estimation in biological material. *J. Pharmacol. Exp. Ther. 118:*46-54, 1956.
28. J. B. Ragland, V. J. Kinross-Wright, and R. S. Ragland, Determination of phenothiazines in biological samples. *Anal. Biochem. 12:*60-69, 1965.
29. W. L. Pacha, A method for the fluorimetric determination of thioridazine (Mellaril) or mesoridazine (Lidanil) in plasma. *Experientia 25:*103, 1969.
30. P. N. Kaul, M. W. Conway, and M. L. Clark, Sensitive quantitative determination of chlorpromazine metabolites. *Nature 226:*372-373, 1970.
31. P. Kaul, M. Clark, M. Conway, and J. Huffine, Chlorpromazine metabolism, I: Quantitative fluorimetric method for eleven chlorpromazine metabolites. *J. Pharm. Sci. 59:*1745, 1970.
32. P. N. Kaul, M. W. Conway, M. K. Ticku, and M. L. Clark, Chlorpromazine metabolism, II: Determination of non conjugated metabolites in blood of schizophrenic patients. *J. Pharm. Sci. 61:*581-585, 1972.
33. P. N. Kaul, L. R. Whitfield, and M. L. Clark, Chlorpromazine metabolism, VII: New quantitative fluorimetric determination of chlorpromazine and its sulphoxide. *J. Pharm. Sci. 65:*689, 1976.
34. G. M. Simpson, R. Lament, T. B. Cooper, J. H. Lee, and R. B. Bruce, The relationship between blood levels of different forms of butaperazine and clinical response. *J. Clin. Pharmacol. 13:*288-297, 1973.
35. D. H. Manier, J. Sekerke, J. V. Dingell, and M. K. El-Yousef, A fluorimetric method for the measurement of butaperazine in human plasma. *Clin. Chem. Acta 57:*225, 1974.
36. D. L. Garver, H. Dekirmenjian, J. M. Davis, B. Casper, and S. Ericksen, Neuroleptic drug levels and therapeutic response: Preliminary observations with red blood cell bound butaperazine. *Amer. J. Psychiat. 134:*304, 1977.
37. J. M. Davis, D. S. Janowsky, H. J. Sekerke, H. Manier, and M. K. El-Yousef, The pharmacokinetics of butaperazine in serum. *Advan. Biochem. Psychopharmacol. 9:*433, 1974.
38. N. R. West, M. P. Rosenblum, H. Sprince, S. Gold, D. A. Boehme, and W. H. Vogel, Assay procedures for thioridazine, trifluoperazine, and their sulphoxides and determination of urinary excretion of these compounds in mental patients. *J. Pharm. Sci. 63:*417-420, 1974.

39. M. Shostak, Immunological properties of some phenothiazines. *Advan. Biochem. Psychopharmacol. 9:*365, 1974.
40. S. Spector, Development of antibodies to chlorpromazine. *Advan. Biochem. Psychopharmacol. 9:*363, 1974.
41. K. Kawashima, R. Dixon, and S. Spector, Development of a radioimmunoassay for chlorpromazine. *Eur. J. Pharmacol. 32:*195, 1975.
42. D. H. Wiles, and M. Franklin, Radioimmunoassay for fluphenazine in human plasma. *Brit. J. Clin. Pharmacol. 5:*265-268, 1978.
43. W. Reiss, Drug assay by radioactive reagents. In *The Poisoned Patient: The Role of the Laboratory.* Ciba Foundation Symposium 26. Amsterdam, ASP Elsevier, 1974, pp. 139-154.
44. J. P. Coghlan and B. A. Scoggins, Measurement of aldosterone in peripheral blood of man and sheep. *J. Clin. Endocrinol. Metab. 27:*1470-1486, 1967.
45. D. H. Efron, L. E. Gaudette, and S. R. Harris, A new method for measuring minute amounts of chlorpromazine and some of its metabolites in plasma. *Agressologie 9:*103, 1968.
46. D. H. Efron, A. A. Manian, and S. R. Harris, The simultaneous measurement of chlorpromazine, chlorpromazine sulphoxide, and their demethylated analogs in plasma by radioactive derivative formation. *Psychopharmacol. Bull. 6:*73, 1970.
47. D. H. Efron, S. R. Harris, A. A. Manian, and L. E. Gaudette, Radioassay of chlorpromazine and its metabolites in plasma. *Psychopharmacologia 9:*207, 1971.
48. V. Clarke and E. R. Cole, A colour reaction for psychotropic drugs on thin layer chromatograms. *J. Chromatogr. 24*(1):259, 1966.
49. J. Kofoed, C. Fabierkiewicz, and G. H. Lucas, A study of the conversion of phenothiazine derivatives to the corresponding sulphoxides on thin layer plates. *J. Chromatogr. 23*(3):410, 1966.
50. C. L. Huang, Isolation and identification of urinary chlorpromazine metabolites in man. *Int. J. Neuropharmacol. 6:*1-13, 1967.
51. M. B. Wechsler, R. N. Wharton, E. Tanaka, and S. Malitz, Chlorpromazine metabolite pattern in psychotic patients. *J. Psychiat. Res. 5:*327-333, 1967.
52. H. R. Steinberg and J. Robinson, Nor-2-chlorpromazine sulphoxide and 3,4-dimethoxyphenethylamine. *Nature 217:*1054-1055, 1968.
53. R. J. Coumbis, C. C. Fulton, J. P. Calise, and C. Rodriguez, The necessity of elution and identification of drugs indicated by thin-layer chromatography. *J. Chromatogr. 54:*245-250, 1971.
54. J. C. Garriott and A. Stolman, Detection of some psychotherapeutic drugs and their metabolites in urine. *Clin. Toxicol. 4:*225-243, 1971.
55. P. Turano, W. J. Turner, and A. A. Manian, Thin layer chromatography of chlorpromazine metabolites: Attempt to identify each of the metabolites appearing in blood, urine, and faeces of chronically medicated schizophrenics. *J. Chromatogr. 75:*277-293, 1973.
56. N. C. Jain, W. J. Leung, R. D. Budd, and T. C. Sneath, Thin layer chroma-

tographic identification of phenothiazines in urine specimens. *Amer. J. Med. Technol. 41:*322-326, 1975.

57. J. J. Weir and J. Sanford, Metabolism and excretion of promazine by the horse. *J. Pharm. Pharmacol. 21:*169-173, 1969.
58. A. Jorgensen, V. Hansen, U. D. Larsen, and A. R. Khan, Metabolism, distribution, and excretion of flupenthixol. *Acta Pharmacol. Toxicol. 27:* 301-313, 1969.
59. J. Dreyfuss and A. I. Cohen, Identification of 7-hydroxyfluphenazine as major metabolite of fluphenazine-14C in the dog. *J. Pharm. Sci. 60:*826-828, 1971.
60. I. Zingales, Systematic identification of psychotropic drugs by thin layer chromatography, I. *J. Chromatogr. 31:*405-419 (1968).
61. I. Zingales, Systematic identification of psychotropic drugs by thin layer chromatography, II. *J. Chromatogr. 34:*44-51, 1968.
62. I. A. Zingales, Detection of chlorpromazine and thioridadine metabolites in human erythrocytes. *J. Chromatogr. 44:*547-562, 1969.
63. B. Arons, J. C. Kosek, and I. S. Forrest, Chlorpromazine therapy in a female albino mental patient: Clinical, histochemical, and biochemical observations. *Life Sci. 7:*1273-1280, 1968.
64. P. Turano, J. E. March, W. J. Turner, and S. Merus, Qualitative and quantitative report on chlorpromazine metabolites in plasma, erythrocytes, and erythrocyte washings from chronically medicated patients. *J. Med.* (Basel) *3:*109-120, 1972.
65. P. Turano and W. J. Turner, Quantitation of chlorpromazine and its metabolites by two dimensional thin-layer chromatography and direct scanning microdensitometry. *J. Chromatogr. 64:*347-354, 1972.
66. T. L. Chan and S. Gershon, Chlorpromazine metabolism in humans, I: Quantitation of chlorpromazine and its metabolites in human plasma and urine by direct scan spectrodensitometry. *Mikrochim. Acta 3:*435-452, 1973.
67. G. Sakalis, T. L. Chan, G. Sathananthan, N. Schooler, S. Goldberg, and S. Gershon, Relationships among clinical response, extrapyramidal syndrome, and plasma chlorpromazine and metabolite ratios. *Comm. Psychopharmacol. 1:*157-166, 1977.
68. A. J. Kapadia, M. A. Barber, and A. E. Martin, Quantitative determination of butaperazine by TLC. *J. Pharm. Sci. 59:*1476-1479, 1970.
69. U. Breyer and K. Villumsen, Measurement of plasma levels of tricyclic psychoactive drugs and their metabolites by UV reflectance photometry of thin layer chromatograms. *Eur. J. Clin. Pharmacol. 9:*457-465, 1976.
70. R. Whelpton and S. H. Curry, Gas chromatographic separation of chlorpromazine, diazepam, and N-desmethyldiazepam. *J. Pharm. Pharmacol. 27:*970, 1975.
71. S. H. Curry, Gas chromatographic methods for the study of chlorpromazine and some of its metabolites in human plasma. *Psychopharmacol. Comm. 2:*1, 1976.

72. S. H. Curry, Determination of nanogram quantities of chlorpromazine and some of its metabolites in plasma with an electron capture detector. *Anal. Chem. 40:*1251-1255, 1968.
73. S. H. Curry and G. P. Mould, Gas chromatographic identification of thioridazine in plasma, and a method for routine assay of the drug. *J. Pharm. Pharmacol. 21:*674-677, 1969.
74. S. H. Curry, J. M. Davis, D. S. Janowsky, and J. H. Marshall, Factors affecting chlorpromazine plasma levels in psychiatric patients. *Arch. Gen. Psych. 22:*209-215, 1970.
75. C. Korczak-Fabierkiewicz, D. W. Robinson, and G. H. Lucas, Conversion of chlorpromazine sulphoxide to chlorpromazine by use of metals in acid solution. *J. Chromatogr. 31:*538-544, 1967.
76. C. G. Hammar and B. Holmstedt, The identification of chlorpromazine metabolites in human blood by gas liquid chromatography. *Experientia 24:*98-100, 1968.
77. S. H. Curry and J. H. Marshall, Plasma levels of chlorpromazine and some of its relatively non-polar metabolites in psychiatric patients. *Life Sci. 7:* 9-17, 1968.
78. H. M. Berman and M. A. Spirtes, Gas chromatographic analysis of chlorpromazine and its metabolites formed by hepatic microsomes, I: Influence of magnesium. *Biochem. Pharmacol. 20:*2275-2286, 1971.
79. D. R. Flint, C. R. Ferullo, P. Levandoski, and B. Hwang, More sensitive gas-chromatographic measurement of chlorpromazine in plasma. *Clin. Chem. 17:*830-831, 1971.
80. A. A. Manian, D. H. Efron, and S. R. Harris, Appearance of monohydroxylated chlorpromazine metabolites in the central nervous system. *Life Sci. 10:* 679-684, 1971.
81. G. Sakalis, S. H. Curry, G. P. Mould, and M. H. Lader, Physiologic and clinical effects of chlorpromazine and their relationship to plasma level. *Clin. Pharmacol. Ther. 13:*931-946, 1972.
82. G. W. Christoph, D. E. Schmidt, J. M. Davis, and D. S. Janowsky, A method for determination of chlorpromazine in human blood serum. *Clin. Chim. Acta 38:*265-270, 1972.
83. M. A. Spirtes, Artifactual contamination of control serum extracts in gas chromatographic analyses for chlorpromazine. *Clin. Chem. 18:*317-318, 1972.
84. L. Rivera-Calimlim, L. Castaneda, and L. Lasagna, Effects of mode of management on plasma chlorpromazine in psychiatric patients. *Clin. Pharmacol. Ther. 14:*978-986, 1973.
85. S. F. Cooper, J. M. Albert, J. Hillel, and G. Caille, Plasma-level studies of chlorpromazine hydrochloride and chlorpromazine embonate in chronic schizophrenics. *Curr. Ther. Res. 15:*73-77, 1973.
86. S. H. Curry, Chlorpromazine analysis by gas chromatography with an electron capture detector. *Advan. Biochem. Psychopharmacol. 9:*335-345, 1974.

87. S. H. Curry and S. Evans, Assay of 7-hydroxychlorpromazine, and failure to detect more than small quantities, in plasma of responding schizophrenics. *Psychopharmacol. Comm. 1:*481-490, 1975.
88. S. H. Curry and S. Evans, A note on the assay of chlorpromazine N-oxide and its sulphoxide in plasma and urine. *J. Pharm. Pharmacol. 28:*467-468, 1976.
89. M. I. Kelsey, A. Keskiner, and E. A. Moscatelli, Gas liquid chromatographic analysis of fluphenazine and fluphenazine sulphoxide in the urine of chronic schizophrenic patients. *J. Chromatogr. 75:*294-297, 1973.
90. R. Whelpton and S. H. Curry, Methods for the study of fluphenazine kinetics in man. *J. Pharm. Pharmacol. 28:*869-873, 1976.
91. M. Franklin, D. H. Wiles, and D. J. Harvey, Sensitive gas chromatographic determination of fluphenazine in human plasma. *Clin. Chem. 24:*41-44, 1978.
92. E. Martensson and B. E. Roos, Serum levels of thioridazine in psychiatric patients and healthy volunteers. *Eur. J. Clin. Pharmacol. 6:*181-186, 1973.
93. F. A. Vanderheeren and D. J. Theunis, Gas liquid chromatographic determination of perazine, thioridazine, and thioridazine metabolites in human plasma. *J. Chromatogr. 120:*123-128, 1976.
94. E. C. Dinovo, L. A. Gottschalk, B. R. Nandi, and P. G. Geddes, GLC analysis of thioridazine, mesoridazine, and their metabolites. *J. Pharm. Sci. 65:*667-669, 1976.
95. R. Whelpton and S. H. Curry, Chromatographic properties of imines formed from dedimethylchlorpromazine and various aldehydes and ketones. *J. Chromatogr. 121:*88-92, 1976.
96. C. H. Ng and J. L. Crammer, Measurement of thioridazine in blood and urine. *Brit. J. Clin. Pharmacol. 4:*173-183, 1977.
97. N. E. Larsen and J. Naestoft, Determination of perphenazine and fluphenazine in whole blood by gas chromatography. *Med. Lab. Technol. 30:* 129-132, 1973.
98. C. E. Hansen and N. E. Larsen, Perphenazine concentrations in human whole blood: A pilot study during anti-psychotic therapy using different administration forms. *Psychopharmacologia 37:*31-36, 1974.
99. N. E. Larsen and J. Naestoft, Determination of perphenazine and its sulphoxide metabolite in human plasma after therapeutic doses by gas chromatography. *J. Chromatogr. 109:*259-264, 1975.
100. A. De Leenheer and A. Heyndrickx, Methotrimeprazine and its sulphoxide and desmethyl metabolites in urine of psychiatric patients. *J. Pharm. Sci. 61:*914-917, 1972.
101. S. G. Dahl and S. Jacobsen, GLC determination of methotrimeprazine and its sulphoxide in plasma. *J. Pharm. Sci. 65:*1329-1333, 1976.
102. J. S. Noonan, J. W. Blake, P. W. Murdick, and R. S. Ray, Bromination of phenothiazine tranquilisers: A method for sensitive and specific detection. *Life Sci. 2:*363-373, 1972.

103. A. De Leenheer, Gas liquid chromatography of phenothiazine derivatives and related compounds. *J. Chromatogr. 77:*339-350, 1973.
104. A. P. De Leenheer, Identification and quantitative determination of phenothiazine drugs in urine samples of psychiatric patients. *J. Pharm. Sci. 63:*389-394, 1974.
105. P. F. Dixon, M. S. Stoll, and C. K. Lim, High pressure liquid chromatography in clinical chemistry. *Ann. Clin. Biochem. 13:*409-432, 1976.
106. J. H. Knox, High speed liquid chromatography. *Ann. Rev. Phys. Chem. 24:*29, 1973.
107. R. G. Muusze and J. F. K. Huber, Evaluation of liquid-liquid systems for the chromatographic separation of the psychotropic drug thioridazine and its metabolites. *J. Chromatogr. 83:*405-420, 1973.
108. R. G. Muusze and J. F. K. Huber, Determination of the psychotropic drug thioridazine and its metabolites in blood by means of high pressure liquid chromatography in combination with fluorimetric reaction detection. *J. Chromatogr. Sci. 12:*779-787, 1974.
109. D. H. Rodgers, Separation and analysis of psychopharmacologic drugs by high efficiency liquid chromatography. *J. Chromatogr. Sci. 12:*742-746, 1974.
110. J. H. Knox and J. Jurand, Separation of tricyclic psychosedative drugs by high-speed ion-pair partition and liquid-solid adsorption chromatography. *J. Chromatogr. 103:*311-326, 1975.
111. J. Lankelma and H. Poppe, Design and characterization of a coulometric detector with a glassy carbon electrode for high performance liquid chromatography. *J. Chromatogr. 125:*375-388, 1976.
112. U. Tjaden, J. Lankelma, H. Poppe, and R. G. Muusze, Anodic coulometric detection with a glassy carbon electrode in combination with reversed-phase high performance liquid chromatography: Determination of blood levels of perphenazine and fluphenazine. *J. Chromatogr. 125:*275-286, 1976.
113. D. C. Williams and R. W. Burnett, A reversed phase liquid chromatographic method for the determination of therapeutic levels of phenothiazines in serum. *Clin. Chem. 23:*1139, 1977.
114. A. G. Butterfield and R. W. Sears, High performance liquid chromatographic determination of perphenazine and amitriptyline hydrochloride in two-component tablet formulations. *J. Pharm. Sci. 66:*1117-1119, 1977.
115. B. B. Wheals and I. Jane, Analysis of drugs and their metabolites by high performance liquid chromatography. *Analyst 102:*625-644, 1977.
116. C. G. Hammar, B. Holmstedt, and R. Ryhage, Mass fragmentography: Identification of chlorpromazine and its metabolites in human blood by a new method. *Anal. Biochem. 25:*532-548, 1968.
117. G. Alfredsson, B. Wode-Helgodt, and G. Sedvall, A mass fragmentographic method for the determination of chlorpromazine and two of its active metabolites in human plasma and CSF. *Psychopharmacol. 48:*123-131, 1976.

118. W. J. Turner, P. Turano, and S. Badzinski, An attempt to establish quality control in determination of plasma chlorpromazine by a multi-laboratory collaboration. In *Pharmacokinetics of Psychoactive Drugs* (L. Gottschalk and S. Merlis, eds.). New York, Spectrum, 1976, pp. 33-43.
119. R. E. Lehr and P. N. Kaul, Chlorpromazine metabolism, IV: Quaternisation as a key to determination of picomoles of chlorpromazine and other tertiary amine drugs. *J. Pharm. Sci. 64:*950-953, 1975.
120. W. Soudijn, J. Van Wijngaarden, and F. Allewijn, Distribution, excretion, and metabolism of neuroleptics of the butyrophenone type, I: Excretion and metabolism of haloperidol and nine related butyrophenone-derivatives in the Wistar rat. *Eur. J. Pharmacol. 1:*47, 1974.
121. A. Forsman, G. Folsch, M. Larsson, and R. Ohman, On the metabolism of haloperidol in man. *Curr. Ther. Res. 21:*606-661, 1977.
122. P. J. A. W. Demoen, Properties and analysis of haloperidol and its dosage forms. *J. Pharm. Sci. 50:*350-353, 1961.
123. A. Haemers and W. Van Den Bossche, A note on the colourimetric determination of butyrophenones with 3,5-dinitrobenzoic acid. *J. Pharm. Pharmacol. 21:*531-532, 1969.
124. I. A. Zingales, A gas chromatographic method for the determination of haloperidol in human plasma. *J. Chromatogr. 54:*15-24, 1971.
125. F. Marcucci, E. Mussini, L. Airoldi, R. Fanelli, A. Frigerio, F. DeNadai, A. Bizzi, M. Risso, P. L. Morselli, and S. Garattini, Analytical and pharmacokinetic studies on butyrophenones. *Clin. Chim. Acta 34:*321-332, 1971.
126. A. Forsman, E. Martensson, G. Nyberg, and R. Ohman, A gas chromatographic method for determining haloperidol. *Arch. Pharmacol. 286:*113-124, 1974.
127. J. Rosenfeld, M. Kawai, J. R. Rigg, and J. K. Khandelwai, Gas chromatographic method for the analysis of butyrophenones based on the Hofmann degradation reaction. *J. Chromatogr. 129:*387-392, 1976.
128. B. R. Clark, B. B. Tower, and R. T. Rubin, Radioimmunoassay of haloperidol in human serum. *Life Sci. 20:*319-325, 1977.
129. B. S. Finkle, E. J. Cherry, and D. M. Taylor, A GLC based system for the detection of poisons, drugs, and human metabolites encountered in forensic toxicology. *J. Chromatogr. Sci. 9:*393-419, 1971.
130. J. E. Wallace, Ultraviolet spectrophotometric determination of chlorprothixene in biologic specimens. *J. Pharm. Sci. 56:*1437-1441, 1967.
131. L. G. Allgen, B. Jonsson, B. Nauckhoff, M. Andersen, I. Huus, and I. M. Nielsen, On the elimination of chlorprothixene in rat and man. *Experientia 16:*325, 1960.
132. H. Christensen, Chlorprothixene and its metabolites in blood, liver, and urine from a fatal poisoning. *Acta Pharmacol. Toxicol. 34:*16-26, 1974.
133. T. Mjorndal and L. Oreland, Determination of thioxanthenes in plasma at therapeutic concentrations. *Acta Pharmacol. Toxicol. 29:*295-302, 1971.

134. R. Bergling, T. Mjorndal, L. Oreland, W. Rapp, and S. Wold, Plasma levels and clinical effects of thioridazine and thiothixene. *J. Clin. Pharmacol. 15:*178-186, 1975.
135. D. G. Hobbs, W. M. Welch, M. J. Short, W. A. Moody, and C. D. Van der Velde, Pharmacokinetics of thiothixene in man. *Clin. Pharmacol. Ther. 16:* 473-478, 1974.
136. C. K. Wong, C. M. Cohen, and K. P. Munnelly, High-pressure liquid chromatographic determination of thiothixene in pharmaceutical formulations. *J. Pharm. Sci. 65:*1090-1092, 1976.
137. J. D. Robinson and D. Risby, Radioimmunoassay for flupenthixol in plasma. *Clin. Chem. 23:*2085-2088, 1977.
138. D. M. Hailey, Chromatography of the 1,4-benzodiazepines. *J. Chromatogr. 98:*527-568, 1974.
139. D. J. Greenblatt and R. I. Shader, Detection and Quantitation. In *Benzodiazepines in Clinical Practice.* New York, Raven Press, pp. 17-42, 1974.
140. J. M. Clifford and W. Franklin-Smyth, The determination of some 1-4 benzodiazepines and their metabolites in body fluids: A review. *Analyst 99:*241-272, 1974.
141. S. L. Tompsett, Extraction procedures in chemical toxicology. *Analyst 93:*740-748, 1968.
142. H. F. Proelss and H. J. Lohmann, Profile of sedatives and tranquilizers in serum as measured by gas liquid chromatography. *Clin. Chem. 17:*222-228, 1971.
143. W. Muller and U. Wollert, Characterisation of the binding of benzodiazepines to human serum albumin. *Nauyn-Schmiedebergs Arch Pharmakol. Exp. Pathol. 280:*229-237, 1973.
144. J. A. F. de Silva and C. V. Puglisi, Determination of medazepam (nobrium), diazepam (valium), and their major biotransformation products in blood and urine by electron capture gas liquid chromatography. *Anal. Chem. 42:* 1725-1736, 1970.
145. J. M. Fujimoto and R. I. H. Wang, A method of identifying narcotic analgesics in human urine after therapeutic doses. *Toxicol. Appl. Pharmacol. 16:*186-193, 1970.
146. S. J. Mulé, M. L. Bastos, D. Jukofsky, and E. Saffer, Routine identification of drugs of abuse in human urine, II: Development and application of the XAD-2 resin column method. *J. Chromatogr. 63:*289-301, 1971.
147. M. L. Bastos, D. Jukofsky, E. Saffer, M. Chedekel, and S. J. Mulé, Modifications of the XAD-2 resin column method for the extraction of drugs of abuse from human urine. *J. Chromatogr. 71:*549-553, 1972.
148. L. B. Hetland, D. A. Knowlton, and D. Douri, A method for the detection of drugs at therapeutic dosages in human urine using adsorption column chromatography and thin layer chromatography. *Clin. Chim. Acta 36:* 473-478, 1972.
149. P. A. F. Pranitis, J. R. Milzoff, and A. Stolman, Extraction of drugs from biofluids and tissues with XAD-2 resin. *J. Forens. Sci. 19:*917-926, 1974.

150. H. Sawada, A. Hara, S. Asano, and Y. Matsumoto, Isolation and identification of benzodiazepine drugs and their metabolites in urine by use of Amberlite XAD-2 resin and thin layer chromatography. *Clin. Chem. 22:* 1596-1603, 1976.
151. J. Meola and M. Vanko, The use of charcoal in the qualitative and quantitative analysis of drugs. *Clin. Chem. 18:*713, 1972.
152. J. Grove and P. A. Toseland, The gas-liquid chromatography of hydroxyamylobarbitone in plasma and urine. *Clin. Chim. Acta 29:*253-260, 1970.
153. M. L. Bastos, G. K. Kananen, R. M. Young, J. R. Montforte, and I. Sunshine, Detection of basic organic drugs and their metabolites in urine. *Clin. Chem. 16:*931-940, 1970.
154. M. G. Horning, P. Gregory, J. Nowlin, M. Stafford, K. Lertrantanangkoon, C. Butler, W. G. Stillwell, and R. M. Hill, Isolation of drugs and drug metabolites from biological fluids by use of salt-solvent pairs. *Clin. Chem. 20:*282-287, 1974.
155. J. Barrett, W. F. Smyth, and I. E. Davidson, An examination of the acid-base equilibria of 1,4-benzodiazepines by spectrophotometry. *J. Pharm. Pharmacol. 25:*387-393, 1973.
156. P. Jatlow, Ultraviolet spectrophotometric measurement of chlordiazepoxide in plasma. *Clin. Chem. 18:*516-518, 1972.
157. J. H. Riddick, An ultraviolet and visible spectrophotometric assay method for chlordiazepoxide. *Clin. Biochem. 6:*189-199, 1973.
158. N. Gallo, V. D. Bianco, S. Doronzo, and P. D. Laforgia, A new spectrophotometric determination of nitrazepam. *Experientia 30:*439-440, 1974.
159. A. C. Bratton and E. K. Marshall, A new coupling component for sulfanilamide determination. *J. Biol. Chem. 128:*537-550, 1939.
160. L. O. Randall, Pharmacology of chlordiazepoxide (Librium). *Dis. Nerv. System, Suppl. 22*(7):1-9, 1961.
161. J. Baumler and S. Rippstein, Uber den Nachweis von "Methamino diazepoxid" (Librium) und seiner Metaboliten. *Helv. Chim. Acta 44:*2208-2210, 1961.
162. K. H. Beyer and W. Sadee, Spectrophotometric determination of 5-phenyl-1,4-benzodiazepine-derivatives and studies on metabolism of nitrazepam, V: Chemistry and analytics of benzodiazepine derivatives. *Arzneim.-Forsch. 19:*1929-1931, 1969.
163. K. Besserer, S. Henzler, E. Kohler, and H. J. Mallach, Microchemical determination of chlordiazepoxide and medazepam in pharmacokinetic studies. *Arzneim.-Forsch. 21:*2003-2006, 1971.
164. C. S. Frings and P. S. Cohen, Rapid colorimetric method for the quantitative determination of Librium (chlordiazepoxide hydrochloride) in serum. *Amer. J. Clin. Pathol. 56:*216-219, 1971.
165. A. M. Diab, Colorimetric estimation of nitrazepam and metabolites in formulations and in blood and urine samples. *Pharmazie 29:*746, 1975.
166. I. Ganescu, C. Varhelyi, G. Grinzan, and I. Boboc, Thiocyanato chromium (III) complexes in chemical analysis, XXV: Oxydometric and spectro-

photometric determination of diazepam with Reinecke salt-like compounds. *Pharmazie 31:*259, 1976.
167. I. Ganescu, C. Varhelyi, G. Brinzan, and L. Boboc, Thiocyanato chromium (III) complexes in chemical analysis, XXVI: Oxidimetric and spectrophotometric determination of chlordiazepoxide and tetrathiocyanatodiamine-chromates. *Pharmazie 32:*53, 1977.
168. B. A. Koechlin and L. D'Arconte, Determination of chlordiazepoxide (Librium) and of a metabolite of lactam character in plasma of humans, dogs, and rats by a specific spectrofluorometric micro method. *Anal. Biochem. 5:*195-207, 1963.
169. M. A. Schwartz and E. Postma, Metabolic N-demethylation of chlordiazepoxide. *J. Pharm. Sci. 55:*1358-1362, 1966.
170. J. A. F. De Silva and N. Strojny, Determination of flurazepam and its major biotransformation products in blood and urine by spectrophotofluorometry and spectrophotometry. *J. Pharm. Sci. 60:*1303-1314, 1971.
171. J. Rieder, A fluorimetric method for determining nitrazepam and the sum of its main metabolites in plasma and urine. *Arzneim-Forsch. 23:*207-211, 1973.
172. J. C. Valentour, J. R. Monforte, B. Lorenzo, and I. Sunshine, Fluorometric screening method for detecting benzodiazepines in blood and urine. *Clin. Chem. 21:*1976-1979, 1975.
173. J. T. Stewart and J. L. Williamson, Fluorometric determination of chlordiazepoxide in dosage forms and biological fluids with fluorescamine. *Anal. Chem. 48:*1182-1185, 1976.
174. K. B. Alton, R. M. Grimes, C. Shaw, J. E. Patrick, and J. L. McGuire, Biotransformation of a 1,5-benzodiazepine, triflubazam, by man. *Drug Metab. Dispos. 3:*352-360, 1975.
175. F. Weist and E. Schmid, Rapid thin layer chromatography demonstration of tranquilizers of the benzodiazepine series and thymoleptic series. *Med. Welt 7:*369-372, 1969.
176. B. R. Manno, J. R. Baker, J. E. Manno, and J. R. Hughes, Identification of flurazepam (Dalmane) and a primary metabolite in urine by thin-layer-chromatography. *J. Forens. Sci. 20:*38-44, 1975.
177. H. D. Beckstead and S. J. Smith, Detection of impurities in medical 1,4-benzodiazepines and related compounds by thin-layer chromatography. *Arzneim.-Forsch. 18:*529-535, 1968.
178. P. Haefelfinger, Sensitive method for the detection of substances containing primary amino groups on thin-layer plates. *J. Chromatogr. 48:*184-190, 1970.
179. S. N. Tewari and S. K. Shukla, Paper electrophoretic detection and separation of some psychotropic drugs of 1,4-benzodiazepine series in autopsy material. *Pharmazie 32:*243, 1977.
180. S. N. Tewari and S. K. Shukla, Separation and identification of 1,4-benzodiazepine drugs present in the biological fluids by two dimensional t.l.c. *Pharmazie 32:*536, 1977.

181. D. Schutz and H. Schutz, Rapid detection of Lorazepam (Tavor), a new benzodiazepine tranquilizer. *Arch. Toxicol. 30:*183–186, 1973.
182. R. D. Maier and K. H. Wehr, The detection of prazepam, a new benzodiazepine tranquilizer. *Arch. Toxicol. 32:*341–345, 1974.
183. S. Lauffer and E. Schmid, Thin-layer chromatographic-spectrophotofluorimetric determination of 7-chlor-2,3-dihydro-1-methyl-5-phenyl-1H,1,4-benzodiazepine (medazepam). *Arzneim.-Forsch. 19:*740–741, 1969.
184. J. A. De Silva, I. Bekersky, and C. V. Puglisi, Spectrofluorodensitometric determination of flurazepam and its major metabolites in blood. *J. Pharm. Sci. 63:*1837–1841, 1974.
185. P. Haefelfinger, Determination of nanogram amounts of primary aromatic amines and nitro compounds in blood and plasma. *J. Chromatogr. 111:* 323–329, 1975.
186. N. Wad, H. Rosenmund, and E. Hanifl, A simplified quantitative method for the simultaneous determination of diazepam and its metabolites in serum by thin layer chromatography. *J. Chromatogr. 128:*231–234, 1976.
187. N. T. Wad and E. J. Hanifl, Simplified thin-layer chromatographic method for the simultaneous determination of clonazepam diazepam, and their metabolites in serum. *J. Chromatogr. 143:*214–218, 1977.
188. A. C. Moffat and K. W. Smalldon, Optimum use of paper, thin layer, and gas liquid chromatography for the identification of basic drugs, II: Paper and thin-layer chromatography. *J. Chromatogr. 90:*9–17, 1974.
189. K. K. Kaistha, R. Tadrus, and R. Janda, Simultaneous detection of a wide variety of commonly abused drugs in a urine screening program using thin-layer identification techniques. *J. Chromatogr. 107:*359–379, 1975.
190. N. Stronjny, K. Bratin, M. A. Brooks, and J. A. De Silva, Determination of chlordiazepoxide, diazepam, and their major metabolites in blood or plasma by spectrophotodensitometry. *J. Chromatogr. 143:*363–374, 1977.
191. S. R. Sun, Quantitative determination of chlordiazepoxide and its metabolites in serum by fluorescence TLC-densitometry, *J. Pharm. Sci. 67:*639–641, 1978.
192. P. J. Van der Merew and J. M. Steyn, Thin-layer chromatographic method for determination of diazepam and its major metabolite, N-desmethyldiazepam, in human serum. *J. Chromatogr. 148:*549–552, 1978.
193. C. G. Scott and P. Bommer, The liquid chromatography of some benzodiazepines. *J. Chromatogr. Sci. 8:*446–451, 1970.
194. D. J. Weber, High pressure liquid chromatography of benzodiazepines: Analysis of ketazolam. *J. Pharm. Sci. 61:*1797–1800, 1972.
195. R. E. Huettemann and A. P. Shroff, High-pressure liquid chromatographic analysis of triflubazam and its metabolites in human and animal blood and urine. *J. Pharm. Sci. 64:*1339–1342, 1975.
196. A. Bugge, Quantitative high-performance liquid chromatography of diazepam and N-desmethyldiazepam in blood. *J. Chromatogr. 128:*111–116, 1976.

197. B. Moore, G. Nickless, C. Hallett, and A. G. Howard, Analysis of nitrazepam and its metabolites by high-pressure liquid chromatography. *J. Chromatography. 137:*215-217, 1977.
198. T. B. Vree, B. Lenselink, E. Van der Kleijn, and G. M. Nijhuis, Determination of flunitrazepam in body fluids by means of high-performance liquid chromatography. *J. Chromatogr. 143:*530-534, 1977.
199. M. D. Osselton, M. D. Hammond, and P. J. Twitchett, The extraction and analysis of benzodiazepines in tissues by enzymic digestion and high-performance liquid chromatography. *J. Pharm. Pharmacol., 29:*460-462, 1977.
200. P. M. Kabra, G. L. Stevens, and L. J. Marton, High-pressure liquid chromatographic analysis of diazepam, oxazepam, and N-desmethyldiazepam in human blood. *J. Chromatogr. 150:*355-360, 1978.
201. R. R. Brodie, L. F. Chasseaud, and T. Taylor, High performance liquid chromatographic determination of benzodiazepines in human plasma. *J. Chromatogr. 150:*361-366, 1978.
202. B. J. Gudzinowicz and M. J. Gudzinowicz, *Analysis of Drugs and Metabolites by Gas Chromatography-Mass Spectrometry,* vol. 2: *Hypnotics, Anticonvulsants, and Sedatives.* New York, Marcel Dekker, 1977, pp. 277-320.
203. W. Sadee and E. Van der Kleijn, Thermolysis of 1,4 benzodiazepines during gas chromatography and mass spectrometry. *J. Pharm. Sci. 60:* 135-137, 1971.
204. A. Berlin, B. Siwers, S. Agurell, A. Hiort, F. Sjöqvist, and S. Strom, Determination of bioavailability of diazepam in various formulations from steady state plasma concentration data. *Clin. Pharmacol. Ther. 13:*733-744, 1972.
205. A. G. Howard, G. Nickless, and D. M. Hailey, A rapid gas chromatographic method for the determination of diazepam and metabolites in body fluids. *J. Chromatogr. 90:*325-329, 1974.
206. E. Arnold, A simple method for determining diazepam and its major metabolites in biological fluids: Application in bioavailability studies. *Acta Pharmacol. Toxicol. 36:*335-352, 1975.
207. M. Linnoila and F. Dorrity, Rapid gas chromatographic assay of serum diazepam N-desmethyldiazepam, and N-desalkylflurazepam. *Acta Pharmacol. Toxicol. 41:*458-464, 1977.
208. E. Rey, J. M. Turquais, and G. Olive, Micromethod for determination of diazepam by electron-capture gas-liquid chromatography. *Clin. Chem. 23:*1338-1339, 1977.
209. J. M. Steyn and H. K. L. Hundt, Quantitative gas chromatographic determination of diazepam and its major metabolite in human serum. *J. Chromatogr. 107:*196-200, 1975.
210. A. Viala, J.-P. Cano, J.-P. Reynier, and R. Rispe, Determination of N-desmethyldiazepam in plasma by gas chromatography with an internal standard. *J. Chromatogr. 147:*349-357, 1978.

211. D. M. Rutherford, Rapid micro-method for the measurement of diazepam and desmethyldiazepam in blood plasma by gas-liquid chromatography. *J. Chromatogr. 137:*439-448, 1977.
212. R. E. Weinfeld, H. N. Posmanter, K. C. Khoo, and C. V. Puglisi, Rapid determination of diazepam and nordiazepam in plasma by electron capture gas liquid chromatography: Application in clinical pharmacokinetic studies. *J. Chromatogr. 143:*581-595, 1977.
213. D. J. Greenblatt, Determination of desmethyldiazepam in plasma by electron-capture GLC: Application to pharmacokinetic studies of clorazepate. *J. Pharm. Sci. 67:*427-429, 1978.
214. R. Dixon, M. A. Brooks, E. Postma, M. R. Hackman, S. Spector, J. D. Moore, and M. A. Schwartz, N-desmethyldiazepam: A new metabolite of chlordiazepoxide in man. *Clin. Pharmacol. Ther. 20:*450-457, 1976.
215. A. G. De Boer, J. Rost-Kaiser, H. Bracht, and D. D. Breimer, Assay of underivatised nitrazepam and clonazepam in plasma by capillary gas chromatography applied to pharmacokinetic and bioavailability studies in humans. *J. Chromatogr. 145:*105-114, 1978.
216. G. P. Beharrell, D. M. Hailey, and M. K. McLaurin, Determination of nitrazepam (Mogadon) in plasma by electron capture gas-liquid chromatography. *J. Chromatogr. 70:*45-52, 1972.
217. K. M. Jensen, Determination of nitrazepam in serum by gas-liquid chromatography: Application in bioavailability studies. *J. Chromatogr. 111:* 389-396, 1975.
218. L. Kangas, Comparison of two gas-liquid chromatographic methods for the determination of nitrazepam in plasma. *J. Chromatogr. 136:*259-270, 1977.
219. J. P. Cano, A. M. Baille, and A. Viala, Determination of bromazepam in plasma with an internal standard by gas-liquid chromatography. *Arzneim.-Forsch. 25:*1012-1016, 1975.
220. J. A. De Silva, I. Bekersky, M. A. Brooks, R. E. Weinfeld, W. Glover, and C. V. Puglisi, Determination of bromazepam in blood by electron capture GLC and of its major urinary metabolites by differential pulse polarography. *J. Pharm. Sci. 63:*1440-1445, 1974.
221. I. A. Zingales, Determination of chlordiazepoxide plasma concentrations by electron capture gas-liquid chromatography. *J. Chromatogr. 61:*237-252, 1971.
222. J. Vessman, M. Johansson, P. Magnusson, and S. Stromberg, Determination of intact oxazepam by electron capture gas chromatography after an extractive alkylation reaction. *Anal. Chem. 49:*1545-1549, 1977.
223. J. A. Knowles and H. W. Ruelius, Absorption and excretion of 7-chloro-1,3-dihydro-3-hydroxy-5-phenyl-2H-1,4-benzodiazepin-2-one (oxazepam) in humans: Determination of the drug by gas-liquid chromatography with electron capture detection. *Arzneim.-Forsch. 22:*687-692, 1972.
224. M. S. Greaves, Quantitative determination of medazepam, diazepam, and nitrazepam in whole blood by flame-ionization gas-liquid chromatography. *Clin. Chem. 20:*141-147, 1974.

225. E. S. Baird, D. M. Hailey, and S. Malcolm, A gas chromatographic assay for medazepam and its major metabolites in plasma. *Clin. Chim. Acta 48:*105-108, 1973.
226. D. M. Hailey, Gas chromatographic analysis of medazepam and its metabolites using an electrolytic conductivity detector. *J. Chromatogr. 100:*49-54, 1974.
227. B. E. Pape and M. A. Ribick, Analysis of medazepam, diazepam, and metabolites in plasma by gas-liquid chromatography with an electrolytic conductivity detection. *J. Chromatogr. 136:*127-139, 1977.
228. J. A. De Silva, C. V. Puglisi, M. A. Brooks, and M. R. Hackman, Determination of flurazepam (Dalmane) and its major metabolites in blood by electron-capture gas-liquid chromatography and in urine by differential pulse polarography. *J. Chromatogr. 99:*461-483, 1974.
229. M. A. Brooks, M. R. Hackman, R. E. Weinfeld, and T. Macasieb, Determination of clorazepate and its major metabolites in blood and urine by electron capture gas-liquid chromatography. *J. Chromatogr. 135:*123-131, 1977.
230. D. J. Hoffman and A. H. Chun, G.L.C. determination of plasma drug levels after oral administration of clorazepate potassium salts. *J. Pharm. Sci. 64:*1668-1671, 1975.
231. J. P. Cano, J. Guintrand, C. Aubert, and A. Viala, Determination of flunitrazepam, desmethyl-flunitrazepam, and clonazepam in plasma by gas-liquid chromatography with an internal standard. *Arzneim.-Forsch. 27:*338-342, 1977.
232. D. B. Faber, B. M. Kok, and E. M. Dijk, Quantitative gas chromatographic analysis of flunitrazepam in human serum with electron-capture detection. *J. Chromatogr. 133:*319-326, 1977.
233. P. J. Howard and W. Toner, Plasma lorazepam estimation in neonates. *Anaesthesia 32:*767, 1977.
234. G. De Groot, R. A. Maes, and H. H. Lemmens, Determination of lorazepam in plasma by electron capture GLC. *Arch. Toxicol. 35:*229-234, 1976.
235. G. M. Pacifici and G. F. Placidi, Rapid and sensitive electron-capture gas chromatographic method for the determination of pinazepam and its metabolites in human plasma, urine, and milk. *J. Chromatogr. 135:*133-139, 1977.
236. J. A. De Silva, I. Bekersky, C. V. Puglisi, M. A. Brooks, and R. E. Weinfeld, Determination of 1,4-benzodiazepines and diazepin-2-ones in blood by electron-capture gas-liquid chromatography. *Anal. Chem. 48:*10-19, 1976.
237. F. Marcucci, R. Fanelli, and E. Mussini, A method for gas chromatographic determination of benzodiazepines. *J. Chromatogr. 37:*318-320, 1968.
238. R. C. Baselt, C. B. Stewart, and S. J. Franch, Toxicological determination of benzodiazepines in biological fluids and tissues by flame-ionisation gas chromatography. *J. Anal. Toxicol. 1:*10-13, 1977.

239. A. Forgione, P. Martelli, F. Marcucci, R. Fanelli, E. Mussini, and G. C. Jommi, Gas liquid chromatography and mass spectrometry of various benzodiazepines. *J. Chromatogr. 59:*163-168, 1971.
240. W. Sadee and E. Van der Kleijn, Thermolysis of 1,4-benzodiazepines during gas chromatography-mass spectroscopy. *J. Pharm. Sci. 60:*135-137, 1971.
241. T. T. Chang, C. F. Kuhlman, R. T. Schillings, S. F. Sisenwine, C. O. Tio, and H. W. Ruelius, Identification of oxazepam and lorazepam glucuronides by chemical ionisation mass spectrometry. *Experientia 29:*653-655, 1973.
242. A. J. Clatworthy, L. V. Jones, and M. J. Whitehouse, The gas chromatography mass spectrometry of the major metabolites of flurazepam. *Biomed. Mass Spectrom. 4:*248-254, 1977.
243. F. Marcucci, R. Bianchi, L. Airoldi, M. Salmona, R. Fanelli, C. Chiabrando, A. Frigerio, E. Mussini, and S. Garattini, Gas chromatographic-mass spectrometric determination of intact C3-hydroxylated benzodiazepine glucuronides in urine. *J. Chromatogr. 107:*285-293, 1975.
244. A. Trebbi, G. B. Gervasi, and V. Comi, Determination of pinazepam and its metabolites in serum, urine, and brain by gas-liquid chromatography and mass spectrometry. *J. Chromatogr. 110:*309-319, 1975.
245. M. C. Sanchez, J. Colome, and E. Gelpi, Electron capture and multiple ion detection of benzodiazepine esters in pharmacokinetic studies. *J. Chromatogr. 126:*601-613, 1976.
246. B. Peskar and S. Spector, Quantitative determination of diazepam in blood by radioimmunoassay. *J. Pharmacol. Exp. Ther. 186:*167-172, 1973.
247. H. P. Gelbke, H. J. Schlicht, and G. Schmidt, Radioimmunological screening and gas chromatographic identification of diazepam in blood and serum. *Arch. Toxicol. 38:*295-305, 1977.
248. W. R. Dixon, J. Earley, and E. Postma, Radioimmunoassay of chlordiazepoxide in plasma. *J. Pharm. Sci. 64:*937-939, 1975.
249. H. Oelschlager, J. Volke, C. T. Lim, and R. Spang, Reduction of oxazepam on Hg-drip-electrode, X: Drug analysis by polarography and oscillopolarography. *Arch. Pharm. 302:*946-951, 1969.
250. H. Oelschlager and H. P. Oehr, Polarographic determination of medazepam (Nobrium), XII: Drug analysis by polarography and oscillopolarography. *Pharm. Acta Helv. 45:*708-716, 1970.
251. D. J. Berry, The cathode-ray polarographic determination of diazepam, 7-chloro-1,3-dihydro-1-methyl-5-phenyl-2H-1,4-benzodiazepine-2-one, in human plasma. *Clin. Chim. Acta 32:*235-241, 1971.
252. S. Halvorsen and E. Jacobsen, Electroreduction and polarographic determination of nitrazepam in serum. *Anal. Chim. Acta 59:*127-136, 1972.
253. E. Jacobsen, T. V. Jacobsen, and T. Rojahn, The determination of diazepam in serum by differential pulse polarography. *Anal. Chim. Acta 64:*473-476, 1973.

254. M. R. Hackman, M. A. Brooks, and J. A. De Silva, Determination of chlordiazepoxide hydrochloride (Librium) and its major metabolites in plasma by differential pulse polarography. *Anal. Chem. 46:*1075-1082, 1974.
255. M. A. Brooks and M. R. Hackman, Trace level determination of 1,4-benzodiazepines in blood by differential pulse polarography. *Anal. Chem. 47:*2059-2062, 1975.
256. M. A. Brooks, L. D'Arconte, M. R. Hackman, and J. A. F. De Silva, Toxicological analysis of 1,4-benzodiazepines, I: Differential pulse polarography. *J. Anal. Toxicol. 1:*179-188, 1977.

4

Pharmacokinetics of Tricyclic Antidepressants

Lars F. Gram* / *Western Psychiatric Institute and Clinic, University of Pittsburgh, Pittsburgh, Pennsylvania, United States*

*Present affiliation: Department of Clinical Pharmacology, Institute of Pharmacology, Odense University, Odense, Denmark.

I. INTRODUCTION

Tricyclic antidepressants (TCA) exhibit three distinct pharmacokinetic characteristics:

1. High degree of tissue binding with high apparent volume of distribution
2. Efficient and almost complete elimination by metabolism in the liver, with high clearance
3. Pronounced interindividual variations in pharmacokinetics—in particular, elimination—resulting in large differences in steady-state plasma concentrations between individuals on identical doses.

The possible practical significance of this variability in terms of clinical effect has been the matter of research by several groups in recent years. There is evidence from different groups indicating that the plasma concentrations of the active compounds of TCA are in fact important determinants of their therapeutic and to some extent toxic effects [1,2]. The use of plasma level monitoring as an aid in the control of TCA therapy thus may become part of clinical practice within some years [1].

The rational use of plasma level monitoring requires a certain knowledge of the relevant pharmacokinetics of the compounds. Early research on TCA pharmacokinetics mainly dealt with metabolism, metabolite formation, etc., whereas recent research, by the introduction of methods for assay of TCA in plasma, has focused more on the quantitative aspects of TCA kinetics. The extensive literature on TCA metabolism has been reviewed in detail earlier [3], and these aspects will only be summarized here. The recent quantitative data on TCA require a more detailed discussion in relation to the general pharmacokinetic principles related to plasma level monitoring of drugs [1].

II. PHARMACOKINETIC PRINCIPLES

The theoretical basis of controling TCA therapy by measuring plasma levels is the assumption that the effect is mediated by a reversible binding of active compounds to the receptors, and that a given effect requires a certain drug concentration at the receptor site to be maintained for a certain period of time. Since the drug concentration cannot be measured at the receptor site, measurements at a certain reference point have to be used, and for convenience measurements in plasma are usually used. For such measurements to be valid, it must be required that the plasma drug level reflect the receptor drug level in a reproducible way with no or small variability within individuals with time and between individuals. These factors will be influenced by the rate of absorption and distribution as well as by the intra- and interindividual variations in drug binding to plasma proteins: Only when distributional equilibrium has been reached within the body can the plasma

Table 1 Pharmacokinetic Measurements Obtained by Dividing the Absolute Measurements by the Drug Plasma Concentration

Absolute measurement	Concentration-independent measurement
Amount of drug in the body (unit: mg)	Apparent volume of distribution (unit: liter)
Amount of drug eliminated per unit time (unit: $mg\text{-}h^{-1}$)	Clearance (unit: $liter\text{-}h^{-1}$)

concentration of free, unbound drug be expected to reflect the receptor drug concentration in a reproducible way. The total plasma concentration (free + bound drug), which is the usual measurement obtained, may be a poor reflection of the receptor drug concentration if there are pronounced intra- or interindividual variations in the degree of drug protein binding in plasma [1].

During repeated administration of TCA the amount of drug in the body gradually will increase until a plateau, the *steady-state level,* is reached (Fig. 1). At this point the rate of drug administration equals the rate of drug elimination. The present evidence [4-9] indicates that the kinetics of TCA are dose and concentration independent, at least within the usual therapeutic ranges. Accordingly there will be a proportionality between dose and corresponding steady-state drug levels within a given subject.*

The amount of drug in the body and the rate of elimination cannot be measured directly, but the corresponding concentration-independent measurements—apparent volume of distribution (Vd) and clearance (Cl)—can be determined directly and are immediately applicable in practice (Table 1). *The apparent volume of distribution* is a theoretical term that ideally should be determined as dose divided by plasma concentration at instantaneous distribution and equilibrium of drug in the body. The term expresses the amount of drug present in the body relative to the plasma concentration. In practice, Vd may be calculated as

$$Vd_\beta = \frac{\text{dose}}{AUC_{sd}\,\beta} \qquad (1)$$

where β is the rate constant calculated from the final slope of the single-dose curve, and AUC_{sd} is the total area under the plasma concentration-time curve after a single dose (sd). This equation is applicable whether the drug distributes according to a one- or two-compartment model. *Clearance* may be determined according to the equation

*Whereas steady-state measurements of nortriptyline have shown proportionality between dose and plasma concentrations [116], recent data on imipramine given to elderly patients have shown marked disproportional rise in the plasma level of the metabolite desipramine when the imipramine dose was increased [117].

$$Cl = \frac{\text{dose}}{AUC_{sd}} \tag{2}$$

The clearance determines the average steady-state concentration ($\bar{C}_\infty$) which is reached after repeated administration of a given dose, according to the equation

$$\bar{C}_\infty = \frac{\text{dose/time}}{Cl} \tag{3}$$

The half-life ($T_{1/2}$) is physiologically a function of both volume of distribution and clearance, as seen from the following equation:

$$T_{1/2} = \frac{\ln 2}{\beta} = \ln 2 \ \frac{Vd_\beta}{Cl} \tag{4}$$

The average steady-state level ($\bar{C}_\infty$) thus is determined only by the rate of drug administration and clearance, and is independent of volume of distribution, whereas the half-life ($T_{1/2}$) is determined both by clearance and volume of distribution. The *time* it takes to reach steady state during multiple dosing is directly related (proportionally) to the half-life (Fig. 1). When repeated doses have been given for a period corresponding to 4-5 half-lives, the plasma level has reached 94-96% of the final theoretical steady-state level.

III. ABSORPTION AND BIOAVAILABILITY

Absorption kinetics usually describe the mechanisms, site, rate, and extent of absorption. Bioavailability usually represents the quantitative description of rate and the fraction of drug that is transferred from the site of administration to a certain reference point, e.g., the systemic circulation (systemic availability).

Clinically, the rate of appearance of drug in blood after oral administration of tablets will be a function of the dissolution rate of the tablets, the passage of drug through the gastrointestinal tract to the site of absorption, which for TCA will be the intestines, as well as the absorption process itself. TCA will be totally ionized in the stomach, and no absorption will take place until the drug reaches the basic milieu of the intestines. After single oral doses of various TCA (imipramine, IP; nortriptyline, NT; desipramine, DMI) administered as tablets or in solution, the peak concentration in plasma is obtained after 2-10 h [5-8,10,11]. After multiple administration of IP, peak values were found 2-6 h after drug administration at steady state [12]. Estimates of the absorption rate constant of NT range from 0.25 to 0.70 h^{-1} [5,8], corresponding to a total duration of the

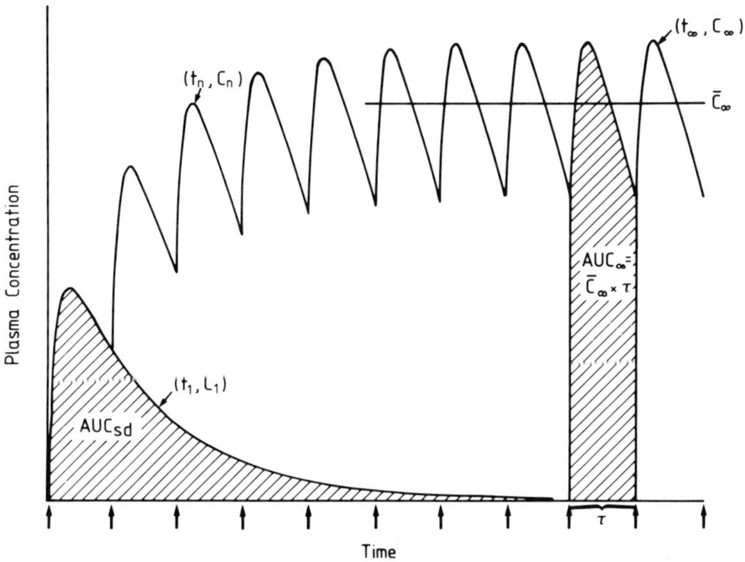

Figure 1 Theoretical plasma concentration-time curves after single (- - -) and multiple (——) oral drug administration. The calculations have been made for a drug with an absorption rate constant approximately 10 times higher than the elimination rate constant, and with dose interval (τ) = elimination half-life; AUC_{sd} = area under concentration-time curve after single dose; AUC_∞ = area under concentration-time curve through one-dose interval at steady state; t_1, t_n, t_∞ = time from dose administration to blood sampling after first dose (single dose), nth dose, and at steady state, respectively; C_1, C_n, C_∞ = concentration after first dose (single dose), nth dose, and at steady state; $\bar{C}_\infty$ = average steady-state concentration; ↑ = oral drug administration.

absorption phase of 4-12 h. However, interference with the distributional changes which take place at the same time and the relatively few samples drawn in these studies make these estimates somewhat uncertain. Administration of the drug in solution does not necessarily increase the rate of absorption, since dissolved TCA may exert a stronger, direct anticholinergic effect on the stomach, causing delayed emptying. After administration of IP or NT in solution, a 30-60-min delay before the drug appeared in the systemic circulation was seen in several cases [7,8]. Food intake immediately prior to the drug administration may delay the absorption [11], whereas food or liquid intake concomitant to drug administration may facilitate the passage of drug to the site of absorption. Concomitant measurements of drug concentration in portal and cubital vein indicated that peak concentration in portal blood appears about 30 min earlier than in the systemic circulation [13]. This may be an effect of the distribution of IP into a large distributional volume in the liver, lung, etc. before reaching the venous part of the vascular system. Studies with radiolabeled TCA given as single oral and intravenous (i.v.) doses have shown that the orally administered TCA is completely absorbed from the gut [7,8], and the same amount of radioactivity is ultimately recovered in the urine after oral and i.v. administration. Parenteral drug administration has traditionally been considered more reliable and reproducible than oral administration. However, recent research has shown that the absorption of various drugs including TCA after intramuscular (i.m.) and even i.v. administration may be incomplete and variable. Reduced availability of i.m. administered NT and DMI have been strongly indicated in several single-dose studies [10,14, 15]. IP and clomipramine (CIP) appear to be completely absorbed after i.m. administration [10,16]. Single-dose studies with i.v. administration indicate that NT but not IP may have reduced availability and cause local phlebitis, unless it is infused in a fairly large volume [7,8,10].

IV. FIRST-PASS ELIMINATION

TCA is eliminated from the body almost entirely by metabolism in the liver [3]. This mechanism of elimination is very efficient, and each time an amount of TCA passes through the liver, 30-70% will be extracted and metabolized. After oral administration, the whole dose will pass via the portal vein through the liver and a 30-70% fraction will be eliminated before reaching systemic distribution. Compared to an i.v. dose, an oral dose of TCA thus will result in lower concentrations of the parent compound in the systemic circulation and a more rapid appearance of metabolites in blood and urine [7,8]. The total amount of metabolites formed, however, will be the same after oral and i.v. administration of identical doses. Therefore, the effect of changing from oral to parenteral drug administration during continuous therapy will be that the average steady-state level of parent compound will increase, whereas the average steady-state level of metabolites will remain unchanged. Recent data on IP and CIP have generally confirmed this [16]. When IP was given orally, there was no sign of metabolism in the gut or gut wall, as judged from the appearance of IP but no DMI, the major metabolite of IP, in the portal vein immediately after administration [13]. The extent of first-pass elimination may be quantified by using the general equation for systemic availability:

$$f'f'' = \frac{AUC_{oral}/dose_{oral}}{AUC_{i.v.}/dose_{i.v.}} \tag{5}$$

where f′ represents the bioavailability factor due to possible incomplete absorption, and f″ represents the first-pass elimination [17]. As a consequence of the first-pass elimination, different terms of clearance should be used for different routes of administration:

$$\text{Systemic clearance } Cl_s = \frac{\text{dose}_{i.v.}}{AUC_{i.v.}} \tag{6}$$

$$\text{Intrinsic or oral clearance } Cl_o = \frac{\text{dose}_{oral}}{AUC_{oral}} \tag{7}$$

The oral clearance accounts for the reduced systemic availability following the first-pass elimination and is the term to be used when predicting steady-state levels during multiple oral drug administration (cf. Eq. 3). A consequence of the high hepatic extraction of TCA is that the elimination is influenced by both the hepatic enzyme activity and blood flow. Systemic clearance thus will increase with increasing flow, whereas the relationship between hepatic blood flow and oral clearance (and thereby steady-state levels–cf. Eq. 3) as yet is not fully understood [17].

V. METABOLISM

Metabolism, mainly by oxidation and conjugation, is the main route of elimination of TCA, and only 1-3% is eliminated unchanged through the kidney [8,18, 19]. The metabolism takes place in the liver, whereas extrahepatic metabolism probably is negligible in man [13,20]. The major metabolic pathways of TCA are demethylation, hydroxylation, and glucuronide coupling. N-Oxidation and dealkylation are minor metabolic pathways [3,18,19]. The main metabolic pathways are shown schematically for IP in Figs. 2 and 3. The different metabolic events, demethylation, hydroxylation, and glucuronide coupling, thus take place in sequence, and it has been shown in first-pass studies that an IP molecule may pass through all three metabolic steps–methylation, hydroxylation, glucuronide coupling–during one passage through the liver [7]. This probably reflects the close functional and anatomical link between the microsomal cytochrome P_{450}-dependent drug oxidation enzyme system which mediates demethylation and hydroxylation, and the UDP-glucuronyltransferase enzyme system that mediates the glucuronide coupling of the hydroxymetabolites [21,22]. First-pass studies also indicate that 60-85% of the first-pass elimination of IP is demethylation [7, 17]. A fraction of IP and probably most of the formed DMI is eliminated by

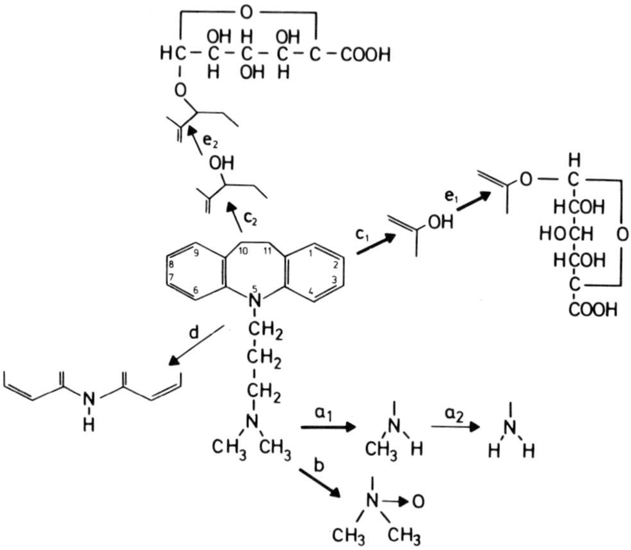

Figure 2 Pathways of imipramine metabolism, where a = demethylation of tertiary (a_1) and secondary (a_2) amine; b = N-oxide formation; c_1 = 2-hydroxylation; c_2 = 10-hydroxylation; d = dealkylation; e_1 = 2-O-glucuronide formation; e_2 = 10-O-glucuronide formation.

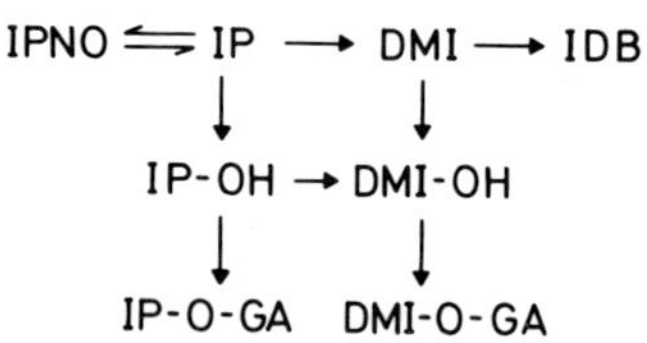

Figure 3 The pathways of imipramine metabolism in schematic form. Symbols are defined in the text.

aromatic ring hydroxylation in the 2-position and subsequent glucuronide coupling. 10-11-Hydroxylation is a minor pathway of IP-DMI metabolism.

Amitriptyline (AT) and NT differ from IP and DMI by being hydroxylated mainly by aliphatic hydroxylation in the 10-11-position and subsequent glucuronide coupling [19,23,24]. It has been shown that NT is hydroxylated to two isomers with a constant ratio [25]. Demethylation of the secondary amine to primary amine appears to be somewhat more pronounced for NT compared to DMI [18,19,26]. N-Oxide formation from IP or AT has been described in several works on urinary metabolites [18,27-29], where the N-oxide formation was found to be pronounced only during the first 12 h after administration. In plasma drawn 12 h after IP administration, IP-N-oxide (IPNO) was found in concentrations of only 5-10% of the corresponding IP levels [30]. Fifty to eighty percent of the total urinary excretion after radiolabeled single doses [7,8,18] represents known metabolites, whereas the rest appears to be polar metabolites that cannot be extracted, even after enzymatic hydrolysis of the urine [18]. After single doses about 40% of the dose appears in the urine in the first 24 h [18], and after a week, 70-100% of the dose (^{14}C-labeled IP or NT) can be recovered in urine [7,8], and only minor amounts (5-20%) are recovered in feces in man [31].

The metabolism of TCA other than IP, DMI, AT, and NT has been much less studied. Protriptyline (PT) appears to be metabolized as NT [32], and CIP follows the pattern of IP (Christiansen, unpublished data). IPNO, which is available as an antidepressant drug in several countries, is kinetically different from the other TCA. The first step in its metabolism is reduction to IP. This reduction appears to take place mainly intracellularly in the erythrocytes, brain tissue, and possibly other cells [33-35]. IPNO is apparently not metabolized in the liver to any major extent, as indicated by a high clearance and no first-pass metabolism [34]. The formed IP is subsequently metabolized as described above.

VI. ACTIVE METABOLITES

Relatively soon after IP and AT had been introduced as antidepressants, their demethylated metabolites DMI and NT were shown to have antidepressant activity of their own [36,37]. Indeed, DMI once was suspected to be the active principle of IP [38], but this can hardly be proven clinically, since IP treatment will result in significant levels of both IP and DMI in the body. In terms of therapeutic effect there is no definite difference between the tertiary and secondary amines, although there have been some indications that DMI had a weaker antidepressive effect than IP [39]. Since these conclusions were based on studies not involving plasma level monitoring, they are of somewhat limited value. The measurement of plasma levels of the assumed active compounds, and the fact that there are considerable individual variations in the ratio between tertiary and secondary amines, in particular for IP/DMI [12], makes it theoretically possible to analyze the relative contribution of each compound to the overall antidepressant effect [40]. In animal models the tertiary and secondary amines of TCA have clearly different effects [41,42], and if these model effects are at all related to the antidepressive effect, this should be reflected in the plasma level-effect relationship. Such analyses have, so far, only been attempted in a few studies. Some data thus suggest that antidepressive effect only is obtained when the plasma levels of both

IP and DMI are above certain limits [43,44]. Other analyses, assuming that IP and DMI are acting qualitatively similar, have suggested that IP is about twice as potent as DMI relative to the plasma levels [40,45]. During AT therapy the AT/NT ratio is much less variable [46], and therefore a differentiation between the effect of these two compounds is even more difficult. Demethylation of DMI appears to be negligible [18] and demethylation of NT is probably limited [28, 47], and the plasma levels of these compounds have not been studied in relation to therapy control. Recently several groups have reported measurable plasma concentrations of the hydroxy metabolites of TCA. Ziegler and others [48] and Kragh-Sørensen and others [49] thus found plasma levels of nonconjugated 10-hydroxy-NT ranging from 2/3 to 3 times the corresponding NT-levels. Preliminary data on 2-hydroxy-IP and 2-hydroxy-DMI in IP-treated patients indicated that the hydroxy metabolite levels generally were lower than the corresponding nonhydroxylated compounds IP and DMI, and among individuals there was a positive correlation between IP and 2-OH-IP levels and DMI and 2-OH-DMI levels, respectively [30]. The possible clinical significance of these metabolites is as yet unknown since no data on their plasma protein binding or clinical effects are available. In experiments on dogs it was found that 2-OH-IP was clearly more toxic on the myocardium than IP or any of the other metabolites (DMI, 2-OH-DMI) [50]. Recently Wilkerson [51] showed that 2-OH-IP also was more potent than IP and DMI in counteracting digoxin-induced cardiac arrhythmias in dogs. These studies thus indicate that some hydroxy metabolites may be related to some of the cardiac effects of TCA. It appears less likely that the hydroxy metabolites are involved in the therapeutic effect, since they do not reach the brain in appreciable amounts [52,53].*

IPNO appears to be of little quantitative significance during IP treatment [30], but when given as the parent drug it reaches significant levels in blood and brain [34]. Extended clinical studies are needed to determine the possible significance of measuring these different metabolites in relation to therapy and toxicity.

VII. DISTRIBUTION AND PROTEIN BINDING

TCA is characterized by being lipophilic and by passing biological membranes, including the blood-brain barrier, very easily. TCA thus appears in the most vascularized tissues very rapidly after administration [52,54,55]. Clinical studies with intravenous administration of single doses of various TCA (IP, AT, NT) have shown a biexponential plasma concentration-time curve compatible with a two-compartment distribution model [9,56,57]. TCA thus is rapidly distributed to

*Recently it has been shown [118] that 10-hydroxy nortriptyline is present in appreciable amounts in cereberspinal fluid, and also has the same effect on neurotransmittors as nortriptyline, indicating that the hydroxymetabolites might contribute to the therapeutic effect.

a central compartment, probably representing well-vascularized tissues such as liver, lung, heart, and brain, and more slowly to other parts of the body (peripheral compartment). Of the total amount of drug in the body, 15-40% was found in the central compartment. The tissue concentration of TCA is much higher than the concentration in blood or plasma, as reflected by the high values of apparent volume of distribution (Vd_β = 10-20 liters/kg—see Table 3). Less than 1% of the total amount of TCA in the body therefore will be present in the blood. This clearly influences the elimination of TCA from the body, since only a very small fraction of drug in the body is available for elimination per unit time. Even with the high hepatic extraction ratio (about 50%) of TCA, the elimination *rate* thus will be relatively low, and the half-life accordingly relatively long.

There are significant differences in Vd_β between different TCAs (see Table 3) [57], but the present data are insufficient for analyses of possible systematic relationships between chemical structure and distribution kinetics of TCA. IPNO differs from other TCA by distributing according to a one-compartment model and by having a comparatively small volume of distribution [34]. As seen from Table 3, interindividual variations in Vd_β with a factor 1.5-2.0 have been found in most studies. This variability may relate to variations in binding in the tissues, variations in elimination kinetics [58,59], and variations in binding to plasma constituents.

Various studies employing different methods have shown a relatively high degree of binding of TCA to plasma proteins, usually in the range of 80-95% (Table 2). Particularly for IP there is some disagreement as to the degree of binding, but it is difficult to assess if this represents true differences between different patient materials or if methodological factors play a role. Plasma protein binding of TCA has been assessed by two principles: either in vitro measurements involving the use of radiolabeled compounds and ultrafiltration or equilibrium dialysis, or a more physiological approach with simultaneous measurement of TCA concentrations in cerebrospinal fluid (CSF) and plasma. The results obtained by ultrafiltration or equilibrium dialysis may be influenced by factors as pH, temperature, sampling and storing procedures, and impurities of the radiolabeled material [70]. The use of CSF drug concentration as a measurement of free drug concentration in plasma will involve a systematic error if there are drug-binding proteins present in the CSF or if the CSF belongs to a peripheral distributional compartment not in equilibrium with the central compartment at the time of sampling. Since there are no reports on direct, within-subject comparisons of methods, it is not possible at the present time to evaluate if there are such systematic differences between different principles or methods of protein binding measurement.

Borgå and others [60] found a significantly higher degree of plasma protein binding of the tertiary amines IP and AT than that of their corresponding secondary amines DMI and NT. In accordance with this, Muscettola and others

Table 2 Results from Studies on Plasma Protein Binding of Tricyclic Antidepressants in Humans

TCA	Method[a]			n	Free fraction (% total)		Reference
					Mean	Range	
IP	UF		20°C	5	4.2 ± 0.8[b]	?	[60]
	5-HT uptake inhibition		?	?	23.8	18.5-30.4[c]	[61]
	ED		37°C	8	13.7	?	[62]
	ED		37°C	26	15	5-23	[63]
	ED		?°C	19	14.8	?	[64]
	ED		37°C	23	7.9	6.1-11.1	[65]
		CSF		12	9.5	4.4-12.9	[66]
DMI	UF		20°C	5	8.4 ± 0.9[b]	?	[60]
	UF		20°C	41	10	5-13	[4]
		CSF		12	12.9	7.7-17.2	[66]
AT	UF		20°C	5	3.6 ± 0.8[b]	?	[60]
NT	UF		20°C	5	5.5 ± 0.6[b]	?	[60]
	ED		?	5	5.8	3.2-9.6	[67]
		CSF		15	6.6	3-11	[4]
		CSF		8	9.2	5.3-14.2	[68]
		CSF		13	7.0	4.7-11.5	[69]

[a]UF = ultrafiltration; ED = equilibrium dialysis; CSF = concurrent measurement of drug concentration in plasma and cerebrospinal fluid.
[b]Mean ± SD.
[c]95% fiducial limits.

[66] found lower CSF/plasma concentration ratio of IP than of DMI (Table 2).

In all studies an interindividual variation in percentage of free fraction with a factor 2-3 have been found. In several studies the distribution was fairly close to normal [4,63, 69, 71], and relatively few subjects will have markedly high or low degree of protein binding. This interindividual variability is small compared to the interindividual variability in total plasma concentration TCA, and it is therefore not surprising that Muscettola and others [66] found a high degree of correlation between CSF and plasma levels of IP and DMI in spite of a variation in CSF/plasma concentration ratio with a factor 2-3. Whereas Borgå and others [60] and Alexanderson and Borgå [72] found only small intraindividual day-to-day variations in protein binding, the CSF/plasma ratios calculated from the data of Muscettola and others [66] showed intraindividual variations of the same magnitude as the interindividual variations. In the light of the distribution patterns discussed above, one may expect that plasma protein binding measurements as a supplement to plasma level monitoring only will be needed in a certain smaller number of patients. Besides being genetically determined [72], abnormal protein binding may be related to age, sex, pregnancy, disease, stress, etc.

Relatively few data are available on the qualitative aspects of the protein binding of TCA. Pruitt and Dayton [62] reported a 50-60% binding of IP to commercial 1% human α-globulin, and similar results for β-globulins. Borgå and others [71] found that IP binds to albumin, α_1-acid-glycoprotein, and lipoproteins. In studies on fresh plasma it was shown that the degree of protein binding of IP correlated well to the concentration of α_1-acid-glycoprotein, but not to the albumin concentration [65]. Variations in α_1-acid-glycoprotein concentration thus explained about 60% of the total variability in IP binding.

Spuriously low total plasma levels of TCA may be seen in blood samples drawn in vacutainers [73]. A substance in the stopper of these tubes (tris-2-butoxyethylphosphate) causes this effect by an apparently selective displacement of TCA from the binding to α_1-acid-glycoproteins [71]. α_1-Acid-glycoprotein is one of the "acute phase" proteins that may rise in various stress situations after physical exercise etc. [74]. Such effects thus appear to be obvious explanations of the day-to-day fluctuations in total concentrations of TCA seen in most steady-state studies [44,75-77].

Variations or changes in the plasma protein binding may have some effects on the kinetics of the drug. The total amount of TCA in the body will not be influenced by changes in plasma protein binding, since TCA in plasma is only a very small fraction of the total amount. Apparent volume of distribution (Vd_β, Eq. 1) may for obvious reasons be influenced by the degree of protein binding. Indeed, it has been suggested [78] that individual variations in Vd_β may be explained by corresponding variations in plasma protein binding, but direct evidence of this is lacking. The hepatic extraction of TCA involves both the free and bound fraction in blood, and most likely the proteins can be considered as a transport vehicle, facilitating the transport of drug from the tissues to the site of elimination.

VIII. CLEARANCE, HALF-LIVES, AND STEADY-STATE LEVELS

Following the development of methods for quantitative determination of TCA in plasma or blood, several groups have attempted to characterize the quantita-

Table 3 Pharmacokinetic Measurements of Tricyclic Antidepressants Obtained from Single-Dose Studies in Healthy Volunteers[a]

TCA	Systemic clearance $Cl_s = \frac{dose}{AUC_{i.v.}}$ (liters/min)	Oral clearance $Cl_o = \frac{dose}{AUC_o}$ (liters/min)	First-pass elimination $1 - f = 1 - \frac{AUC_o}{AUC_{i.v.}}$	Apparent volume of distribution $Vd_\beta = \frac{dose}{\beta \cdot AUC_{i.v.}}$ (liters/kg)	Half-life $T_{1/2} = \frac{\ln 2}{\beta}$ (h)	No. of subjects—male + female	Reference
IP	*1.17* (0.83-1.47)	*2.31* (1.43-3.79)	*0.44* (0.21-0.64)	*11.5* (9.2-14.9)	*8.6* (6.0-11.2)	5 + 0	[57][b]
	1.10 (0.70-1.70)	*2.52* (0.91-3.54)	*0.49* (0.23-0.71)	*17.5* (14.3-21.0)	*11.7* (8-14)	1 + 2	[7]
	1.03 (0.56-1.52)	*3.08* (1.08-5.00)	*0.39* (0.29-0.52)	*15.4* (10.7-22.1)	*10.2* (7.5-13.8)	1 + 4	[10][c]
DMI	–	*2.15* (1.33-3.36)	–	–	*17.1* (12.5-24.7)	5 + 3	[6][d]
AT	*0.46* (0.32-0.64)	–	–	*8.9* (6.4-11.3)	*17.1* (15.5-19.5)	4 + 0	[9]
	–	*2.47* (0.97-3.41)	–	–	*36.1* (31.0-46.6)	3 + 1	[79]
NT	–	*0.84* (0.52-1.30)	–	–	*26.8* (18.2-35.0)	5 + 3	[6][d]
	0.53 (0.32-0.68)	*1.04* (0.64-1.42)	*0.48* (0.41-0.51)	*19.1* (15.1-23.1)	*33.3* (17.8-57.8)	5 + 0	[57][b]
	–	*2.87* (0.93-4.24)	–	–	*15* (6-28)	10 + 0	[11]
CIP	*0.39* (0.31-0.48)	*1.07* (0.59-1.99)	*0.52* (0.22-0.81)	*11.9* (7.1-19.8)	*24.7* (20.1-39.6)	4 + 1	[16][c]
IPNO	*0.85* (0.66-0.98)	*0.84* (0.73-1.17)	*0.04* (−0.33-0.16)	*2.5* (1.9-3.4)	*2.3* (2.0-2.5)	3 + 2	[34]
PT	–	*0.26* (0.14-0.40)	–	–	*78.4* (54.6-124.0)	5	[80][e]
	–	*0.34* (0.17-0.51)	–	–	*74.3* (53.6-91.7)	6 + 2	[81]
Doxepine	*4.95* (1.87-10.28)	–	–	–	*16.8* (8.2-24.5)	6 + 1	[82]

[a]Figures in italic type (e.g., *1.17*) indicate the mean; figures in roman type (e.g., 0.83-1.47) indicate the range.
[b]Same subjects in IP and NT studies.
[c]Systemic clearance determined after intramuscular administration.
[d]Same subjects in DMI and NT studies.
[e]Subjects' sex not indicated.

tive aspects of their kinetics. Table 3 shows comparable kinetic data obtained from single-dose studies in healthy volunteers aged 20-40 years. Generally there is good agreement between different studies on the same drug, and only a few discrepancies require further studies to be fully understood. For example, a recent study by Nakano and Hollister [11] showed clearly shorter half-lives and higher oral clearance of NT than that found in earlier studies [6,8,57]. One possible explanation is that the use of vacutainers in the study of Nakano and Hollister [11] has resulted in spuriously low and variable plasma concentration measurements [71,73]. The estimated half-lives of AT were shorter after intravenous (i.v.) single doses [9] than found after oral single doses [79] or after multiple dosing [83]. Difficulties in determining the final slope after the relatively small i.v. dose of AT (15-mg AT base) may be an explanation of these findings.

Following i.v. administration of IP, the IP concentration could be determined until 30-48 h [57]. After the initial distribution phase lasting 3-6 h, a final slope could be identified with half-lives of 6-11 h, and there was no sign of a later slower elimination phase. Data from steady-state studies indicate that some patients may have longer IP half-lives [12]. The difference in age between depressed patients and healthy volunteers appears to be the most likely explanation of this discrepancy.

Apart from these possible shortcomings the considerable amount of data summarized in Table 3 form a good pharmacokinetic basis for plasma level monitoring, and they also permit some analyses of systematic differences in kinetics of different TCA: In two crossover studies, the kinetics of NT were compared with the kinetics of DMI and IP, respectively: NT had significantly lower oral clearance and longer half-lives than DMI [6], and compared to IP, NT had lower systemic and oral clearance, higher apparent volume of distribution, and consequently much longer half-lives [57]. The reported half-lives of DMI are generally longer than those of IP [6,10,57], which is consistent with data from steady-state studies [12]. The difference in oral clearance between NT and DMI corresponded well to the higher steady-state levels of NT compared to DMI obtained in the same subjects given the same multiple oral doses of the two drugs [6]. The differences in oral clearance between IP and CIP (Table 3) is consistent with the corresponding differences in steady-state level/dose ratios found in studies on patients [12,84]. The low oral clearance of PT (Table 3) is also consistent with the very high steady-state level/dose ratio seen in patients [85,86].

The interindividual variability of the oral clearance is generally more pronounced than that of the systemic clearance (Table 3), but for NT a significant correlation ($r = 0.93$, $n = 6$) between the two measurements was found, and accordingly the first-pass elimination showed small variations [8]. IP and CIP, on the other hand, show pronounced interindividual variations in first-pass elimination [7,16,57]. The present data are insufficient to determine if this represents a systematic difference between secondary and tertiary amines. In general, more studies in crossover design are needed before a systematic analysis of the relation-

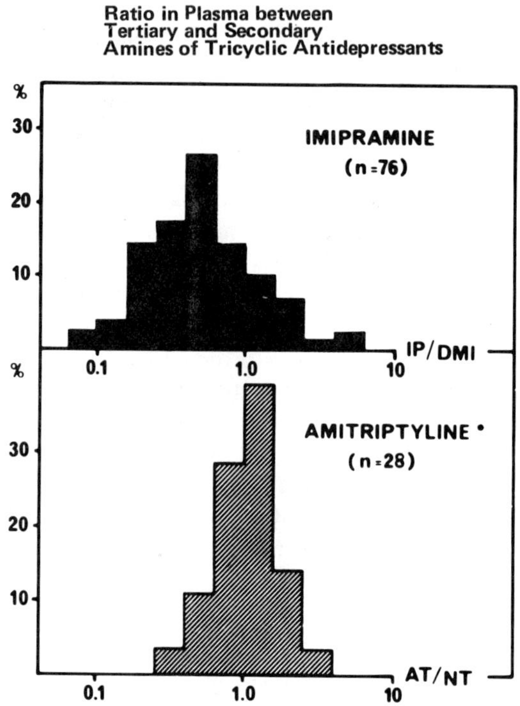

Figure 4 Distribution histograms (log-scale) of steady-state imipramine/desipramine ratio in 76 imipramine-treated patients and steady-state amitriptyline/nortriptyline ratio in 28 amitriptyline-treated patients. (*Source:* Refs. 12 and 87).

ship between chemical structure and pharmacokinetic properties of TCA can be carried out. As discussed in previous sections, the kinetics of IPNO differs markedly from other TCA by the lack of first-pass elimination and with almost all elimination taking place extrahepatically [34,35].

Steady-state kinetics point out other interesting differences between TCA analogues. When comparing IP- and AT-treated patients, it was found that the ratio between the parent compound and the demethylated metabolite (DMI or NT, respectively) was significantly lower for IP than for AT, and that the interindividual variability of this ratio was significantly more pronounced for IP (see Fig. 4) [12,87]. For CIP the ratio between the parent compound and the demethylated metabolite in plasma is even lower than for IP, but the interindividual variability is less pronounced [84]. The pronounced individual variations in IP/DMI ratio indicate that the demethylation and hydroxylation (see Fig. 3) are processes that are varying independently among individuals; perhaps the two types of oxidative biotransformation are mediated by different species of cytochrome P_{450}-microsomal enzymes with different stereospecificity [88-90]. This would also explain why IP and NT clearance showed no significant correlation among individuals [57], whereas the oral clearance of NT and DMI correlated well [6].

IX. DOSE SCHEDULE AND PREDICTION OF STEADY-STATE PLASMA LEVELS

Combining Eqs. (2) and (3) yields

$$\bar{C}_{\infty} = \frac{AUC_{sd}}{\tau} \qquad (8)$$

where τ is the dose interval during multiple-dose administration, and AUC_{sd} represents the area under the plasma concentration-time curve after a single dose of same amount as that given during multiple administration (cf. Fig. 1; $AUC_{sd} = AUC_{\infty} = \bar{C}_{\infty}\tau$). Alexanderson [5,6,91] and recently Braithwaite and others [92] have shown that such prediction of steady-state levels of NT in fact is possible in clinical practice. Nagy and Johansson [10] also found a correlation between AUC_{sd} and C_{∞} of IP, whereas prediction of the plasma levels of the main metabolite DMI was not possible. In these studies the AUC_{sd} was in fact not related to $\bar{C}_{\infty}$, but to a single concentration measurement (C_{∞}) obtained at a certain time (8-12 h) after dose administration during steady state. As shown in Fig. 5, the relationship between AUC_{sd} and C_{∞} is not necessarily constant in all situations. These computed relationships are based on the assumption that Vd_{β} is relatively constant among individuals compared to the variations in clearance, and these curves show that the dose interval (τ), the time of sampling (t_{∞}), and the variations in $T_{1/2}$ in the patient population determine how constant the relationship between AUC_{sd} and C_{∞} will be. With a dose interval (τ) of 24 h and blood sampling in the middle of the dose interval (t_{∞} = 12 h) there will be an almost constant ratio between AUC_{sd} and C_{∞} over a wide range of $T_{1/2}$ from 10 to 100 h, which is about the total variability in $T_{1/2}$ of NT reported by Alexanderson [93]. Figure 5 also shows which single concentration measurements (C_{∞}) most constantly reflect the average steady-state concentration ($\bar{C}_{\infty}$, cf. Eq. 8).

The fluctuations in plasma level through the dose interval are related to the rates of absorption, distribution, and elimination, anf for TCA the last factor is probably the most important one. Different TCAs show different degrees of such fluctuations as a consequence of their different pharmacokinetic properties [12,67,77,94,95]. For practical purposes both in therapy control and prediction the blood sampling should take place not earlier than 8-12 h after last dose, in order to avoid the variability from absorption and distribution.

Recently Braithwaite and others [92] and Cooper and Simpson [96]

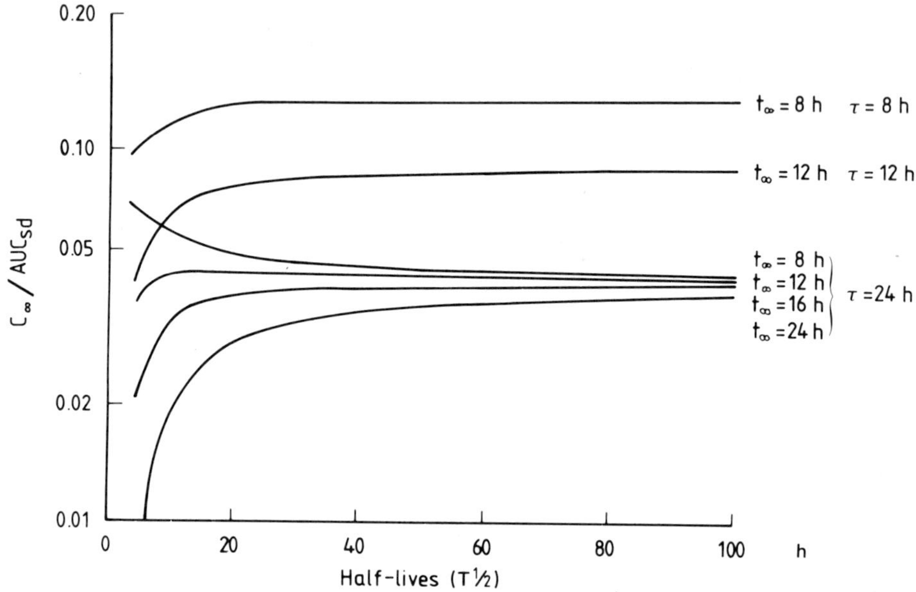

Figure 5 Computed theoretical values of the ratio between the steady-state plasma concentration (C_∞) measured at a certain time (t_∞) after last dose, and the area under the plasma concentration curve after administration of a single dose. The computed curves are based on the assumption that there are no inter-individual variations in apparent volume of distribution and that absorption and distribution have been completed at the time of sampling. The curves show the C_∞/AUC_{sd} for different sampling times (t_∞), dose intervals (τ), and half-lives ($T_{1/2}$).

showed that concentration measurements of NT from 12 to 72 h after a single dose (C_1, Fig. 1) correlated well to concentration measurements obtained at steady state (C_∞, t_∞ = 12-24 h). Figure 6 shows computed correlations between C_1 and C_∞ for different sampling and dose schedules, assuming negligible variability of Vd_β over a simulated range of $T_{1/2}$ (6-120 h). Over a certain range of $T_{1/2}$ variations the correlation between the two measurements may be close to linear, and these theoretical curves are fairly compatible with the clinical data reported by Braithwaite and others [92] and Cooper and Simpson [96]. The reliability of this type of prediction thus depends on the interplay between dose- and blood-sampling schedule and the range of half-lives expected for the given drug in the given population. According to similar principles it should also be possible to use single concentration measurements taken after the second, third, or nth dose (C_n, Fig. 1) for prediction of steady-state concentrations, but clinical data on this are not available. Such a procedure would possibly be more applic-

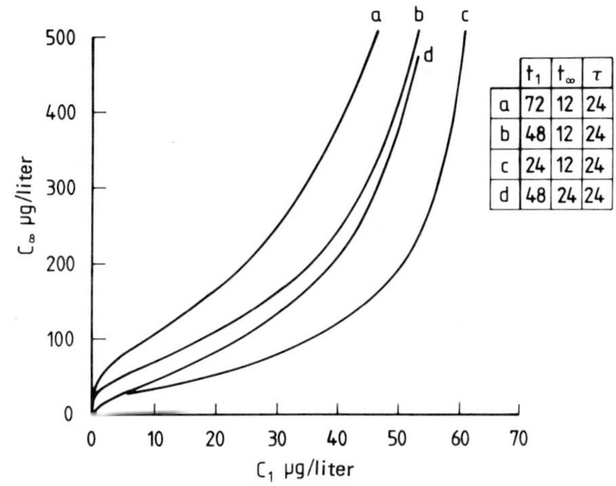

	t_1	t_∞	τ
a	72	12	24
b	48	12	24
c	24	12	24
d	48	24	24

Figure 6 Theoretical correlation between the plasma concentration after a single dose (C_1) and at steady state (C_∞), when different sampling times after the single dose (t_1) and after last dose at steady state (t_∞) and different dose intervals (τ) are used. Values of t_1, t_∞, and τ given in hours. The computed values are based on the assumption that there are no interindividual variations in apparent volume of distribution ($f \cdot dose/Vd_\beta$) = 70 h/liter) or in absorption rate constant ($k_a = 0.5\ h^{-1}$). The curves cover a range of interindividual variations in half-lives from 6 to 120 hours.

able for drugs with active metabolites. After a single dose the levels of the metabolites very often will be too low for making accurate predictions [7,10].

X. FACTORS INFLUENCING THE KINETICS OF TRICYCLIC ANTIDEPRESSANTS

Various factors related to the subject or the milieu or both may influence the kinetics of TCA and be responsible for the inter- and intraindividual variability in kinetics discussed in previous sections. In a study on mono- and dizygotic twins, Alexanderson and others [97] found strong evidence of a genetic control of the variability in steady-state levels of NT. Comparison between subjects exposed and not exposed to other drugs (barbiturates etc.) showed that such exogenous factors also contributed to the total individual variability. Since steady-state levels are determined by the clearance, these data indicate that the hepatic metabolism of NT is both under genetic control and is influenced by concurrent exposure to other xenobiotics. It is not known how the activity of the different species of cytochrome P_{450}-dependent microsomal enxymes discussed in previous sections is genetically determined or related.

In a twin study on single-oral-dose kinetics of NT, the results indicated that both the half-lives ($T_{1/2}$) and the apparent volume of distribution calculated as Cl_o [$T_{1/2}$/(ln 2)] were independently genetically determined [91,93]. Since the first-pass elimination is included in this determination of volume of distribution, it is difficult to assess if there is a true genetically determined variation of distributional volume.

Studies on the plasma protein binding of NT in non-drug-exposed twins showed a significantly lower within-pair variability in monozygotic than in dizygotic twins, pointing to a genetic control of the binding [72]. To which extent this control is associated with quantitative or qualitative properties of particular plasma proteins is not known.

Recently, two independent groups have reported clear age-related differences in TCA kinetics. Nies and others [98] found that in IP-treated patients there was a significant correlation between age and steady-state levels of both IP and DMI. Five patients, 65 years old or more, had significantly higher steady-state levels of both IP and DMI than those found in 5 patients of lower age. After discontinuation of the IP treatment, the disappearance rate of DMI, but not of IP, was significantly lower in the oldest patients. In 12 AT-treated patients there was a similar age correlation for the AT steady-state levels, but interestingly not for the NT levels.

In a study of the steady-state kinetics of IP in 76 patients, 20-65 years old, clear age-related differences in steady-state levels of IP, and to some extent of DMI and IP + DMI, were found (see Fig. 7) [12,40]. This study showed significantly higher steady-state levels with higher age already fromt he 30-39-year age group and upward. These analyses were based on dose- and weight-corrected plasma levels, and this procedure may introduce systematic errors if obesity is more pronounced in certain age groups. However, analyses of dose-corrected but not weight-corrected plasma levels showed the same age-related changes (unpublished data).

It is interesting that in reports on steady-state levels from about 600 patients on NT treatment, no or only weak age correlation was found [78,99,100]. In light of the negative finding concerning NT in the study of Nies and others [98], one might speculate whether NT is different from IP and AT in this respect.*

In 35 AT-treated and 30 NT-treated patients, Ziegler and Biggs [101] found no correlation between age and dose- and weight-corrected steady-state levels of AT + NT and NT, respectively. The few patients in the higher age groups (median age below 40 in both materials) may explain these negative findings. Higher steady-state levels of NT were found in black patients, but the possible effects of differences in obesity in the different groups were not ruled out.

*Kragh-Sørensen and Larsen [116] have recently demonstrated a clear age relationship for nortriptyline steady-state levels in hospitalized patients.

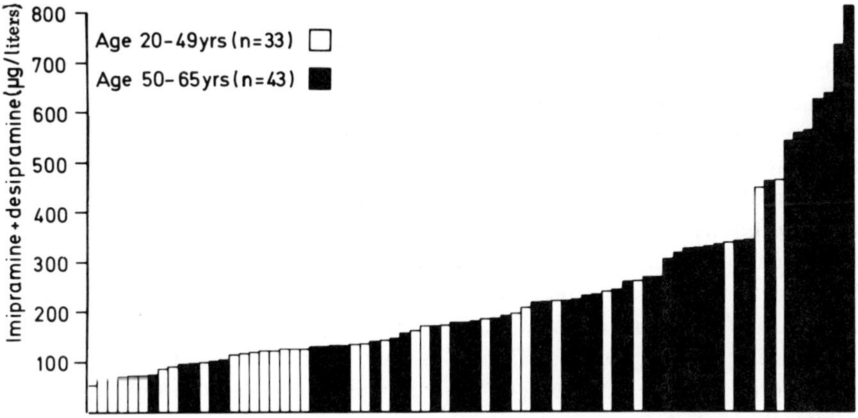

Figure 7 Steady-state plasma levels of imipramine plus desipramine in 76 patients. Concentration measurements corrected for differences in dose and body weight to 3.5 mg/kg/day. (*Source:* Ref. 40.)

The use of weight-corrected dose or weight-corrected plasma level measurements may be a significant problem in studies on sex differences, but the present data indicate that the possible between-sexes variability is insignificant compared to the within-sex group variability whatever procedure is being used for data analysis [12]. In 76 IP-treated patients [12] the interindividual variation in steady-state levels of IP and DMI was *not* reduced by correcting for the individual differences in body weight (unpublished data). The drug elimination (clearance), which is probably determined by liver size, hepatic enzyme activity, and hepatic blood flow, thus is better correlated to age than to body weight.

Various diseases may be expected to influence the kinetics of TCA: liver affection of a certain degree of severity may reduce the hepatic clearance of various drugs [102,103]. Liver blood flow may be influenced by cardiac disease, physical activity, food intake, etc., and thereby the TCA kinetics may be influenced [17]. Infections or stress of different kind may influence the composition of plasma proteins and thereby the drug binding in plasma. However, at the present time no consistent clinical data are available that can elucidate the practical significance of these possibilities.

Among the milieu factors that may influence the kinetics of TCA, interaction with other concurrently administered drugs probably is one of the most likely and relevant factors to be aware of. It has been shown that barbiturates may lower the steady-state levels of TCA [80,97,104], probably through the well-known stimulatory effect of barbiturates on the activity of the microsomal drug oxidation system. Several clinical studies have shown that different neuroleptics, phenothiazines, thioxanthenes, and butyrophenones may inhibit the metabolism of TCA [17,59,105]. The mechanism behind this interaction appears to be a competitive inhibition of the hydroxylation of the TCA [106,107]. The consequence of this inhibitory effect is that the steady-state levels of TCA during therapy will rise if neuroleptics are added [108,109]. For perphenazine a certain relationship between dose and interaction effect has been found in patients [107], and the effect was not seen in patients given relatively low doses (12 mg/day [49]). The interaction effect was found to be reversible even in patients taking neuroleptics for 10-15 years [105]. Methylphenidate has been shown to have a similar inhibitory effect on TCA metabolism, probably by a competitive inhibition of the microsomal drug oxidation [110].

The possible clinical significance of these interactions on TCA elimination and steady-state kinetics should be viewed in relation to the knowledge about the relationship between steady-state levels and clinical effects as discussed in the introduction. These pharmacokinetic interactions thus may influence the clinical effect of TCA both in positive and negative directions depending on drug and patient, and in addition there may be a possibility of pharmacodynamic interactions.

In protein binding studies, Borgå and others [60] found that in vitro addition of various acidic, neutral, and basic drugs in therapeutic concentration caused a statistically signigicant increase in the free fraction of DMI, but in any case not more than by a factor 0.4. A displacement effect of this magnitude probably will be of limited practical significance in therapy control, although it adds to the variability and therefore should be controlled in research projects. More direct clinical data on interactions at the protein binding level with steady-state level measurements etc. are not available.

Several clinical studies have indicated that benxodiazepines have no significant effect on the kinetics of TCA [80,111,112].

Relatively less information is available on the influence of nondrug xenobiotics on the TCA kinetics. Perel and others [113] reported that patients smoking more than 15 cigarettes or 6 cigars per day had significantly lower steady-state plasma levels of IP + DMI than had patients not smoking. Norman and others [114] studying NT and Ziegler and Biggs [101] studying AT and NT found no difference in steady-state levels between nonsmokers and those smoking more than 10 cigarettes per day. To what extent these discrepancies are related to different definitions of smokers or other variables cannot be settled, and more studies in this field are needed.

Steady-state plasma levels of TCA thus may be influenced by a variety of factors, but generally the individual patient retains a certain plasma level on a given dose with only small and nonsystematic fluctuations over months and years [91,115].

In general, more research on the factors influencing the kinetics of TCA should be initiated. The increasing use of plasma level monitoring in TCA therapy certainly offers new possibilities for extending such investigation to a larger patient population. Increased ability to control such kinetic variables, as well as other variables related to patients and environment, should ultimately improve the efficacy and safety in the clinical use of TCA.

REFERENCES

1. L. F. Gram, Plasma level monitoring of tricyclic antidepressants. *Clin. Pharmacokinet. 2:*237-251, 1977.
2. F. Sjöqvist, Monitoring of antidepressant drug plasma levels: The next ten years. In *Perspectives in Psychopharmacotherapy.* International Symposium organized in collaboration with the World Health Organization. Florence, 1977.
3. L. F. Gram, Metabolism of tricyclic antidepressants: A review. *Dan. Med. Bull. 21:*218-231, 1974.
4. F. Sjöqvist, W. Hammer, O. Borgå, and D. L. Azarnoff, Pharmacological significance of the plasma level of monomethylated tricyclic antidepressants. In *The Present Status of Psychotropic Drugs* (Cerletti, ed.). Excerpta Medica International Congress Series no. 180. Amsterdam, Excerpta Medica, 1969, pp. 128-136.
5. B. Alexanderson, Pharmacokinetics of nortriptyline in man after single and multiple oral doses: The predictability of steady-state plasma concentrations from single-dose plasma level data. *Eur. J. Clin. Pharmacol. 4:*82-91, 1972.
6. B. Alexanderson, Pharmacokinetics of desmethylimipramine and nortriptyling in man after single and multiple oral doses. *Eur. J. Clin. Pharmacol. 5:* 1-10, 1972.
7. L. F. Gram and J. Christiansen, First-pass metabolism of imipramine in man. *Clin. Pharmacol. Ther. 17:*555-563, 1975.
8. L. F. Gram and K. Fredricson Overø, First-pass metabolism of nortriptyline in man. *Clin. Pharmacol. Ther. 18:*305-314, 1975.
9. A. Jørgensen and V. Hansen, Pharmacokinetics of amitriptyline infused infused intravenously in man. *Eur. J. Clin. Pharmacol. 10:*337-341, 1976.
10. A. Nagy and R. Johansson, Plasma levels of imipramine and desipramine in man after different routes of administration. *Naunyn-Schmiedebergs Arch. Pharmakol. Exp. Pathol. 290:*145-160, 1975.
11. S. Nakano and L. E. Hollister, No circadian effect on nortriptyline kinetics in man. *Clin. Pharmacol. Ther. 23:*199-203, 1978.
12. L. F. Gram, I. Søndergaard, J. Christiansen, G. Odden Petersen, P. Bech, N. Reisby, I. Ibsen, J. Ortmann, A. Nagy, S. J. Dencker, O. Jacobsen and O. Krautwald, Steady state kinetics of imipramine in patients. *Psychopharmacology 54:*255-261, 1977.
13. H. Dencker, S. J. Dencker, A. Green, and A. Nagy, Intestinal absorption,

demethylation, and enterohepatic circulation of imipramine studied by portal catheterization in man. *Clin. Pharmacol. Ther. 19:*584-586, 1976.
14. B. Alexanderson, O. Borgå, and G. Alván, The availability of orally administered nortriptyline. *Eur. J. Clin. Pharmacol. 5:*181-185, 1973.
15. G. Alván, O. Borgå, M. Lund, L. Palmér, and B. Siwers, First pass hydroxylation of nortriptyline: Concentration of parent drug and major matabolites in plasma. *Eur. J. Clin. Pharmacol. 11:*219-224, 1977.
16. A. Nagy and R. Johansson, The demethylation of imipramine and clomipramine as apparent from their plasma kinetics. *Psychopharmacology 54:* 125-131, 1977.
17. L. F. Gram, Factors influencing the metabolism of tricyclic antidepressants: Studies on interactions and first-pass elimination. *Dan. Med. Bull. 24:*81-89, 1977.
18. J. Christiansen, L. F. Gram, B. Kofod, and O. Rafaelsen, Imipramine metabolism in man. *Psychopharmacologia* (Berlin) *11:*255-264, 1967.
19. B. Alexanderson and O. Borgå, Urinary excretion of nortriptyline and five of its metabolites in man after single and multiple oral doses. *Eur. J. Clin. Pharmacol. 5:*174-180, 1973.
20. R. Minder, F. Schnetzer, and M. H. Bickel, Hepatic and extra-hepatic metabolism of the psychotropic drugs, chlorpromazine, imipramine, and imipramine-N-oxide. *Naunyn-Schmiedebergs Arch. Pharmakol. Exp. Pathol. 268:*334-347, 1971.
21. C. von Bahr, Metabolism of tricyclic antidepressants: Pharmacokinetics and molecular aspects. Doctoral thesis, Karolinska Institute, Stockholm, 1972.
22. M. H. Bickel and H. Börner, Uptake, subcellular distribution, and transfer process of imipramine and its metabolites formed in rat liver perfusion systems. *Naunyn-Schmiedebergs Arch. Pharmakol. Exp. Pathol. 284:*339-352, 1974.
23. C. G. Hammar, B. Alexanderson, B. Holmstedt, and F. Sjöqvist, Gas chromatography-mas spectrometry of nortriptyline in body fluids of man. *Clin. Pharmacol. Ther. 12:*496-505, 1971.
24. O. Borgå and M. Garle, A gas chromatographic method for the quantitative determination of nortriptyline and some of its metabolites in human plasma and urine. *J. Chromatogr. 68:*77-88, 1972.
25. L. Bertilsson and B. Alexanderson, Stereospecific hydroxylation of nortriptyline in man in relation to interindividual differences in its steady-state plasma level. *Eur. J. Clin. Pharmacol. 4:*201-205, 1972.
26. M. H. Bickel, M. Flückiger, and M. Baggiolini, Vergleichende Demethylierung von tricyclischen Psychopharmaka durch Rattenleber-Mikrosomen. *Naunyn-Schmiedebergs Arch. Pharmakol. Exp. Pathol. 256:*360-366, 1967.
27. M. H. Bickel, Liver metabolic reactions: Tertiary amine N-dealkylation, tertiary amine N-oxidation, N-oxide reduction, and N-oxide N-dealkylation. *Arch. Biochem. Biophys. 148:*54-62, 1971.
28. E. Eschenhof and J. Rieder, Untersuchungen uber das Schicksal des Antidepressivums Amitriptylin im Organismus der Ratte und des Menschen. *Arzneim.-Forsch. 19:*957-966, 1969.

29. G. Santagostino, R. M. Facino, and D. Pirillo, Urinary excretion of amitriptyline N-oxide in humans. *J. Pharm. Sci. 63:*1690-1691, 1974.
30. L. F. Gram, Plasma level monitoring of tricyclic antidepressants: Methodological and pharmacokinetic considerations. In *Workshop on Plasma Level Monitoring of Tricyclic Antidepressants* (L. F. Gram, comp.). Eleventh Congress Coll. Int. Neuropsychopharmacol. Vienna, *Comm. Psychopharmacol. 2:*373-380, 1978.
31. J. L. Crammer, B. Scott, H. Woods, and B. Rolfe, Metabolism of ^{14}C-imipramine, I: Excretion in the rat and in man. *Psychopharmacologia* (Berlin) *12:*263-277, 1968.
32. S. F. Sisenwine, C. O. Tio, and S. R. Schrader, The biotransformation of protriptyline in man, pig, and dog. *J. Pharmacol. Exp. Ther. 175:*51-59, 1970.
33. M. H. Bickel, H. J. Weder, and H. Aebi, Metabolic interconversions between imipramine, its N-oxide, and its desmethyl derivative in rat tissues in vitro. *Biochem. Biophys. Res. Comm. 33:*1012-1018, 1968.
34. A. Nagy and T. Hansen, The kinetics of imipramine-N-oxide in man. *Acta Pharmacol. Toxicol. 42:*58-67, 1978.
35. A. Nagy, The kinetics of imipramine-N-oxide in rat. *Acta Pharmacol. Toxicol. 42:*68-72, 1978.
36. J. E. Oltman and S. Fredman, Preliminary investigations of desmethylimipramine. *Amer. J. Psychiat. 119:*370-371, 1962.
37. J. E. Oltman and S. Friedman, Evaluation of nortriptyline in the treatment of affective disorder (and comparison with other drugs). *Amer. J. Psychiatry 119:*988-991, 1963.
38. J. R. Gillette, J. V. Dingell, F. Sulzer, R. Kuntzmann, and B. B. Brodie, Isolation from rat brain of a metabolic product, desmethylimipramine, that mediates the antidepressant activity of imipramine (Tofranil). *Experientia 17:*417-448, 1961.
39. American Medical Association, Council on Drugs, A new antidepressant: Desipramine hydrochloride. *JAMA 194:*82-83, 1965.
40. L. F. Gram, N. Reisby, P. Bech, A. Nagy, and J. Christiansen, Factors influencing pharmacokinetics and clinical effects of tricyclic antidepressants. In *Depressive Disorders* (S. Garattini, ed.). Stuttgart and New York, Schattauer Verlag, 1978, pp. 337-346.
41. A. Carlsson, H. Corrodi, K. Fuxe, and T. Hökfelt, Effect of antidepressant drugs on the depletion of intraneuronal brain 5-hydroxytryptamine stores caused by 4-methyl-α-ethyl-meta-tyramine. *Eur. J. Pharmacol. 5:*357-366, 1969.
42. A. Carlsson, H. Corrodi, K. Fuxe, and T. Hökfelt, Effects of some antidepressant drugs on the depletion of intraneuronal brain catecholamine stores caused by 4-α-dimethyl-meta-tyramine. *Eur. J. Pharmacol. 5:*367-373, 1969.
43. L. F. Gram, N. Reisby, I. Ibsen, A. Nagy, S. J. Dencker, P. Bech, G. O. Petersen, and J. Christiansen, Plasma levels and antidepressive effect of imipramine. *Clin. Pharmacol. Ther. 19:*318-324, 1976.

44. N. Reisby, L. F. Gram. P. Bech, A. Nagy, G. O. Petersen, J. Ortmann, I. Ibsen, S. J. Dencker, O. Jacobsen, O. Krautwald, I. Søndergaard, and J. Christiansen, Imipramine: Clinical effect and pharmacokinetic variability. *Psychopharmacology 54:*263-272, 1977.
45. J. M. Perel, F. Irani, M. Hurwic, A. H. Glassman, and A. A. Manian, Tricyclic antidepressants: Relationship among pharmacokinetics, metabolism and clinical outcome. In *Depressive Disorders* (S. Garattini, ed.). Stuttgart and New York, Schattauer Verlag, 1978, pp. 325-336.
46. D. J. Kupfer, I. Hanin, D. G. Spiker, T. Grau, and P. Coble, Amitriptyline plasma levels and clinical response in primary depression. *Clin. Pharmacol. Ther. 22:*904-911, 1977.
47. F. Sjöqvist, B. Alexanderson, M. Åsberg, L. Bertilsson, O. Borgå, B. Hamberger, and D. Tuck, Pharmacokinetics and biological effects of nortriptyline in man. *Acta Pharmacol. Toxicol.,* Suppl. *29:*255-280, 1971.
48. V. E. Ziegler, T. A. Fuller, and J. T. Biggs, Nortriptyline and 10-hydroxy-nortriptyline in plasma concentrations. *J. Pharm. Pharmacol. 28:*849-850, 1976.
49. P. Kragh-Sørensen, O. Borgå, M. Garle, L. Bovig-Hansen, C. E. Hansen, E. F. Huidberg, N.-E. Larsen, and F. Sjöqvist, Effects of simultaneous treatment with low doses of perphenazine and plasma and urine concentrations of nortriptyline and 10-hydroxy-nortriptyline. *Eur. J. Clin. Pharmacol. 11:* 479-483, 1977.
50. B. S. Jandhyala, M. L. Steenberg, J. M. Perel, A. A. Marian, and J. P. Buckley, Effects of imipramine, chlorimipramine, and its metabolites in the hemodynamics and myocardial contractility of anesthetized dogs. *Eur. J. Pharmacol. 42:*403-410, 1977.
51. R. D. Wilkerson, Antiarrhythmic effects of tricyclic antidepressant drugs in ouabain-induced arrhythmias in the dog. *J. Pharmacol. Exp. Ther. 205:* 666-674, 1978.
52. M. H. Bickel and H. J. Weder, The total fate of a drug: Kinetics of distribution, excretion, and formation of 14 metabolites in rats treated with imipramine. *Arch. Int. Pharmacodyn. 173:*433-463, 1968.
53. J. Christiansen and L. F. Gram, Imipramine and its metabolites in human brain. *J. Pharm. Pharmacol. 25:*604-608, 1973.
54. G. B. Cassano, S. E. Sjöstrand, and E. Hansson, Distribution and fate of C^{14}-amitriptyline in mice and rats. *Psychopharmacologia* (Berlin) *8:*1-11, 1965.
55. G. B. Cassano, S. E. Sjöstrand, and E. Hansson, Distribution of ^{14}C-labeled amitriptyline in the cat brain. *Psychopharmacologia* (Berlin) *8:*12-22, 1965.
56. K. Fredricson Overø, L. F. Gram, and V. Hansen, Kinetics of nortriptyline in man according to a two compartment model. *Eur. J. Clin. Pharmacol. 8:*343-347, 1975.
57. L. F. Gram, P. B. Andreasen, K. Fredricson Overø, and J. Christiansen, Comparison of single dose kinetics of imipramine, nortriptyline, and antipyrine in man. *Psychopharmacology 50:*21-27, 1976.

58. W. J. Jusko and M. Gibaldi, Effects of change in elimination on various parameters of the two compartment open model. *J. Pharm. Sci. 61:*1270-1273, 1972.
59. K. Fredricson Overφ, L. F. Gram, and V. Hansen, Interaction of perphenazine with the kinetics of nortriptyline. *Acta Pharmacol. Toxicol. 40:*97-105, 1977.
60. O. Borgå, D. L. Azarnoff, G. P. Forshell, and F. Sjöqvist, Plasma protein binding of tricyclic antidepressants in man. *Biochem. Pharmacol. 18:* 2135-2143, 1969.
61. I. C. Campbell and A. Todrick, Plasma protein binding of tricyclic antidepressive drugs. *J. Pharm. Pharmacol. 22:*226, 1970.
62. A. W. Pruitt and P. G. Dayton, A comparison of the binding of drugs to adult and cord plasma. *Eur. J. Clin. Pharmacol. 4:*59-62, 1971.
63. A. H. Glassman, N. J. Hurwic, and J. M. Perel, Plasma binding of imipramine and clinical outcome. *Amer. J. Psychiatry 130:*1367-1369, 1973.
64. J. R. Boissier, J. P. Tillement, D. Marxin, and P. Pichot, Effet de la lévoniepromazine sur le métabolisme de l'imipramine chez l'homme. *J. Pharmacol. Clin. 1:*11-15, 1975.
65. K. M. Piafsky and O. Borgå, Plasma protein binding of basic drugs, II: Importance of α_1-acid glycoprotein for individual variation. *Clin. Pharmacol. Ther. 22:*545-549, 1977.
66. G. Muscettola, F. K. Goodwin, W. Z. Potter, M. M. Claeys, and S. P. Markey, Imipramine and desipramine in plasma and spinal fluid. *Arch. Gen. Psychiat. 35:*621-625, 1978.
67. I. H. Stevenson, N. M. Wilson, and A. A. Schift, Implications of dose regimen and protein binding for plasma nortriptyline estimations. *Neuropharmacology 17:*417-431, 1978.
68. G. D. Burrows, B. A. Scoggins, and B. Davies, Plasma nortriptyline and clinical response. In *Classification and Prediction of Outcome of Depression* (J. Angst, ed.). Stuttgart, Schattauer Verlag, 1974, pp. 173-179.
69. P. Kragh-Sφrensen, C. E. Hansen, P. C. Baastrup, and E. F. Hvidberg, Self-inhibiting action of nortriptyline's antidepressive effect at high plasma levels. *Psychopharmacology 45:*305-316, 1976.
70. E. M. Reimann and M. S. Soloff, The effect of radioactive contaminants on the estimation of binding parameters by Scatchard analysis. *Biochim. Biophys. Acta 533:*130-139, 1978.
71. O. Borgå, K. M. Piafsky, and O. G. Nilsen, Plasma protein binding of basic drugs, I: Selective displacement from α_1-acid glycoprotein by tris (2-butoxyethyl) phosphate. *Clin. Pharmacol. Ther. 22:*539-544, 1977.
72. B. Alexanderson and O. Borgå, Interindividual differences in plasma protein binding of nortriptyline in man: A twin study. *Eur. J. Clin. Pharmacol. 4:* 196-200, 1972.
73. D. J. Brunswick and J. Mendels, Reduced levels of tricyclic antidepressants in plasma from vacutainers. *Comm. Psychopharmacol. 1:*131-134, 1977.
74. H. Liesen, B. Dufaux, and W. Hollman, Modification of serum glycopro-

teins the day following a prolonged physical exercise and the influence of physical training. *Eur. J. Appl. Physiol. 37:*243-254, 1977.
75. P. Kragh-Sørensen, M. Åsberg, and C. Eggert-Hansen, Plasma nortriptyline levels in endogenous depression. *Lancet 1:*113-115, 1973.
76. S. Montgomery, R. A. Braithwaite, S. Dawling, and R. McAuley, High plasma nortriptyline levels in the treatment of depression. *Clin. Pharmacol. Ther. 23:*309-314, 1978.
77. V. E. Ziegler, J. W. Knesevick, L. T. Wylie, and J. T. Biggs, Sampling time, dosage schedule, and nortriptyline plasma levels. *Arch. Gen. Psychiat. 34:* 613-615, 1977.
78. F. Sjöqvist, Assessment of antidepressants: Pharmacokinetic aspects. In *Advanced Medicine: Topics in Therapeutics* (A. Breckenridge, ed.). Proceedings of Conference of Royal College of Physicians of London. London, Pitman, 1974, pp. 198-217.
79. V. E. Ziegler, J. T. Biggs, A. B. Ardekani, and S. H. Rosen, Contribution to the pharmacokinetics of amitriptyline. *J. Clin. Pharmacol. 18:*462-467, 1978.
80. J. P. Moody, S. F. Whyte, A. J. McDonald, and G. J. Naylor, Pharmacokinetic aspects of protriptyline plasma levels. *Eur. J. Clin. Pharmacol. 11:* 51-56, 1977.
81. V. E. Ziegler, J. T. Biggs, R. T. Wylie, Wl H. Coryell, K. M. Hanife, D. J. Hawf, and S. H. Rosen, Protriptyline kinetics. *Clin. Pharmacol. Ther. 23:* 580-584, 1978.
82. V. E. Ziegler, J. T. Biggs, and L. T. Wylie, Doxepin kinetics. *Clin. Pharmacol. Ther. 23:*573-579, 1978.
83. R. A. Braithwaite and B. Widdop, A specific gas-chromatographic method for the measurement of "steady-state" plasma levels of amitriptyline and nortriptyline in patients. *Clin. Chim. Acta 35:*461-472, 1971.
84. B. Mellström and G. Tybring, Ion-pair liquid chromatography of steady-state plasma levels of chlorimipramine and demethylchlorimipramine. *J. Chromatogr. 143:*597-605, 1977.
85. J. T. Biggs, W. H. Holland, and W. R. Sherman, Steady-state protriptyline levels in an outpatient population. *Amer. J. Psychiat. 132:*960-962, 1975.
86. S. F. Whyte, A. J. MacDonald, G. J. Naylor, and J. P. Moody, Plasma concentrations of protriptyline and clinical effects in depressive women. *Br. J. Psychiatr. 128:*384-390, 1976.
87. S. Montgomery and R. Braithwaite, The relationship between plasma concentration amitriptyline and therapeutic response. Paper read before the Joint British and Scandinavian Associations of Psychopharmacology Meeting, London, July 1975.
88. S. Orrenius, Reaction mechanisms of cytochrome P-450. In *Proc. 6th Int. Cong. Pharmacol.,* vol. 6 (J. Tuomisto and M. K. Paasonen, eds.). Finnish Pharmacological Society, 1975, pp. 39-53.
89. F. P. Guengerich, Separation and purification of multiple forms of microsomal cytochrome P-450. *J. Biol. Chem. 252:*3970-3979, 1977.
90. A. Küpfer, J. Bircker, and R. Preisig, Stereoselective metabolism, pharma-

cokinetics, and biliary elimination of phenylethylhydantoin (Nirvanol) in the dog. *J. Pharmacol. Exp. Ther. 203:*493-499, 1077.
91. B. Alexanderson, Prediction of steady-state plasma levels of nortriptyline from single oral dose kinetics: A study in twins. *Eur. J. Clin. Pharmacol. 6:*44-53, 1973.
92. R. A. Braithwaite, S. Montgomery, and S. Dawling, Nortriptyline in depressed patients with high plasma levels, II. *Clin. Pharmacol. Ther. 23:* 303-308, 1978.
93. B. Alexanderson, On interindividual variability in plasma levels of nortriptyline and desmethylimipramine in man: A pharmacokinetic and genetic study. Doctoral thesis, Linköping University, Medical Dissertations no. 6, 1972.
94. R. A. Braithwaite, B. R. S. Nakra, and R. Grαind, Steady-state plasma concentration during single and multiple dosage schedules of amitriptyline. *Psychol. Med. 4:*338-341, 1974.
95. V. E. Ziegler, D. A. Meyer, S. H. Rosen, J. W. Knesevick, and J. T. Biggs, Amitriptyline dosage schedule, sampling time, and tricyclic plasma levels. *Brit. J. Psychiatr. 131:*168-171, 1977.
96. T. B. Cooper and G. M. Simpson, Prediction of individual dosage of nortriptyline. *Amer. J. Psychiatr. 135:*333-335, 1978.
97. B. Alexanderson, D. A. P. Evans, and F. Sjöqvist, Steady-state plasma levels of nortriptyline in twins: Influence of genetic factors and drug therapy. *Brit. Med. J. 4:*764-768, 1969.
98. A. Nies, D. S. Robinson, M. J. Friedmann, R. Green, T. B. Cooper, C. L. Ravaris, and J. O. Ives, Relationship between age and tricyclic antidepressant plasma levels. *Amer. J. Psychiatr. 134:*790-793, 1977.
99. M. Åsberg, Treatment of depression with tricyclic drugs: Pharmacokinetic and pharmacodynamic aspects. *Pharmacopsychiatr. 9:*18-26, 1976.
100. M. Åsberg and F. Sjöqvist, On the role of plasma level monitoring of tricyclic antidepressants in clinical practice. In *Workshop on Plasma Level Monitoring of Tricyclic Antidepressants* (L. F. Gram, comp.). Eleventh Congress Coll. Int. Neuropsychopharmacol. Vienna, *Comm. Psychopharmocol. 2:*381-392, 1978.
101. V. E. Ziegler, J. T. Biggs, Tricyclic plasma levels: Effect of age, race, sex, and smoking. *JAMA 238:*2167-2169, 1977.
102. P. B. Andreasen, L. Ranek, B. E. Statland, and N. Tygstrup, Clearance of antipyrine-dependence of quantitative liver function. *Eur. J. Clin. Invest. 4:*129-134, 1974.
103. R. A. Branch, J. A. James, and A. E. Read, The clearance of antipyrine and indocyamine green in normal subjects and in patients with chronic liver disease. *Clin. Pharmacol. Ther. 20:*81-86, 1976.
104. B. R. Ballinger, A. Presley, A. H. Reid, and I. H. Stevenson, The effect of hypnotics on imipramine treatment. *Psychopharmacologia 39:*267-274, 1974.
105. L. F. Gram and K. Fredricson Overφ, Drug interaction: Inhibitory effect

of neuroleptics on metabolism of tricyclic antidepressants in man. *Brit. Med. J. 1:*463-465, 1972.

106. L. F. Gram, J. Christiansen, and K. Fredricson Overø, Pharmacokinetic interaction between neuroleptics and tricyclic antidepressants in the rat. *Acta Pharmacol. Toxicol. 35:*223-232, 1974.

107. L. F. Gram, Effects of perphenazine on imipramine metabolism in man. *Psychopharmacol. Comm. 1:*165-175, 1975.

108. R. Olivier-Martin, D. Marzin, E. Buschenschutz, P. Pichot, and J. Boissier, Concentration plasmatique de l'imipramine et de la desmethylimipramine et effet anti-depresseur au cours d'un traitement controlé. *Psychopharmacologia 41:*187-195, 1975.

109. L. F. Gram, Effects of neuroleptics on the metabolism of tricyclic antidepressants. In *Proc. 10th Cong. Coll. Int. Neuropsychopharm, Quebec, 1976* (C. Radouco-Thomas, ed.). New York, Pergamon, 1977.

110. R. N. Wharton, J. M. Perel, P. G. Dayton, and S. Malitz, A potential clinical use for methylphenidate with tricyclic antidepressants. *Amer. J. Psychiatr. 127:*1619-1625, 1971.

111. G. Silverman and R. A. Braithwaite, Benzodiazepines and tricyclic antidepressant plasma levels. *Brit. Med. J. 3:*18-20, 1973.

112. L. F. Gram, K. Fredricson Overø, L. Kirk, Influence of neuroleptics and benzodiazepines on metabolism of tricyclic antidepressants in man. *Amer. J. Psychiatr. 131:*863-866, 1974.

113. J. M. Perel, M. Shostak, E. Gann, S. J. Kantor, and A. H. Glassman, Pharmacodynamics of imipramine and clinical outcome in depressed patients. In *Pharmacokinetics, Psychoactive Drug Blood Levels, and Clinical Outcome* (L. Gottschalk and S. Merlis, eds.). New York, Spectrum, 1976, pp. 229-241.

114. T. R. Norman, G. D. Burrows, K. P. Maguire, G. Rubinstein, B. A. Scoggins, and B. Davies, Cigarette smoking and plasma nortriptyline levels. *Clin. Pharmacol. Ther. 21:*453-456, 1977.

115. P. Kragh-Sørensen, C. E. Hansen, N.-E. Larsen, J. Naestoft, and E. F. Hvidberg, Long term treatment of endogenous depression with nortriptyline with control of plasma levels. *Psychol. Med. 4:*174-180, 1974.

116. P. Kragh-Sørensen and N. E. Larsen, Factors influencing the steady state kinetics of nortriptyline in patients. To be published.

117. M. Bjerre, L. F. Gram, P. Kragh-Sørensen, C. Bruun Kristensen, O. Lindegaard Petersen, M. Møller, and P. Thayssen, Dose-dependent kinetics of imipramine in elderly patients. To be published.

118. L. Bertilsson, B. Mellström, and F. Sjöqvist, Pronounced inhibition of noradrenaline uptake by 10-hydroxy-metabolites of nortriptyline. *Life Sci. 25:*1285-1292, 1979.

5

Tricyclic Antidepressants
Plasma Levels and Clinical Response

Graham D. Burrows and Trevor R. Norman /
Department of Psychiatry,
University of Melbourne, Parkville, Victoria, Australia

I. INTRODUCTION

Depressive illness is one of the most common psychiatric disorders, affecting 8-10% of a population at any one time [1]. Advances in the treatment of depressive illness in the past 20 years are partly the result of the introduction of the tricyclic antidepressants. These drugs are widely prescribed for therapy of moderate to severe depressive illness. Imipramine, the prototype of the tricyclic antidepressants, was first introduced by Kuhn in 1958. The intervening two decades have seen a proliferation of compounds with antidepressant effects. Despite the wide choice of antidepressants available, imipramine and another early one, amitriptyline, still remain the most widely prescribed tricyclics. There is a need, however, for better antidepressants, since in large-scale clinical trials only a 70-80% response rate is observed [2,3]. To attempt to meet this need, a new generation of antidepressants, the bicyclic and tetracyclic drugs, have recently been introduced. Their efficacy in large patient populations is mostly unproven, but they do appear to offer some clinical advantages over the tricyclics, especially in the nature and severity of the side effects experienced.

Hollister [4] reviewed the clinical use of the antidepressants. Briefly, there are no clear-cut differences between members of the tricyclic antidepressant groups as regards potency, speed of action, and consistency of effect. There is little evidence that these drugs have any difference in their onset of action. Early improvement may be noted not infrequently at the end of the first week, but may become evident after three to six weeks. Amitriptyline, trimipramine, nortriptyline, and doxepin have sedative effects which are useful in agitated depression. Imipramine and desipramine have a less comparable sedative component.

There is good evidence that responses to therapy are in part genetically determined, and evidence of response in previous depressive illness, or in relatives, may help in the choice between the tricyclics and the monoamine oxidase inhibitors.

The most useful therapeutic dosage is 150 mg of the tricyclic drug per day. Higher doses of tricyclic antidepressant drugs in clinical studies have been shown to produce better improvement than the lower doses. Blashki et al. [5] showed that 150 mg/day of amitriptyline produced significantly better results than 75 mg/day.

In some outpatients it may be advisable to begin with a lower dose but to increase to the maximum dose within a week or two at the most, as the patient's tolerance will permit. If adequate use of a tricyclic has failed to relieve the depression, it is unlikely that another of the same group will prove effective. Change to a monoamine oxidase inhibitor may be tried; more commonly, electroconvulsive therapy (ECT) will need to be considered. If the depression is severe and social conditions unfavorable, and where suicide is a possibility, early specialist referral is indicated.

II. PLASMA CONCENTRATIONS OF TRICYCLIC ANTIDEPRESSANTS

Since the initial introduction of the tricyclic antidepressant drugs in the late 1950s and early 1960s, there has been considerable interest and gradual modification in the therapeutic use of these compounds, which has partly resulted from plasma level studies. Until recently the techniques available for measuring plasma psychotropic drug levels, apart from lithium, have been totally inadequate in that they lacked specificity and sensitivity.

The notion of measurement of plasma levels of psychotropic drugs was introduced by Brodie [1] on the basis that differences in patient responses to psychotropic drugs might be related to concentrations of the drug in various body fluids. The value of monitoring plasma levels of drugs has been well documented in other areas of medicine (e.g., anticonvulsants, digitalis). Until recently the methodology for psychotropic drugs has neither been sensitive nor specific enough. Since 1967 techniques with adequate sensitivity, specificity, and precision have been available and are often applied for routine measurement of plasma concentrations. The necessity for such measurements, except in certain well-defined situations, is questionable. The crux of routine measurement of psychotropic drug levels centers on the relationship between plasma concentration and clinical response. The scope of this review is to examine this relationship for the psychotropic drugs in which this has been investigated.

III. FACTORS AFFECTING PLASMA CONCENTRATIONS

Plasma concentrations of a drug reflect the pharmacokinetic parameters of the drug for an individual patient. There are wide interindividual variations in the plasma levels of the psychotropic drugs, and much of this variation is genetically determined. Other factors such as the patient's age, sex, weight, diet, urinary pH, cigarette smoking, and so on may also influence plasma levels. The presence of physical disease, especially hepatic and renal pathology, may affect plasma concentrations. Concomitant administration of other drugs, notably enzyme inducers and inhibitors, may profoundly alter psychotropic drug concentrations [6]. These factors must be taken into account when considering the results of plasma level and clinical response relationships.

A. Plasma Level-Receptor Relationships

Underlying all plasma level clinical response studies is the assumption that plasma concentrations represent, but do not necessarily equal, concentrations of the drug at receptor sites within the central nervous system [7]. For most other psychotropic drugs this has been inferred from studies of cerebrospinal fluid (CSF) concentrations. A linear relationship between plasma and CSF levels of some tricyclics has been observed. The CSF concentrations of the tricyclics average about 10% of that in the plasma. These data suggest that plasma concentrations do reflect levels at receptor sites.

In 1967, Hammer and Brodie reported a technique which involved the acetylation of the secondary amine (desmethylimipramine) with radioactively labeled acetic anhydride. This method was modified for the quantification of nortriptyline by a number of researchers, including Sjöqvist et al. in 1969, Burrows in 1972, and Overø in 1972, and has been used extensively in the investigation of plasma nortriptyline and clinical response. Later methods for quantification of the tricyclics included spectrofluorimetry, gas-liquid chromatography, gas-liquid chromatography with mass spectrometry and densitometry (Chaps. 2 and 3).

Since 1970 research groups in Scandinavia, Europe, Australia, and the United States have published results of investigations which set out to establish the relationship between plasma levels of tricyclic antidepressant drugs and their therapeutic response in depressed patients.

There are more than 40 studies of the relationship between plasma concentrations of tricyclic antidepressants and clinical response. Most of these have concerned amitriptyline/nortriptyline and imipramine/desipramine. Other, less extensively investigated drugs are maprotiline, doxepin, butriptyline, clomipramine, dothiepin, mianserin, and protriptyline. These studies are summarized in Table 1. It is not the intention to discuss all of these studies individually but rather to present an overview of the subject.

B. Interindividual Variations in Plasma Tricyclic Levels

It has been shown by many researchers that patients treated with identical doses of tricyclic antidepressants reveal great interindividual differences in their "steady-state" plasma concentrations. Hammer and Sjöqvist [8] demonstrated a 36-fold difference between the lowest and highest steady-state level of desipramine in patients taking equal amounts of the drug. Others have shown variations of 5-fold [9], 10-fold [10], to 14-fold [11,12].

Most of the variability in steady-state plasma concentrations between individuals was considered to be genetically determined unless they were simultaneously exposed to other drugs. This type of study raised many questions, including: What were the pharmacokinetic mechanisms behind these individual differences and what was their significance in terms of drug response?

Table 1 Plasma Antidepressant Levels and Clinical Response

Reference	Patients (male/female)	Diagnosis (+ duration)	Drug, dose, other drugs	Rating	Plasma level (PL)	Improvement criterion	Conclusion re plasma level and clinical response
			Nortriptyline				
[103]	29 Inpatients (10 M, 19 F)	Endogenous depression (2-wk trial)	75-255 mg/day t.i.d. (barbiturates, glutethimide, diazepam)	Cronholm-Ottosson	32-164 ng/ml mean 90 ± 40	Amelioration score	Therapeutic range 50-140 ng/ml; curvilinear relationship
[11]	32 Inpatients (14 M, 18 F)	Primary depression, severe excluded (4-wk trial)	150 mg/day t.i.d (no other drug)	HDRS	37-592 ng/ml mean 171 ± 19	Amelioration score, -8 significant	No simple relationship
[27]	80 Inpatients (28 M, 52 F)	Primary depression, severe excluded (4-wk trial)	75, 150, 200, 250 mg/day to different groups	HDRS	Means (ng/ml): 65.9 ± 34.3 170.9 ± 108.2 227 ± 108.1 374.8 ± 92.0 Common mean: 172.7 ± 103.0	Percentage change in HDRS	12 patients each respond to individual level; no simple relationship
[33]	40 Inpatients (18 M, 22 F)	Primary depression, severe excluded; pairs matched for age, sex, HDRS (4-wk trial)	Dosage adjusted to give required level	HDRS	Each pair: one 140, one 49	Amelioration score, -8 significant	No simple correlation; no statistically significant difference between high and low

(continued)

Table 1 (continued)

Reference	Patients (male/female)	Diagnosis (+ duration)	Drug, dose, other drugs	Rating	Plasma level (PL)	Improvement criterion	Conclusion re plasma level and clinical response
			Nortriptyline (continued)				
[104]	22 Inpatients (2 M, 20 F)	Primary depressive illness (5-wk duration)	150 mg/day for 14 days; then t.i.d. 50/200 for 7 days; then 200/50 for 7 days; then 150 for 7 days (few nitrazepam)	HDRS	173 ± 15 ng/ml (91 ± 15)/ (286 ± 42) (236 ± 28)/ (88 ± 22) 174 ± 21	Final HDRS, percentage change in HDRS	No simple correlation PL/HDRS
[35]	31 Inpatients (all F)	Endogenous depression (4-wk trial)	150 mg/day (meprobamate, aspirin, and estrogens)	Modified Cronholm-Ottosson	48–238 ng/ml mean 141 ± 48.2	⩽3 Recovered	Best effect below 170 ng/ml; negative correlation between PL and clinical response
[36]	22 Inpatients (all F)	Endogenous depression (4-wk followed up for 20 wk as outpatients)	Dose adjusted, two PL groups (no other drug)	Cronholm-Ottosson	67–181 ng/ml mean 127 ± 35	⩽3 Recovered	High PL decreases therapeutic effect; best response 50–150 ng/ml
[105]	24 Inpatients (5 M, 19 F)	Endogenous depression, mod.-severe (6 wk trial)	50–300 mg/day adjusted for PL	Modified Cronholm-Ottosson	Two groups' plasma levels >180 ng/ml ($\bar{x}$ = 220.3 ± 26.9) and <150 ng/ml ($\bar{x}$ = 114.8 ± 17.1)	⩽3 Recovered	Therapeutic range 50–150 ng/ml

[44]	45 Outpatients (13 M, 32 F)	Depression (2-7 wk trial)	55-200 mg/day	Clinical judgment	20-355 ng/ml	Satisfactory or unsatisfactory	No correlation between dose or PL and response
[106]	36 Inpatients (16 M, 20 F)	Previous treatment by GPs unsuccessful (3-6 wk trial)	75-150 mg/day (lithium and benzodiazepines)	Global	77-684 ng/ml	Pronounced persistent improvement in depressive symptoms	Better response in 50-150-ng/ml range
[107]	18 Outpatients (6 M, 12 F)	Primary or secondary depression (6-wk trial)	Max. 150 mg by day 8 (no sedatives or hypnotics)	HDRS	39-352 ng/ml mean 138 at 6 wk mean dose 127 mg/day	$\leqslant$6 on HDRS, no suicidal ideation	Correlation 50-140 ng/ml; better response
[46]	21 Inpatients (9 M, 12 F); 18 completed trial	Endogenous depression (1-wk placebo, 4-wk drug)	100 mg/day at night (nitrazepam, diazepam, and lithium: 2 patients)	HDRS MADS	120-681 ng/ml mean 290 at week 4	HDRS $\leqslant$ 8 or amelioration score of 12 or more	High PL (>200 ng/ml) associated with poor clinical effect
				Amitriptyline			
[12]	15 (9 Outpatients) (4 M, 11 F)	Depressive illness (6-wk trial)	150 mg/day (nitrazepam)	HDRS	20-278 ng/ml NT 20-228 ng/ml AT	Percentage improvement over baseline	Highly significant correlation; poor response <120 ng/ml
[9]	28 Inpatients (7 M, 21 F)	Endogenous depression (6-wk trial)	150 mg/day (nitrazepam, diazepam)	HDRD	137 ± 60 ng/ml total, 69.5 ± 27.3 ng/ml AT, 67.0 ± 43.2 ng/mg NT	Amelioration score	Better response at mean ± 1 SD than above or below

(continued)

Table 1 (continued)

Reference	Patients (male/female)	Diagnosis (+ duration)	Drug, dose, other drugs	Rating	Plasma level (PL)	Improvement criterion	Conclusion re plasma level and clinical response
			Amitriptyline (continued)				
[50]	18 Outpatients (6 M, 12 F)	Primary or secondary affective disorder (6-wk trial)	50, 100, 150 mg/day as tolerated; mean 120 mg/day for 6 wk	HDRS	52–318 ng/ml total only 1 patient > 250	Hamilton $\leqslant 6$	Negative correlation between rating score/(AT + NT) and AT alone but not NT; percentage recoveries increase as PL rises to 250 ng/ml
[51]	41 Outpatients (14 M, 27 F)	Primary or secondary depression (6-wk trial)	AT n = 22, 150 mg/day; NT n = 19, 150 mg/day (other drugs not stated)	HDRS	AT: AT + NT = 131 ± 20 ng/ml mean dose 119 mg NT: 141 ± 15 ng/ml mean dose 117 mg/day	$\leqslant 6$ HDRS, no suicidal ideation	Positive correlation between PL and Hamilton score in NT patients; negative correlation between PL and Hamilton score in AT patients
[53]	16 Inpatients (9 F, 7 M)	Primary depression (4-wk trial) 11 unipolar, 4 bipolar, 1 schizoaffective	7-day placebo 3-day 50-mg AT 4-day 100-mg AT 7-day 150-mg AT 14-day 200-mg AT	HDRS	Totai AT + NT: 69–538 ng/ml ($\bar{x}$ = 275 ± 155) mean AT 146 ± 86 mean NT 129 ± 90	12/2 (sum of 2 raters)	Negative correlation found between Hamilton and total tricyclic levels; 200 ng/ml total tricyclic separates responders/nonresponders

[54]	54 Inpatients (16 M, 38 F)	Primary depressive illness, no mania (6-wk medication, 7-12-day preliminary period)	75 mg AT 3 days; 150 mg AT until end of 6 wk	HDRS	46-391 ng/ml AT mean 125 39-366 ng/ml NT mean 108	1. ⩽6 recovered, 7-15 improved, ⩾16 not improved 2. % Improvement 3. Amelioration score	No correlation
			Imipramine and Desipramine				
[55]	16 Inpatients (10 M, 6 F)	Endogenous depression	150-225 mg/day or related to body weight (nitrazepam)	HDRS	2.5-71.0 ng/ml IMI mean 33.8	Responders showed 85% reduction of Hamilton score	Responders' PL significantly greater than nonresponders', IMI not DMI-measured
[56]	–	–	DMI (+ antiparkinsonism drugs in some); lower dose if on antiparkinsonism drugs		Mean plasma DMI not significantly different for two groups	–	Significant correlation between PL and rating scales
[57]	31 Inpatients (5 M, 26 F)	Unipolar depression, neurotic depression (3-weeks)	150 mg/day IMI (amylobarbitone nitrazepam)	Global scale and visual analogue scale	IMI + DMI: 100-1400 ng/ml DMI 20-600	Change in rating scale	No significant correlation
[10]	18 Inpatients	Primary affective disorder (7-wk trial including 1-wk placebo)	3.5 mg/kg/day IMI (flurazepam)	Modified HDRS	IMI + DMI: 95-1020 ng/ml mean 210 ± 110	Final Hamilton ⩽9	Sigmoid relationship 180 ng/ml minimum for therapeutic response

(continued)

Table 1 (continued)

Reference	Patients (male/female)	Diagnosis (+ duration)	Drug, dose, other drugs	Rating	Plasma level (PL)	Improvement criterion	Conclusion re plasma level and clinical response
			Imipramine and Desipramine (continued)				
[58]	24 Inpatients	Endogenous depression	150 mg/day IMI	–	108-118 ng/ml IMI 130-160 ng/ml DMI	–	Significant correlation PL/DMI or IMI + DMI, not IMI
		Nonendogenous depression (3-wk trial)	–	–	No correlation	Poorer response	–
[108]	24 Inpatients (10 M, 14 F)	Endogenous depression (4-wk trial, 16 continued to 6 wk)	225 mg/day IMI (nitrazepam)	HDRS	15-312 ng/ml IMI 0-740 ng/ml DMI	⩽8 recovery	No correlation between response and total concentrations but 45 ng/ml IMI + 75 ng/ml DMI needed for recovery
[60]	10 Inpatients (9 M, 1 F)	Depressive illness (4-wk trial)	150 mg/day IMI (nitrazepam)	HDRS, Wakefield scale	75.4 ng/ml IMI 76.7 ng/ml DMI Total 152.1 ng/ml	Change of 4 points on Hamilton scale	Significant negative correlation between IMI and DMI, PL and depression rating
[109]	66 Inpatients (inc. 24 above) (20 M, 46 F)	37 endogenous, 29 nonendogenous (4-wk trial)	225 mg/day IMI (nitrazepam)	HDRS, Beck, WHO Depression scale	1-223 ng/ml IMI 18-675 ng/ml DMI	⩽7 responders 8-15 partial, ⩾16 nonresponders	Endogenous depressions; significant correlations HDRS and total (IMI + DMI); no correlation for nonre-

							sponders; all nonresponders, total PL $<$ 240 ng/ml; no upper limit
[61]	60 Inpatients (18 M, 42 F)	Endogenous depression (4-week trial)	3.5 mg/kg/day IMI (flurazepam: 100-300 mg depending on weight; mean 215 mg)	Depression scale	50-1050 ng/ml mean 200 ± 137	Depression rating scale, mood scale, global rating	Significant linear correlation between PL and clinical response; 17 unipolar delusional patients showed no correlation; 43 nondelusional patients: significant correlation
[23]	7 Inpatients (3 M, 4 F)	"Psychotic" depressions	Increasing doses up to 450 mg/day for 2 wk, then lowered to 150 mg/day (dextroamphetamine, chloral hydrate)	Clinical rating scale	170-750 ng/ml total IMI + DMI	Clinical judgment	Significant correlation between PL and improvement for individuals
				Maprotiline			
[67]	20 Inpatients	Depressive psychosis (4-wk trial)	300 mg/day for 2 days, then 150 mg/nocte or 225 mg/day	HDRS and AMP system	150-mg: 107-892 ng/ml, mean 288 ± 82 225 mg: 165-1277 ng/ml, mean 464 ± 99	Amelioration score	No correlation; speculate high levels resistant, suggesting curvilinear response

(continued)

Table 1 (continued)

Reference	Patients (male/female)	Diagnosis (+ duration)	Drug, dose, other drugs	Rating	Plasma level (PL)	Improvement criterion	Conclusion re plasma level and clinical response
			Maprotiline (continued)				
[70]	10 Inpatients (4 M, 6 F)	Primary depressive illness (4-wk trial)	150 mg/day for 2 wk, adjusted up to 200 mg/day if no response	HDRS	(At 4 wk) 132-378 ng/ml mean 262 ± 87.5	Amelioration score	No simple correlation between PL and clinical response
[68]	14 Outpatients + 15 Outpatients	Depressive illness	25 mg t.d.s., 75 mg for 4 wk	17-Item rating scale	26-168 ng/ml		No significant correlation
[69]	18 Outpatients	Mixed group of endogenous depression and neurotic/reactive depressions	150 mg/day for 5 wk (diazepam, nitrazepam)	Observer rating scale and Wakefield self-rating scale	35-560 ng/ml	Fall in rating scale to ⩽10 recovery	No significant correlation
			Protriptyline				
[76]	28 Inpatients (all F)	Depressive illness (3½-wk trial)	20 mg/day for 3 days, then 40 mg/day for 3 wk (amylobarbitone, nitrazepam)	Global rating scale	120-429 ng/ml	Determined from Global impression	Curvilinear relationship; best response with PL of 150-280 ng/ml
[110]	21 Outpatients (3 M, 18 F)	Primary or secondary depression (4-wk trial)	10 mg/day up to 20 mg/day during week 1, then fixed	HDRS	22-167 ng/ml mean 69	⩽6, no suicidal ideation	Suggested therapeutic range 70-170 ng/ml; positive correlation between PL/clinical response

				Doxepin			
[62]	15 Inpatients (4 M, 11 F) (⩾60 years old)	Primary or secondary affective disorder	50-300 mg nocte	Clinical global impression	9-138 ng/ml mean 81 ± 44 total dox. + desdox	Degree of improvement	Minimum dox. + desdox. = 110 ng/ml required for improvement
[65]	10 Outpatients	Primary depression, mild to moderate (4-wk trial)	10 mg t.i.d.; or 10 mg t.i.d. for 4 days, then 50 mg t.i.d.	HDRS	No details	"Improved" or "unchanged"	Improved patients on higher dose; PL desdox. 20 ng/ml (no relationship to dox.)
[66]	17 Inpatients (6 M, 11 F)	Primary depressive illness	150 mg/day	HDRS	30-118 ng/ml mean 52.3 ± 5.9 total dox. + desdox.	Amelioration score of 8	No simple correlation
				Clomipramine			
[82]	32 GP patients (9 M, 23 F)	Depressive illness (4-wk trial)	9 patients: 10 mg t.i.d.; 9 patients: 30 mg nocte; 9 patients: 25 mg t.i.d.; 5 patients: 75 mg nocte	17-Symptom rating scale	Mean (ng/ml CMI DESCMI 35.3 31.7 22.3 21.9 37.6 71.0 33.1 55.1	Decrease in total symptom score	Response at all levels; no relationship between PL and response; poor responders show higher PL than good responders; no statistical significance of PL of 4 groups
[83]	18 Outpatients (6 M, 12 F)	Depressive illness; 7 reactive, 11 endogenous (4-wk trial)	50 mg nocte	10-Symptom depression scale, rated 0-6 on each item, Visual Analogue scale	14-136 ng/ml CMI mean 55 4-344 ng/ml DESCMI mean 77	Decrease in each item of rating scale monitored	No correlation between PL and clinical response

(continued)

Table 1 (continued)

Reference	Patients (male/female)	Diagnosis (+ duration)	Drug, dose, other drugs	Rating	Plasma level (PL)	Improvement criterion	Conclusion re plasma level and clinical response
				Butriptyline			
[111]	10 Inpatients	Primary depression	50 mg t.i.d.	HDRS, Beck, Carroll, Visual Analogue	35-295 ng/ml mean 139.4 ± 60.8	Amelioration score	No simple correlation between PL and clinical response
				Mianserin			
[79]	17 Inpatients (2 M, 15 F)	Primary depressive illness (1-wk placebo, 6-wk treatment)	60 mg in divided doses	HDRS $\geqslant$16	18.3-72.7 ng/ml mean 36.2	Percentage improvement over baseline scores; Amelioration score	No relationship between PL and therapeutic outcome
[80]	26 Inpatients 24 Outpatients	Moderate to severe depressive illness	60 mg nocte or 60 mg divided doses	HDRS, MADS, Beck self-rating scale	Divided dosage group mean 42.7 ng/ml Nighttime dosage group mean 56.4 ng/ml	Amelioration score	Significant negative correlation between PL and clinical response; suggestion of a curvilinear relationship

				Lofepramine			
[84]	31 In- and Outpatients (10 M, 21 F)	Endogenous and mixed depression (1-wk placebo, 5-wk treatment)	210 mg/day in divided doses (pentobarbital and methaqualone as needed; lithium, oral contraceptives)	Cronholm-Ottosson scale; Zung self-rating scale	4-53 ng/ml mean 11 ± 2 DMI levels 4-184 ng/ml mean 49 ± 10	Amelioration score	No correlation between PL and clinical response
				Dibenzepin			
[77]	12 Patients (all F)	Endogenous depression (22-day trial)	8 mg/kg	–	–	–	Positive correlation between PL of dibenzepin and metabolite levels and clinical response
				Dothiepin			
[78]	16 Inpatients (5 M, 11 F)	Endogenous/psychotic depression, I.C.D. 296 (4-wk trial)	50 mg t.d.s. (nitrazepam as needed)	HDRS	Prothiaden: 26-194 ng/ml mean 105 Northiaden: 15-134 ng/ml mean 51 ng/ml	Amelioration score	No relationship between PL of drug and metabolite and clinical response

IV. PLASMA CONCENTRATIONS AND SIDE EFFECTS

Sjöqvist et al. [13] reported plasma levels of the monomethylated compounds and side effects in man. They studied hospitalized patients with various types of depression arbitrarily allocated to treatment with various types of tricyclic antidepressants. Many of the earlier studies reported much detail of the methodology of plasma measurement, but little concerning the patients or the evaluation of depression and clinical progress.

The "occasional doses of hypnotics by night," glutethimide, meprobamate, chloralhydrate, or methaqualone, were given. Later work demonstrated that concomitant prescribing of drugs may alter steady-state plasma levels [14-16].

Within patients the steady-state plasma level was found to be directly proportional to the administered dose [8,17].

Åsberg et al. [18] studied the occurrence of subjective side effects of nortriptyline in relation to the plasma level of the drug in 40 psychiatric inpatients with depressive disorders. The plasma levels varied widely between individual patients, but in any given patient the plasma level tended to be constant over a period of time. The side effects of nortriptyline diminished significantly with time and in most cases were absent during the fourth week of drug treatment of nortriptyline at 50 mg three times a day. These workers claimed a significant positive correlation between plasma levels of nortriptyline and subjective side effects. Åsberg [19] correlated drug-related side effects to plasma nortriptyline levels and found a significant correlation in patients and in healthy volunteers. Braithwaite [12], Burrows [11], and Gram [20] have been unable to correlate plasma levels with side effects.

V. PLASMA CONCENTRATIONS AND CLINICAL RESPONSE

An early study by Haydu et al. [21] reported that in eight patients on 150 mg/day of imipramine, four responded well while four proved refractory to imipramine therapy. The patients who had high plasma levels of imipramine did not respond to therapy. Yates [22] showed the clinical response to desipramine was poor in two patients with high plasma levels in comparison to four patients with lower levels. In contrast, Zeidenberg and co-workers [23] demonstrated six out of seven severely depressed patients rapidly improved on very high doses of imipramine. There was a close correlation with the blood drug levels, although these levels varied greatly from patient to patient. The plasma levels were characteristic of individual patients rather than of oral dose of the medication.

A. Nortriptyline

1. Plasma Level Studies

The most extensively studied tricyclic is nortriptyline because it was believed that it did not have any active metabolites. Recent studies have shown that this is not true (see below). It was studies with this drug that began the interest in plasma levels and clinical response of tricyclics. The first study was conducted by Åsberg et al. in 1971 and demonstrated a curvilinear relationship, with high and low concentrations of nortriptyline producing a poorer therapeutic response than intermediate concentrations. A therapeutic range was 50-140 ng/ml of the drug.

The Australian group [15,11,24-31] found there was no simple relationship between plasma nortriptyline and clinical response as measured by the Hamilton Depression Rating Scale (HDRS) in a number of separate group studies involving 32, 24, 22, and 80 depressed patients. All patients studied were inpatients who were observed and studied for a drug-free period of 1 week prior to active drug therapy.

In contrast, when individual patients were studied with variations of plasma nortriptyline levels there was a significant relationship. Of the 80 patients who had steady-state nortriptyline levels, 12 were given identical capsules of different potency, either increasing or decreasing their medication [27]. There was an obvious increase in depressive symptomatology as the oral dose and plasma level fell and a clinical improvement as the original dose was reinstated. Calculation of regression coefficients showed a positive relationship between clinical change and plasma nortriptyline levels in all these 12 patients. Comparison of the regression coefficients showed that they differed significantly among themselves and were not related to age or sex. The original study [11] has been censured on two points [19,32]. The patient selection was criticized on the grounds that the more seriously ill patients received treatment with ECT and were excluded from the drug studies. The classification of the patients into primary depressive illness where there was a primary mood disorder and not into the classification of endogenous and other types of depression was criticized. This has been answered in that the patients studied were those that normally would be given tricyclic antidepressant therapy. Burrows et al. [33] also tested the hypothesis that levels of nortriptyline greater than 140 ng/ml would lead to a greater clinical improvement than plasma levels of less than 40 ng/ml. In a sequential skew-restricted design, 20 paired depressed patients were studied. On analysis at the end point indication showed that it was highly unlikely that if the study had continued a significant difference between the therapy regimes would be found.

In a further study over 5 weeks of 22 depressed patients treated with nortriptyline, significant changes in plasma levels both elevated and reduced were deliberately produced in the third and fourth weeks of each patient's treatment [34]. The results of this study show that while significant differences in plasma levels were obtained, no correlations with clinical response, either in the group as a whole or in individual patients, were found [29]. This data along with the previous studies from the Australian group failed to demonstrate any tendency to lesser response at plasma levels about 175 ng/ml, as proposed by the Scandinavian group [35,36].

The study of the clinical data from these patients collected independently at the same interview by six psychiatrists [37] showed that all psychiatrists considered 10 patients to be "reactive depressives" and four "endogenous." In 8 patients there was disagreement, or the patients were labeled "indeterminate." The initial mean and percentage change in Hamilton Depression Rating scores of these three groups of patients were 24.8 and 63.3%, 23.4 and 56.3%, and 29.4 and 57.5%, respectively. There was no evidence from this study that the so-called reactive depressions respond poorly to tricyclic medication.

The original paper [11] was also criticized on methodological reasons. There were high fluctuations in the steady-state levels of a few patients. The correlation between plasma level and receptor site concentration depends largely upon the assumption of true steady state. Factors in variation of steady state have been thoroughly investigated [30]. In particular, it was shown that between-individual variations in steady-state plasma levels are large. Between-day within-individual variation at a steady-state plasma level is 15-20%. Once again, there is considerable variation between individuals. Dosage regime, time of sampling after the last oral dose, the method of plasma handling, and the analytical methods were considered unlikely to be responsible for the differences in interpretation between the different research groups. Within an individual the oral dose, duration of treatment, and concomitant drug treatments are all important determinants of the steady-state plasma level.

The individual variability in plasma levels is mainly due to variations in the hepatic metabolism of these drugs [20,38-40]. Differences in distribution of binding to tissue and plasma proteins may add to the variability. Borgå et al. [41] stated that only 5% of the total drug is "free." Glassman et al. [42] claimed that plasma binding was not constant between individuals and reported a fourfold difference of 5.4-23% in the amount of "free" imipramine available to different patients. Maclean [43] found a variability of protein binding of 75-89% bound when receiving nortriptyline. The variability in hepatic metabolism is due to both hepatic enzyme activity and hepatic blood flow.

Lyle et al. [44] in a U.K. study of 45 patients attending six different hospitals reported plasma nortriptyline estimations performed at the same laboratory. No statistically significant correlation could be discerned between oral dose or plasma level and clinical response. The uncontrolled study was aimed at demonstrating whether or not "spot" determination of plasma nortriptyline would be useful as a guide to dosage requirements. Criticisms of this study might also include the lack of controls for concomitant medication, length of drug treatment, and patient compliance.

Another study, involving 150 outpatients receiving tricyclics, including nortriptyline, designed to test the practicality of routine plasma measurements by Biggs et al. [45], reported a number of individual case studies. These authors claimed that plasma analysis revealed both the failure to ingest prescribed medication and also the abuse of medication. They also reported that "some patients simply do not respond to antidepressant therapy even in the presence of plasma levels which have proven adequate in most other patients." Not enough detail of the depressed patients is given to draw any definite conclusions.

Montgomery et al. [46] studied 18 patients with endogenous depression for 4 weeks. All patients received a single oral dose of 100 mg of nortriptyline at night. Patients were rated using the Hamilton Depression Scale at weekly intervals, and plasma nortriptyline levels were determined by gas chromatography at the same time. A sixfold variation in plasma levels was observed. Patients with plasma levels above 200 ng/ml showed significantly poorer clinical response than those below this value. The study thus provides support for a curvilinear relationship between plasma levels and clinical response.

2. Critique

Each of these studies has been criticized on methodological grounds. In Åsberg's study the hypothesis tested was derived from inspection of the data. Burrows' studies did not include the more severely ill patients who were given ECT, and the fluctuations in steady-state levels were high in some patients. Lyle's study lacked controls for concomitant medication, length of treatment, and patient compliance. Both primary and secondary depressives were included in Ziegler's study and it was conducted on outpatients. Only one-third of Kragh-Sørensen's patients fulfilled the trial protocol, and 11 of those withdrawn received ECT. These criticisms highlight the problems of drug trials designed to investigate plasma level and clinical response relationships. It should be kept in mind that the data concerning optimal nortriptyline levels has, for the most part, been gathered from a small (<400 patients), highly selected (possibly atypical) population. As far as clinical management is concerned, satisfactory therapeutic response can be obtained with nortriptyline in the majority of patients with recommended daily doses and without the benefit of plasma level determinations.

B. Amitriptyline and Plasma Level Studies

This drug presents an additional factor to the plasma level-response relationship. It is a tertiary amine and is metabolized to a secondary amine (nortriptyline), which is itself an active antidepressant. A further complicating factor is that the tertiary amine tricyclics are believed to exert their antidepressant effects by inhibition of serotonin reuptake, while the secondary amines act mainly on noradrenaline reuptake [47]. The relative contributions of parent drug and metabolite to the clinical response observed cannot be distinguished. Accordingly, most authors have correlated clinical outcome with the plasma concentration of either amitriptyline or nortriptyline or the sum of both components.

An English group, Braithwaite et al. [12], in 1972 measured plasma amitriptyline and nortriptyline concentrations in 15 depressive patients who were treated with 150 mg of amitriptyline daily for 6 weeks. There was a considerable variation in plasma levels of both amitriptyline and its metabolite, nortriptyline, in these depressed patients. The researchers claimed a highly significant positive correlation between plasma levels of both compounds and clinical improvement. Patients who had plasma concentrations of amitriptyline and nortriptyline below 120 ng/ml showed a poor clinical response. They showed a simple linear relationship between increasing plasma levels and improved clinical response. The raw data from this study was later reanalyzed by Gruvstad [48], who considered after using a ranking technique that the antidepressant effect was greater in those patients with "intermediate" plasma levels (70-180 ng/ml).

Kane et al. [49] using a multiple regression approach reanalyzed Braithwaite's data. They confirmed the findings of a significant positive correlation between total drug plasma level and clinical response. The original study may be criticized as 9 of the 15 "depressed" were outpatients and control for medication and time of dosage interval would be lacking. These authors also collected plasma samples 19 hours after the last dose.

In a further study by this group [9] plasma amitriptyline and nortriptyline concentrations were measured in a group of 28 patients suffering from endogenous depressions treated with 150 mg/day of amitriptyline for 6 weeks. The mean amelioration scores for these patients within 1 standard deviation of the mean plasma concentration of amitriptyline and nortriptyline (137 ± 60.2 ng/ml) were compared to those above and below this range. The amelioration score appeared much better in those patients with "intermediate" plasma levels.

A U.S. study by Ziegler et al. [50] reported 18 depressed outpatients treated for 6 weeks with amitriptyline. For the 17 patients having total tricyclic plasma levels between 0 and 250 ng/ml, there was a negative correlation between the Hamilton Depression Rating score and the mean total tricyclic level of amitriptyline and nortriptyline ($P < .01$) and amitriptyline level ($P < .005$). The mean nortriptyline level did not significantly correlate with the Hamilton score. They claimed that the percentage of recovered patients increases significantly as the plasma levels rise to 250 ng/ml, the maximum plasma level considered in their study. They considered that further studies were required to clarify the upper range. In a second study the same group proposed a therapeutic range of 95-299 ng/ml for amitriptyline level and 50-139 ng/ml for nortriptyline [51]. In both studies the subjects were a heterogenous diagnostic group of outpatients of mixed race. Recent studies suggest an influence of race on plasma levels [52]. Kupfer et al. [53] studied 16 patients and found that a total tricyclic concentration of 200 ng/ml could be used to distinguish responders from nonresponders. A correlation between plasma levels and clinical response was found. A collaborative study, carried out under the auspices of the World Health Organization, found no correlation between clinical response and either total or individual tricyclic levels [54]. This study has been criticized as atypical because of the very poor response rate of the patients.

It has been argued that the studies of nortriptyline and amitriptyline are not comparable. Amitriptyline and the other tertiary amine tricyclic antidepressants are thought to inhibit mainly serotonin reuptake, while the secondary amines like nortriptyline inhibit noradrenaline reuptake.

As with data for nortriptyline, *no clear picture has emerged for amitriptyline.* Again the data have been gathered in relatively few patients (<200), and if the response of these patients is atypical, then it is perhaps because they are atypical patients. Most patients with depressive illness are treated successfully by their general practitioner. Those patients in whom treatment is not successful are referred on to the psychiatrist, and it is most probable that it is on this biased population that research studies are conducted.

C. Imipramine and Desipramine and Plasma Level Studies

Imipramine is the only other drug which has been investigated in detail. About 300 patients have been studied with this tertiary amine tricyclic. Some authors suggest that the antidepressant effect of imipramine is due to its metabolite desipramine (desmethylimipramine). Most studies have determined plasma level-clinical response relationships on the total tricyclic levels. The first studies involved plasma determinations using nonspecific analytical techniques. A high negative correlation between the therapeutic response to imipramine and Hamilton Depression Rating Scale and plasma concentration of the drug was shown by Walter [55] in 16 patients. Eight patients received 150-225 mg/day and the other eight received a dose related to their body weight. He reported a positive correlation between plasma levels of imipramine and the incidence of side effects. Zeidenberg et al. [23] found no relationship between total tricyclic levels and clinical response for the group as a whole, but found a relationship for individuals.

In a study of 13 patients suffering from Parkinson's disease treated with desipramine, Muscettola et al. [56] claimed a significant correlation between plasma levels and clinical rating scales. The patients had not responded to other therapies and several were receiving anti-Parkinson drugs as well. The authors thought there might be some drug interaction of anti-Parkinson drugs with tricyclics, as the mean plasma values were not significantly different despite the fact those on anti-Parkinson drugs received lower dosages of the desipramine. Ballinger et al. [57] found no correlation. More intensive studies of imipramine have been carried out since the early 1970s using analytical techniques specific for the parent drug and its metabolites. The overall pattern that has emerged from these studies is that there is a relationship between plasma levels and clinical response, but the exact nature of the relationship varies according to the author!

Gram et al. [40] studied the relationship between the antidepressive effect of imipramine and the plasma concentrations of imipramine and the active metabolite, desipramine, in 24 patients suffering from endogenous depression. Patients received imipramine, 150-225 mg, on a divided three-times-per-day basis. Of 12 patients who responded, 11 had plasma concentrations greater than or equal to 45 ng/ml of imipramine and 75 ng/ml of desipramine. In contrast, the 12 patients not responding satisfactorily all had concentrations of imipramine or desipramine or both below these limits. These researchers reported that there were no clear indications that high plasma concentrations reduced the antidepressant effect. The stated that "imipramine and desipramine have different effects and . . . both are needed for the antidepressive action." They suggest that in patients where imipramine levels are adequate, but desipramine levels are low, desipramine could be administered concomitantly. If demethylation was rapid, administration of imipramine parentally may be indicated to eliminate the "first-pass" effect. Gram and Christiansen [20] showed that "first-pass" effect through the liver of amitriptyline can result in 30-70% demethylation.

Olivier-Martin et al. [58] found a significant correlation between the degree of clinical improvement in endogenous depressions and desipramine level and imipramine and desipramine level, but not imipramine alone. Six patients diagnosed as neurotic depressives did not improve.

Perel et al. [10] studied 29 hospitalized depressed patients treated with imipramine 3.5 mg/kg/day for 4 weeks. Clinical ratings included a modified Hamilton Rating Scale for depression, a global rating scale, and the Raskin Mood Scale. They excluded the delusional patients, and 12 of the 18 improved and were discharged. Five of the six drug failures had total imipramine plus desipramine plasma levels below 180 ng/ml.

In contrast, 10 of the 12 responders had levels above 180 ng/ml. No further data were presented on actual plasma levels or clinical ratings. There was not enough data available to critically review this study. Total plasma imipramine plus desipramine were in the range 95-1020 ng/ml, with a steady state of 210 ± 110 ng/ml. A prospective study initially excluding delusional people would be necessary rather than post hoc evaluation of results, as occurred here.

Simpson et al. [59], however, have also confirmed that depressed patients with delusions are "markedly unresponsive" to tricyclics.

Plasma imipramine and plasma desipramine were correlated negatively with depression rating scores in another study of 10 patients [60]. Glassman et al. [61] studied a group of 60 endogenously depressed inpatients for 4 weeks. A significant linear correlation between plasma level and clinical response was observed in 43 nondelusional patients. No correlation was found in 17 unipolar delusional patients. Again it is clear that *no consistent findings have emerged from these studies.*

D. Other Antidepressants

1. Doxepin

Friedel and Raskind [62], in a study of 15 elderly depressed patients given doxepin in a single nightly dose of 50-300 mg, reported plasma levels of doxepin and desmethyldoxepin. These averaged 60 ng/ml (24-118 ng/ml) in the 7 patients who experienced little or no therapeutic benefit. In contrast, the 8 patients with marked to moderate improvement had a mean level of 111 ng/ml (53-138 ng/ml). The mean daily dose of doxepin in the two groups was 104 mg (50-250 mg/day) in the nonresponders and higher at 164 mg (50-300 mg/day) in the responders. One patient required 400 mg/day and achieved a blood level of 281 ng/ml when marked improvement occurred, having experienced no improvement at 250 mg/day with plasma levels of 107 ng/ml.

Burrows et al. [63] compared the cardiac effects of 150 mg/day of nortriptyline and doxepin in a crossover comparative study. High-fidelity rapid-recording surface electrocardiography, a noninvasive technique, allowed for accurate measurement of the QRS width at either 200 or 500 mm/s.

After three weeks on 150 mg/day of either tricyclic, 6 out of 17 patients on nortriptyline showed more than 25% prolongation of the QRS complex. Only one of the patients had significance prolongation while receiving doxepin. Plasma levels of doxepin were measured by gas-liquid chromatography with protriptyline as an internal standard. Nortriptyline was analyzed by double-isotrope derivative dilution procedures [31]. The group of patients when receiving nortriptyline had a mean plasma level of 196 ± 29 ng/ml, but while on doxepin a mean plasma level of 52 ± 6 ng/ml was obtained. The level of doxepin compares with those of Friedel and Raskind [62] and that of 55 ng/ml of O'Brien and Hinsvark [64].

Another study found no relationship with plasma doxepin levels [65,66], but suggested that 20 ng/ml of desmethyldoxepin was necessary for response [65].

2. Maprotiline

The results of all the published studies are consistent: there is no relationship between plasma level of maprotiline and clinical response [67-70]. A total of 80 patients have been studied, but only 30 of these have been inpatients. More trials are needed to assess the relationship for this drug.

Fischbach [71] reported mean therapeutic maprotiline plasma levels in depressed patients of 200-300 ng/ml. Higher levels produced more marked and frequent side effects without increase in antidepressant effects. In a study of 25 healthy volunteers [72] there was no correlation between steady-state levels of the drug (60-600 ng/ml) and side effects. Angst and Rothweiler [67] studied 20 patients suffering from depressive psychosis (I.C.D. 296) receiving maprotiline for 4 weeks. The patients received 300 mg/day for 2 days and then were randomly assigned to two groups. One group received 150 mg/day and the other 225 mg/day, and on the 10th day the mean plasma levels were 228 ± 82 ng/ml and 464 ± 99 ng/ml, respectively. There was no significant correlation between clinical response and plasma levels by days 20 and 30. When they excluded patients from each group with excessively high plasma levels, these authors claimed statistically significant correlations between blood levels and clinical effect. Exclusion of these 2 patients could be criticized, as one showed significant improvement on day 30 and because of the authors' later manipulation of data after the initial agreed study criteria. This study, therefore, shows no significant correlation between plasma level and clinical response, although the authors speculate that excessively high levels may be resistant to therapy, suggesting a curvilinear response.

In a 1-year trial in 39 patients with affective disorders, Coppen et al. [73] found a significant negative correlation between plasma maprotiline which averaged 225 ng/ml (144-420 ng/ml) and body weight.

3. *Protriptyline*

Biggs et al. [74] measured steady-state protriptyline levels in 12 outpatients treated for depression with daily dosage of 10-70 mg. Plasma protriptyline values ranged from 24 to 434 ng/ml. An earlier study, Moody et al. [75], treated 9 patients with 40 mg daily. The mean ratio of their plasma level to daily dose was 3.02, which compared with the mean ratio of 6.4 of Biggs and co-workers. These levels were comparatively higher than other tricyclic plasma levels.

Whyte et al. [76] reported the relationship between side effects, clinical outcome, and drug plasma levels in 28 female depressed patients treated with protriptyline. After 3½ weeks treatment, patients with plasma levels within a median range of 189-270 ng/ml showed the best response. There was no statistically significant correlation between plasma levels and side effect scores or "corrected" side effect scores for the group. A positive correlation for the "neurotic" subgroup, after 14 and 21 days of treatment, though not after 17 days, between the plasma levels and the "corrected" scores (that is, after subtracting pretreatment values) was shown.

The authors considered that further studies were necessary to confirm their findings and to define more precisely the therapeutic range. The paradoxical association between high protriptyline levels (270 ng/ml) and poor clinical response needs further investigation from both a clinical and biochemical viewpoint.

4. Dibenzepin

In a study of 22 endogenously depressed female inpatients Modestin [77] found a positive correlation between therapeutic response and plasma dibenzepin levels. Plasma levels of dibenzepin plus its major metabolite were also correlated with therapeutic response. Sixteen depressed inpatients treated with dothiepin for 4 weeks showed no relationship between plasma concentration of the parent drug and its metabolite northiaden and clinical response at 4 weeks [78].

5. Mianserin

Two studies with mianserin have produced conflicting results. In a group of 17 inpatients suffering from primary depressive illness, there was no relationship between the plasma concentration of mianserin and therapeutic outcome after 6 weeks treatment [79]. A significant negative correlation between plasma mianserin levels and clinical response was observed in a group of 50 patients with primary depressive illness [80]. A trend for patients with low plasma levels to respond poorly, suggestive of a curvilinear response, was also found. In this study both inpatients and outpatients were included, which may lead to unreliable drug taking and large variations in plasma levels.

For butriptyline [81], clomipramine [82,83], and lofepramine [84] limited studies have found no relationship between plasma level and clinical response.

VI. PSYCHOTROPIC DRUGS IN THE ELDERLY

Despite the widespread use of psychotropic drugs in all age groups, relatively little is known about their pharmacokinetics in the elderly. Very few studies have been carried out in the elderly either to assess pharmacokinetic data or to establish the relative efficacies of drugs to treat psychiatric disorders. Clearly, more research is required in this area.

A review of the literature showed that for a few drugs detailed pharmacokinetic investigations in the elderly have been carried out [85]. Potentially the aging process can affect absorption, distribution, metabolism, or excretion of drugs to bring about observed pharmacokinetic and pharmacodynamic changes.

There is little evidence to suggest significant changes in the rate of absorption of drugs from the gastrointestinal tract of the elderly compared with the young [85]. The validity of this observation is due to lack of systematic research. A number of factors such as the increase in gastric pH with age, reduction in intestinal blood flow, and decrease in gastrointestinal motility may all act to modify absorption rates with age [86]. Many drugs are absorbed by passive diffusion, and aging probably has no effect on these processes.

Changes in body composition in the elderly can affect drug distribution. On average, elderly patients are smaller than younger patients. Total body water and lean body mass decrease with age, while body fat increases in both men and women [87]. Plasma protein concentrations are also altered with aging: albumin level falls while the gamma globulin rises [88]. This may be of significance for the psychotropic drugs, as the tricyclic antidepressants, for example, are greater than 90% bound to plasma proteins. Small changes in protein binding can result in large variations of drug concentrations at receptor sites. Changes in the volume of distribution of some drugs have been observed with age, but no consistent pattern has emerged [85]. Biologically these factors may contribute to altered rates of elimination and be important determinants of drug effects.

Animal studies have shown a reduction in the activity of liver microsomal drug metabolizing enzymes with age [89], but no comparable studies have been done with human liver samples. Studies of plasma half-lives of drugs indicate some reduction in the metabolic ability of the elderly. This finding, though not universal, is the most consistent [85]. Generally, the rate of drug metabolism for the elderly patient is likely to be comparable to that of the younger adult, if the patient has normal hepatic function [90].

A consistent functional decline in glomerular filtration rate occurs with age. The implications for drug excretion are consistent with the change in renal physiology, viz., drugs excreted by the kidneys without prior metabolism persist at higher concentrations and for longer times in the blood and tissues of the elderly [90].

The generally acknowledged increased susceptibility of the elderly to drugs may in part be due to altered pharmacokinetics.

A. Tricyclic Antidepressant Plasma Levels in the Elderly

Raskin [91] was among the first to study the effects of age and sex as factors in the response to antidepressant drugs. The study showed significant differences in response to imipramine treatment between young (<40 years) and old (>40 years) males and between young and old females. Sex was also a significant factor in determining response to the drug regimen. No plasma levels were recorded.

Perhaps the most studied antidepressant from a pharmacokinetic viewpoint is nortriptyline. A study of the genetic control of nortriptyline kinetics in man revealed no evidence of major alterations with increasing age [92]. Subsequent clinical trials have confirmed that steady-state plasma levels of nortriptyline are not influenced by either age or sex of the patients [11,27]. A reanalysis of this data showed that age was positively correlated with plasma level, but stepwise multiple regression analysis showed that this correlation was not significant when corrected for the effects of sex and smoking status [93]. Other studies have found a positive but not significant correlation between plasma nortriptyline level and age [94].

Imipramine steady-state kinetics have been studied by Gram and colleagues [95]. A comparison of age-sex groups showed significantly different steady-state levels of imipramine. Women in the age group 30-39 years had lower steady-state levels than women in the other age groups examined: 20-29, 40-49, 50-59. Similarly, men aged 30-39 years had lower levels than those aged 50-65. Gram has attributed the tendency toward higher steady-state plasma levels in the aged to decreased hepatic elimination rates. The bimodal distribution of female plasma levels clearly points to a more complex mechanism. A significant positive correlation between steady-state imipramine concentrations and age was observed by Nies et al. [94]. This group were unable to demonstrate any significant differences between the mean plasma half-life of imipramine for young and old patients (19.0 vs. 23.8 h). Sex was not considered as a variant in this study.

Age-related differences in the steady-state plasma levels of both men and women have been observed for desipramine [94,95]. Older patients tended to have higher steady-state levels. A prolonged plasma half-life in aged compared with young patients was observed (75.8 vs. 34.2 h) [94]. This has been taken to indicate a decreased hepatic elimination rate, but changes in the volume of distribution, an important determinant of drug elimination, were not recorded.

Very few systematic studies have been carried out on the other available antidepressants. Most clinical trials suggest that the antidepressants are well tolerated by the aged. Accordingly, steady-state plasma butriptyline concentrations were not influenced by age or sex [81]. On the other hand, amitriptyline steady-state plasma levels show significant differences between young and old patients, older patients exhibiting higher levels [94]. Doxepin plasma levels have been studied in elderly patients and show a 15-fold variation in the levels achieved [62]. The effect of age on plasma concentrations was not studied. These data when combined with those of Burrows [63] showed no significant correlation between age and plasma level nor any significant differences between young (<65 years) and old (>65 years) patients. Recent studies in our unit suggest that age and sex have no effect on the steady-state plasma levels of maprotiline [67].

B. Conclusions

It appears that the elderly may have a decreased rate of elimination of antidepressants compared with younger people. As a consequence, the elderly will attain higher steady-state plasma concentrations on normal therapeutic doses, which will result in an increased susceptibility to side effects, especially those of a cardiovascular nature. Of course, prescribing lower-than-normal doses would tend to alleviate this problem. Alternatively, treatment could be initiated with a drug in which age-related effects are not pronounced, as in nortriptyline, doxepin, or maprotiline. Where cardiovascular problems are suspected, doxepin [26], mianserin [96] or nomifensine [96] may be the drug of choice.

VII. SUMMARY

It can be stated that *no consensus exists on the relationship between plasma levels and clinical response of the tricyclic antidepressants.*

The reasons for the discrepancies between studies may be harder to identify. A number of factors can affect steady-state plasma levels of tricyclics. Some are beyond the control of the investigator, but others, such as the concomitant administration of other drugs, should be controlled. Many of the studies used other drugs, thereby invalidating "between-trial" comparisons. Recent studies suggest that the hydroxylated metabolites of the tricyclics are as potent inhibitors of noradrenaline and serotonin reuptake as the parent compounds themselves [97]. Furthermore, these compounds cross the blood-brain barrier [98], and studies of the relationship must take this into account. Plasma protein binding is another factor which has been overlooked in the current studies. Individual differences have been observed in this parameter, and a small change in binding can bring about large changes in free drug concentrations [61]. Assay methodology has been criticized by some authors as the major source of variation between studies. While this may be a factor in some of the earlier studies, utilizing such nonspecific techniques as apectrofluorimetry, later papers have concentrated on the use of gas-liquid chromatography, double-isotope derivative dilution analysis, and mass fragmentography, which are specific, sensitive analytical techniques. In the absence of standard materials, cross-validation of assays between laboratories is essential to establish theri reliability [99]. The influence of nonpharmacological factors on treatment response has been described [100]. Between-study differences may arise from this source. Other reasons for the discrepancies may be the atypical (more resistant) patients studied, the lack of homogeneity of the illness, and the recurrent problems of relating the more sensitive plasma levels to crudely estimated changes in depressive symptomatology and of measuring plasma levels at different intervals after ingestion [101].

Future studies should be carried out in patients with recurrent depressive illnesses which have responded to tricyclic antidepressant treatment in the past. Rather than use standard doses, plasma levels of the parent drug should be adjusted within the so-called therapeutic range and clinical response ascertained.

The plasma level could be raised or lowered beyond the therapeutic range randomly and response measured again after steady-state levels were achieved. In this way it could be delineated for a sufficiently large population to ascertain the therapeutic range within the general community. Collaborative multicenter trials, although they present enormous logistical problems, offer the possibility of overcoming problems of diagnosis and the measurement of clinical response. Trials must include a 5-7-day placebo period, not only to "wash out" the effects of previous drug treatments, but also to remove from the trial responders to nonpharmacological treatments. This practice is widely accepted and practiced in antidepressant trials. A minimum of 4 weeks active drug treatment is needed to properly assess antidepressant effects. A standard time of drug sampling in such a study would be desirable. Gram [101] has suggested *10-15 hours* after the last dose, to avoid the plasma peaks after dosing. Some of the variation of "steady-state" levels in certain reported trials to date might be due to sampling too soon after the last dose. A reliable method for drug assay should be used. It should not only be precise and accurate but also specific. An assay based on gas chromatography, isotope derivative dilution analysis, or mass fragmentography, would appear to be the most reliable. Standardized measures of clinical response should be used in these studies. Finally, use of the appropriate statistical tests should be made in the analysis of the data.

The question of the routine analysis of plasma concentrations of tricyclic antidepressants has caused considerable debate. *In the light of the above discussion, routine monitoring does not appear warranted.* It is disturbing to find editorials [102] of prestigious medical journals advocating the "translation of these research findings into routine clinical practice" and increasing "efficacy of nortriptyline at least by monitoring plasma concentrations." Isolated plasma level determinations may aid, but cannot substitute for, sound clinical judgment. If an upper concentration limit of tricyclic antidepressants does exist, then it is most likely to be determined by their toxic effects rather than by other pharmacological factors. In this respect the findings of Burrows et al. [63,99] are of interest. Above levels of 200 ng/ml nortriptyline had significant cardiotoxicity in patients as evidenced by changes in their His bundle electrogram before and during treatment. In some patients levels of nortriptyline up to 500 ng/ml were observed, which produced satisfactory clinical response, but did not produce any significant changes in the cardiological parameters studied. The changes seen in some patients may be irreversible following chronic administration.

Routine monitoring of tricyclic antidepressant plasma levels may be indicated in therapeutic failure, where a low level may indicate poor compliance or rapid metabolism, and a need to increase the dosage. This applies particularly in the management of troublesome or potentially troublesome side effects, especially when cardiac abnormalities exist prior to therapy. Other indications include the management of overdoses; where many drugs are prescribed concomitantly, where drug interactions may cause anomalies in plasma levels; and in patients with physical illnesses, especially hepatic and renal disease where dangerously high plasma levels may appear.

REFERENCES

1. B. B. Brodie, Physicochemical and biochemical aspects of pharmacology. *JAMA 202:*600-609, 1967.
2. I. F. Bennet, Is there a superior antidepressant? In *Antidepressant Drugs* (S. Garattini and M. N. G. Dukes, eds.). Amsterdam, Excerpta Medica, 1967, pp. 375-393.
3. A. Coppen and C. Perris, Trials with antidepressants reassessed. *Int. Pharmacopsychiatry 11:*175-180, 1976.
4. L. E. Hollister, The clinical use of psychotherapeutic drugs, I: Antidepressants. *Curr. Therapeut.*, 65-89, October 1972.
5. T. G. Blashki, R. Mowbray, and B. Davies, Controlled trial of amitriptyline in general practice. *Brit. Med. J. 1:*133-138, 1971.
6. G. D. Burrows, Plasma tricyclic levels, clinical response, and drug interactions. In *Handbook of Studies on Depression* (G. D. Burrows, ed.). Amsterdam, Excerpta Medica, 1977, pp. 173-194.
7. S. H. Curry, Plasma level studies in psychotropic drug evaluation. *Brit. J. Clin. Pharmacol., Suppl., 3:*20-28, 1976.
8. W. Hammer and F. Sjöqvist, Plasma levels of monomethylated tricyclic antidepressants during treatment with imipramine-like compounds. *Life Sci. 6:*1895-1903, 1967.
9. S. Montgomery, R. Braithwaite, and A. Coppen, The relationship between plasma concentrations and amitriptyline and therapeutic response. Paper read to the British Academy of Psychopharmacology, London, July 1, 1975.
10. J. M. Perel, M. Shostak, E. Gann, S. J. Kantor, and A. H. Glassman, Pharmacodynamics of imipramine and clinical outcome in depressed patients. In *Pharmacokinetic Psychoactive Drug Blood Levels and Clinical Outcome.* (L. Gottschalk and S. Merlis, eds.). New York, Spectrum, 1975.
11. G. D. Burrows, B. Davies, and B. A. Scoggins, Plasma concentration of nortriptyline and clinical response in depressive illness. *Lancet 2:*619-623, 1972.
12. R. A. Braithwaite, R. Goulding, G. Theano, J. Bailey, and A. Coppen, Plasma concentrations of amitriptyline and clinical response. *Lancet 1:* 1297-1300, 1972.
13. F. Sjöqvist, W. Hammer, C. M. Ideström, M. Lind, D. Tuck, M. Åsberg, Plasma level of monomethylated tricyclic antidepressants and side-effects in man. In *Proc. Eur. Soc. Study Drug Toxic.* (Paris). Amsterdam, Excerpta Medica, 1968.
14. B. A. Alexanderson, D. A. Price-Evans, and F. Sjöqvist, Steady-state plasma levels of nortriptyline in twins: Influence of genetic factors and drug therapy. *Brit. Med. J. 4:*764-768, 1969.

15. G. D. Burrows and B. Davies, Antidepressants and barbiturates. *Brit. Med. J. 4:*113, 1971.
16. L. F. Gram and K. F. Overø, Drug interaction: Inhibitory effect of neuroleptics on metabolism of tricyclic antidepressants in man. *Brit. Med. J. 1:* 463-465, 1972.
17. F. Sjöqvist, W. Hammer, O. Borgå, and D. L. Azarnoff, Pharmacological significance of the plasma level of monomethylated tricyclic antidepressants. *Excerpta Med. ICS 180:*128-136, 1969.
18. M. Åsberg, B. Cronholm, F. Sjöqvist, and D. Tuck, Correlation of subjective side effects with plasma concentrations of nortriptyline. *Brit. Med. J. 4:*18-21, 1970.
19. M. Åsberg, P. Kragh-Sørensen, L. Bertilsson, B. Cronholm, C. Eggert-Hansen, F. Sjöqvist, and J. R. Tuck, Studies of relationship between plasma level and clinical effects of nortriptyline: Methodological problems. In *Symp. Med. Hoechst.* Stuttgart, Schattauer, 1973.
20. L. F. Gram and J. Christiansen, First-pass metabolism of imipramine in man. *Clin. Pharmacol. Ther. 17:*555-563, 1975.
21. G. G. Haydu, A. Dhrymiotis, and G. P. Quinn, Plasma imipramine levels in syndromes of depression. *Amer. J. Psychiatry 119:*574-575, 1962.
22. C. M. Yates, A. Todrick, and A. C. Tait, Aspects of the clinical chemistry of desmethylimipramine in man. *J. Pharm. Pharmacol. 15:*432-439, 1963.
23. P. Zeidenberg, J. M. Perel, M. Kanzler, R. N. Wharton, and S. Malitz, Clinical and metabolic studies with imipramine in man. *Amer. J. Psychiatry 127:*1321-1326, 1971.
24. G. D. Burrows, L. R. Turecek, and B. Davies, Studies of plasma tricyclic levels. CINP, 8th Cong. Copenhagen, August 1972.
25. G. D. Burrows, Clinical and pharmacological studies in depressive illness. M.D. thesis, University of Melbourne, 1973.
26. G. D. Burrows, B. Davies, and B. A. Scoggins, Plasma tricyclic levels and drug interactions. In CINP, 9th Cong., Paris. *J. Pharmacol. 5, Suppl. 2:* 1974.
27. G. D. Burrows, B. A. Scoggins, L. R. Turecek, and B. Davies, Plasma nortriptyline and clinical response. *Clin. Pharmacol. Ther. 16:*639-644, 1974.
28. V. Davies, G. D. Burrows, P. Dumovic, J. Vohra, D. Hunt, and J. G. Sloman, Effects on the heart of different tricyclic antidepressants. In *Sinequan (Doxepin HCl): A Monograph of Recent Clinical Studies* (J. Mendels, ed.). Amsterdam, Excerpta Medica, 1975, pp. 54-58.
29. B. Davies, G. D. Burrows, and B. A. Scoggins, Plasma nortriptyline and clinical response. Paper read to the British Academy of Psychopharmacology, London, July 1, 1975.
30. B. A. Scoggins, J. P. Coghlan, K. Maguire, G. D. Burrows, and B. Davies, The measurement of plasma levels of tricyclic antidepressant drugs. *Aust. N.Z. J. Psychiatr. 10:*7-12, 1976.
31. K. P. Maguire, G. D. Burrows, J. P. Coghlan, and B. A. Scoggins, Rapid radioisotopic procedure for determination of nortriptyline in plasma. *Clin. Chem. 22:*761-764, 1976.

32. P. Kragh-Sørensen, M. Åsberg, and C. Eggert-Hansen, Plasma nortriptyline levels in endogenous depression. *Lancet 1:*113-115, 1973.
33. G. D. Burrows, L. R. Turecek, B. Davies, R. Mowbray, and B. Scoggins, A sequential trial comparing two plasma levels of nortriptyline. *Aust. N.Z. J. Psychiatry 8:*21-23, 1974.
34. G. D. Burrows, Plasma nortriptyline and clinical response: A study using changing plasma levels. In *Plasma Nortriptyline and Lorazepam.* Presented at CINP meeting, Quebec, 1976.
35. P. Kragh-Sørensen, C. E. Hansen, and M. Åsberg, Plasma levels of nortriptyline in the treatment of endogenous depression. *Acta Psychiatr. Scand. 49:* 444-456, 1973.
36. P. Kragh-Sørensen, C. Eggert-Hansen, N. Larsen, J. Naestoft, and E. F. Hvidberg, Long-term treatment of endogenous depression with nortriptyline with control of plasma levels. *Psychol. Med. 4:*174-180, 1974.
37. A. Verghese, G. D. Burrows, G. Foenander, J. Stevenson, and B. Davies, Observer variation and depressive phenomenology. *Psychol. Med. 6:*587-590, 1976.
38. B. Alexanderson and O. Borgå, Urinary excretion of nortriptyline and five of its metabolites in man after single and multiple oral doses. *Eur. J. Clin. Pharmacol. 5:*174-180, 1973.
39. J. L. Crammer, B. Scott, and B. Rolfe, Metabolism of ^{14}C-imipramine, II. Urinary metabolites in man. *Psychopharmacologia* (Berlin) *15:*207-225, 1969.
40. L. Gram and K. F. Overø, First-pass metabolism of nortriptyline in man. *Clin. Pharmacol. Ther. 18:*305-314, 1975.
41. O. Borgå, D. L. Azarnoff, G. Plym Forshell, and F. Sjöqvist, Plasma protein binding of tricyclic antidepressants in man. *Biochem. Pharmacol. 18:* 2135-2143, 1969.
42. A. H. Glassman, M. J. Hurwic, and J. Perel, Plasma binding of imipramine and clinical outcome. *Amer. J. Psychiatry 130:*1357-1369, 1973.
43. A. R. Maclean, Plasma protein binding of the tricyclic antidepressants. M.Sc. thesis, University of Melbourne, 1974.
44. W. H. Lyle, P. W. Brooks, D. F. Early, W. P. Leggett, G. Silverman, R. A. Braithwaite, J. M. Cuthill, R. Goulding, I. B. Pearson, R. P. Snaith, and G. E. Strang, Plasma concentration of nortriptyline as a guide to therapy. *Postgrad. Med. J. 50:*282-287, 1974.
45. J. T. Biggs, S. S. Chang, W. R. Sherman, and W. H. Holland, Measurement of tricyclic antidepressant levels in an outpatient clinic. *J. Nerv. Ment. Dis. 162:*46-51, 1976.
46. S. Montgomery, R. Braithwaite, S. Dawling, and R. McAuley, High plasma nortriptyline levels in the treatment of depression. *Clin. Pharmacol. Ther. 23:*309-314, 1978.
47. D. Luchins and J. Ananth, Therapeutic implications of tricyclic antidepressant plasma levels. *J. Nerv. Ment. Dis. 162:*430-436, 1976.
48. M. Gruvstad, Plasma levels of antidepressants and clinical response. *Lancet 1:*95-96, 1973.

49. J. Kane, A. Rifkin, F. Quitkin, and D. Klein, In *Progress in Psychiatric Drug Treatment,* vol 2 (D. F. Klein and R. Gittelman-Klein, eds.). New York, Brunner-Mazel, 1976.
50. V. E. Ziegler, B. T. Co, J. R. Taylor, P. J. Clayton, and J. T. Biggs, Amitriptyline plasma levels and therapeutic response. *Clin. Pharmacol. Ther. 19:*795-801, 1976.
51. V. Ziegler, P. J. Clayton, and J. T. Biggs, A comparison study of amitriptyline and nortriptyline with plasma levels. *Arch. Gen. Psychiatry 34:*607-612, 1977.
52. V. E. Ziegler and J. T. Biggs, Tricyclic plasma levels: Effect of age, race, sex, and smoking. *JAMA 238:*2167-2169, 1977.
53. D. J. Kupfer, I. Hanin, D. G. Spiker, T. Grau, and P. Coble, Amitriptyline plasma levels and clinical response in primary depression. *Clin. Pharmacol. Ther. 22:*904-911, 1977.
54. A. Coppen, K. Ghose, S. A. Montgomery, V. A. Ramo Rao, J. Bailey, J. Christiansen, P. L. Mikkleson, H. M. van Praag, F. van de Poel, E. J. Minsker, V. G. Kozulja, N. Matussek, G. Kunghunz, and A. Jorgensen, Amitriptyline plasma-concentration and clinical effect. *Lancet 1:*63-66, 1978.
55. C. J. S. Walter, Drug plasma levels and clinical effects. *Proc. Roy. Soc. Med. 64:*282-285, 1971.
56. G. B. Muscettola, M. Giovannucci, R. Montanani, P. L. Morselli, and S. Garattini, Relationship between desipramine plasma levels and the effect in Parkinson's syndrome. *Rev. Eur. Etudes Clin. Biol. 17:*375-379, 1972.
57. B. R. Ballinger, A. Presly, A. H. Reid, and I. H. Stevenson, The effects of hypnotics on imipramine treatment. *Psychopharmacologia 39:*267-274, 1974.
58. R. Olivier-Martin, D. Marzin, E. Buchsenschutz, P. Pichot, and A. J. Boissier, Concentrations plasmatiques de l'imipramine et de la desmethylimipramine et effet anti-depresseur au cours d'un traitment controlé. *Psychopharmacologia* (Berlin) *41:*187-195, 1975.
59. G. M. Simpson, T. B. Cooper, and J. H. Lee, In *Depression: Behavioural, Biochemical, Diagnostic, and Treatment Concepts* (D. M. Gallant and G. M. Simpson, eds.). New York, Spectrum, 1975.
60. S. Bhanji and M. H. Lader, The electroencephalographic and psychological effects of imipramine in depressed inpatients. *Eur. J. Clin. Pharmacol. 12:*349-354, 1977.
61. A. H. Glassman, J. M. Perel, M. Shostak, S. J. Kantor, and J. L. Fleiss, Clinical implications of imipramine plasma levels for depressive illness. *Arch. Gen. Psychiatry 34:*197-204, 1977.
62. R. O. Friedel and M. A. Raskind, Relationship of blood levels of Sinequan to clinical effects in the treatment of depression in aged patients. In *Sinequan (Doxepin HCl) A Monograph of Recent Clinical Studies* (J. Mendels, ed.). Amsterdam, Excerpta Medica, 1975, pp. 51-53.
63. G. D. Burrows, J. Vohra, P. Dumovic, K. Maguire, B. A. Scoggins, and B. Davies, Tricyclic antidepressant drugs and cardiac conduction. *Progr. Neuro-Psychopharmacol. 1:*329-334, 1977.

64. J. O'Brien and O. Hinsvark, GLC determination of doxepin plasma levels. *J. Pharm. Sci. 65:*1068, 1976.
65. N. S. Kline, T. Cooper, and B. Johnston, Doxepin and desmethyldoxepin serum levels and clinical response. In *Pharmacokinetics of Psychoactive Drugs: Blood Levels and Clinical Response* (L. A. Gottschalk and S. Merlis, eds.). New York, Spectrum, 1976.
66. G. D. Burrows, T. R. Norman, K. P. Maguire, B. A. Scoggins, and J. M. E. Wurm, Plasma doxepin levels and clinical response (Unpublished data.)
67. J. Angst and R. Rothweiler, Blood levels and clinical effects of maprotiline. In *Classification and Prediction of Outcome of Depression.* Symposia Medica Hoechst 8 (J. Angst, ed.). Stuttgart, Schattauer-Verlag, 1973, pp. 237-244.
68. P. Miller, G. Beaumont, J. Seldrup, V. John, D. K. Luscombe, and R. Jones, Efficacy, side-effects, plasma, and blood levels of maprotiline (Ludiomil). *J. Int. Med. Res., Suppl. (4) 5:*101-111, 1977.
69. L. Mulgirigama, C. M. Pare, P. Turner, R. S. B. Ehsanullah, and D. Witts, An assessment of uptake inhibition of 5-hydroxy-tryptamine, dopamine, and nor-adrenaline in a double blind clinical trial of clomipramine and maprotiline in depressed outpatients. (Unpublished data, 1978.)
70. T. R. Norman, G. D. Burrows, K. P. Maguire, B. A. Scoggins, and B. M. Davies, Maprotiline plasma levels and clinical response. Presented at 11th CINP Congress, Vienna, 1978.
71. R. Fischbach, Die Bedeutung von Ludiomil. In *Die Depression in der Sicht des praktischen Arztes* (Lenz, ed.). Vienna, Ciba-Geigy, 1974, pp. 67-71.
72. N. Matussek and M. Aarons, Wirkung akuter und chronisher Applikation von Maprotilin und ihre Berziehung zum Plasmaspiegel bei gesunden Versuchspersonen. *Arzneim.-Forsch. 24:*1107-1111, 1974.
73. A. Coppen, S. A. Montgomery, R. K. Gupta, and J. E. Bailey, A double-blind comparison of lithium carbonate and maprotiline in the prophylaxis of the affective disorders. *Brit. J. Psychiatry 128:*479-485, 1976.
74. J. T. Biggs, W. H. Holland, and W. R. Sherman, Steady-state protriptyline levels in an outpatient population. *Amer. J. Psychiatry 132:*960-962, 1975.
75. J. P. Moody, S. F. Whyte, and G. J. Naylor, A simple method for the determination of protriptyline in plasma. *Clin. Chem. Acta 43:*355-359, 1973.
76. S. F. Whyte, A. J. MacDonald, G. J. Naylor, and J. P. Moody, Plasma concentrations of protriptyline and clinical effects in depressed women. *Brit. J. Psychiatry 128:*384-390, 1976.
77. J. Modestin, The relationship between the clinical effects of dibenzepin (Noveril) and its plasma concentration. *Pharmakopsychiatry 6:*28-38, 1973.
78. E. B. Gordon, Clinical response and blood levels of dothiepin in the treatment of depression. Presented at 11th CINP Congress, Vienna, 1978.
79. A. Coppen, R. Gupta, S. Montgomery, K. Ghose, J. Bailey, B. Burns, and

J. J. de Ridder, Mianserin hydrochloride: A novel antidepressant. *Brit. J. Psychiatry 129:*342-345, 1976.

80. S. Montgomery, R. McAuley, and D. B. Montgomery, Relationship between mianserin plasma levels and antidepressant effect in a double-blind trial comparing a single night-time and divided daily dose regimens. *Brit. J. Clin. Pharmacol. 5:*71S-76S, 1978.
81. G. D. Burrows, T. R. Norman, K. P. Maguire, G. Rubinstein, B. A. Scoggins, and B. M. Davies, A new antidepressant, butriptyline: Plasma levels and clinical response. *Med. J. Aust. 2:*604-606, 1977.
82. P. Miller, D. K. Luscombe, R. B. Jones, J. Seldrup, G. Beaumont, and V. John, Relationships between clinical response, plasma levels, and side-effects of clomipramine (Anafranil) in general practitioner trials. *J. Int. Med. Res., Suppl. (1) 5:*108-118, 1977.
83. M. Gringras, D. K. Luscombe, R. B. Jones, G. Beaumont, J. Seldrup, and V. John, A clinical trial of a 50 mg formulation of clomipramine (Anafranil) with steady-state plasma level measurements. *J. Int. Med. Res., Suppl. (1) 5:*119-124, 1977.
84. R. Siwers, S. Borg, G. D'Elia, G. Lundlin, G. Plym-Forshell, H. Raotma, and G. Roman, Comparative clinical evaluation of lofepramine and imipramine. *Acta Psychiatr. Scand. 55:*21-31, 1977.
85. J. Crooks, K. O'Malley, and I. H. Stevenson, Pharmacokinetics in the elderly. *Clin. Pharmacokin. 1:*280, 1976.
86. A. D. Bender, Effect of age on intestinal absorption: Implications for drug absorption in the elderly. *J. Amer. Geriatr. Soc. 16:*1331, 1968.
87. I. S. Edelman and J. Liebman, Anatomy of body water and electrolytes. *Amer. J. Med. 27:*256, 1959.
88. E. Woodford-Williams, A. S. Alvarez, D. Webster, B. Landless, and M. P. Dixon, Serum protein patterns in normal and pathological ageing. *Gerontologia 10:*86, 1964.
89. R. Kato, P. Vassanelli, G. Frontino, and E. Chiesara, Variation in the activity of liver microsomal drug-metabolising enzymes in rats in relation to age. *Biochem. Pharmacol. 13:*1037, 1964.
90. R. H. Briant, Drug treatment in the elderly: Problems and prescribing rules. *Curr. Therapeut. 18:*41, 1977.
91. A. Raskin, Age-sex differences in response to antidepressant drugs. *J. Nerv. Ment. Dis. 59:*120, 1974.
92. M. Åsberg, D. A. Price-Evans, and F. Sjöqvist, Genetic control of nortriptyline kinetics in man: A study of relatives of propositi with high plasma concentrations. *J. Med. Genet. 8:*129, 1971.
93. T. R. Norman, G. D. Burrows, K. P. Maguire, G. Rubinstein, B. A. Scoggins, and B. Davies, Cigarette smoking and plasma nortriptyline levels. *Clin. Pharmacol. Ther. 21:*453, 1977.
94. A. Nies, D. S. Robinson, M. J. Friedman, R. Green, T. B. Cooper, C. L. Ravaris, and J. D. Ives, Relationship between age and tricyclic antidepressant plasma levels. *Amer. J. Psychiatry 134:*790, 1977.

95. L. F. Gram, I. Sondergaard, J. Christiansen, G. O. Peterson, P. Bech, N. Reisby, I. Ibsen, J. Ortmann, A. Nagy, S. J. Dencker, O. Jacobsen, and O. Krautwald, Steady-state kinetics of imipramine in patients. *Psychopharmacol. 54:*255, 1977.
96. G. D. Burrows, J. Vohra, D. Hunt, J. G. Sloman, B. A. Scoggins, and B. Davies, Cardiac effects of different tricyclic antidepressant drugs. *Brit. J. Psychiatry 129:*335-341, 1976.
97. W. Z. Potter and F. K. Goodwin, Antidepressant drug levels and clinical response. *Lancet 1:*1049, 1978.
98. J. Christiansen and L. F. Gram, Imipramine and its metabolites in human brain. *J. Pharm. Pharmacol. 25:*604-608, 1973.
99. G. D. Burrows, B. Davies, K. Maguire, T. R. Norman, B. A. Scoggins, R. P. Hullin, and J. Burch, Interlaboratory comparison of nortriptyline levels. *Biochem. Med. 20:*125-127, 1978.
100. K. Rickels, *Non-specific Factors in Drug Therapy.* Springfield, Ill. Thomas. 1968.
101. L. F. Gram, Plasma level monitoring of tricyclic antidepressant therapy. *Clin. Pharmacokin. 2:*237-251, 1977.
102. Tricyclic antidepressant concentrations and clinical response (editorial). *Brit. Med. J. 2:*783-784, 1978.
103. M. Åsberg, B. Cronholm, F. Sjöqvist and D. Tuck, Relationship between plasma level and therapeutic effect of nortriptyline. *Brit. Med. J. 3:*331-334, 1971.
104. G. D. Burrows, K. P. Maguire, B. A. Scoggins, J. Stevenson, and B. Davies. Plasma nortriptyline and clinical response—a study using changing plasma levels. *Psychol. Med. 7:*87-91, 1977.
105. P. Kragh-Sørensen, C. E. Hansen, P. C. Braastrup, and E. F. Hvidberg, Self-inhibiting action of nortriptyline's antidepressive effect at high plasma levels. *Psychopharmacologia 45:*305-312, 1976.
106. S. A. Montgomery, R. A. Braithwaite, and J. L. Crammer, Routine nortriptyline levels in treatment of depression. *Brit. Med. J. 2:*166-167, 1977.
107. V. E. Ziegler, P. J. Clayton, J. R. Taylor, B. T. Co, and J. T. Biggs, Nortriptyline plasma levels and therapeutic response. *Clin. Pharmacol. Ther. 20:*458-463, 1976.
108. L. F. Gram, N. Reisby, I. Ibsen, A. Nagy, S. J. Dencker, P. Bech, G. O. Petersen, and J. Christiansen, Plasma levels and antidepressive effects of imipramine. *Clin. Pharmacol. Ther. 19:*318-324, 1976.
109. N. Reisby, L. F. Gram, P. Bech, A. Nagy, G. O. Petersen, J. Ortmann, I. Ibsen, S. J. Dencker, O. Jacobsen, I. Sondergaard, and J. Christiansen, Imipramine, clinical effects and pharmacokinetic variability. *Psychopharmacologia 54:*263-272, 1977.
110. J. T. Biggs and V. E. Ziegler, Protriptyline plasma levels and antidepressant response. *Clin. Pharmacol. Ther. 22:*269-273, 1977.
111. G. D. Burrows, T. R. Norman, K. P. Maguire, G. Rubinstein, B. A. Scoggins, and B. Davies, A new antidepressant butriptyline—plasma levels and clinical response. *Med. J. Aust. 2:*604-606, 1977.

6

Zimelidine Pharmacology, Pharmacokinetics, and Clinical Response

Sven-Ove Ögren / *Astra Läkemedel AB, Research and Development Laboratories, Södertälje, Sweden*

Jan Lundström / *Astra Läkemedel AB, Research and Development Laboratories, Södertälje, Sweden*

George Moore / *Astra Pharmaceuticals Pty. Ltd., Medical Department, Sydney, New South Wales, Australia*

I. INTRODUCTION

Studies in man suggest that there may exist a reduced noradrenaline (NA) and/or 5-hydroxytryptamine (5-HT) transmission in depressive disorders. In certain groups of depressive patients a reduction of the cerebrospinal fluid (CSF) concentration of 5-hydroxyindoleacetic acid (5-HIAA), the major metabolite of 5-HT, has been observed [1]. The concentration of 3-methoxy-4-hydroxyphenylethylglycol (MHPG), the main metabolite of NA, has also been reported to be low in some depressed patients [2].

The observations that the tricyclic antidepressants inhibit the neuronal uptake of NA and 5-HT [3-6] suggested that their therapeutic effect may be due to enhancement of NA or 5-HT activity in the brain [7-9]. Most tricyclic antidepressants have been found to affect the uptake of NA. Some tricyclic antidepressants–in particular the tertiary amine analogues, e.g., chlorimipramine–inhibit also the uptake of 5-HT [6]. However, chlorimipramine, although being the most potent of the tricyclics on 5-HT uptake, is not particularly selective since it produces an equal inhibition of NA and 5-HT uptake under in vivo conditions in rats [10].

It has been suggested that the different action of the tricyclic antidepressants on NA and 5-HT uptake may be important for their therapeutic efficacy in depression. Thus, inhibition of NA uptake has been linked to psychomotor activation, whereas inhibition of 5-HT uptake may be important for the alleviation of mood [6]. Work in several laboratories has therefore been directed toward the development of more selective 5-HT uptake inhibitors.

In this chapter we describe zimelidine [(Z)-3(4-bromophenyl)-N,N-dimethyl-3-(3-pyridyl)allylamine] (Fig. 1), a new antidepressant, acting primarily on central 5-HT mechanisms. Zimelidine has in animal studies been shown to be a potent and selective 5-HT uptake inhibitor. Clinical studies suggest that zimelidine may be an effective antidepressant.

II. ANIMAL PHARMACOLOGY

A. Inhibition of Monoamine Uptake

The effects of zimelidine on neuronal uptake of 5-HT and NA has been evaluated in mice and rats. In some studies the ability of zimelidine and tricyclic antidepressants to inhibit the uptake of [^{14}C] 5-HT and [^{3}H] (-)NA was compared in slices or homogenates prepared from various regions of mouse and rat brain. When slices of mouse brain were incubated with the drugs in vitro, zimelidine and chlorimipramine were about 20 times more active in blocking the uptake of [^{3}H] 5-HT than that of [^{3}H] (-)NA [11]. Chlorimipramine was more active as a

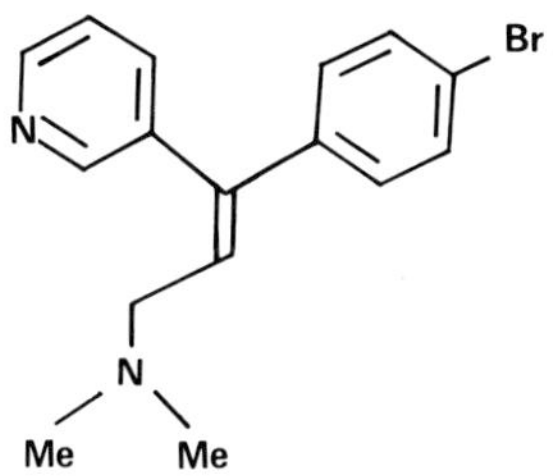

ZIMELIDINE

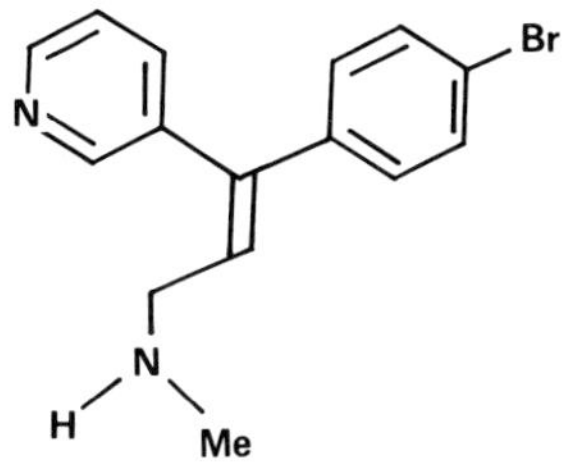

NORZIMELIDINE

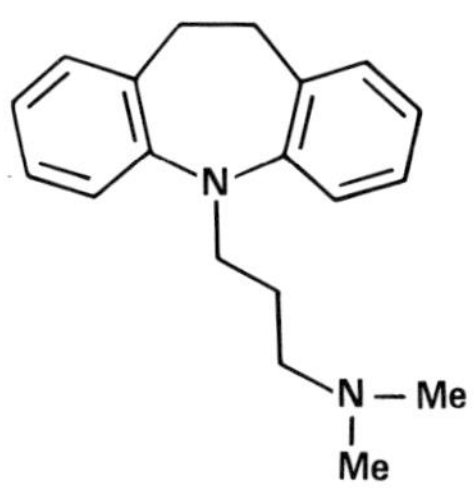

IMIPRAMINE

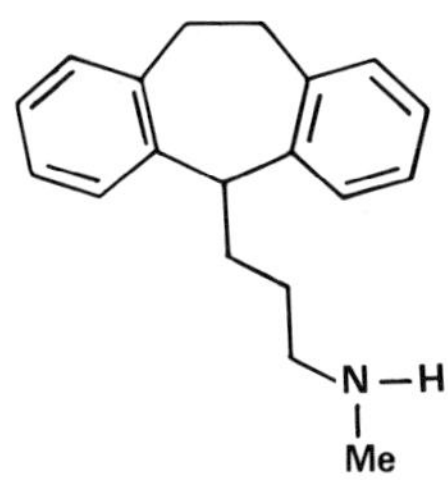

DESIPRAMINE

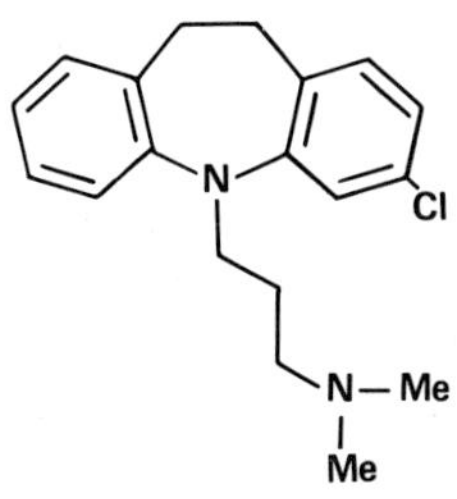

CHLORIMIPRAMINE

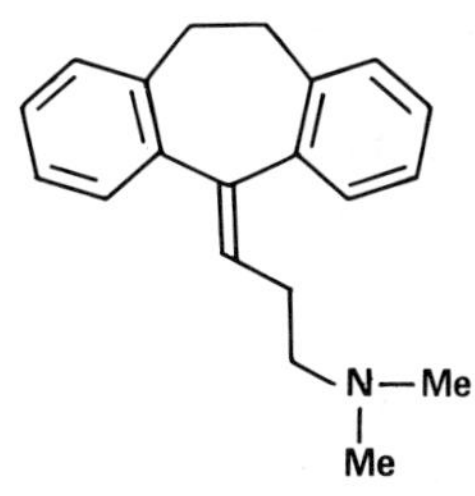

AMITRIPTYLINE

Figure 1 Structures of zimelidine and its main metabolite norzimelidine together with common tricyclic antidepressants.

Table 1 Inhibition of the Accumulation of NA and 5-HT in Rat Hypothalamic Slices after the Administration of the Compounds in Vivo[a]

	ED_{50} (mg/kg)			
	[^{3}H] 1-NA		[^{14}C] 5-HT	
Compound	i.p.	Oral	i.p.	Oral
Zimelidine	>20	25	5.5	7
Norzimelidine	38	57	5	5.4
Imipramine	6	8	50	50
Desipramine	10	8	>40 (15%)	>50
Chlorimipramine	25	20	10	35

[a]The rats were sacrificed 1 h after i.p. and 2 h after oral administration. Slices (60 mg) of hypothalamus were incubated with 1×10^{-7} M of the labeled amines in 2.0-ml buffer for 5 min. ED_{50} values were determined from log dose-response curves based on at least 3 doses with 4 animals in each dose

Source: Results from Refs. 10 and 12.

5-HT inhibitor than zimelidine in vitro. Subsequent studies in rats showed that the secondary amine of zimelidine, norzimelidine, was considerably more potent than zimelidine to inhibit 5-HT uptake in vitro [12].

When uptake was measured in vivo in mouse brain slices prepared from animals given the drugs intraperitoneally (i.p.), zimelidine produced a preferential inhibition of 5-HT uptake with a slight effect on NA uptake [11]. Chlorimipramine was less selective than zimelidine and also markedly affected the uptake of NA.

The selectivity of zimelidine for 5-HT uptake was further demonstrated after oral and i.p. administration to rats. As shown in Table 1, zimelidine was about equally potent in inhibiting 5-HT uptake after oral and i.p. administration. Norzimelidine was equipotent with zimelidine. Zimelidine was, after oral administration to rats, about 7 times more potent than imipramine and 5 times more potent than chlorimipramine in blocking 5-HT uptake. After both i.p. and oral administration imipramine and desipramine preferentially inhibited NA uptake. Chlorimipramine was somewhat more active in blocking NA than 5-NT uptake when given orally.

In the uptake studies the metabolic fate of the drugs has to be considered. In the rat both imipramine and chlorimipramine form demethylated metabolites which are both potent inhibitors of NA uptake. Thus, the discrepancy between the in vitro and in vivo activity of chlorimipramine on 5-HT uptake is largely due to the formation of chlordesipramine, a NA uptake inhibitor [10]. Recent studies have demonstrated that chlorimipramine also in man is about equally active in blocking NA and 5-HT uptake [13]. The high potency of zimelidine as a 5-HT uptake inhibitor under in vivo conditions is largely due to the formation of the active metabolite norzimelidine. Inhibition of the formation of norzimelidine by the metabolic inhibitor proadifene (SKF 525A) reduced markedly the inhibitory effect of zimelidine on 5-HT uptake [12]. The inhibition of 5-HT uptake in the rat has also shown to be related to the concentration of norzimelidine. Zimelidine produced a rather long-lasting inhibition of 5-HT uptake in the rat brain which was correlated to the concentration of norzimelidine in the brain [12]. Administration of zimelidine and norzimelidine produced an almost identical inhibition of 5-HT uptake and also about equal concentrations of norzimelidine in the brain of rats. Thus, in contrast to chlorimipramine-chlordesipramine, norzimelidine, although being more potent, shares qualitatively the same properties as zimelidine.

The effects of the drugs on the 5-HT uptake was also evaluated in vivo by studying their ability to counteract 5-HT depletion induced by 4-methyl-α-ethyl-m-tyramine (H75/12). This drug is supposed to use the membrane pump to enter the 5-HT neurons, and the blockade of this uptake mechanism will prevent the depletion of 5-HT stores induced by H75/12 [6]. Zimelidine in contrast to desipramine and amitriptyline caused a marked protection of the 5-HT stores from depletion in the cortical regions, striatum, hypothalamus, and the spinal cord (Table 2). These findings suggest that zimelidine is about equally potent in blocking 5-HT uptake in both ascending and descending 5-HT terminal systems under in vivo conditions.

B. Effects on Turnover of Monoamines

The effects of zimelidine on 5-HT turnover and synthesis has also been examined. Zimelidine produced after acute administration a reduction of 5-HT synthesis in the rat brain in the same dose range as inhibition of 5-HT uptake [15]. Zimelidine did not influence the concentration of tryptophan in the rat brain. Zimelidine was found to only slightly affect NA synthesis even when given in high doses [15] and exerted a very weak α-receptor blocking activity in vitro in contrast to tricyclic antidepressants (Table 3). Zimelidine exerted also a negligible effect on dopamine (DA) uptake [12] and did not exhibit any direct DA receptor blocking action in vitro and in vivo (Table 3). Zimelidine was, however, observed to reduce DA turnover at a rather low dose (3 mg/kg), particularly in the limbic DA system [17]. Also, amitriptyline and desipramine reduced DA turnover at 3 mg/kg i.p. in some limbic structures [17].

Table 2 Inhibition of 5-HT Uptake in Vivo: Effect of Zimelidine on the H75/12-Induced Depletion in Cortex Cerebri, in Hypothalamus, and in the Spinal Cord[a]

	Inhibition of Uptake, ED_{50}, H75/12 (mg/kg i.p.)		
Compound	Cortex cerebri	Hypothalamus	Spinal cord
Zimelidine	6	5.5	5
Amitriptyline	>30 (25%)	>30 (44%)	>30
Desipramine	>30 (25%)	>30 (33%)	>30

[a]The drugs were given i.p. 30 min before the injection of H75/12 (50 mg/kg i.p.), 2 h before killing. ED_{50} values were determined by log dose-response curves and are based on 4 dose levels with 5-6 animals per dose level. Percentages refer to inhibition at the highest dose tested.

Source: Data from Ref. 14.

Table 3 Effects of Zimelidine on Postsynaptic Central Noradrenergic and Dopaminergic Receptors in the Rat Brain[a]

Compound	Displacement of [^{3}H] WB-4101 (α receptor binding) IC_{50} (μM)	Displacement of [^{3}H] spiroperidol (DA receptor binding) IC_{50} (μM)	Apomorphine antagonism ED_{50} (mg/kg i.p.)
Zimelidine	1.18	14.4	>40
Norzimelidine	0.95	40.8	>40
Amitriptyline	0.022	1.07	–
Desipramine	0.25	5.03	>30

[a]IC_{50} values refer to the concentration which inhibits by 50% the specific binding of [^{3}H]-WB-4101 to α-adrenergic receptors in the cortex cerebri and [^{3}H] spiroperidol to DA receptors in the striatum. IC_{50} values were determined by log-probit analysis. The ability of the drugs to block stereotypes induced by the DA agonist apomorphine (1 mg/kg s.c.) was tested in the rat.

Source: Results from Ref. 16.

C. Effects on Pituitary Hormones

The neuroendocrine action of zimelidine was evaluated in male rats. Zimelidine caused a trend for an increase in serum prolactin levels, a dose-related reduction in serum growth hormone levels, and in the low dose of 3 mg/kg a slight increase in the levels of luteinizing hormone (LH) [17].

D. Peripheral and Central Anticholinergic Action

It is well known that tricyclic antidepressants exert rather potent central and peripheral anticholinergic effects. Tricyclic antidepressants antagonize the pharmacological effects of acetylcholine and of cholinergic agonists such as oxotremorine. In contrast to amitriptyline and imipramine, zimelidine was shown to have very weak anticholinergic effects in the guinea pig ileum preparation (Table 4). Peripheral and central anticholinergic effects in vivo were measured by the ability to block oxotremorine-induced salivation and tremor, respectively. Zimelidine did not block oxotremorine-induced salivation and tremor even when given in a high dose. Zimelidine produced in vitro a weak displacement of [^{3}H]-QNB, a potent cholinergic antagonist, which binds to muscarinic receptors [19]. It is concluded (see Table 4) that zimelidine has very weak peripheral and central anticholinergic properties compared to the tricyclic antidepressants.

E. Behavioral Effects

Both zimelidine and norzimelidine enhanced central 5-HT activity in mice as evidence by a marked potentiation of the behavioral effects of 5-hydroxytryptophan (5-HTP), the precursor of 5-HT. After oral administration to mice zimelidine was about 7 times more potent than chlorimipramine [20].

Behavioral studies in rats and mice show clear differences between zimelidine and tricyclic antidepressants. The tricyclics are characterized by their ability to inhibit reserpine-induced hypothermia, by their rather strong sedative effect (decrease of locomotor activity), and by a marked potentiation of amphetamine. Zimelidine failed to inhibit reserpine-induced hypothermia [11], and zimelidine produced in mice much less sedation than tricyclic antidepressants (Table 5). Zimelidine did not increase spontaneous activity in mice in the lower dose range in contrast to nomifensine [21] and did not enhance the central stimulant action of amphetamine in mice. Zimelidine, however, blocked the decrease in avoidance performance caused by p-chloroamphetamine in the rat [22]. Zimelidine did not by itself affect a learned avoidance response in the rat. Zimelidine reduced markedly aggressive behavior in isolated mice in a nonsedative dose range well related to its effect on 5-HT uptake. Aggressive behavior in mice is strongly blocked by anxiolytics such as diazepam.

After treatment with zimelidine there was no protection against convulsions induced by pentylenetetrazole (metrazole), isoniazide, picrotoxin, and bicuculline in mice (unpublished data). Zimelidine did not change the convulsive threshold for metrazole in mice.

F. Drug Interactions

Studies on the interaction between zimelidine and sedative/hypnotic drugs were performed in mice. Zimelidine caused a very slight interaction with hexobarbital

Table 4 The Antimuscarinic Potency of Zimelidine and Some Tricyclic Antidepressants[a]

	Central anticholinergic effect		Peripheral anticholinergic effect	
Compound	Displacement of [^{3}H] QNB IC_{50} (μM)	Block of oxotremorine tremor ED_{50} (mg/kg i.p.)	Block of acetylcholine (guinea pig ileum) IC_{50} (μM)	Block of oxotremorine salivation ED_{50} (mg/kg i.p.)
Zimelidine	33.7	>80	41	>80
Norzimelidine	19.8	>80	34	>80
Amitriptyline	0.069	2.6	0.4	5.6
Desipramine	0.848	44.2	4.4	43.8
Imipramine	0.181	15.2	3.5	26.4

[a]IC_{50} values refer to the concentration which inhibits by 50% the specific binding of [^{3}H] QNB to muscarinic receptors in the cortex cerebri of rats and blocks contractions induced by acetylcholine in the guinea pig ileum preparation. Block of oxotremorine-induced tremor and salivation was performed in mice.

Source: Results from Ref. 18.

Table 5 Effect of Zimelidine on Locomotor Activity in Mice[a]

Compound	Decrease of motor activity by 50%, ED_{50} (mg/kg i.p.)	(μmol/kg i.p.)
Zimelidine	86	210
Norzimelidine	92	232
Amitriptyline	34	110
Chlorimipramine	56	159
Desipramine	46	152

[a]Locomotor activity was measured for 10 min in automatic activity cages. ED_{50} determined by regression analysis refers to the calculated dose which lowers spontaneous locomotion by 50% compared with saline controls. ED_{50} values are based on 5-6 dose levels with 12 animals per dose level.

Source: Results from Ref. 21.

in contrast to amitriptyline and imipramine. Zimelidine did not potentiate the sedative/hypnotic effects of ethanol, diazepam, and nitrazepam.

G. Cardiovascular Effects

Tricyclic antidepressants produce several cardiovascular side effects which are clinical problems, particularly in the treatment of the elderly and people with heart disease. The tricyclics induce change in the electrocardiogram such as PR and QT prolongations, widening of the QRS complex, as well as tachycardia. Some of these effects, e.g., tachycardia, appear to be associated with the anticholinergic properties of the tricyclics.

In the rat the tricyclic drugs amitriptyline, imipramine, and chlorimipramine caused ECG changes in a rather low dose range in contrast to zimelidine (Table 6). Similar results were obtained in the anesthetized dog [24]. In the anesthetized dog, amitriptyline produced a clear and prominent tachycardia, whereas imipramine caused a biphasic effect: Tachycardia in a low dose range followed by bradycardia. Zimelidine did not affect heart rate. The contractile force of the myocardium was also very little affected by zimelidine in contrast to imipramine and chlorimipramine (Table 7).

The general, pharmacodynamic properties of zimelidine are summarized in Table 7. It can be seen that zimelidine exerts slight effects on cardiovascular functions. Contrary to the tricyclics, zimelidine does not antagonize the tyramine pressor response.

Table 6 Effect of Antidepressants on Blood Pressure, Heart Rate, and ECG Parameters in Unanesthetized Rats[a]

Compound	Lethal dose (mg/kg)	Blood pressure		Heart rate		PR prolongation	QRS widening	QT prolongation
		Increase	Decrease	Increase	Decrease			
Zimelidine	64	–	16	2	32	–	16	4
Amitriptyline	16-32	0.5	8	0.5	16	4	0.5	0.5
Chlorimipramine	16-32	2	4	4	8	4	2	2
Desipramine	32	0.1	8	–	8	4	0.5	0.5
Imipramine	16-32	0.5	8	1	8	8	1	2

[a]Doses in mg/kg. Groups of 5 rats were given drugs i.v. at increasing doses (0.001, 0.01, 0.1, 0.5, 1.2, 4,8,16,32,64 mg/kg) with 5-15-minute intervals. For the mean arterial blood pressure the doses which caused a change of at least 10 mm Hg are given. For all other parameters the doses which caused statistically significant (P = .05) changes are given.

Source: Results from Ref. 23.

Table 7 General Pharmacodynamic Properties of Zimelidine in Rats and Dogs

ECG:	
PR prolongation	None or small
QRS widening	At high doses
QT prolongation	At moderate to high doses
Heart rate	Small increase (<10% at 2 mg/kg; transient decrease at 32 mg/kg in unanesthetized rats; no change in anesthetized dogs given 0.5 mg/kg/min i.v. for 40 minutes
Blood pressure	Transient decrease at high doses in unanesthetized rats; no change in anesthetized dogs
Isometric contractible force of myocardium	No change in anesthetized dogs given 0.5 mg/kg/min for 40 minutes
Interactions:	
Noradrenaline	No potentiation
Adrenaline	No potentiation
Vagal stimulation	No blockade until high doses
Acetylcholine	No blockade until high doses
Tyramine	No blockade until high doses

Source: Results from Refs. 23 and 24.

III. BIOTRANSFORMATION AND EXCRETION PRODUCTS

The importance of the in vivo demethylation of zimelidine to norzimelidine became evident during the pharmacological testing. In the rat the formation of norzimelidine is very rapid (Fig. 2) and pharmacological effects of zimelidine must be related to norzimelidine at least after oral and intraperitoneal administration.

The metabolism of zimelidine has been investigated with the use of ^{14}C-labeled material [25]. The major metabolic routes as found in rat and dog are shown in Fig. 3. In these species, most of the administered radioactivity was excreted into urine (~65%) where the predominant metabolites were the acrylic acid derivative (V), the N′-oxide of zimelidine (IV), and the N′-acetyl conjugate of the primary amine (VI). These metabolites have also been detected in urine from a patient receiving zimelidine, and there appear to be similar metabolic pathways in man and these experimental animals. Metabolites IV and V are present in plasma from the investigated animals as well as from man.

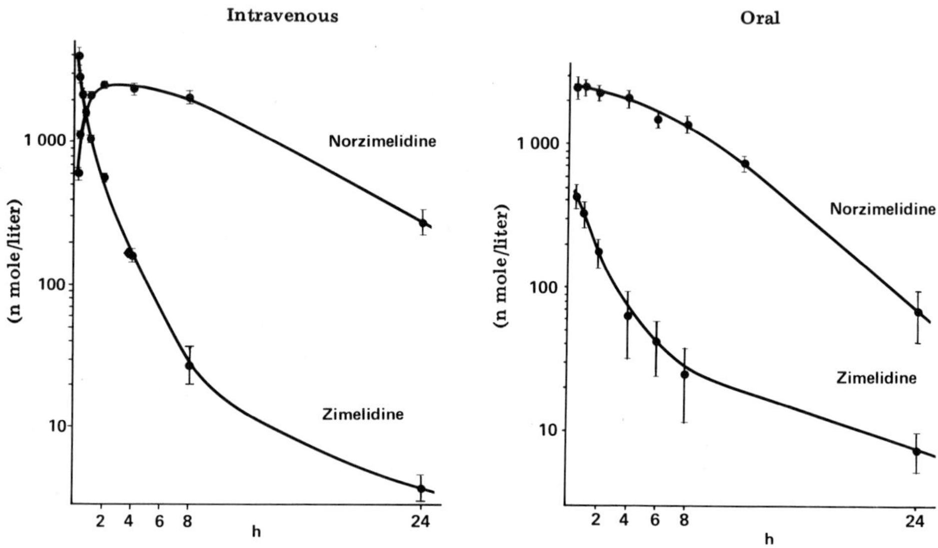

Figure 2 Plasma levels (mean ± SEM, n = 6) of zimelidine and norzimelidine in rats after administration of zimelidine 10 mg/kg.

However, the primary amine (III) has so far only been detected in human plasma.

The pharmacological activity of norzimelidine compared to zimelidine has already been described above. Among the metabolites the primary amine (III) has only a weak 5-HT uptake blocking activity. The N′-oxide (IV) is, under in vivo conditions in rats, equipotent to zimelidine. However, it is inactive in vitro, and its activity in vivo is most likely a result of its reduction to the parent amine, primarily in the liver. The other two metabolites V and VI are inactive.

IV. CLINICAL PHARMACOLOGY

A. The Action of Zimelidine and 5-HT System in Man

The assessment of the antidepressant effects in patients of new drugs is difficult, and various biochemical tests have been used in attempts to correlate the results in animal experiments with the response in man. Such methods include the inhibition of uptake of NA and 5-HT into rat brain slices incubated in plasma from treated patients [27], inhibition of uptake of 5-HT into blood platelets from depressed patients [28], and the measurement of monoamine metabolites in

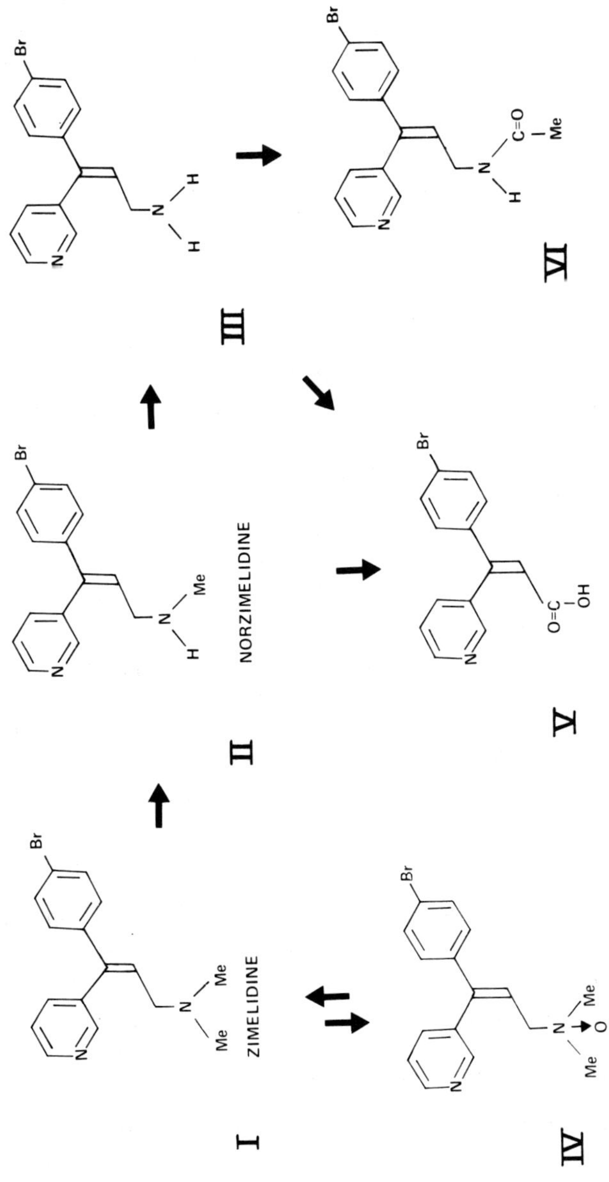

Figure 3 Major metabolic routes of zimelidine.

cerebrospinal fluid (CSF) [29]. Two recent studies have shown that plasma samples from patients treated with zimelidine effectively inhibited 5-HT uptake into rat brain slices [13,30]. The uptake inhibition was significantly correlated to the concentration of norzimelidine in the plasma samples. Plasma from patients on zimelidine treatment inhibited the uptake of NA less than plasma from chlorimipramine treated patients [13].

As reported by Siwers et al. [30] and Bertilsson et al. [13], zimelidine treatment significantly decreased the concentration of 5-hydroxyindoleacetic acid (5-HIAA) and increased slightly the level of indoleacetic acid (IAA) in CSF of depressed patients. The decrease of 5-HIAA may be interpreted as a result of uptake inhibition of 5-HT at central neurons which then by a negative feedback reduces the synthesis of 5-HT [31]. The increase of IAA in CSF may be a result of decreased activity of tryptophan-5-hydroxylase. The observed weak decrease of the levels of the NA metabolite 3-methoxy-4-hydroxyphenylglycol (MHPG), and the unaffected levels of the DA metabolite homovanillic acid (HVA) [30], support the finding in animals that zimelidine predominantly affects 5-HT systems.

The accumulation of 5-HT in human platelets has been employed as a model for the neuronal uptake of 5-HT, since this uptake mechanism is very similar to that in the 5-HT neurons as regards the sensitivity to inhibitors [28]. The 5-HT occurring in blood is almost exclusively located in the platelets, and since 5-HT is not synthesized in the platelets, their content of 5-HT is dependent on uptake of 5-HT formed in other tissues. Inhibition of the membrane uptake mechanism results therefore in a decrease in 5-HT in the platelets and in the blood. It was found that zimelidine (150 mg daily) or chlorimipramine (100 mg daily) produced a pronounced decrease in the 5-HT concentration in blood [32]. The accumulation of [^{14}C] 5-HT in platelet-rich plasma from patients treated with zimelidine (200 mg daily) or chlorimipramine (100 mg daily) was strongly reduced, whereas desipramine (150 mg daily) had only a partial effect [46]. Thus, zimelidine, like chlorimipramine, appears to inhibit the 5-HT uptake also in man under clinical conditions.

Coppen et al. [33] have also reported on the significantly reduced 5-HT uptake into blood platelets of depressive patients treated with zimelidine. However, no significant relationship could be detected between the degree of inhibition of uptake and clinical outcome.

B. Pharmacokinetics in Healthy Volunteers

Primary pharmacokinetic characteristics of zimelidine have been evaluated in two studies in healthy volunteers. In the first study the relationship between plasma levels and doses of different size was investigated. Zimelidine (tablets) was administered to each of 9 volunteers (aged 22-50 years) in single oral doses of 25, 75, and 150 mg. Plasma concentrations determined by the method of Westerlund et al. [26] revealed a rapid and extensive absorption with peak levels of zimelidine usually within 1.5 h (Fig. 4). Also, norzimelidine appeared rapidly in plasma with peak levels about 3 h after the zimelidine administration. The expected slower elimination of norzimelidine was confirmed in this study. The terminal plasma half-life of zimelidine was 6.3, and the apparent half-life of norzimelidine after oral administration of zimelidine was 17 h. The total area under the plasma concentration-time curve (AUC) for both zimelidine and norzimelidine showed a linear increase with increasing dose (Fig. 5). There was no significant intrasubject variation in the estimated plasma half-lives of the two compounds within this dosage interval. The results of this investigation suggest therefore that the pharmacokinetics of zimelidine administered in single oral doses of 25-150 mg is not dose dependent.

In a second study both zimelidine and norzimelidine were administered intravenously and orally to 6 healthy volunteers [34]. The plasma levels obtained in this study are exemplified in Fig. 6 by the results obtained in one of the volunteers. The half-lives in plasma after intravenous administration were in agreement with those observed earlier (Table 8). The different plasma elimination rates can be explained by the difference in distribution volumes (Table 8). Norzimelidine is less bound to plasma proteins (~85%) than zimelidine (~95%) and is therefore more available for uptake in peripheral tissues.

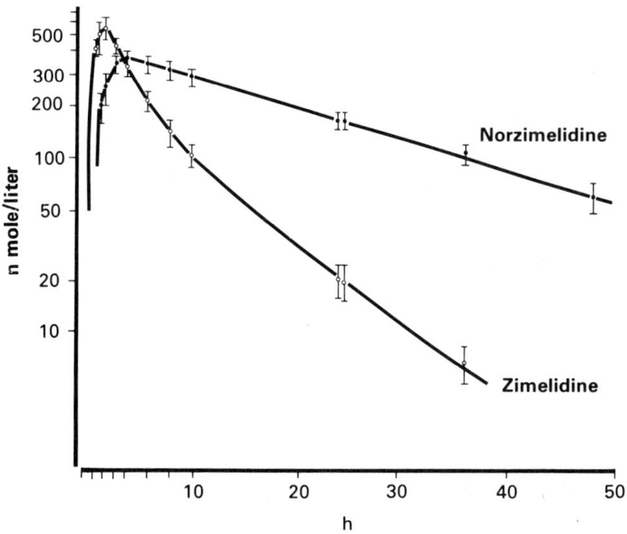

Figure 4 Plasma levels in healthy volunteers after a single oral dose of zimelidine 150 mg. (Mean values ± SEM, n = 9.)

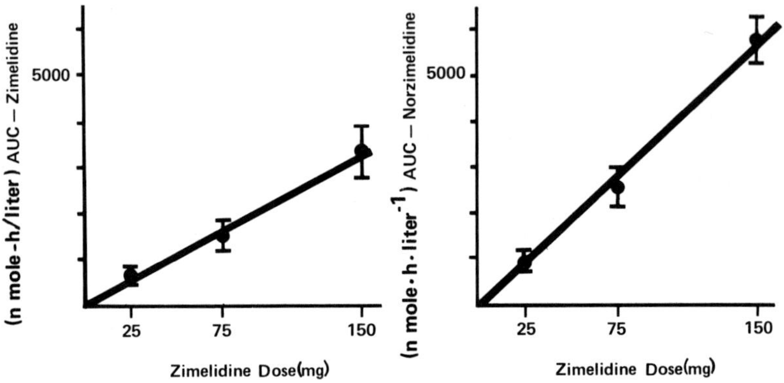

Figure 5 AUC-dose relationships after administration of zimelidine to nine healthy volunteers in single oral doses. Mean values ± SEM.

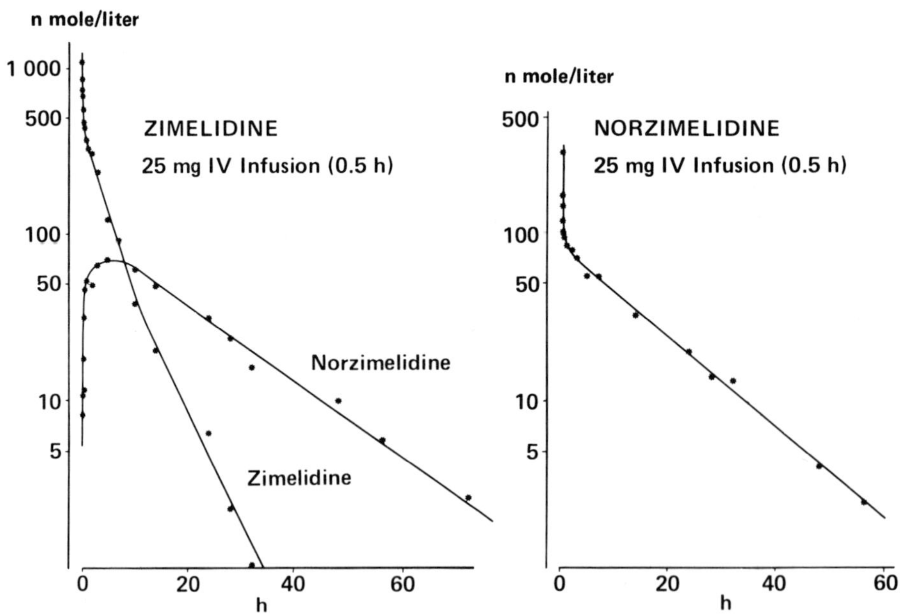

Figure 6 Examples of plasma levels obtained after intravenous administration to a healthy volunteer.

Table 8 Model-Independent Pharmacokinetic Constants after Intravenous Infusion to Six Healthy Volunteers: Mean Values ± SD

	Administered compound	
	Zimelidine 25 mg	Norzimelidine 25 mg
Half-life, $T_{1/2}$ (h)	5.1 ± 0.6	15.5 ± 5.0
Plasma clearance (ml/min/kg)	6.9 ± 2.0	8.0 ± 2.9
Volume of distribution (liters/kg)	3.2 ± 1.3	9.4 ± 1.2

Table 9 Area under Plasma Concentration-Time Curves Following Oral and Intravenous Administration of Zimelidine and Norzimelidine to Six Healthy Volunteers: Mean Values ± SD

		AUC (μmol-h-liter^{-1})	
Administration		Zimelidine	Norzimelidine
Zimelidine 25 mg	Oral	0.5 ± 0.1	1.6 ± 0.7
	Intravenous	2.2 ± 1.0	2.0 ± 0.7
Norzimelidine 25 mg	Oral	–	1.3 ± 0.3
	Intravenous	–	2.2 ± 1.0

The major object of this combined intravenous and oral investigation was to evaluate the bioavailability of the two compounds. Zimelidine appeared to have a mean bioavailability of 23% as determined from the ratio of the AUC values after oral and intravenous administrations (Table 9). However, a measure of the availability of norzimelidine may be more relevant. It is very interesting to note that the mean AUC value for norzimelidine after oral administration of zimelidine is higher than after oral administration of norzimelidine itself (difference not significant). Consequently, zimelidine is a very good prodrug of norzimelidine, the metabolite responsible for the major part of the effect.

C. Pharmacokinetics in Depressed Patients on Chronic Oral Dosing

The pharmacokinetics of zimelidine and norzimelidine have been studied [35] in 12 therapy-resistant patients diagnosed as endogenously depressive [36]. The hospitalized patients were treated with zimelidine in an open study designed primarily to evaluate its safety properties. After a 5-day placebo washout, patients

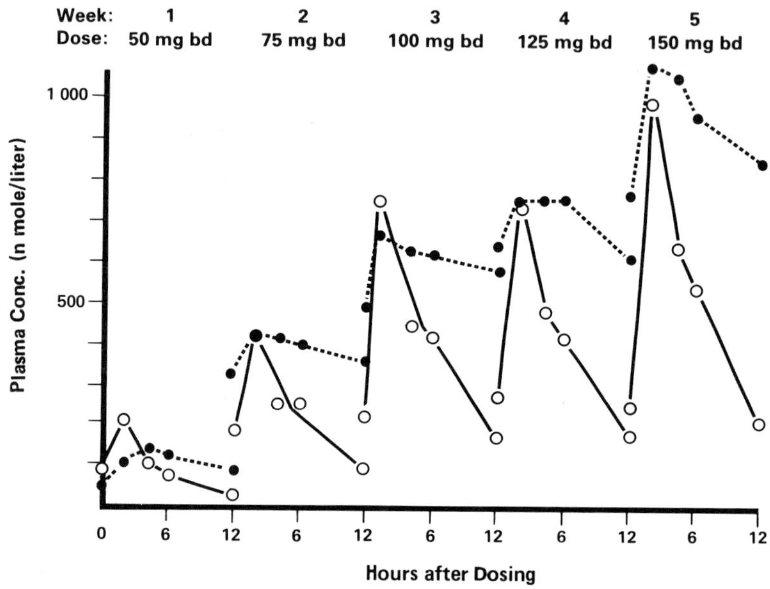

Figure 7 Typical plasma concentration-time profile for zimelidine and norzimelidine over a 5-week dosage interval for patients on oral zimelidine. —○—○— zimelidine, ---●---●--- norzimelidine.

received zimelidine in two doses a day (8:00 A.M. and 8:00 P.M.) for at least 5 weeks. The dose was incremented from 2 X 50 mg/day up to a maximum of 2 X 150 mg/day.

Each week during the active treatment, the plasma concentration of zimelidine and norzimelidine was determined using a method based on high-performance liquid chromatography [37]. A typical example of the plasma concentration time (C_P-t) data for one patient is presented in Fig. 7. This data enabled the determination of a number of parameters for zimelidine and norzimelidine at steady state for a range of doses of zimelidine.

The maximum plasma concentration ($C_{P_{max}}$) of zimelidine usually occurred within 2 h of dosing, while the $C_{P_{max}}$ for norzimelidine occurred between 2 and 6 h after dosing. The $C_{P_{max}}$ data for zimelidine and norzimelidine at steady state in Table 10 indicate that their interpatient variation is considerably less than the 20-30-fold variation between patients in the steady-state plasma levels of other tricyclic antidepressant compounds [38].

It was not possible to obtain an accurate estimate of terminal phase half-life ($T_{1/2}$) of zimelidine with the limited blood sampling schedule used in these

Table 10 Summary of Steady-State Plasma Concentration Data (nmole/liter) for Zimelidine and Norzimelidine in Patients on Oral Zimelidine

Compound	Dose at steady state (mg)			
	50	75	100	150
Zimelidine Cp_{max}				
n	7	11	7	12
Mean	290	490	1,110	2,260
SD	180	220	490	960
Range	130-570	170-870	590-1,700	980-4,650
Norzimelidine Cp_{max}				
n	1	9	4	10
Mean	790	750	1,050	1,640
SD	–	280	400	330
Range	–	400-1,280	540-1,500	970-1,990

patients. There did not, however, appear to be any consistent intrapatient trend in the value of $T_{1/2}$ with time. The value of $T_{1/2}$ appeared to vary between 3 and 7 h for zimelidine. No estimate of norzimelidine $T_{1/2}$ was possible.

Of the 12 patients studied, the area under the zimelidine plasma concentration-time curve at steady state (Z-AUC_{ss}) was obtained at more than one dosage level in all patients. There appeared to be a linear relationship between Z-AUC_{ss} and dose for 8 of the 12 patients (Fig. 8, patients 8 and 12). For the remaining 4 patients, Z-AUC_{ss} at the highest dose was greater than that predicted from data at lower doses (Fig. 8, patient 10).

The area under the norzimelidine plasma concentration-time curve at steady state (NZ-AUC_{ss}) was obtained at more than one dosage level in 6 patients. In none of these cases was there any marked deviation from linearity in the relationship between NZ-AUC_{ss} and dose, even for those cases where there was nonlinearity for Z-AUC_{ss} (Fig. 8).

D. Age and Bioavailability

Age appeared to be a factor contributing to the nonlinearity in Z-AUC_{ss} at high doses. The incidence of nonlinear increases in Z-AUC_{ss} with dose was higher (3/6) in the patients more than 60 years of age than that (1/6) in the patients less than 60 years old. The amount of zimelidine reaching the systemic circula-

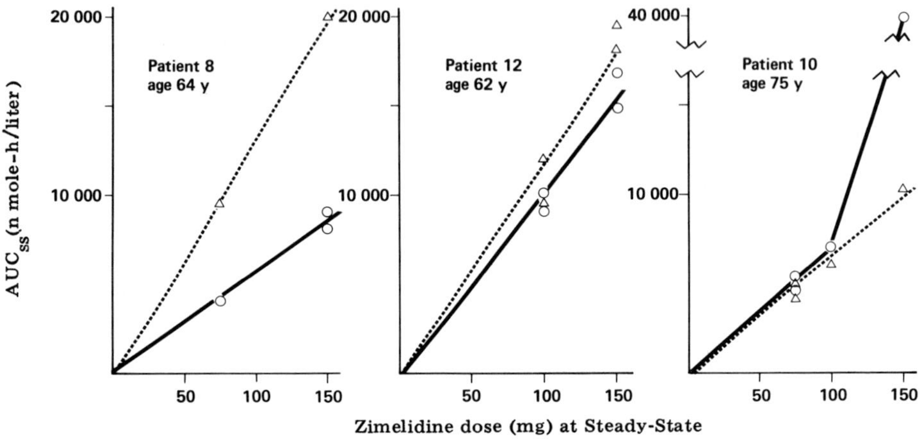

Figure 8 Examples of patient data on the relationship between Z-AUC$_{SS}$ and NZ-AUC$_{SS}$ and dose. —○—○— zimelidine, ---△---△--- norzimelidine.

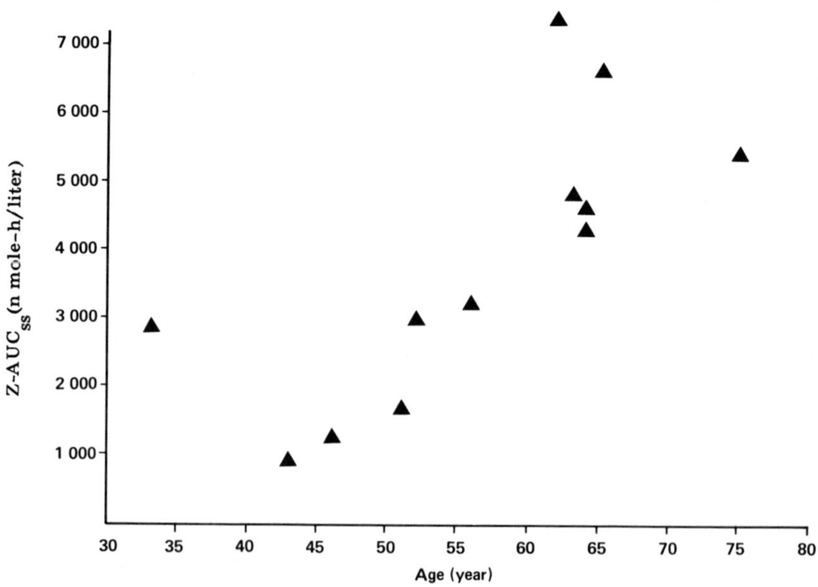

Figure 9 Plot of Z-AUC$_{SS}$ for a 75-mg dose versus patient age indicating the high positive rank-order correlation of these two variables. Spearman's rank correlation = .8, significant at $P = .01$.

tion after oral administration was also markedly influenced by the age of the patient, since there was a highly significant positive correlation between Z-AUC_{ss} and age (Fig. 9). There was an approximate 7-fold variation in the estimate of Z-AUC_{ss} for a 75-mg dose among the patients. There was, however, no correlation between NZ-AUC_{ss} and age.

These effects of age on the systemic availability of zimelidine and norzimelidine after the administration of oral zimelidine are similar to those reported for amitriptyline-nortriptyline and imipramine-desimipramine [39]. These authors found that older patients treated with imipramine or amitriptyline developed significantly higher steady-state plasma concentrations of both parent drugs, but the age effect was not as definite for their mono-N-dealkylated metabolites. No correlation was found between age and steady-state nortriptyline plasma levels, but there was a significant, though weak, correlation ($r = .30, P = .05$) between desipramine plasma levels at steady state and age.

The increasing systemic availability after oral administration of imipramine, amitriptyline, and zimelidine with age may be caused by a decrease in the "first-pass" metabolism in the liver of the elderly. In healthy young subjects, these three compounds have in common some important pharmacokinetic characteristics, e.g., a relatively high hepatic clearance that results in a high hepatic extraction ratio and hence a low, and usually variable, oral bioavailability [40] (see above for references on zimelidine).

E. Plasma Concentration of Zimelidine and Norzimelidine and Clinical Response

An evaluation of relationship between plasma concentration and clinical response for zimelidine is complicated by the presence of significant concentrations of the active metabolite, norzimelidine, in the systemic circulation. If a single blood sample is to be taken within a dosage interval for the purpose of monitoring plasma levels, then the timing of this sample will be important, since zimelidine has a relatively short half-life (~5 h) compared to norzimelidine (~17 h). The zimelidine/norzimelidine plasma concentration ratio varies considerably, therefore, within a dosage interval.

Different antidepressant potencies for zimelidine and norzimelidine might further complicate attempts to establish a relationship between clinical response and plasma level of the active components. Several studies of the inhibition of 5-hydroxytryptamine uptake in rat brain slices [13,30] and in homogenates and slices of the rat hypothalamus [12] have suggested that norzemelidine is more potent than zimelidine in these models.

Of the 12 patients in the open study described above [35], four showed good improvement (final Hamilton Rating Scale, HRS $\leqslant$ 10) and two improved moderately (final HRS $\leqslant$ 15). There was no difference between the responders and nonresponders in the final estimates of Z-AUC_{SS}, NZ-AUC_{SS}, or the sum of these. No simple relationship could be found between any of these estimates and the onset of clinical improvement. No correlations were found for Z-AUC_{SS} and/or NZ-AUC_{SS} and any of the side effects observed among these patients. The higher plasma levels of zimelidine observed in older patients were not consistently associated with any adverse reactions.

In another reported open trial by Åberg and Holmberg [42], 11 out of 15 patients with depression of endogenous type improved markedly during zimelidine treatment. Also, in this study only few, mild side effects were observed. Particularly, the frequency of anticholinergic side effects appeared to be very low. These authors conclude that steady-state plasma levels 5 h after dosing should reach at least 250 nmole/liter (zimelidine) and 500 nmole/liter (norzimelidine) to obtain the desired effect of the drug. A general dosage of 100 mg twice daily is recommended to reach these levels.

The limitations of the open study design for the evaluation of clinical efficacy is well recognized. Controlled double-blind studies are a more suitable setting for evaluating possible relationships between plasma levels of the active agents and clinical response. Although several such studies on zimelidine are in progress, preliminary data is presently available only from two controlled double-blind trials [43,44]. In both these studies zimelidine in doses of 200 mg/day was as effective as 150 mg amitriptyline and with significantly less anticholinergic side effects.

In the study of Coppen et al. [44] steady-state plasma levels of zimelidine and norzimelidine were determined 13 h after the evening dose. Steady-state levels were achieved within the second week of treatment. The levels at the end of the treatment period were (6th week, mean ± SEM, n = 15) for zimelidine 453 ± 68 nmole/liter and for norzimelidine 856 ± 81 nmole/liter. There was about a 30-fold range for zimelidine plasma levels and a 5-fold range for norzimelidine during steady state. The plasma levels of zimelidine and norzimelidine were, however, not significantly correlated with the therapeutic outcome in this study.

The side effects in the reported studies have generally been few and mild, and the very low frequency of anticholinergic side effects is especially notable. In a separate study by Burgess et al. [45] the cardiovascular effect of zimelidine was shown to be small compared to amitriptyline. Data in the report of Coppen et al. [44] indicate that patients treated with zimelidine did not show a weight increase, which might be another advantage over the tricyclic antidepressants.

V. SUMMARY

Zimelidine, (Z)-3-(4-bromophenyl)-N,N-dimethyl-3-(3-pyridyl)allylamine, is a new antidepressant compound primarily acting on central 5-hydroxytryptamine

(5-HT) mechanisms. After oral administration to rats zimelidine is about 5 times more potent than chlorimipramine in inhibiting 5-HT uptake. Zimelidine is rapidly demethylated in vivo to norzimelidine, the secondary amine derivative. Norzimelidine is responsible for the major part of the pharmacological activity of zimelidine in vivo and exhibits a similar specificity for inhibiting 5-HT uptake. In contrast to tricyclic antidepressants, zimelidine has very low peripheral and central anticholinergic effects. Zimelidine exerts only slight effects on cardiovascular functions, in particular ECG. Contrary to the tricyclic drugs, zimelidine does not potentiate the noradrenaline and adrenaline pressor response and does not antagonize the tyramine pressor response.

The plasma half-life of zimelidine in man is 5-7 h, and the apparent half-life of norzimelidine after oral zimelidine administration is about 17 h. The systemic availability of norzimelidine after oral administration of zimelidine is equal to that after administration of norzimelidine itself (65%). No dose dependency was observed in the pharmacokinetics after single oral administration in the range of 25-150 mg to healthy volunteers. It also appears that linear kinetics prevail for zimelidine and norzimelidine in the majority of patients aged less than 60 years on chronic oral therapy in the dose range of 100-300 mg/day. In older patients, however, nonlinear increases in the plasma concentrations of zimelidine may be observed at higher oral doses (300 mg/day).

In the few open and controlled clinical trials, zimelidine has proved to be an effective antidepressant. Also, zimelidine appears to exert a rather selective action on central 5-HT mechanisms in man. The studies in man have largely confirmed the animal studies showing a notably low frequency of anticholinergic side effects and very slight effects on cardiovascular functions. An understanding of the relationship between plasma levels of active agents and clinical response awaits the results of further controlled double-blind studies.

REFERENCES

1. M. Åsberg, P. Thorén, L. Träskman, L. Bertilsson, and V. Ringberger, Serotonin depression: A biochemical subgroup within the affective disorders? *Science 191:*478, 1976.
2. R. M. Post, E. K. Gordon, F. K. Goodwin, and W. E. Bunney, Central norepinephrine metabolism in affective illness: MHPG in the cerebrospinal fluid. *Science 179:*1002, 1973.
3. J. Glowinski and J. Axelrod, Inhibition of uptake of tritiated noradrenaline in the intact rat brain by imipramine and structurally related compounds. *Nature 204:*1318, 1964.
4. K. J. Blackburn, P. C. French, and R. J. Merrills, 5-Hydroxytryptamine uptake by rat brain in vitro. *Life Sci. 6:*1635, 1967.

5. S. B. Ross and A. L. Renyi, Inhibition of the uptake of tritiated 5-hydroxytryptamine in brain tissue. *Eur. J. Pharmacol. 7:*270, 1969.
6. A. Carlsson, H. Corrodi, K. Fuxe, and T. Hökfelt, Effects of antidepressant drugs on the depletion of intraneuronal brain 5-hydroxytryptamine stores caused by 4-methyl-α-ethyl-metatyramine. *Eur. J. Pharmacol. 5:*357, 1969.
7. A. Coppen, The biochemistry of affective disorders. *Br. J. Psychiatry 113:* 1237, 1967.
8. J. J. Schildkraut, The catecholamine hypothesis of affective disorders. A review of supporting evidence. *Am. J. Psychiat. 122:*509, 1965.
9. H. M. van Praag, Towards a biochemical typology of depression? *Pharmakopsychiatry 7:*281, 1974.
10. S. B. Ross and A. L. Renyi, Tricyclic antidepressant agents, II: Effect of oral administration on the uptake of ^{3}H-noradrenaline and ^{14}C-5-hydroxytryptamine in slices of the midbrain-hypothalamus region of the rat. *Acta Pharmacol. Toxicol. 36:*395, 1975.
11. S. B. Ross, S. O. Ögren, and A. L. Renyi, (Z)-Dimethylamino-1-(4-bromophenyl)-1-(3-pyridyl)propene (H102/09), a new selective inhibitor of the neuronal 5-hydroxytryptamine uptake. *Acta Pharmacol. Toxicol. 39:*152, 1976.
12. S. B. Ross and A. L. Renyi, Inhibition of the neuronal uptake of 5-hydroxytryptamine and noradrenaline in rat brain by (Z)- and (E)-3-(4-bromophenyl)-N,N-dimethyl-3-(3-pyridyl) allylamines and their secondary analogues. *Neuropharmacology 16:*57, 1977.
13. L. Bertilsson, I. Tuck, and B. Siwers, Neuronal effects of zimelidine in man. *Eur. J. Clin. Pharmacol.* Submitted 1980.
14. S. O. Ögren, Effects of the 5-HT uptake inhibitors zimelidine and alaproclate on the regional uptake of 5-HT in the rat. To be published, 1980.
15. A. Carlsson and M. Lindqvist, Effects of antidepressant agents on the synthesis of brain monoamines. *J. Neural. Transm. 43:*73, 1978.
16. H. Hall and S. O. Ögren, Effects of antidepressant drugs on different receptors in the brain. Submitted, *Eur. J. Pharmacol.*
17. K. Fuxe, S. O. Ögren, B. J. Everitt, L. F. Agnati, P. Eneroth, J. Å. Guftafsson, G. Jonsson, P. Skett, and A. C. Holm, The effect of antidepressant drugs of the imipramine type on various monoamine systems and their relation to changes in behaviour and neuroendocrine function. In *Depressive Disorders* (S. Garattini, ed.). Stuttgart and New York, F. K. Schattauer, 1978.
18. S. O. Ögren and H. Hall, Peripheral and central anticholinergic properties of the 5-HT uptake inhibitors zimelidine and alaproclate. *J. Neurol. Transm.* Submitted 1980.
19. S. H. Snyder and H. I. Yamamura, Antidepressants and the muscarinic acetylcholine receptor. *Arch. Gen. Psychiatry 34:*236, 1977.
20. S. O. Ögren and A. C. Holm, Effects of the 5-HT uptake inhibitors zimelidine and alaproclate on central 5-HT activity in mice. To be published, 1980.

21. M. Toneby and S. O. Ögren, Effects of the 5-HT uptake inhibitors zimelidine and alaproclate on motor activity in mice. To be published, 1980.
22. S. O. Ögren, S. B. Ross, A. C. Holm, and L. Baumann, 5-Hydroxytryptamine and avoidance performance in the rat: Antagonism of the acute effect of p-chloroamphetamine by zimelidine, an inhibitor of 5-hydroxytryptamine uptake. *Neurosci. Lett. 7:*331, 1977.
23. L. O. Lindbom and T. Forsberg, Cardiovascular effects of zimelidine and other antidepressants in conscious rats. *Acta Psych. Scand.* In press, 1980.
24. J. Malatray, L. O. Lindbom, and S. O. Ögren, Cardiovascular effects of zimelidine and tricyclic antidepressants in anaesthetized dogs. To be published, 1981.
25. J. Lundström, T. Gosztonyi, and T. de Paulis, Major metabolites of zimelidine, a new antidepressant, in rat, dog, and man. To be published, 1981.
26. D. Westerlund, L. B. Nilsson, and Y. Jaksch, Straight-phase ion-pair chromatography of zimelidine and similar divalent amines. *J. Liq. Chromatogr. 3:*373, 1979.
27. I. R. Tuck and G. Punell, Uptake of ^{3}H-5-hydroxytryptamine and ^{3}H-noradrenaline by slices of rat brain incubated in plasma from patients treated with chlorimipramine, imipramine, or amitriptyline. *J. Pharm. Pharmacol. 25:*573, 1973.
28. J. M. Sneddon, Blood-platelets as a model for monoamine-containing neurons. *Prog. Neurobiol. 1:*151, 1973.
29. M. Åsberg, V. A. Ringberger, F. Sjöqvist, P. Thorén. L. Träskman, and J. R. Tuck, Monoamine metabolites in cerebrospinal fluid and serotonin uptake inhibition during treatment with chlorimipramine. *Clin. Pharmacol. 21:*201, 1977.
30. B. Siwers, V. Ringberger, J. R. Tuck, and F. Sjökvist, Initial clinical trial based on biochemical methodology of zimelidine (a serotonin uptake inhibitor) in depressed patients. *Clin. Pharmacol. Ther. 21:*194, 1977.
31. H. Corrodi and K. Fuxe, Decreased turnover in central 5-HT nerve terminals induced by antidpresssant drugs of the imipramine type. *Eur. J. Pharmacol. 7:*56, 1969.
32. S. B. Ross, S. Jansa, L. Wetterberg, B. Fyrö, and B. Hellner, Decreased blood level of 5-hydroxytryptamine by inhibitors of the membranal 5-hydroxytryptamine uptake. *Life Sci. 19:*205, 1976.
33. A. Coppen, V. A. Rama Rao, C. Swade, and K. Wood, Inhibition of 5-hydroxytryptamine reuptake by amitriptyline and zimelidine and its relationship to their therapeutic action. *Psychopharmacol. 63:*125, 1979.
34. D. Brown, D. H. T. Scott, D. B. Scott, M. Meyer, D. Westerlund, and J. Lundström, Pharmacokinetics of zimelidine. Systemic availability of zimelidine and norzimelidine in human volunteers. *Eur. J. Clin. Pharmacol. 17:*111, 1980.
35. R. G. Moore, B. Love, D. Cooke, and L. G. Kiloh, Plasma levels of zimelidine and norzimelidine in depressed patients on incrementing oral doses of zimelidine. *Eur. J. Clin. Pharmacol.* In press, 1980.

36. C. Gurney, M. Roth, R. F. Garside, T. A. Kerr, and K. Schapira, Studies in the classification of affective disorders. *Brit. J. Psychiatry 121:*162, 1972.

37. B. Emanuelsson and R. G. Moore, Quantitation of zimelidine and norzimelidine in plasma using high-performance liquid chromatography. *J. Chromatogr. Biomed. Appl. 146:*113, 1978.

38. B. Alexanderson and F. Sjöqvist, Individual differences in the pharmacokinetics of monomethylated tricyclic antidepressants: Role of genetic and environmental factors and clinical importance. *Ann. N.Y. Acad. Sci. 179:* 739, 1971.

39. A. Nies, D. S. Robinson, M. J. Friedman, R. Green, T. B. Cooper, C. L. Ravaris, and J. O. Ives, Relationship between age and tricyclic antidepressant plasma levels. *Am. J. Psychiatry 134:*790, 1977.

40. L. F. Gram and J. Christiansen, First-pass metabolism of imipramine in man. *Clin. Pharmacol. Ther. 17:*555, 1975.

41. M. Hamilton, A rating scale for depression. *J. Neurol. Neurosurg. Psychiatry 23:*56, 1960.

42. A. Åberg and G. Holmberg, Preliminary clinical test of zimelidine (H 102/09): A new 5-HT uptake inhibitor. *Acta Psychiatr. Scand. 59:*45, 1979.

43. S. Montgomery, R. McAuley, G. Rani, and D. B. Montgomery, A double blind comparison of antidepressant efficacy of zimelidine, a new 5-HT uptake inhibitor, with amitriptyline. *Abstr. 7th Int. Cong. Pharmacol.* (Paris) *246:* 1978

44. A. Coppen, V. A. Rama Rao, C. Swade, and K. Wood, Zimelidine: A therapeutic and pharmacokinetic study in depression. To be published, 1979.

45. C. Burgess, S. Montgomery, and J. Wadsworth, Cardiovascular effects of amitriptyline, mianserine, and zimelidine in depressed patients. *Abstr. 7th Int. Cong. Pharmacol.* (Paris) *830:* 1978.

46. S. B. Ross, B. Aperia, J. Beck-Friis, S. Jansa, L. Wetterberg, and A. Åberg, Inhibition of 5-hydroxytryptamine uptake in human platelets by antidepressant agents in vivo. *Psychopharmacology 67:*1, 1980.

7

Antimanic Agents

Lithium and Mania: Plasma Levels and Response

William J. Annitto / *Second Annex Community Unit, Fair Oaks Hospital, Summit, New Jersey, and New Jersey Medical School, Newark, New Jersey, United States*

Samuel Gershon / *Department of Psychiatry, School of Medicine, New York University Medical Center, New York, New York, United States*

I. INTRODUCTION

Since Cade [1] introduced lithium into psychiatry in 1949, the biological treatment of mental illness has dominated the psychotherapeutic scene. Lithium has become a specific pharmacologic treatment for manic-phase manic-depressive illness [2-5]. It has opened new areas of research [3] and forced psychiatry to reevaluate its nosology [6]. It also has been claimed to be effective in chronic schizophrenics (when added to the neuroleptic regimen) [7], aggression syndromes [8,9], and alcoholism [10]. As time passes, more researchers slowly add more subgroups to the category of affective disorders, thereby justifying the administration of lithium [11]. The logic is, of course, that since lithium is specific, if we can broaden the category—affective disorder—we can treat more people. This attitude, however, may lead to a loss of nosologic clarity, while perhaps affording atypical patients clinical relief.

II. REVIEW OF LITERATURE

A. Lithium in Mania

The studies of lithium in mania demonstrate a clear level of consistency in concluding that this ion is therapeutic for the majority of manic patients. However, methodological difficulties arise, even in studies with "typical" manic patients. There is diagnostic confusion [12], lack of rating scales, deficient drug washouts, concomitant use of other drugs, and the self-limiting recurrent nature of the disease itself [5]. Nonetheless, these studies give an improvement rate of 60-100% in mania treated with lithium. This effect is independent of age, sex, and duration of illness [13]. It is suggested by these studies that lithium, although slower in onset of action, is more specific for "pure" mania than neuroleptics; while as more schizoaffective features are added, lithium becomes less effective.

1. Lithium versus Placebo

Gerbino et al. [5] have thoroughly reviewed the five studies comparing lithium to placebo in mania: Schou et al. [14], Maggs [15], Bunney et al. [16], Goodwin et al. [17], and Stokes et al. [18]. They conclude "that lithium is superior to placebo in the acute treatment of mania." Although serum levels were adjusted in these studies (ranging from 0.5 to 2.0), only Bunney and Goodwin noted that there was a correlation between worsening of manic symptoms and fall in serum lithium level.

2. Lithium versus Neuroleptics

Six studies have compared these two modalities in treating mania: Johnson et al. [19], Spring et al. [20], Platman [21], Prien et al. [22], Shopsin et al. [23], and

Stokes et al. [24]. Shopsin et al. compared haloperidol, chlorpromazine, and lithium in double-blind fashion, while the other groups employed only chlorpromazine as the neuroleptic standard. Stokes et al. used various neuroleptics for unspecified lengths of time during their study.

Johnson et al. [19] found that lithium produced highly significant improvement in their manic-depressives. Serum levels were maintained between 1.0 and 2.5 meq/liter. They made no correlation of response with levels. Spring et al. [20] found no significant difference in the manics' response to either lithium or chlorpromazine. Two chlorpromazine failures responded positively to lithium. They found that all patients who responded to lithium had serum levels less than 1.3 meq/liter.

Platman [21] found, in 23 manics studies, that lithium response (mean serum level 0.8 meq/liter) was superior to chlorpromazine on all evaluation scales. However, here too there was neither statistical significance nor correlation of response and plasma levels.

Prien et al. [22], using data generated in a large collaborative Veterans Administration-National Institute of Mental Health study, addressed specifically the question of serum lithium level and clinical response. A discussion of methodological differences has been described elsewhere [5]. Prien found that "serum lithium levels of 1.4 meq/liter are adequate for treating acute mania." More significantly, they state that "patients with levels exceeding 1.4 meq/liter showed no greater improvement than patients on [sic] lower levels." Moreover, Prien found that complete remission of manic symptoms was not achieved with levels below 0.9 meq/liter. Even in their "mildly active" group they found that serum lithium levels of 0.5 meq/liter may be too low to "provide optimal benefit."

Shopsin et al. [23] used rating scales and discharge rate to compare the aforementioned three antimanic agents. They were concerned that the earlier studies using lithium and neuroleptics had failed to show a statistically significant difference in these treatment modalities.

They found a general trend (not statistically significant) that both lithium and haloperidol were superior to chlorpromazine and that qualitative differences between lithium and haloperidol, although clinically apparent, fail to be measurable on existing rating scales. Lithium, while slower in onset, exerted a more complete and specific effect on the manic symptomatology. Seven patients of ten treated with lithium were able to be discharged after 3 weeks of active treatment; only two patients receiving haloperidol and one receiving chlorpromazine were clinically ready for discharge after 3 weeks. Although this study used serum lithium levels between 1.0 and 2.0 meq/liter, no correlations were made between response and these levels.

The most recent study, Stokes et al. [24], examined the relationship between three separate lithium chloride dosing schedules, steady-state serum lithium levels, and clinical response. They attempted also to correct for the fact that some patients also received neuroleptics "to control agitated or assaultive behavior" by showing nonsignificant differences in response to their high- and low-dose lithium alone vs. lithium plus neuroleptic groups. They found that higher serum lithium levels were significantly correlated with higher improvement rates. However, in order to avoid toxicity, they had few treatment periods with serum levels greater than 1.4 meq/liter. Thus, they could not address the issue raised by Prien et al. [22] that levels greater than 1.4 meq/liter offered no increase in responsiveness.

Stokes et al. [24] suggested that their preliminary data may show that more severe manics may have lower serum lithium levels at a given dose. These would be original and intriguing data; however, they remain only suggestive and preliminary. Baldessarini and Stephens [25], in fact, found no relationship between serum lithium levels and affective status in 22 patients on a fixed-dosage schedule.

In summary, one can say that, indeed, lithium has efficacy and perhaps specificity, for acute mania. One must add that haloperidol (and possibly other neuroleptics) also is an acceptable somatic treatment for mania, at least in the acute phase. Moreover, although there are indications that serum levels of lithium must be at least between 0.9 and 1.4 meq/liter, and that positive response continues to increase, at least, to 1.2 meq/liter in positive responders, there are no data that specifically compare clinical response or nonresponse and these levels. We cannot state categorically whether a lithium nonresponder at one serum level would become a positive responder at a higher level. Amdisen [26] recommends that relapses at one level should not be considered nonresponders until a new, higher steady state has been achieved and maintained "for some length of time."

3. Intravenous Lithium

Apparently there is one article in English which deals with intravenous (i.v.) lithium salts, blood levels attained, and clinical response. Rimón and Räkkö-läinen [27] in 1968 attempted to reproduce earlier Russian work that they review. The Russian investigators administered 0.5-1 g of i.v. lithium iodide to patients with "different kinds of psychotic disturbances" and got "highly favourable" effects within 7-15 days. Unfortunately, they mention no serum levels; moreover, none of their patients had affective psychosis.

In Rimón's study, 1 g of lithium iodide was given intravenously for 7 days. Two cases needed increases to 1.3 g in order to attain serum levels greater than 0.6 meq/liter. Thirty patients diagnosed as "confusional psychotics" were studied. Half received the lithium. Of these, nine patients has no effect "whatsoever"; four patients had alleviation of psychomotor agitation, insomnia, and aggressiveness, with decreased delusions and hallucinations, but in "lesser degree" than those on neuroleptic. After 7 days, all patients had serum levels of 0.6

meq/liter. After 2 days mean level was 0.34 meq/liter; after 4 days it was 1.2 meq/liter. They note no increased incidence or severity in side effects. However, the study did not use manics, the topic of this chapter. The important clinical aspect is that, apparently, serum lithium levels depend not only on dose and mode of administration, but probably on duration of administration of the salt.

B. Lithium as Prophylaxis in Mania

There are no studies specifically relating plasma levels of lithium to clinical response in the prophylaxis of recurrent mania. Confounding the issue is the dearth of information concerning patients diagnosed as manic-phase manic-depressive illness, as opposed to depressed-phase. Still, studies do exist which respond to the more general question of this section, i.e., whether lithium is effective in recurrent mania: Hartigan [28], Baastrup et al. [29], Baastrup and Schou [30], Melia [31], Coppen et al. [32], Prien et al. [33], Persson [34], Hullin et al. [35].

In 1951 Noack and Trautner [36] reported that in 30 cases of mania, lithium was effective in terminating and preventing the manic phase in recurrent mania [5]. Since then, lithium has been found to decrease the duration and severity of the attacks [29,30], reduce the time in hospital [35], and increase the duration of normal interphase [32].

Spring et al. [20] placed 10 of their 12 positive lithium responders on prophylaxis with lithium. Interestingly, 5 of the 10 had relapsed, all with serum lithium levels greater than 0.6 meq/liter. Unfortunately, they give no data as to further response, or lack of it, with increased blood levels.

As Gershon [37] has noted, other reviewers of the literature have drawn quite contrary conclusions. He recommends Shull and Sapira [38] or Blackwell and Shepard [39] for those interested in the alternate point of view, i.e., that these studies, due to various experimental design inadequacies, neither prove nor disprove the efficacy of lithium in recurrent mania.

III. SIDE EFFECTS AND SERUM LITHIUM LEVELS

A. Mild to Moderate Toxic Effects

Patients ingesting lithium will most commonly complain of anorexia, transient nausea, gastric discomfort, diarrhea, vomiting, thirst, polyuria, and hand tremor [3,37,40]. These effects usually diminish or disappear even without reduction of dose. Although they occur at serum lithium levels usually greater than 1.0 meq/liter, they may be more related to the steepness of the rise of the lithium level than to the absolute level attained. With persistent symptoms, a reduction in dosage or change to another lithium preparation may generally alleviate the problem [3]. Again we must note the inconsistency of the serum levels of lithium. There is no evidence available that correlates level with side effects.

Baldessarini and Stephens [25] found that none of 15 minor side effects occurred at elevated or rapidly increasing serum lithium levels. Generally, he found minor side effects occurred at the beginning of lithium therapy or during a phase of rapid increase of dose.

Persson [41] briefly reviews this area. He finds that tremor is related to higher doses, to higher concentrations of lithium in plasma, and to steeper increases of lithium in plasma. Nausea may be related to higher gradients. Both abdominal pain and loose stools showed no relation to doses, levels, or gradients.

B. Serious Neurotoxic Side Effects

These effects include muscle fasciculation and twitching, hyperactive deep tendon reflexes, ataxia, dysarthia, confusion, lethargy, seizures, and finally, coma. Lithium-induced delirium has also been reported [3]. These are accompanied by reversible electroencephalographic changes including altered α-activity, diffuse slowing, accentuation of focal abnormalities, or appearance of previously absent focal changes. Moreover, Shopsin et al. [42] have noted the induction of a toxic-confusional state in schizophrenics treated with lithium at levels of 0.75 meq/liter.

Many authors [40,22], describing these side effects in manics, state that they occur at serum Li^+ levels of 1.5 meq/liter and greater. Others [3] use 2.0 meq/liter as the upper limit, below which one can generally be secure from intoxication. However, the literature is replete with individual case reports of severe toxic reactions at almost any level postulated [42]. In short, it may be that the absolute serum level is not the optimal indicator for prognosticating toxicity.

Elizur et al. [43] found that the red blood cell (RBC) concentration of lithium was an indicator of clinical status and impending toxicity. Thus, the clinician may be confronted by the following dilemma: A manic patient stabilized at 1.2 meq/liter serum level of lithium develops a recrudescence of tremor, polyuria, and fatigue. Repeat serum determination is stable while the RBC level has doubled! Thus, one is faced with lowering the absolute dose of lithium in order to lower the intracellular levels of the ion.

Again, it must be stressed that few statistically meaningful studies have been done correlating side effects with plasma level (or intraerythrocyte level) of lithium.

IV. DIFFERENTIAL RETENTION OF LITHIUM IN MANIA

Fyrö and Sedvall [44] reviewed this area in Johnson's [45] text, *Lithium Research and Therapy*. They report four studies since 1968, all of which confirm the earliest work by Trautner et al. [46], which showed that manics excreted a lower percentage of ingested lithium in their urine than did healthy persons. They state that manic patients distribute lithium in the tissues differently from healthy subjects and that the serum concentration does not differentiate retainers from nonretainers.

Alternately, they review the literature which is contrary to Trautner et al. Six papers are reviewed. They then state that "we still do not know for sure whether lithium is excreted less readily by manics as compared to other patients." More importantly, they point out the shortcomings in all the studies which should be controlled, before definitive results can be evolved. These include: diet, including electrolytes and fluid intake, lithium doses, time for collection, concomitant medications, and correlation of results with clinical state, motor activity, sex, and age. One will find, clinically, that the intraindividual variations of response, serum level, and side effects are myriad.

V. NEUROLEPTICS AND MANIA

It is obvious from the studies reviewed in Sec. II.B that neuroleptics certainly control the acute-phase manic patient. Shopsin et al. [23], however, raise the important issue of whether this is merely symptom specific, and not, in fact, disease specific, as lithium may be. Notwithstanding, neuroleptics, including thioridazine, thioproperazine, chlorpromazine, and thioxanthenes have all been found useful [13]. Moreover, the butyrophenone haloperidol is specifically recommended for mania by Mayer-Gross et al. [47] and Garfinkel [48]. However, Klein and Davis [49] do not recommend this same butyrophenone as specifically useful in mania.

Summarizing, one can suggest that any neuroleptic may control the behavioral aspects of mania, enabling patients to be "quietly manic" [5]. In fact, the neuroleptics act more rapidly on these aspects of mania. However, lithium may be clinically more specific and efficacious (in terms of dischargeability) [23] than the less specific, but more sedating, neuroleptics.

VI. CONCLUSION

As the research and clinical studies have indicated, lithium is a powerful pharmacologic agent in the treatment of affective illness. Newer areas of study—neurendocrine provocative testing, genetics, histocompatibility studies, membrane electrophysiology, and RBC/lithium ratio—are beginning to clarify many of the questions surrounding bipolar and unipolar disease. It may well be that subgroups of patients exist in which cell membrane defects are the etiopathogenetic cause for affective illness [50]. Thus, the efficacy of lithium would be explained by electrophysiologic changes occurring on a subcellular level. Rybakowski [51], following the work of many others, has confirmed the finding of Lyttkens et al. [52] that women have higher mean RBC/lithium indices than men. Rybakowski has also observed a higher incidence of affective illness in first-degree relatives of patients with high RBC/lithium ratio. We do not know if this line of hypothesizing will lead to a genetic "answer."

As noted by Annitto et al. [12], one of the major problems with much of present research in affective disorder is simply that the vast majority of the research has been carried on in either the normothymic or the depressive phase of the bipolar illness. Neuropsychopharmacological findings in the depressive phase may not be 100% transposable to the manic phase of the illness, as they are unlikely to be polar opposites neurochemically. For our purposes this would mitigate against any simple reductionistic view of serum lithium levels and clinical response—already self-evident in fact, since lithium appears prophylactic in both phases of the illness.

Moreover, the clinical studies described here are mainly done at large university-centered medical facilities. The clinical psychiatrist, alone in his office but for the patient, must continue to satisfy himself with the art of medicine. If in "the end," plasma lithium levels prove grossly unrelated to clinical response (which seems unlikely given the known, accepted therapeutic range), our lone clinician must harken to the signs and symptoms of health and toxicity, i.e., he will elicit appropriate history, observe speech and motor coordination, and elicit appropriate physical signs. Perhaps, then, it is best, this lack of a "perfect level," this confusing array of individual responses; perhaps this is the answer, beyond the sought-after measurable fact. Like Ozymandias, will we have to warn our followers to look on these works and despair? Perhaps there is no homogeneity in man.

The multitude of variables that go into the distribution of lithium in the body, from sex to drug formulation, renal clearance, severity of illness, etc., may preclude the codifying of specific interindividual levels and expected results. The *art* will remain in giving the patient the opportunity to perform at his peak, whether this depends on a low or high serum lithium level.

REFERENCES

1. J. Cade, Lithium salts in the treatment of psychotic excitement, *Med. J. Aust. 36:*349-352, 1949.
2. A. Gattozzi, *Lithium in the Treatment of Mood Disorders,* National Clearinghouse for Mental Health Information, Publication No. 5033. Washington, D.C., U.S. Government Printing Office, 1970.

3. S. Gershon and B. Shopsin, eds., *Lithium: Its Role in Psychiatric Research and Treatment.* New York, Plenum Press, 1973.
4. R. Baldessarini and J. Lipinski, Lithium salts, 1970-1975. *Ann. Intern. Med. 83:*527-533, 1975.
5. L. Gerbino, M. Oleshansky, and S. Gershon, The clinical use and mode of action of lithium. In *Psychopharmacology: A Generation of Progress* (M. Lipton, A. DiMascio, and K. Killian, eds.). New York, Raven Press, 1978.
6. R. Baldessarini, Frequency of diagnoses of schizophrenia versus affective disorders from 1944 to 1968. *Amer. J. Psychiatry 127:*59-63, 1970.
7. J. Small, J. Kellams, V. Milstein, and J. Moore, A placebo-controlled study of lithium combined with neuroleptics in chronic schizophrenic patients. *Amer. J. Psychiatry 132:*1315-1317, 1975.
8. A. Rifkin, F. Quitkin, C. Carillo, A. Blumberg, and D. F. Klein, Lithium in emotionally unstable character disorder. *Arch. Gen. Psychiatry 27:*519-523, 1972.
9. M. H. Sheard, J. L. Marini, C. I. Bridges, and E. Wagner, The effect of lithium on impulsive aggressive behaviour in man. *Amer. J. Psychiatry 133:*1409-1412, 1976.
10. N. S. Kline, J. C. Wren, T. B. Cooper, E. Varga, and O. Canal, Evaluation of lithium therapy in chronic and periodic alcoholism. *Amer. J. Med. Sci. 268:*15-19, 1974.
11. M. Akiska, M. Djenderedjan, R. Rosenthal, and M. Khani, Cyclothymic disorder: Validating criteria for inclusion in the bipolar affective group. *Amer. J. Psychiatry 134:*1227-1233, 1977.
12. W. Annitto and B. Shopsin, Neuropharmacology of mania. In *Manic Illness* (B. Shopsin ed.). New York, Raven Press, 1979.
13. B. Shopsin and S. Gershon, Chemotherapy of manic-depressive disorder. In *Brain Chemistry and Mental Disease* (B. T. Ho and W. M. McIsaac, eds.). New York, Plenum Press, 1971.
14. M. Schou, N. Juel-Nielsen, E. Stromgren, and H. Voldby, The treatment of manic psychoses by the administration of lithium salts. *J. Neurol. Neurosurg. Psychiatry 17:*250-260, 1954.
15. R. Maggs, Treatment of manic illness with lithium carbonate. *Brit. J. Psychiatry 109:*56-65, 1963.
16. W. E. Bunney, F. K. Goodwin, J. M. Davis, and J. A. Fawcett, A behavioural-biochemical study of lithium treatment. *Amer. J. Psychiatry 125:*499-512, 1968.
17. F. K. Goodwin, D. L. Murphy, and W. E. Bunney, Lithium carbonate treatment in depression and mania. *Arch. Gen. Psychiatry 21:*486-496, 1969.
18. P. E. Stokes, P. M. Stoll, C. A. Shamoian, and M. J. Patton, Efficacy of lithium as acute treatment of manic-depressive illness. *Lancet 1:*1319-1325, 1971.
19. G. Johnson, S. Gershon, and L. J. Hekimian, Controlled evaluation of

lithium and chlorpromazine in the treatment of manic states: An interim report. *Compr. Psychiatry 9:*563-573, 1968.

20. G. Spring, D. Schweid, C. Gray, J. Steinberg, and M. Horowitz, a double-blind comparison of lithium and CPZ in the treatment of manic states. *Amer. J. Psychiatry 126:*1306-1309, 1970.
21. S. R. Platman, A comparison of lithium carbonate and chlorpromazine in mania. *Amer. J. Psychiatry 127:*351-353, 1970.
22. R. Prien, E. Caffey, and C. Klett, Relationship between serum lithium level and clinical response in acute mania treated with lithium. *Brit. J. Psychiatry 120:*409-414, 1972.
23. B. Shopsin, S. Gershon, H. Thompson, and P. Collins, Psychoactive drugs in mania. *Arch. Gen. Psychiatry 32:*34-42, 1975.
24. P. Stokes, J. Kocsis, and O. Arcuni, Relationship of lithium chloride dose to treatment response in acute mania. *Arch. Gen. Psychiatry 33:*1080-1084, 1976.
25. R. Baldessarini and J. Stephens, Lithium carbonate for affective disorders. *Arch. Gen. Psychiatry 22:*72-77, 1970.
26. A. Amdisen, Serum level monitoring and clinical pharmacokinetics of lithium. *Clin. Pharmacokinetics 2:*73-92, 1977.
27. R. Rimon and V. Räkköläinen, Lithium iodide in the treatment of confusional states. *Brit. J. Psychiatry 114:*109-110, 1968.
28. G. P. Hartigan, The use of lithium salts in affective disorders. *Brit. J. Psychiatry 109:*810-814, 1963.
29. P. C. Baastrup, J. C. Poulsen, M. Schou, K. Thomsen, and A. Amdisen, Prophylactic lithium: Double-blind discontinuation in manic-depressive and recurrent depressive disorders. *Lancet 2:*326, 1970.
30. P. C. Baastrup and M. Schou, Lithium as a prophylactic agent: Its effect against recurrent depressions and manic-depressive psychosis. *Arch. Gen. Psychiatry 16:*162-172, 1967.
31. P. I. Melia, A pilot trial of lithium carbonate in recurrent affective disorders. *J. Irish Med. Assoc. 60:*160-170, 1967.
32. A. Coppen, R. Noguera, J. Bailey, Prophylactic lithium in affective disorders. *Lancet 2:*275-279, 1971.
33. R. F. Prien, E. M. Caffey, Jr., and C. J. Klett, Prophylactic efficacy of lithium carbonate in manic-depressive illness. *Arch. Gen. Psychiatry 28:*337-341, 1973.
34. G. Persson, Lithium prophylaxis in affective disorders: An open trial with matched controls. *Acta Psychiatr. Scand. 48:*462-467, 1972.
35. R. P. Hullin, R. McDonald, and M. N. E. Allsopp, Prophylactic lithium in recurrent affective disorders. *Lancet 1:*1044-1046, 1972.
36. C. H. Noack and E. M. Trautner, The lithium treatment of maniacal psychosis. *Med. J. Aust. 2:*219-222, 1951.
37. S. Gershon, Lithium. In *American Handbook of Psychiatry,* 2nd ed., vol 5. New York, Basic Books, 1975.
38. W. Shull, and J. Sapira, Critique of studies of lithium salts in the treatment of mania. *Amer. J. Psychiatry 127:*136-140, 1970.

39. B. Blackwell and M. Shepard, Prophylactic lithium: Another therapeutic myth? An Examination of the Evidence to Date. *Lancet 1:*968-971, 1968.
40. S. Gershon, Lithium. In *Psychotherapeutic Drugs,* vol. 2 (E. Usdin and I. Forrest, eds.). New York, Marcel Dekker, 1976.
41. G. Persson, Lithium side effects in relation to dose and to levels and gradients of lithium in plasma. *Acta Psychiatr. Scand. 55:*208-213, 1977.
42. B. Shopsin, G. Johnson, and S. Gershon, Neurotoxicity with lithium: Differential drug responsiveness. *Int. Pharmacopsychiatry 5:*170, 1970.
43. A. Elizur, B. Shopsin, and S. Gershon, Intraextra cellular lithium ratios and clinical course in affective states. *Clin. Pharmacol. Ther. 13:*947-952, 1972.
44. B. Fyrö and G. Sedvall, The excretion of lithium. In *Lithium Research and Therapy* (F. N. Johnson, ed.). New York, Academic Press, 1975.
45. F. N. Johnson, ed., *Lithium Research and Therapy.* New York, Academic Press, 1975.
46. E. Trautner, R. Morris, C. Noack, and S. Gershon, The excretion and retention of ingested lithium and its effect on the ionic balance of man. *Med. J. Aust. 2:*200-291, 1955.
47. W. Mayer-Gross, E. Slater, and M. Roth, *Clinical Psychiatry,* 3rd ed. Baltimore, Williams & Wilkins, 1969.
48. P. Garfinkel, Efficient management of the acute psychotic patient: Stabilization and maintenance with haloperidol. *Proc. Roy. Soc. Med.,* Suppl. (1) *69:*26-31, 1976.
49. D. Klein and J. Davis, eds., *Diagnosis and Drug Treatment of Psychiatric Disorders.* Baltimore, Williams & Wilkins, 1969.
50. A. Sen, R. Murthy, H. Stancer, A. Awad, D. Godse, and P. Grof, The mechanism of action of lithium ion in affective disorders: A new hypothesis. In *Membranes and Disease* (L. Bolis, J. F. Hoffman, and A. Leaf, eds.). New York, Raven Press, 1976.
51. J. Rybakowski, Pharmacogenetic aspect of red blood cell lithium index in manic-depressive psychosis. *Biol. Psychiat. 12:*425-429, 1977.
52. L. Lyttkens, R. Soderberg, and L. Wetterberg, Relationship between erythrocyte and plasma lithium concentrations as an index in psychiatric disease. *Ups. J. Med. Sci. 81:*123-238, 1976.

8

Antipsychotic Agents

Chlorpromazine: Pharmacokinetics, Plasma Levels, and Clinical Response

Stephen H. Curry* / *Department of Pharmacology and Therapeutics, The London Hospital Medical College, London, England*

*Present affiliation: College of Pharmacy, University of Florida, Gainesville, Florida, United States.

I. INTRODUCTION

Chlorpromazine, the prototype neuroleptic phenothiazine, has been a source of continuous fascination to scientists and clinicians for nearly 30 years. First, its introduction accompanied, or perhaps caused, a revolution in the treatment of schizophrenia. Secondly, studies of its properties have been the subject of innumerable papers by pharmacologists. Thirdly, its metabolism and pharmacokinetic properties have been vigorously investigated. This chapter is concerned with the third of these areas of research, metabolism and pharmacokinetics, but particularly in relation to clinical response.

Up to the mid-1960s, metabolic and pharmacokinetic studies with chlorpromazine were largely pursued for two purposes: (1) basic research; (2) in the search for methods of detecting drug-taking reliability in psychiatric patients. It is in this second context that the excellent work of Forrest and her colleagues [1,2] was pursued. More recently, attention has been directed toward plasma level variation as a possible factor in patient response. This has arisen from the general interest of Brodie [3] in this field and also from his particular interest in chlorpromazine [4-6].

Progress with research into chlorpromazine metabolism and pharmacokinetics has always been dependent on development of analytical methods for the drug and its metabolites, so this chapter is initially concerned with assays. The assay methods for phenothiazines and their metabolites were recently reviewed in considerable detail [7].

II. ANALYTICAL METHODS

The specific analysis of chlorpromazine is complicated by the scale of metabolic conversion which occurs. The drug is known to undergo sulfoxidation, N-oxidation, demethylation, and hydroxylation with subsequent conjugation (Fig. 1) [8-10]. Deamination probably also occurs, and it is further believed that other, as yet unidentified, routes may be important. The reactions occur in combination, yielding vast numbers of metabolites. Even the old idea of a possible 168 metabolites must now be considered an underestimate. Assays specific for any

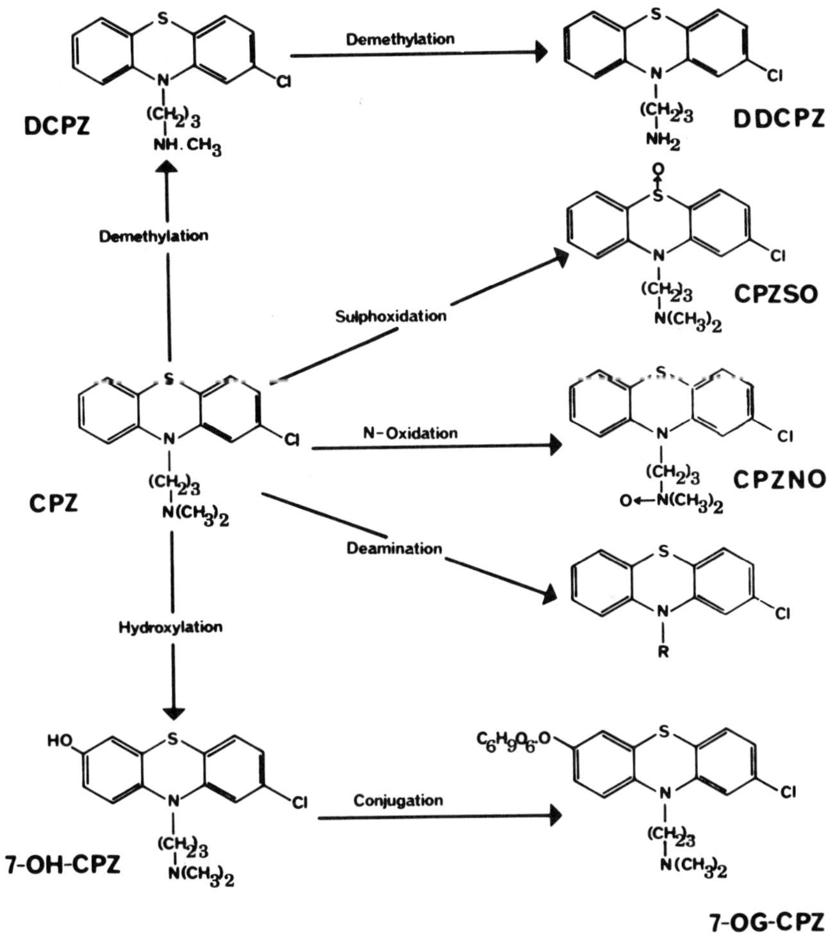

Figure 1 Metabolic reactions of chlorpromazine (CPZ). Abbreviations: DCPZ = demonomethylchlorpromazine; DDCPZ = dedimethylchlorpromazine; 7-OH-CPZ = 7-hydroxychlorpromazine; CPZSO = chlorpromazine sulfoxide; CPZNO = chlorpromazine N-oxide; 7-OG-CPZ = 7-hydroxychlorpromazine glucuronide. (From Ref. 45).

one compound are difficult to devise, and it is not surprising that metabolites have often been discovered when they emerged as complicating factors in what were at one time considered to be specific assays.

A wide variety of chromatographic and extraction techniques have been applied to chlorpromazine analysis, but the most important development from the point of view of measuring concentrations of specific compounds in plasma was the application of solvent extraction followed by gas-liquid chromatographic (GLC) examination of the extracts [6,11-17]. The success of this can be related to the relative lipid solubilities of the compound and its metabolites. The approximate rank order of lipid solubilities of some of the compounds was determined by means of partitioning into a hexane-hexanol solvent mixture from pH 7.4 buffer, and found to be: chlorpromazine (most lipid soluble), demonomethylchlorpromazine, dedimethylchlorpromazine, 7-hydroxychlorpromazine, 7,8-dihydroxychlorpromazine, chlorpromazine N-oxide, 2-chlorophenothiazine 10-propionic acid, 7-hydroxydemonomethylchlorpromazine, 7-hydroxydedimethylchlorpromazine, chlorpromazine sulfoxide, 7-hydroxychlorpromazine sulfoxide, chlorpromazine N-oxide sulfoxide, demonomethylchlorpromazine sulfoxide, 7-hydroxydemonomethylchlorpromazine sulfoxide, dedimethylchlorpromazine sulfoxide, 7-hydroxydedimethylchlorpromazine sulfoxide, 2-chlorophenothiazine 10-propionic acid sulfoxide, and glucuronides (most polar) [18]. The GLC retention times relate approximately to this rank order of lipophilicities, and metabolism leads to decreased lipophilicity, which facilitates renal excretion. Solvent extraction schemes are based on relative lipophilicities, because a good extraction scheme for a particular compound involves choice of a solvent and pH for extraction which leads to adequate separation of the compound from a mixture containing it and other related compounds.

The breakthrough in chlorpromazine analysis was achieved when solvent extraction with n-heptane, GLC on OV-17 columns, and electron capture detection (ECD) were successfully applied to plasma estimations [6,11]. This was the beginning of high-quality plasma studies in man, although a number of somewhat dubious papers preceded this development [19,20]. An assay specific for known compounds and capable of assaying chlorpromazine when present at 10 ng/ml or more in 5-ml plasma samples became available. Concentrations in clinical samples were found to range from 0 to 1000 ng/ml. Since the publication of this method in 1968 a number of modifications and alternatives have emerged, [21-29], and the method has been widely criticized, not least by its originator [30,31], but it is now widely used throughout the world.

It is worth pointing out in this review that in applying the GLC-ECD technique certain special factors can influence data. These are discussed in the following sections.

A. Other Drugs

The sole interfering drug known is diazepam, the retention time of which is within 10% of that of chlorpromazine. The use of OV-225 columns, or careful observation, overcomes this problem [13]. One investigator believed that there was widespread interference from other drugs until he scrupulously cleaned the chlorpromazine residues in his laboratory ware [32].

B. Chlorpromazine Metabolites

As already mentioned, chlorpromazine and its metabolites have different retention times on OV-17 columns, so in theory a nonspecific extraction followed by GLC of the extract should be adequate. A suitable nonspecific extracting solvent is ether. However, the compounds *must* be assayed in at least three groups; (1) chlorpromazine, plus its demethylated analogues, and the sulfoxides; (2) an analogous series based on 7-hydroxychlorpromazine; and (3) chlorpromazine N-oxide and N-oxide sulfoxide. Those in group 1 are best separated by extraction into heptane. Those in groups 2 and 3 are *then* extracted into ether. A specific assay for chlorpromazine must involve separation from chlorpromazine N-oxide, as any chlorpromazine N-oxide in the ether extract is reduced to three products, chlorpromazine, demonomethylchlorpromazine, and N-allyl 2-chlorophenothiazine, in the GLC analysis. Thus ether extracts, when used for chlorpromazine and demonomethylchlorpromazine, can produce inflated data, and this has serious implications for some of the clinical studies mentioned later in this chapter.

C. Gas-Liquid Chromatography Detection

Generally speaking, the electron capture detector is needed. This provides sensitivity but relatively poor stability. The more stable flame ionization detector can be used at higher levels. The alkali flame detector (nitrogen sensitive) may prove satisfactory in the future.

D. Internal Standards

It has been suggested that dichlorpromazine should be added to clinical samples for workup alongside the chlorpromazine, as an internal standard technique, which is common practice with other GLC methods [23]. It has also been suggested that traces of radioactive chlorpromazine should be used similarly [30]. While favoring the use of high-specific-activity radioactivity for this purpose, in the opinion of this writer the use of dichlorpromazine is fallacious for two reasons. First, its validity depends on linearity of electron capture detector response, which is never ensured. Secondly, there is no reason to suppose that the assay of the internal standard itself will be more reliable than that of the chlorpromazine, and so there is a 50-50 chance of compounding error by use of the internal standard.

E. Extraction with Isopropanol/Heptane

This has the advantage of precipitating protein and possibly increasing extraction yields thereby [33]. However, 100% extraction of both free and bound drug is obtainable without protein precipitation, so isopropanol is probably unnecessary.

Against this, there is a risk of loss on the protein plug. In this regard, yields are greater when oxalate or citrate (rather than heparin) is the anticoagulant, and this renders recovery correction unnecessary.

F. Other Approaches to Assay of Chlorpromazine in Plasma

There are a number of reports of isotope derivative [22], radioimmunoassay [25], and combined GLC-mass spectrometry techniques [21,26], and the last of these methods has been applied in a recent study of the relation between plasma levels and effect. However, these methods have not been used outside the laboratories of their originators, and so remain in a sense unproved. In addition, one group has devised a comprehensive system employing thin-layer chromatographic (TLC) separation of chlorpromazine and its metabolites, followed by chemical reaction leading to fluorescent products, which are assessed quantitatively for an indication of the concentrations of the compound of interest [29]. This method is considered again later. Furthermore, two groups have devised TLC-microdensitometric techniques independently of each other, and these are also considered further in later sections of this chapter [27,28].

G. Storage of Samples

Chlorpromazine and its metabolites are stable if stored in the dark. Storage below room temperature is also valuable. Freezing of plasma samples can, surprisingly, cause difficulty, as it has been shown that repeated freezing and thawing of samples can lead to reduced extraction yields. Additionally, storage under nitrogen can cause reduction of chlorpromazine N-oxide. All things considered, storage at 4°C for the minimum of time after collection into oxalate or citrate tubes is recommended.

H. Quality Control

The results of an attempt to assess interlaboratory variation in assay of chlorpromazine and its metabolites were published in 1976 [34]. This praiseworthy experiment concerned chlorpromazine, chlorpromazine sulfoxide, demonomethylchlorpromazine, and dedimethylchlorpromazine. Identical samples were prepared with blank bovine plasma in one laboratory and analyzed in that laboratory and five others. The originating group assayed for all four compounds by GLC and also for chlorpromazine itself by TLC-densitometry. Of the five collaborating groups, four used GLC-ECD and one used TLC with fluorescence derivatization. Unfortunately, the results of this study are not easily evaluated from the published report, as the tables in the paper lack important annotation, for example, in regard to identification of precise methods used and meanings of symbols in tables. However, the data show that the GLC-ECD approach to the assay of chlorpromazine itself generally gave good precision. As to accuracy, two of the groups reported significantly low data. In contrast, the GLC metabolite assays were less satisfactory. The TLC-densitometry approach gave the answer believed to be correct for chlorpromazine alone (metabolites not attempted). The TLC-fluorescence technique gave data of good precision and of reasonable accuracy for both chlorpromazine and the metabolites. However, there was an anomaly in that while the values from the TLC-fluorescence work for one of the two experimental solutions of the demethylated compounds were close to the values believed to be correct, the other five investigators were unanimous in reporting values of approximately 30% of the nominal value. A 5-to-1 vote in favor of a systematic error, and against TLC-fluorescence, was thus recorded. This study has been criticized for using "spiked" bovine plasma, for using freeze-dried solutions, and for using samples without the full set of metabolites, known and unknown, which can occur in plasma when a person or animal is *dosed* with chlorpromazine. However, without doubt the study demonstrated that reliable data for the unchanged drug can be obtained when care is exercised. That, at least, is reassuring. The anomaly, particularly with the didemethylated metabolite, can probably be ignored, as this metabolite has proved to be of little pharmacological importance.

The significance of such work cannot be overemphasized, as good analytical work is crucial. The GLC-ECD method was undoubtedly a major success. However, as already stated, it was widely criticized, and there definitely were research groups who failed in their attempts to apply it. This resulted from insensitive detectors, impure solvents, wholesale laboratory contamination, etc. Adverse literature comments appeared to cast doubt on the validity of clinical data obtained with the method, but since in most cases the authors commenting adversely have later drawn their own conclusions from the data obtained in other laboratories using the GLC-ECD method, the users of this method can draw comfort from the thought that the adverse comments have concerned the ability of imitators to match the achievements of the original investigators. This is a modest claim compared with claims of some of the detractors. Complete confidence can in fact be placed in plasma chlorpromazine data reported since 1968, *provided* that the data is reported with details of precision and accuracy in the laboratory concerned, and provided the factors mentioned in this review have been considered.

III. BASIC PLASMA LEVEL DATA

Only one group of workers has systematically examined chlorpromazine plasma levels as a function of route of administration, dose, dosage regime, etc., even though such research is fundamental to understanding the drug [35-45].

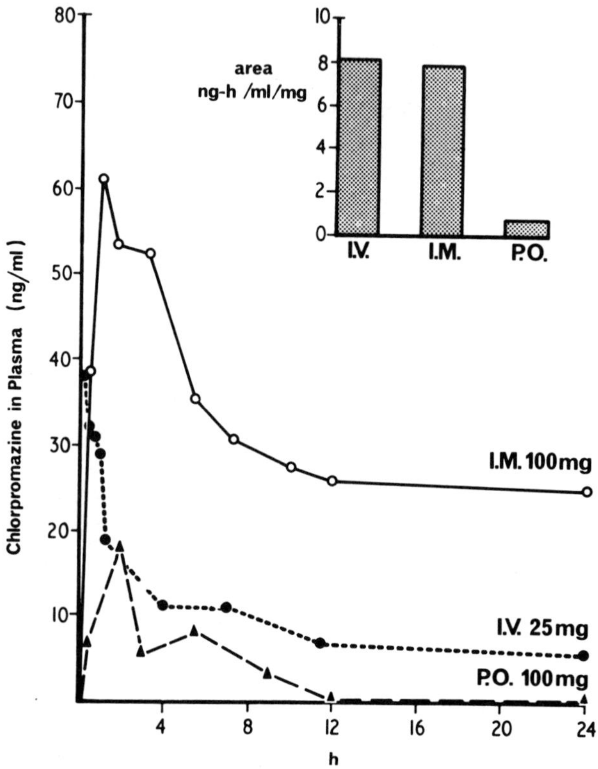

Figure 2 Plasma concentrations of chlorpromazine following three doses in a single previously untreated individual. Inset: area under the curve per mg dose. (From Ref. 45.)

A. Intravenous Doses

Following intravenous (bolus) doses the concentration in plasma declines rapidly at first and then more slowly. There are at least two phases and probably three, perhaps four, in the decay curve. As one example, a subject who received 25 mg provided data which could be adequately described by either of the two equations which follow (Fig. 2):

$$Cp_t = 0.077e^{-0.33t} + 0.060e^{-0.043t} \tag{1}$$

$$Cp_t = 0.077e^{-0.33t} + 0.056e^{-0.043t} + 0.004e^{-0.0005t} \tag{2}$$

This indicates distribution through either a two- or three-compartment system. Additionally, these equations fail to take into account data in the first 30 minutes following the intravenous dose, when decay is exceptionally rapid, so decay occurs in at least three and probably four phases. A more recent and extensive pharmacokinetic review has been conducted by Whitfield and his colleagues [46] who consider that there are three phases, one of them being indicated by the very early data, and the other two being indicated by data analogous to the components of Eq. (1) [46]. Whitfield and his colleagues have used both their data and that of this writer [43] in reaching this conclusion. So there is important disagreement concerning the existence of the third component in Eq. (2) and the half-life of the terminal phase, which is 16.1 hours in Eq. (1) and approximately 60 days in Eq. (2). Further light is shed on this problem by means of measurements on cessation of dosing after long-term treatment (see below).

B. Intramuscular and Oral Doses

These show the anticipated rise and fall consequent upon domination of the plasma level pattern by absorption at first and elimination in later stages. The peak after oral doses is at approximately 2 hours. Absorption is generally believed to follow first-order kinetics, but it has recently been suggested that zero-order kinetics are followed.

C. Area under the Curve

Areas under the plasma level curves per unit of dose following intravenous (i.v.) and intramuscular (i.m.) doses are comparable, indicating complete absorption of the i.m. dose (Fig. 2). The area under an oral curve is less by as much as 90%, indicating inefficient transfer from the gastrointestinal tract to the general circulation from which plasma samples are taken. This results from a pronounced "first-pass" effect—metabolism of the oral dose to a product or products, within the gut lumen, gut wall, or portal circulation, with the metabolites passing into the general circulation. All the evidence points to first-pass formation of chlorpromazine N-oxide and/or sulfoxide. In spite of this, the absorption that does occur can be considered as "rapid."

Patients treated for long periods with oral chlorpromazine show the characteristic rise and fall after each dose, plus an overall rise and fall, with the highest concentrations on or about the eighth day of treatment [47] (Fig. 3). The fall results from enzyme induction (in patients reliably taking their medicines) and from the consequent increased rate of conversion of chlorpromazine to metabolites. This fall has been verified in several studies [33,47,48], all published in the same journal. It can be presumed to be one of the reasons for increased dosage in long-term patients. The pattern at 6 weeks after initiation of treat-

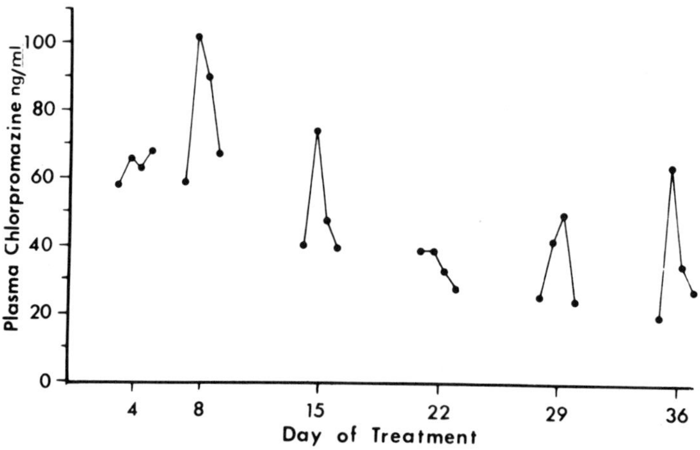

Figure 3 Mean plasma concentrations of chlorpromazine in a group of patients treated for 36 days with 100 mg three times daily, and sampled at four times following the first dose on the days indicated. (From Ref. 47. George Sakalis, Stephen H. Curry, Graham P. Mould, and Malcolm H. Lader, Physiologic and clinical effects of chlorpromazine and their relationship to plasma level. *Clin. Pharmacol. Ther. 13:*931-946 (1972.)

ment, including the rise and fall after each dose, is reproduced at long times such as 2 years. Thus the popular concept of "steady state" is not applicable with this drug. It is not known whether enzyme induction of "first-pass" metabolism occurs, or whether this "pharmacokinetic tolerance" applies only to systemically available chlorpromazine.

Withdrawal of treatment results in an immediate drop from the peak resulting from the final dose, to the predosage concentration, as would have occurred if dosing had been continuing. Decline thereafter is very slow indeed. Mean concentrations in one study indicated a terminal phase half-life of approximately 60 days, (Fig. 4), agreeing with the pharmacokinetic conclusion of this writer [44]. However, this observation has been disputed by others [49] who could not detect chlorpromazine in plasma beyond the eighth day after stopping treatment, with methodology sensitive to 3 ng/ml. Their terminal half-life was 2 days, which more or less agrees with the pharmacokinetic conclusion of Whitfield. There can in fact be no dispute that chlorpromazine is retained in the body for periods as long as 2 years, and this has been verified by several excretion studies. Since the plasma is the transport system of the body, it seems inevitable that storage in tissues and later excretion must involve a finite amount of the drug being present in plasma for long periods, so the long half-time of 60 days seems more likely to be correct, especially as it is based on positive data.

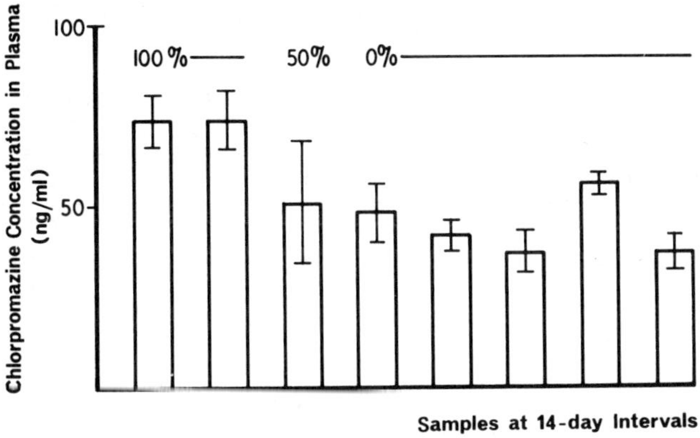

Figure 4 Mean (± SE) plasma chlorpromazine in a group of patients during treatment with a variety of doses (100% dosage) and following halving of dosage (50% dosage) and termination (0% dosage) of chlorpromazine treatment. (From Ref. 44.)

There is an anomaly in the withdrawal data (Fig. 4). Plasma levels rose at about 8 weeks after stopping dosage. It is not clear whether this occurred because of sudden release of the drug from tissues at this point, or because of illicit administration of doses. It is of interest that the increase coincided with a time when many patients whose treatment has ceased show clinical relapse. The 60-day half-life conclusion was based on data collected before this point.

Doubling or halving of the dose in individual subjects treated for long periods leads to doubling or halving of plasma levels (Table 1). In contrast, when a large group of patients was sampled, the increment per unit of doses was minimal (Table 2). It should be emphasized that the data in Table 2 were obtained from patients for whom the psychiatrist concerned had chosen doses in accord with clinical needs.

IV. TISSUE CONCENTRATIONS

Chlorpromazine penetrates tissues, presumably by passive diffusion across lipid membranes. Tissue concentrations exceed plasma concentrations because of binding. However, exchange between plasma and most tissue is rapid, as it is a function of vascularity. In particular, brain is highly vascular, and concentrations of chlorpromazine in brain therefore change in parallel with those in plasma [50] (Fig. 5). A very high correlation between plasma concentrations and cerebrospinal fluid (CSF) concentrations has been shown, with a ratio of concentrations

Table 1 Plasma Levels of Chlorpromazine as a Function of Dose in Three Male Patients[a]

Dose	Time after dose (h)	Plasma chlorpromazine (ng/ml)	
		Mean	SE
Control	0	16.7	5.4
	2	44.0	21.4
	4	29.8	11.9
+50%	0	17.9	5.9
	2	75.0	38.1
	4	39.2	9.5
–50%	0	11.9	3.6
	2	23.8	2.4
	4	20.8	3.0

[a]Patients were treated for more than six months at standard dosage (control), increased dosage (+50%), and reduced dosage (–50%) at three time points. Dosage was changed on one occasion only for each level, with test doses one week apart.

Table 2 Plasma Levels of Chlorpromazine as a Function of Dose in 51 Male Patients[a]

Dose (mg)	Number of patients	Time after dose (h)	Plasma chlorpromazine (ng/ml)	
			Mean	SE
25	18	0	20.5	3.5
		2	23.5	2.3
		4	20.0	4.0
50	16	0	27.0	9.0
		2	40.0	6.0
		4	28.3	5.7
100	11	0	39.1	10.0
		2	45.0	10.0
		4	55.2	14.6
200	6	0	58.5	21.5
		2	65.6	19.6
		4	67.8	17.3

[a]Patients treated for more than six months with 3 times the stated dose each day, and receiving no other drugs.

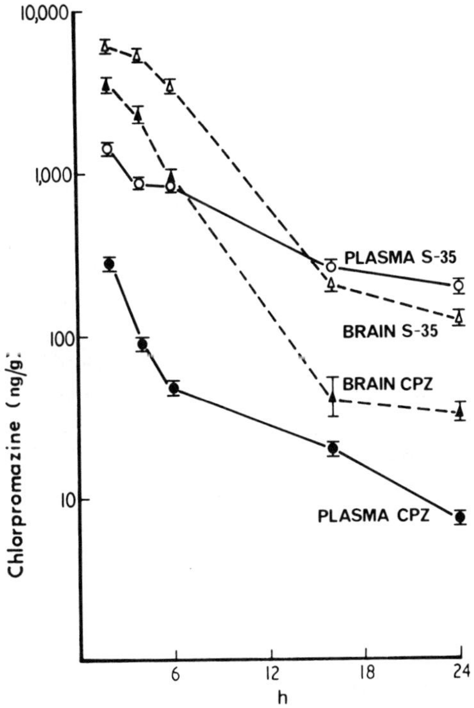

Figure 5 Mean (± SE) brain and plasma concentrations of chlorpromazine and total radioactivity (S-35 assessed as chlorpromazine) in rats given intraperitoneal doses of 10 mg-kg^{-1} of chlorpromazine (S-35). (From Ref. 44.)

between the two media reflecting exactly the binding of chlorpromazine to plasma proteins [51]. It has been shown that the drug has the same half-life in brain and plasma of rats [50]. It has been calculated, on the basis of tissue studies in rats and plasma binding studies in three species, including man, that whole brain concentrations in man exceed plasma concentrations by a factor of 7 [42,50]. It has been suggested by one group, however, that there is an increase in the brain-to-plasma concentration ratio during multiple dosing, but unfortunately the only evidence for this comes from an experiment in which the assay was not specific for chlorpromazine [52]. The assay in question was the long-established heptane extraction and ultraviolet absorption spectrophotometry method devised for chlorpromazine and chlorpromazine sulfoxide before the discovery of the demethylated metabolites, which interfere with assays of both compounds in this method [5].

V. METABOLITES IN PLASMA AND BRAIN

Chlorpromazine sulfoxide reaches substantial concentrations in human plasma, its concentrations occasionally exceeding those of chlorpromazine [35].

There is disagreement about other metabolites. In the earlier studies only the demethylated derivatives were examined, and they were found in quantities less than 10% of those of the unchanged drug [35]. More recently, a similar observation was made concerning 7-hydroxylated analogues [14]. Other authors have found larger quantities of demonomethylchlorpromazine and 7-hydroxychlorpromazine in human plasma [53]. There are at least two possible reasons for this disagreement. First, patient groups vary, and positive metabolite reports are confined generally, but not always, to long-term treatment groups. Detection of metabolites after single doses is not common. Secondly, there could be analytical errors. Demonomethylchlorpromazine has generally been detected with ether extracts, and so *could* have resulted from N-oxide reduction [54] (see above). The N-oxide has in fact been found in plasma when looked for, but actually in quantities insufficient to account for all of the apparent demonomethylchlorpromazine in plasma [16].

A major contribution in this regard was made by Turner and his colleagues [55,56]. They found substantial quantities of 7-hydroxychlorpromazine and other hydroxylated metabolites in erythrocytes, so that the whole blood concentrations of these compounds were higher than their plasma concentrations. In contrast, the nonhydroxylated compounds were not found in red cells to the same extent, so that whole blood concentrations of chlorpromazine, and its demethylated and sulfoxidized metabolites were less than concentrations in plasma. Thus the possibility cannot be ignored that workers finding substantial quantities of 7-hydroxychlorpromazine in plasma have inadvertently detected this compound released from erythrocytes as the result of hemolysis during sample handling. Furthermore, the implications for those who use whole blood, and even worse for investigators using the terms *plasma, blood,* and *serum* with no regard for the precise medium assessed, are obvious.

In fact, the consensus view is quite clear that the sulfoxide often approaches concentrations similar to those of chlorpromazine, while 7-hydroxychlorpromazine sometimes reaches these levels. The concentrations of the demethylated derivatives of chlorpromazine are only rarely above 10% of the concentrations of the unchanged drug. The only other metabolite usually occurring in more than trace quantities is the glucuronide (or glucuronides of 7-hydroxychlorpromazine. There is one report of possibly important quantities of a compound with the properties of 7,8-dihydroxychlorpromazine. This compound has been included in very few studies.

As to metabolites in brain, the sulfoxidized and demethylated group cross the blood-brain barrier. The group based on 7-hydroxychlorpromazine also cross to an extent [57]. Presumably the glucuronides do not. Total radioactivity, which is largely metabolites, is cleared from brain more rapidly, but from the plasma more slowly, than is the unchanged drug (fig. 5).

VI. PLASMA LEVELS AND RESPONSE

The relation between levels and response has been examined by several research groups during the last 10 years. Reports from these groups have ranged from anecdotal descriptions of patients with particular responses and levels to accounts of well-designed clinical trials. This research is considered partly in chronological order, and partly by research group, in this section.

Soon after the GLC methods were published, it was noted that (1) wide variations in chlorpromazine concentrations occurred and that these variations might account for at least some of the variations in response, in that two of the first six patients studied had relatively low levels and relatively poor response; (2) initial doses in previously untreated patients caused postural hypotension and sedation at plasma concentrations lower than those exerting no such effects at a later time in treatment, and (3) the lowest effective plasma level might be around 30 ng/ml. These anecdotal reports confirmed the need for studies with higher levels of experimental control in later years, [35,37,38].

At about the same time as the early plasma level work was conducted, a group in Oklahoma organized the first behavioral dose-response study with chlorpromazine [58]. Doses were randomly assigned to patients. A dose of 150 ng/ml was found to be more effective than placebo. Doses of 300 and 600 mg/day both gave better clinical responses, but there was little difference *between* these two higher doses in this regard. However, "side effects" were more prevalent at the 600-mg/day dose. This study was well designed with, for example, matched groups of patients. It involved the use of the Lorr Inpatient Multidimensional Psychiatric Scale (IMPS) and the Brief Psychiatric Rating Scale (BPRS).

Another important result of this study was the observation that clinical improvement reached its maximum by approximately 12 weeks after initiation of treatment, with very little change thereafter. The rate of achievement of this response was greater with the 600-mg/day regime, so it was suggested that early treatment with a higher dose, once the very early problems of somnolence and postural hypotension had been overcome, combined with later maintenance with an intermediate dose was desirable. This dosage regime is used empirically by some prescribers, in spite of the enzyme induction problems mentioned earlier.

It is interesting to compare these dosage observations with those on plasma levels from other groups. As mentioned earlier, the increment on changing dosage in each individual is proportional to the change in dose, but within a population patients adjusted to receiving higher doses do not attain proportionately higher plasma levels. However, in any population the patients will have been prescribed increasing doses until just below the threshold for unwanted drug effects. Thus the two observations, behavioral and pharmacokinetic, were not derived from analogous studies. Clark and his co-workers appear to have found the maximum response on a dose-response curve, and, with a fixed regimen, it is probable that the concentrations were in proportion to the dose. It is also of interest to note the time scale of response in relation to the plasma level pattern in Fig. 3, which is considered again later.

The first attempt to study the relation between plasma levels and response in a systematic way was published in 1970 [39]. The study in question was primarily an assessment of chlorpromazine dosage forms. However, data was obtained on frequency of occurrence of 10 symptoms and signs, including drowsiness, dry mouth, changes in pulse, etc., at four time intervals following doses in tablet, solution, sustained-release capsule, and intramuscular injection form. The symptoms and signs were recorded with frequencies matching the plasma levels attained, with highest levels and frequencies after the intramuscular doses, with lowest levels and frequencies after sustained-release capsules, and with tablets and solution preparations intermediate by all criteria. Thus in a general way, and assessing responses not really connected with the antipsychotic action of the drug, levels and effects were related.

The study of Sakalis and his colleagues [47] conducted when Sakalis was working in London, and mentioned earlier as characterizing unequivocally the time course of plasma levels of chlorpromazine, also involved assessment of a range of responses over the first 36 days of treatment in newly referred schizophrenics receiving no other drugs. The chlorpromazine was given in solution form, on a fixed regimen 100 mg every 8 hours. Testing was before starting and on days 4, 8, 15, 22, 29, and 36 of treatment. As stated before, plasma chlorpromazine was assessed at four points after the morning dose on these days. Physiological measures were of blood pressure, pulse rate, pupil size, sweat gland activity, electroencephalogram (EEG), EEG-evoked response, salivary secretion, auditory reaction time, handwriting, and clinical rating. There was wide interpatient variation in drug concentrations, and the marked overall increase and decrease in concentrations shown in Fig. 3 were also recorded.

The relation between effects and levels in this study was complex. Changes in most peripheral nervous system phenomena correlated well with plasma levels, although blood pressure results were erratic. In contrast, EEG data were generally disappointing. Most striking, however, was the clinical response relation, which showed a steady decline in pathology over the 36 days (Fig. 6). This occurred against an overall rise in plasma chlorpromazine at first, then against a fall, and this must be considered as a key observation in relation to plasma levels and ef-

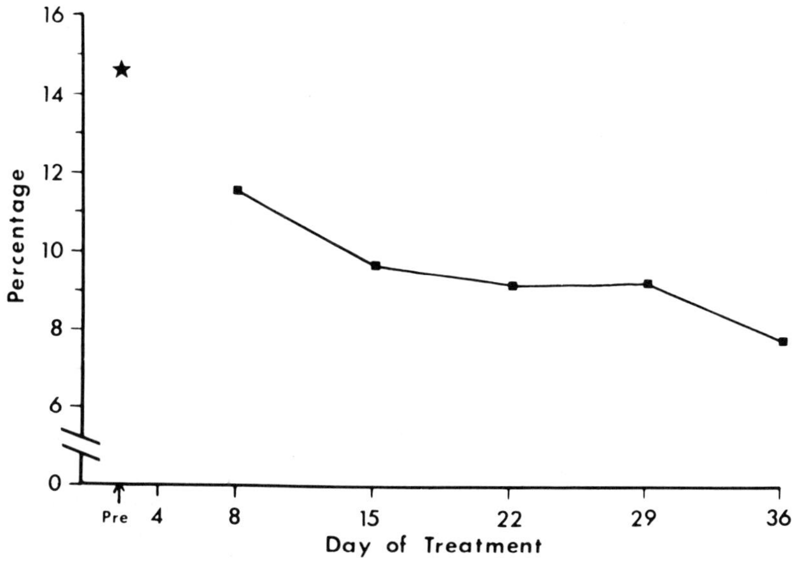

Figure 6 Clinical rating (IMPS scale) in the patients of Fig. 3 (* indicates pre-treatment score). (From Ref. 47, George Sakalis, Stephen H. Curry, Graham P. Mould, and Malcolm H. Lader, Physiologic and clinical effects of chlorpromazine and their relationship to plasma level. *Clin. Pharmacol. Ther. 131*:931-946 (1972).

fect. There are at least three possible explanations for this observation: (1) mediation of the effect through an active metabolite; (2) an unexplored tissue distribution phenomenon; and (3) a bona fide lack of relationship. These possibilities are considered again later.

Essentially similar observations were made by Rivera-Calimlim and her colleagues [33]. This second study employed the slightly modified assay procedure involving the use of isopropanol as a protein precipitant, but this has not been proved to be essential. It is not considered that this modification of the technique would affect data obtained in the sense of leading to conclusions different from those of other workers, although the lowest detectable level in this study was approximately 30 ng/ml. In eight of the patients, plasma chlorpromazine concentrations showed the same rises and falls observed earlier, although in contrast with the earlier study, this was observed in patients receiving a variety of different treatment regimens including electroconvulsive therapy (erratically), trifluoperazine in varied dosage, trihexyphenidyl at various times, and changes in chlorpromazine dosage. The BPRS was used to show the course of clinical treatment at the same time as the biochemical measurements were taken, and all of the patients showed the expected significant trend toward clinical improvement.

Five of the patients failed to show plasma chlorpromazine levels above 30 ng/ml. Three of these patients showed significant trends to clinical improvement, but the other two failed to show a significant trend. This was the basis for an unjustified conclusion that "schizophrenic patients with negligible plasma levels of chlorpromazine [less than 30 ng/ml] are not likely to improve clinically." The data presented just do not support this. Indeed, a proportion of schizophrenics improve on placebo, or drugs other than chlorpromazine, although the authors of this paper presumably intended "within the context of chlorpromazine therapy." In spite of this, a 30-ng/ml lower limit, originally suggested in the earliest phase of this research, has been defined in a study to different standards (see below).

In this study, two patients received massive chlorpromazine dosage complicated in one by a mixture of other drugs, and these patients experienced one or more of tremors, convulsions, facial twitching, and limb twitching/grasping. Plasma levels of chlorpromazine were very high (750-1000 ng/ml), and not surprisingly the patients improved on reducing dosage and bringing the plasma levels to below 350 ng/ml. This was taken as evidence of the rather obvious fact that too much chlorpromazine is dangerous.

The next study was an isolated examination of chlorpromazine-induced sleep changes with plasma level measurement [59]. The study was with only a small group of patients, but a crossover design was used, comparing morning and evening administration of daily doses and placebo. This plan was designed to facilitate study of sleep with high drug concentrations (evening dose) and low concentrations (morning dose with sleep at normal time). This, however, could have been achieved just by changing the dose at bedtime. The more subtle design was devised additionally to examine the possibility that long-term tissue retention could be a factor in the chlorpromazine sleep response, as suggested by other workers. In the event, a reversal of chlorpromazine effects was noted, in that the evening dose improved sleep while the morning dose adversely affected sleep. This could have resulted from (1) a dose-related or plasma level-related effect, with low doses/plasma levels exerting a "stimulant" effect; or (2) the soporific effect of chlorpromazine administered in the morning rendering the patient less in need of sleep at bedtime. The evidence supported a contribution from both phenomena, and also showed conclusively that the effect on sleep declined with the decline in plasma, in keeping with knowledge about retention in brain, thus ruling out a controlling influence of any long-term tissue retention of chlorpromazine or its metabolites on the sleep response.

The most specialized study in this series was a comparison of chlorpromazine kinetics and cerebral effects in relation to cirrhosis. Dosage was 25 mg intravenously and the subjects were in three groups: (1) controls; (2) patients with cirrhosis previously treated with a variety of drugs known to be enzyme inducers; and (3) patients with cirrhosis not treated with such drugs. The concentrations of chlorpromazine in plasma declined in at least two phases, as described earlier. No differences in chlorpromazine kinetics could be detected in the three groups. The drug caused drowsiness in all subjects, with EEG changes. The greatest change in EEG occurred in patients with a past history of encephalopathy in whom the pretreatment observations were abnormal. This study showed that the patients responded differently to the drug independently of pharmacokinetic factors. Thus the existence of pharmacodynamic variation was emphasized. This pharmacodynamic variation could have resulted from blood-brain barrier differences, but since baseline EEG records varied, it probably reflected differences in end organ response—sensitivity of cerebral neurons or some such phenomenon. The failure to demonstrate differences between patients with hepatic impairment and controls in regard to drug metabolism is of course in keeping with the majority of studies in the field.

The possible role of the *metabolites* in plasma was first considered by a group in New York [53]. Eight male adult schizophrenics undergoing chronic chlorpromazine treatment were assessed globally in relation to concentrations of chlorpromazine and eleven of its metabolites, measured by direct scanning of thin-layer chromatograms. The patients judged to be responding well had the higher concentrations of chlorpromazine and of 7-hydroxychlorpromazine, and those classified as nonresponders had high concentrations of chlorpromazine sulfoxide. The cautious conclusion was drawn that "these preliminary findings support the hypothesis that chlorpromazine metabolites play an important role in determining clinical response to treatment."

This conclusion has been quite influential in the field, and the study must be given careful examination. It can be criticized for a number of reasons: (1) the clinical rating was no more than a psychiatrist's opinion whether or not the patient was sufficiently improved, as the result of the treatment, to be discharged; (2) the biochemical techniques used are unique to this group, and they have been verified by no other workers, as the group concerned did not participate in the multicenter quality control study mentioned earlier; (3) the eight patients in the study divided into two very small groups of four, and these two groups differed markedly in size and timetable of dosage; (4) although mean concentrations of the three compounds in question showed the relation discussed above, three of the four nonresponders had plasma chlorpromazine concentrations equal to or above the lowest responder level, all had plasma 7-hydroxychlorpromazine concentrations equal to or above the lowest responder level, and one responder had a plasma chlorpromazine sulfoxide concentration above the lowest level in the nonresponder group. No statistical tests were performed.

This study shows an extraordinary lack of finesse. The design satisfies no clinical trial criteria, and the results are clearly nonsignificant from a statistical point of view.

The metabolite question was next taken up by a group in Cambridge (U.K.) [54]. Blood samples were obtained from 86 chronic schizophrenics receiving a wide range of oral doses of chlorpromazine. The gas chromatographic method, with modifications, was used to assess chlorpromazine and its sulfoxide, in all patients, and 7-hydroxychlorpromazine in 23 of them, and relationships with dose and "global clinical control" were sought. Wide variation in all scores was observed.

In this study the clinical methods used were very weak. Nurses "to whom the patients were well known" were asked to rate the patients for global control of schizophrenic symptomatology within one of three grades–good, moderate, or poor. However, there was a highly significant correlation between plasma chlorpromazine, plasma chlorpromazine sulfoxide, and dose, except above 400 mg/day. Mean plasma concentrations of chlorpromazine and 7-hydroxychlorpromazine were not significantly different in the three clinical groups. Mean plasma chlorpromazine sulfoxide concentrations were highest in the "poor" group and lowest in the "good" group. Much was made by the authors of nonsignificant trends, and significance was contrived by the calculation of ratios. The ratio 7-hydroxychlorpromazine/chlorpromazine sulfoxide gave figures with means significantly lower in the "poor" group and significantly high in the "good" group. Similar ratios 7-hydroxychlorpromazine/chlorpromazine gave ratios with no significant differences. This was used as evidence that conversion to 7-hydroxychlorpromazine is desirable for successful treatment.

This approach is statistically unsound [60]. Chlorpromazine molecules can be converted either to chlorpromazine sulfoxide or to 7-hydroxychlorpromazine (or to other products), so the concentrations of the two metabolites, and of the unchanged drug, are not independent. The use of such variables in which no significant difference has been found to contrive a significant ratio of the two variables cannot be condoned.

The only significant observation in this study is the difference in chlorpromazine sulfoxide concentrations. Judging from other studies, it seemed likely that these reflected the higher dosage likely to be given to nonresponders, who apparently tolerate these higher doses because of enhanced ability to convert chlorpromazine to its sulfoxide by means of first-pass effects. Although the mean doses in the three groups in this study were not published, they were in fact the same in the three groups (Mackay, personal communication). Even so, others have shown this type of relationship when "poor" responding groups had appreciably higher doses.

A major criticism of this work concerns the chemical methods used. Mackay and his colleagues have used ether extracts to assess chlorpromazine. As mentioned before, ether also removes chlorpromazine N-oxide, which shows as chlorpromazine on GLC columns, inflating data for the unchanged drug. The possibility must be considered that the data for chlorpromazine in Mackay's study is inflated, particularly in the "poor" group, who received higher doses. In addition to excessive conversion to the sulfoxide, there is excessive conversion to chlorpromazine N-oxide as a result of the first-pass effect in patients on high doses.

Three or four years after their first communication on the possible role of metabolites, the New York group produced their second and third preliminary communications in 1976 and 1977 [61,62]. These workers have now adopted the concentration ratio technique examined earlier, but with a significant and alarming modification: The ratio

$$\frac{\text{Chlorpromazine} + \text{7-hydroxychlorpromazine}}{\text{Chlorpromazine sulfoxide}}$$

is now used, on the basis that the two compounds in the top line are "active" and the sulfoxide is "inactive." In fact, clinical trials have shown the sulfoxide to have one-seventh the activity of chlorpromazine in man, although not necessarily when assessed for specific antipsychotic effect, and activity of 7-hydroxychlorpromazine is by no means proved. Notwithstanding this, the ratio now includes three variables dependent on each other combined in an artificial manner.

The study differs from that of other groups in a number of ways: (1) dosage is massive—for most patients a fixed regimen reaching 1000 mg/day by the seventh day of treatment; (2) chloral hydrate, a known enzyme inducer, is used for night sedation; and (3) the group continues to use its own spectrodensitometric method. Clinical methods in this study are now better, employing acceptable scales. However, the paper in question includes no details of clinical results, with no more than a grouping into (A) patients developing micrographia; and (B) patients in whom micrographia was never detected. In group A, 6 patients "responded well to treatment" while 3 "did not." Group B showed "excellent response" (all 9 patients). The concentrations of 7-hydroxychlorpromazine were higher in group A, and in most of these patients they exceeded concentrations of the unchanged drug, which were in the range reported by other workers. The ratios were not different in the two groups, but in a larger group, 13 out of 15 "good" responders had ratios above unity.

This study does support one idea, that the occurrence of extrapyramidal effects relates closely to the formation of 7-hydroxychlorpromazine, detected by micrographia. However, micrographia has also occurred in other studies without detection of significant levels of this metabolite. Even so, it has been reported that direct administration of the compound to primates leads to reproducible occurrence of dyskinesia (I. S. Forrest, personal communication).

This group appears to have exploited direct scan microdensitometry with great elegance, in that their technique purportedly measures unchanged chlorpromazine and as many as 18 metabolites in each sample. Evidence has been provided that only 7-hydroxychlorpromazine of the nonconjugated metabolites reaches anywhere near the concentrations of chlorpromazine, most being less than 10% of the concentrations of the unchanged drug. However, the glucuronide of 7-hydroxychlorpromazine has been shown also to reach concentrations comparable with those of the unchanged drug. These investigators have also confirmed the overall rise and fall of chlorpromazine in plasma and shown that 7-hydroxychlorpromazine concentrations rise slowly over 28 days, showing that long-term high-dose treatment is the regimen most likely to lead to accumulation of this compound in plasma. Because of this, the New York group has rightly criticized the idea of a steady state with chlorpromazine. The group has in fact been uninhibited in proclaiming that its own methods are the only good ones and in condemning the work of all others in the field, even though there has been cross-participation of one worker in both praised and condemned groups. The fact is, the work of the New York group is at its best when condemning its own earlier work, in criticizing the classification of patients as responders and nonresponders, and in dismissing "global rating." It is also statistically weak in that data are reported with standard deviations in excess of means. This occurs when the range is very great and the distribution is heavily skewed—just the situation in which statisticians advise against the use of parametric statistics.

The Cambridge group has extended its work in a study with superior control [63]. A modification of the Present State Examination, which is primarily a diagnostic test, has been developed. The modification has permitted the test to be used for rating. Nine acute patients have been assessed by this scale and with a nurses rating scale. The biochemical measures were of chlorpromazine, the sulfoxide, demonomethylchlorpromazine, and 7-hydroxychlorpromazine. As in previous studies, plasma chlorpromazine changes did not parallel the clinical observations. The sulfoxide concentrations were appreciable, and in this case they rose with time as clinical improvement was seen. Concentrations of demonomethylchlorpromazine were trivial, while concentrations of 7-hydroxychlorpromazine rose, especially in the third to sixth weeks after admission to the study, and so clinical improvement was seen against a pattern of rising concentrations of this metabolite. Once again, the misleading ratio of 7-hydroxychlorpromazine concentration to chlorpromazine sulfoxide concentration was derived, but in this case it was not needed, as the 7-hydroxychlorpromazine concentrations were in themselves significant. They were however, still less than the concentrations of chlorpromazine. The correlations between the concentrations of the 7-hydroxylated metabolite and response were most obvious with symptoms of high diagnostic significance for schizophrenia and in scores for perceptual disorders.

The question of hydroxylated metabolites was next taken up in London [14]. Workers in the same group had earlier established the fact that among the heptane-extractable metabolites, relatively large concentrations of chlorpromazine sulfoxide and relative small concentrations of demonomethylchlorpromazine and dedimethylchlorpromazine constituted the standard pattern. The sulfoxide concentrations were similar to those of chlorpromazine. The concentrations of demethylated derivatives rarely exceeded 10% of those of the unchanged drug.

The hydroxylated metabolites were examined in ether extracts. An exhaustive search revealed only traces of hydroxylated metabolites in patients showing a definite clinical response. The patients included both newly diagnosed outpatient schizophrenics and long-established inpatients. Possibilities for analytical errors or other false conclusions were systematically considered, and the data were taken as evidence that the hydroxylated metabolites of chlorpromazine are not essential to its action. This did not mean that they are inactive. If present in sufficient quantities they would contribute an action and could still have potential therapeutic value if administered directly. The observation was merely that some patients could show good response without accumulation of hydroxylated metabolites in plasma.

A series of papers on the relation between chlorpromazine concentrations and indices of endocrinological or physiological function have emerged from a group in Oxford (U.K.) [64-68]. The objective appears to have been to search for a useful index of pharmacological effect of chlorpromazine for time-course studies. The group first examined platelet aggregation, as an in vitro test supposedly related to pharmacology in vivo [64]. The aggregation response induced in platelets by 5-hydroxytryptamine was greatly increased in blood from psychiatric patients receiving chlorpromazine (compared with normal volunteers and psychiatric patients not receiving chlorpromazine). When chlorpromazine treatment was stopped, the platelet response required three weeks for return to normal. At the same time, chlorpromazine concentrations fell to below the limit of sensitivity of the analytical method, as used in the laboratory in question, within one week. The enhanced responses returned when chlorpromazine therapy was reinstated, with chlorpromazine again detectable in plasma.

These workers also detected chlorpromazine sulfoxide and demonomethylchlorpromazine in their extracts. As in other investigations, the sulfoxide concentration was much higher than that of the demethylated metabolite. In this case both were well below that of chlorpromazine, and the metabolite concentrations fell and were reinstated on the same time course as that of chlorpromazine. Thus the delayed return to normal platelet aggregation could not be ascribed to prolonged persistence of metabolites in particular.

Platelet responses are seemingly very complex, as chlorpromazine added to blood in vitro, rather than by dosage in vivo followed by analysis in vitro, *inhibits* platelet aggregation responses. This also occurs with a wide range of chlorpromazine metabolites. Thus it is not surprising that Boullin and his colleagues [65] concluded, "Only further investigation will show whether the effect of chlorpromazine *in vivo,* apparent as enhancement of 5-hydroxytryptamine induced platelet aggregation, will correlate with its [chlorpromazine's] effect in psychoses."

The Oxford group then turned its attention to prolactin. The significance of prolactin is that (1) plasma prolactin rises in human subjects given single doses of chlorpromazine; (2) circulating levels of prolactin are elevated in psychiatric patients receiving phenothiazines and other neuroleptics; and (3) prolactin release relates to function of dopaminergic nerves (in the hypothalamus), and other dopaminergic nerves may well be important in psychoses, and certainly are important in extrapyramidal effects of chlorpromazine (the latter in the basal ganglia). Chlorpromazine of course blocks dopamine receptors. The questions arose: (1) Is the prolactin response related either to chlorpromazine dose or plasma concentration? (2) Is it related to clinical effects of neuroleptics?

In their first prolactin paper the Oxford group showed no relationship between chlorpromazine dose and prolactin levels, but did show a positive correlation ($r = .67, P < .01$) between mean plasma prolactin and mean plasma chlorpromazine in a group of newly diagnosed schizophrenics. They also showed that none of the patients whose mean plasma prolactin remained below 35 ng/ml before or after the morning dose of the drug showed extrapyramidal symptoms, while all patients with higher levels did show symptoms. Mean levels of chlorpromazine were also higher in patients with extrapyramidal side effects. However, neither the therapeutic effect nor autonomic side effects seemed to be related to prolactin levels.

In their second series, the Oxford group extended their investigations to the metabolites chlorpromazine sulfoxide, demonomethylchlorpromazine, and 7-hydroxychlorpromazine and to various additional measures of endocrine function. The clinical assessment was, as in many other studies, quite weak. Although details of clinical methods involving the BPRS and various other rating measures were given in the paper, the results were finally expressed only in terms of "response" or "nonresponse." Six of the seven patients who showed no clinical improvement had plasma chlorpromazine levels equal to or higher than those who improved. Nonresponders had more of the sulfoxide. The occurrence of extrapyramidal side effects was greatest with patients in whom plasma chlorpromazine exceeded 50 ng/ml, with plasma prolactin over 30 ng/ml, but the onset of the side effects lagged two weeks behind elevation of prolactin. Again, the correlation between plasma prolactin and plasma chlorpromazine was stressed. It was suggested that the prolactin response might prove a useful index of the central antidopaminergic effect of neuroleptic drugs, but now the observations do not add up, as the previous paper showed no relation between plasma prolactin and clinical response, and clinical response is believed by many investigators to relate to changes in central dopaminergic function. There may be a false conclusion in the data.

The concentrations of chlorpromazine sulfoxide were about half those of chlorpromazine, and the concentrations of demonomethylchlorpromazine and 7-hydroxychlorpromazine were less than 10% of those of chlorpromazine in keeping with observations of most other workers. No particular interpretation was placed on these figures, except a repetition of the error discussed earlier, of calculating a ratio of the sulfoxide to the chlorpromazine concentration, which indicates only the previously known fact, that sulfoxide concentrations are higher in nonresponding patients, who usually receive higher doses. This is not to say that chlorpromazine sulfoxide is "psychotoxic." It arises in those particular non-responding patients who tolerate high doses because of their capacity to form the sulfoxide in large quantities.

In the third of these studies, the Oxford group studied a group of 18 chronic schizophrenics. The picture was now complicated by a miscellany of other drugs and the diffuse pathology of chronic disease, and the relationships of the acute study now disappeared. Plasma chlorpromazine concentrations in the acute and chronic groups were similar, and so the clinical differences were ascribed to acquired tolerance to the antidopaminergic effects of the drug.

There is one important weakness in the biochemical work of the Oxford group. As with some others, in their desire to measure chlorpromazine *and* its metabolites the investigators have used ether extracts, which include chlorpromazine N-oxide if present. The problems this raises have now been mentioned at least twice in this chapter, and are freely acknowledged by the group concerned. In fact, concentrations of the N-oxide in plasma are quite low, and the very low concentrations recorded of demonomethylchlorpromazine (which would also have been inflated by the N-oxide complication) provide evidence that, in this series at least, the chlorpromazine measurements were not adversely affected.

The Oklahoma group [69-72] has pursued an independent line using its own methods. Like the members of the New York group, these workers have not hesitated to criticize scathingly the work of other workers, and have even accused these other workers of condemning their own methods! Indeed, these two groups appear to be competing for the largest self-awarded laurels. Yet Kaul and his team have made fundamental errors in their work and have placed their own interpretations on condemned work when it suited them.

The Kaul analytical approach is to extract and then react the tertiary amine drug (chlorpromazine) with 9-bromomethylacridine. This generates a reaction product which is separated from other materials by TLC. The TLC spot is eluted, and the eluate is assessed for chlorpromazine content by further reaction and spectrophotofluorometry. This in itself is a valid approach and it has shown itself to have good precision and accuracy within certain limits. A similar approach, with a different reagent, is applied to metabolites with primary or secondary amine groups and/or ring hydroxyl substituents. Comments were made about assays of dedimethylchlorpromazine by this method in an earlier section. The criticisms of this approach are as follows: (1) it is promoted as a method more rapid than extraction and GLC, yet it includes a 16-20 h chemical reaction step; (2) it is stated to be applicable to as low as 20-30 ng/ml, easily achieved by GLC; (3) the published standard curve really *is* a curve, with linearity above 40 ng/ml, but significant deviation toward parallelism with the concentration axis below that level, Kaul and his colleagues having conveniently ignored all scientific convention by leaving out the lowest concentration point in drawing their calibration graphs and extrapolating a straight line from three higher points to meet the concentration axis at a false intercept [69].

Kaul and his colleagues in a preliminary report on a small number of subjects in a clinical/chemical correlation study reported "significant effect" in high dose (600 mg/m^2/day) and less effect in a similar group on lower doses (200 mg/m^2/day). In a representative subgroup, plasma chlorpromazine was reported as higher in the high-dose subjects, and in addition the "response index," a composite score based on six rating scales, was higher in the higher-"blood"-level subjects. So on a small sample evidence was presented of plasma chlorpromazine influencing response. This work is marred by poor scientific method: (1) the analytical weaknesses were considered earlier; (2) the persistence (alone in the chlorpromazine field) in using the "steady-state" idea with concentration data, even though in Kaul's own studies the plasma concentration rose by approximately 300% (without taking into account graphing of only seven-eighths of the available data) in the 2 hours after the dose in a chronically treated patient; (3) changes of as much as 100% up or 50% down on repeated sampling in individual patients over a 12-week study, including data as low as 12.5 ng/ml, well below the authors' own limit of sensitivity of their method; and (4) imprecise use of the terms *blood* and *plasma* with a drug for which red cell localization, or lack of it, is important.

More recently, Kaul et al. extended their study to a total of 13 chlorpromazine-treated and 7 placebo-treated patients. Two types of relationship were examined: (1) the relationship between the "fast" changes (within 12 hours of dosing) in chlorpromazine and chlorpromazine sulfoxide "blood" concentrations after single doses and changes in blood pressure, pulse rate, and sedation in the same 12 hours; and (2) the relationship between "slow" changes in behavior (after 12 weeks of treatment) and "steady-state" chlorpromazine and chlorpromazine sulfoxide "blood" concentrations during treatment with "high" and "low" doses of chlorpromazine. The results showed acute-dose cardiovascular and sedation data with the same time course as blood chlorpromazine and chlorpromazine sulfoxide. This led to the recording of highly significant correlation coefficients between pulse rate, blood pressure, and the two compounds. At 12 weeks, the blood pressure changes were much weaker and the correlations were nonsignificant, although some of the pulse rate changes were maintained. In contrast, sedation still showed the correlation with concentration, but at an overall higher level. This is a fine demonstration of the tolerance to cardiovascular and sedative effects which develops to chlorpromazine. This is *not* a pharmacokinetic tolerance in the sense of the effect disappearing as a result of reduced plasma levels consequent on enzyme induction. This is also a fine demonstration of how easy it is to obtain significant correlations for concentration and drug effect with compounds which most investigators consider active (chlorpromazine) and inactive (chlorpromazine sulfoxide).

In contrast with the above, Kaul et al. were unable to show any significant correlation between 12th-week behavioral changes on any of their scales [BPRS, NOSIE, global, or response index (RI)] and drug concentrations, expressed as both steady-state and ratio figures, although dose showed a significant correlation with clinical RI ($r = .80$, $P < .01$). These investigators have not so far published data on correlations with metabolites other than chlorpromazine sulfoxide.

Two other studies complete the examples of clinical-pharmacokinetic correlations. In the first of these a Japanese group [73] examined the possibility of predicting treatment outcome on the basis of initial test doses. *Serum* samples were examined by the GLC method for chlorpromazine and the heptane-extractable metabolites. A difference in half-time between patients and volunteer subjects, even with the first dose, was noted, with the half-time measurements less in the patients. As in other studies, patients showing high levels of chlorpromazine tended to achieve poorer results. In addition, demethylated metabolites were included with the sulfoxide in this relationship in this study. On this basis, it was suggested that the metabolite conversion status of each patient could be used to predict response. In this study, the metabolite ratio techniques was used, which is not satisfactory, but clinical outcome was well assessed, with the BPRS. All in all, the study, in relation to others, showed that patients with a high first-pass effect have a poor chance of successful chlorpromazine therapy. This has emerged from several studies. As an aside, it is of interest that this work does not support any active metabolite theory, although there was no direct correlation between unchanged chlorpromazine and effect, yet it has actually been quoted by one group as providing justification for a belief in assessment of active and inactive metabolites by a concentration ratio technique.

Finally, Wode-Helgodt [51] has proved to be the first investigator to genuinely show a positive correlation between plasma chlorpromazine (unchanged drug) and clinical effects. A mass fragmentographic method was used, as was a newly developed rating scale. This was in the study quoted earlier as yielding correlated plasma and CSF data, so effects were also positively correlated with CSF concentrations. Extrapyramidal symptoms showed a delay compared with antipsychotic effect, and hence a poorer correlation with plasma chlorpromazine. This study confirmed the basic need for a concentration of at least 30-40 ng/ml for successful treatment in patients needing, and responding to, chlorpromazine, and was taken as indicating a predictive value for pharmacokinetic measurements. The status of this study in the total picture will emerge in due course. The total picture is of no interpatient correlation between clinical effect and plasma measurements.

VII. PHARMACOKINETICS OF EFFECTS

Fascinating pharmacological data has been presented by Smolen and his colleagues [74-78], who have recently made use of the established relation between pupil size and plasma chlorpromazine in an elegant logical extension of the principle of a pharmacokinetic/pharmacodynamic link. This group has investigated the pharmacokinetics of many drug responses, and has become interested in chlorpromazine in recent years because its diverse pharmacology makes it a good model compound. As they rightly argue, it is the time course of effect that matters, and this extends to bioavailability work, a major reason for the existence for pharmacokinetics. Smolen and his group, having noted the observation of others that certain peripheral pharmacological effects of chlorpromazine correlated with disposition pharmacokinetics measured from plasma levels, proceeded to assess bioavailability of this drug in man from pupil size, intraocular pressure by tonometry, resting heart rate, and body temperature. The work has also been extended to miotic response and rectal temperature in rabbits.

The results contain some fascinating observations. For example, changes in pupil size were accurately assessed at doses as low as 10 mg per 70 kg. Plasma measurements cease to be possible with oral doses much below 100 mg per 70 kg. Secondly, the average maximum miotic response was delayed for some 1-1½ h beyond the end of a 30-min intravenous infusion time, possibly resulting from the inevitable penetration time of the drug from blood to receptors. This delay was not noted with oral studies, because of "smoothing out," so that pupil measurements can be taken as correlated with plasma levels for studies of bioavailability of oral preparations. Thirdly, pupil data in particular lends itself to large numbers of measurements, far in excess of those obtained in plasma studies, so Smolen et al. were able to derive accurate estimates of area under the curve of response, in addition to peak time and peak intensity measurements. This made accurate dose-effect relationships possible, and, interestingly, linearity of response (not log dose) over a wide range was demonstrated.

The interpretation of tonometry data was more complex. The response was less clearly defined than the pupil response, and variance was greater. A wide range of similar values for peak time and intensity of response was seen, coinciding with pupil and (implied) plasma chlorpromazine. In addition, Smolen et al. have noted contrasting data from humans, rabbits, and cats. In humans and rabbits, chlorpromazine is miotic. In cats it is mydriatic. In all three species, intraocular pressure falls. It is suggested that this must mean that the two effects are mediated by different chemicals, i.e., at least one by a chlorpromazine metabolite. On this basis, the tonometric data is thought to be analogous to nonspecific chemical assay.

This may be so, but chlorpromazine is both anticholinergic and antiadrenergic. Mydriasis is an anticholinergic effect, while miosis is a result of α-adrenoceptor blocking. It is surprising, but the sympatholytic effect apparently predominates in man in this case. It could be that the more normal physiology of parasympathetic dominance is seen in the cat with this drug. A species difference in active or inactive metabolites would then not be needed, and this would make more acceptable the similar time courses of the two effects and plasma chlorpromazine. Metabolites generally have time courses different from that of the parent drug.

Effects on intraocular pressure are a function of drainage, affected by pupil diameter, and fluid input into the eye, which is affected by at least carbonic anhydrase. Inhibitors of this enzyme reduce intraocular pressure. Since intraocular pressure falls in different species in which dilation and constriction are seen, an effect on fluid input must at least be considered. This should not be taken as a suggestion that chlorpromazine does in fact affect carbonic anhydrase in particular.

Additional light might be shed on this problem by the use of chlorpromazine applied direct to the eye. Although not used as a mydriatic, chlorpromazine is known to dilate the pupil when administered in eyedrops.

Smolen and his colleagues have also considered heart rate and body temperature in detail. Intravenous dosing had little if any effect on resting heart rate but produced an immediate dose-dependent effect on body temperature. Oral dosing, however, caused a time- and dose-dependent tachycardia, with body temperature unaffected. It appeared, therefore, that there was a qualitative difference in the effects of the drug given by the two routes. It was suggested that this difference related to the formation of chlorpromazine sulfoxide when the drug is given orally, this change occurring to a much lesser extent when the drug is given intravenously. This plausible but unproved explanation deserves considerable investigation, possibly by the direct administration of the sulfoxide. If true, this would lead to a reappraisal of the activity of this compound, studied unsuccessfully many years ago for effects in the brain, but never objectively evaluated for cardiovascular effects. Even so, it should be noted that in all tests in animals, chlorpromazine sulfoxide has shown considerably less activity than the parent drug.

Another point to consider is the relation between the conditions of oral and intravenous study. In fact, the data show a general heart rate effect, except for one dose level which has complicated the statistics, and could be a rogue point. Chlorpromazine given orally has only one-tenth of the activity of an equivalent intravenous dose, because of the first-pass effect. It may be that not enough was given by the one route for a temperature effect, this being small and difficult to measure anyway. Pulse did in fact change in the dosages used, and it must be remembered that any effect on temperature is a result of a complex mixture of effects on the central nervous system and peripheral blood vessels. Tachycardia is an uncomplicated anticholinergic effect.

VIII. ACTIVITY OF CHLORPROMAZINE METABOLITES

It must be obvious by this point that the activity of chlorpromazine metabolites and their possible role in the effects of the drug have been questions of great interest for a long time. With no drug in the history of pharmacology has there been such a scientific investment in attempts to assess the role of metabolites.

In this regard, much of the early urinary excretion work was done in the hope of finding particular metabolic routes associated with particular responses. However, over a long period of time Turner and his colleagues [79] have systematically examined plasma, erythrocytes, urine, and feces for concentrations of chlorpromazine and its identifiable metabolites. This work has been performed in healthy volunteers, and in patients at the start and after several years of long-term therapy. From a vast amount of data examined by a variety of statistical methods, Turner and his colleagues have reached the conclusion that there is no "evidence of occurrence of an individual compound or group of compounds which would distinguish those who improved from those who did not. The variance between individuals in each group was so great that we could construct no hypothesis to predict response to CPZ [chlorpromazine] from [the] metabolic pattern in urine" [79]. This confirmed the conclusion of the Oklahoma group, which provided data in a brief abstract reporting "significant negative correlations between amount [of mixed chlorpromazine metabolites] excreted and degree of psychopathology in 48 chronic female schizophrenics in three dose groups [150, 300, and 600 mg/day]" [80]. In addition, this group said that no particular metabolite seems particularly responsible for whether or not the patients responded. Placed together, these observations must actually mean that there was some difference between the groups, as they were all in steady state, with input equaling output, but the difference would have to relate to undetected metabolites, and it still does not support the idea of qualitative differences in metabolic routes in patients showing different responses.

It does now seem that interest in chlorpromazine metabolites as pharmacologically significant molecules (as opposed to molecules significant in elimination) can be confined to the two demethylated metabolites (and probably then only to demonomethylchlorpromazine), 7-hydroxychlorpromazine, chlorpromazine sulfoxide, and 7,8-dihydroxychlorpromazine.

For metabolites to be important in the action of a drug they must (1) have activity; and (2) be present in the body following administration of the drug. The metabolites of chlorpromazine do have activity. They have been assessed in some 25 pharmacological tests in animals. Almost without exception, the metabolites have less activity than the parent drug [81-96]. The only major exception is 7,8-dihydroxychlorpromazine, which has effects in vitro on adenosine triphosphatase at 10^{-12} molar, and so may be dramatically more potent than any other compound in this test (the unchanged drug remains untested) [2]. The activity of these metabolites generally relates to lipid solubility, which, as mentioned earlier, is progressively reduced on metabolism.

The metabolites are sometimes present in the body, but the demethylated derivatives are always much below the unchanged drug in concentration, and 7-hydroxychlorpromazine concentrations vary from similar to those of the unchanged drug down to 0. Chlorpromazine sulfoxide occurs in important concentrations, while 7,8-dihydroxychlorpromazine has been tentatively identified by only one group. However, for the presence of those compounds to be important it seems that their concentrations should *exceed* those of the unchanged drug, which they rarely do, because of their lesser potency. Higher concentrations would also be needed to offset a reduced ability to cross the blood-brain barrier and more rapid removal from the brain. It seems therefore that the metabolites do not reach concentrations high enough to play a major part in the pharmacology. They probably make a contribution but do not *dominate* the response.

Of particular interest is the relation between lipophilic properties of chlorpromazine and its metabolites and inhibition of dopamine-sensitive adenylate cyclase in brain slices. This is shown in Fig. 7, which shows the relationship between activity and partition ratio measured with a relatively unusual solvent. The relationship between activity and partition ratio (P) into heptane is

$$\log (1/IC_{50}) = 4.68 + .48 \log P \quad (r = .994)$$

and similarly for octanol:

$$\log (1/IC_{50}) = 2.80 + .51 \log P \quad (r = .926)$$

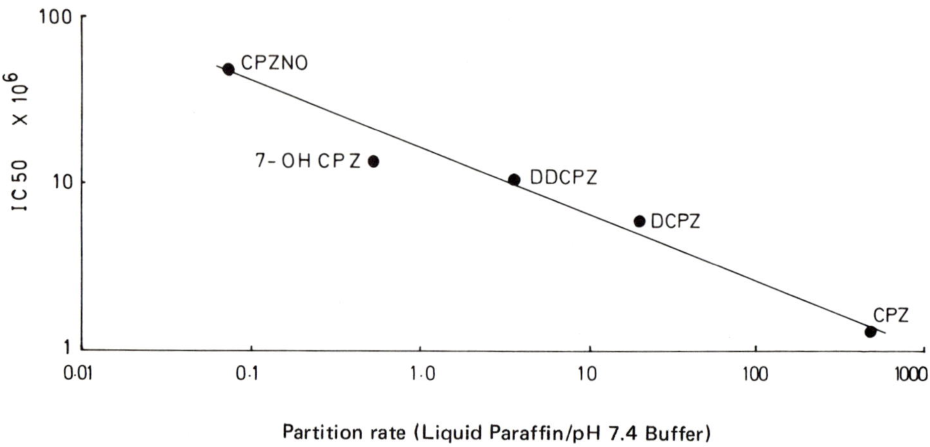

Figure 7 Relation between IC_{50} for inhibition of dopamine-stimulated adenylate cyclase of rat striatum, and partition ratio between liquid paraffin and pH 7.4 buffer. (Data from Refs. 18 and 96.)

Effects on dopamine receptors are suggested as a possible mechanism of chlorpromazine antipsychotic action, although this idea is disputed by others. It was mentioned earlier in this chapter in relation to prolactin, and it is obvious that a great deal of work must still be done before the biochemistry of psychoses and antipsychotic drug action is understood. Nevertheless, it seems that a simple lipophilicity-related binding model may account for the relative actions of chlorpromazine and its metabolites, in which case reduced action on metabolism is not surprising. Even so, 7,8-dihydroxychlorpromazine deserves further investigation.

Some other comments in relation to chlorpromazine metabolite activity are in order:

1. Conversion down a particular route could not be essential as there is no metabolic route common to all neuroleptics; in particular, thioxanthenes do not form 7-hydroxylated metabolites, and no phenolic butyrophenone has shown useful activity.
2. Only one metabolite (chlorpromazine sulfoxide) has been evaluated in man, and its activity was one-seventh or one-eighth that of chlorpromazine.
3. Against this, 7-hydroxychlorpromazine has shown activity, but less than that of standard reference drugs, in tests for imipraminelike activity. It is unique among the chlorpromazine metabolites in doing this, and this has led to the idea that it might be an antidepressant neuroleptic.

Thus, whatever the circumstances of other studies, the active metabolite theory fails to account for the observation of increased response with reduced plasma levels discussed earlier. Since there appears to be no tissue retention without detection in plasma, of the possibilities mentioned for accounting for this, it is necessary to fall back on a nonpharmacological relationship. This should not surprise anyone. As has been said before, the antipsychotic drugs "arrest the progress of psychotic disorders which, if allowed to continue, would lead to further impairment of the patient's contact with reality. They interrupt a vicious circle [of self-perpetuating pathology] and allow the patient's CNS [central nervous system] to function in a more normal manner" [97]. To do this, early treatment with a high dose or high plasma levels would arrest progress of the illness, permitting the all-important nonpharmacological factors in treatment to exert an ever-increasing influence, with the vicious circle eventually going into reverse, so that normality might finally be achieved with no continuing treatment. The time course of treatment would thus lead to a time-dependent relation between kinetics and effect, and such a relation would be so complex as to be undetectable.

IX. PLASMA LEVEL MONITORING

All this research raises the question of whether the measurement of plasma chlorpromazine can be of any use in controlling therapy. Two studies remain to be considered. The first of these was an investigation of the response of patients in whom the first-pass effect is great when treated with the chlorpromazine analogue fluphenazine, which is marketed chiefly as its long-acting injectable decanoate ester. This is primarily designed to overcome the problem of treatment defaulting, but by virtue of its being an antipsychotic phenothiazine delivered more directly into body, it also overcomes problems arising from metabolism in the gastrointestinal tract and liver before the drug arrives in the general circulation. This was proved in a clinical trial, in which the patients were assessed by the BPRS [98-100]. In fact, the BPRS data itself showed only a tenuous relationship between response and chlorpromazine level, although the patients appeared to be in two groups with an important subgroup with concentrations below 30 ng/ml. These patients were selected in the trial for fluphenazine treatment. However, all were poorly responsive, so the other group, in whom plasma levels were above 30 ng/ml, were probably nonresponsive for pharmacodynamic reasons. This illustrates yet another aspect of the difficulty in obtaining and interpreting data. The implication is that nonresponders *may* have low plasma levels, and treatment efficiency will then be improved as the result of pharmacokinetic monitoring.

The relation between plasma chlorpromazine and clinical effect in the most

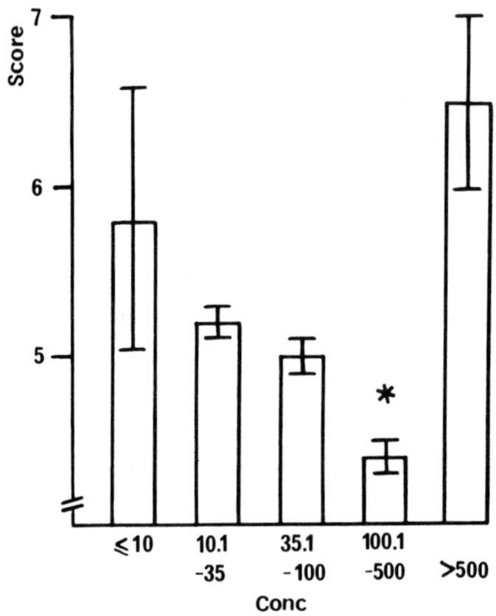

Figure 8 U-shaped relation between plasma chlorpromazine and clinical rating on a global 7-point scale in a large group of long-term patients. (*Source:* Ref. 17.)

general way is shown in Fig. 8. The response to chlorpromazine, and plasma chlorpromazine levels, were assessed in 30 long-term patients, who were rated on one of the two seven-point scales used in the early National Institute of Mental Health trials of phenothiazine drugs [101]. To the question, "Considering your total experience, how mentally ill is this patient at this time?" the psychiatrist answered: (1) normal, not ill at all; (2) borderline mentally ill; (3) mildly ill; (4) moderately ill; (5) markedly ill: (6) severely ill; or (7) among the most extremely ill. All the patients had started treatment in group 7, and were considered to be showing at least some response to their drug treatment. Plasma levels (conc.) were determined at three times and averaged for each patient. The patients were placed in five groups according to their plasma levels. Mean illness scores (range 3-7) were calculated for each group and plotted with standard errors. The asterisk in the figure indicates significance ($P < .001$) of the difference between the mean score of this and all other groups.

This study can of course be criticized on methodological grounds. For example, the use of a global scale in research is crude, but it does reflect what many psychiatrists are obliged to do instinctively. The use of a global scale probably leads to incorporation of unwanted drug effects into scores (particularly high ones), but such reactions are inevitably an influence in the success or otherwise of treatments. The patients were grouped on plasma levels in an uneven distribution, but population plasma levels do show a skewed distribution. Also, ratings on a discontinuous scale have been evaluated for means with standard errors.

This study, like all others in the field, fails to take into account protein binding. Binding of chlorpromazine varies at least from 91.0 to 99.0% of the plasma content. If, for the sake of argument, the binding was least in patients with higher plasma levels, then the range of free concentration would vary over a massive range (1-36 ng/ml) in the total range 100-400 ng/ml. If the binding was least in patients with lower plasma levels, the unbound range would be 4-9 ng/ml. In fact, binding does not vary systematically within the concentration range seen in patients, and the variation clearly indicates patient characteristics. It seems unlikely, therefore, that protein binding measurements would lead to a better correlation between plasma level and effect, but a study should still be done to test this.

In spite of all that has been said, a very general U-shaped relation is evident in Fig. 8, saying no more than too little is too little, too much is too much, and there is a wide intermediate optimum concentration range (30-400 ng/ml). Within this, fluctuation in clinical response will not follow fluctuations in concentration. This will apply even with drugs interacting by affecting chlorpromazine plasma levels [102]. Also, there will *still* be some patients responsive at low concentrations and others unresponsive at high concentrations, and some will develop unwanted effects at low concentrations while others will tolerate and need high concentrations. However, adjustment of dosage to bring plasma levels into the intermediate range will lead to greater confidence that the patient is receiving, in adequate amounts, the drug he or she is thought to need. Maintenance of concentrations in this middle range will hopefully lead to gradual improvement over an extended period of time. The vicious circle of pathology will be put into reverse, as an environment amenable to psychotherapy will be created. The contrast between observations made repeatedly in individuals and observations across populations should especially be noted, as patients may need less at later stages of treatment.

In patients with high concentrations of 7-hydroxychlorpromazine this metabolite will contribute to the response, changing the relationship a little, although as yet we do not know to what extent, as the relative weighting to be given to the plasma levels to account for differential antipsychotic potency is not known.

Finally, what of the old premise that pharmacokinetic research will eventually aid the detection of drug-taking reliability? It is now apparent that this problem will *not* be efficiently studied from plasma, as wide variations occur in plasma levels even with similar consumption of doses. Drug-taking reliability is best studied from 24-h urine samples, provided urine sampling is itself efficient, which can be checked by other biochemical measures. Daily excretion of di-

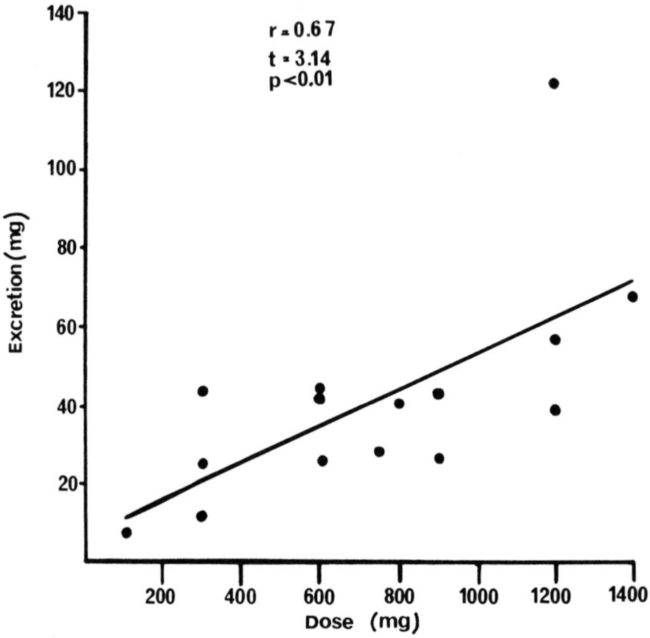

Figure 9 Excretion of relatively nonpolar chlorpromazine metabolites, assessed as chlorpromazine, in relation to dose. (Data from Ref. 103.)

chloromethane-extractable metabolites in urine accounts for 5-10% of daily dose (Fig. 9). This is best studied by means of colorimetric assays [103,104].

RECENT DEVELOPMENTS

The literature survey for this review terminated in February 1978. Since that date the most important development in this field has been the use of radioreceptor assay techniques for the measurement of "total neuroleptic content" of plasma [105,106,107]. This has been reviewed [108]. Additionally, the use of the thermionic sensitive detector (nitrogen sensitive) and high-pressure liquid chromatography with various detectors for phenothiazine drug assays is growing (Curry and Brown, unpublished results). Finally, a meeting in 1979 considered protein binding of centrally acting drugs in detail [109], and subcellular distributions in the brain [110] and red cells [111] have been further studied.

ACKNOWLEDGMENTS

I am grateful to the large number of collaborators who have assisted with chlorpromazine investigations conducted in my own department, and to the large number of workers in other departments who provided data, published and unpublished, for inclusion in this review. Analytical work with chlorpromazine and its metabolites has been greatly facilitated during the last 20 years by the generous provision of a wide range of reference compounds, synthesized for the U.S. National Institute of Mental Health, and all investigators involved are grateful to Dr. A. A. Manian for making this possible.

REFERENCES

1. I. S. Forrest and D. E. Green, Phenothiazines: Metabolism and analytical detection. *J. Forensic Sci. 17:*592-617, 1972.
2. I. S. Forrest, C. J. Carr, and E. Usdin, eds. *Phenothiazines and Structurally Related Compounds.* New York, Raven Press, 1974.
3. B. B. Brodie, Physicochemical and biochemical aspects of pharmacology. *JAMA 202:*600-609, 1967.
4. N. P. Salzman, N. C. Moran, and B. B. Brodie, Identification and pharmacological properties of a major metabolite of chlorpromazine. *Nature 176:* 1122-1123, 1955.
5. N. P. Salzman and B. B. Brodie, Physiological disposition and fate of chlorpromazine and a method for its estimation in biological material. *J. Pharmacol. Exp. Ther. 118:*46-54, 1956.
6. S. H. Curry and B. B. Brodie, Estimation of nanogram quantities of chlorpromazine (CPZ) in plasma using gas-liquid chromatography (GLC) with an electron capture detector. *Fed. Proc. 26:*761, 1967.
7. E. Usdin, The assay of chlorpromazine and metabolites in blood, urine, and other tissues. *CRC Crit. Rev. Clin. Lab. Sci. 2:*347-391, 1971.
8. C. J. Carr and C. Karel, Metabolic studies and analytical methods for phenothiazine derivatives of psychopharmacological interest. *Psychopharmacology Serv. Cent. Bull. 2:*71-106, 1973.
9. J. L. Emerson and T. S. Miya, Metabolism of phenothiazine drugs. *J. Pharm. Sci. 52:*411-419, 1963.
10. R. T. Williams and D. V. Parke, The metabolic fate of drugs. *Ann. Rev. Pharmacol. 4:*85-114, 1964.
11. S. H. Curry, Determination of nanogram quantities of chlorpromazine and some of its metabolites in plasma using gas-liquid chromatography with an electron-capture detector. *Anal. Chem. 40:*1251-1255, 1968.
12. S. H. Curry, The determination and possible significance of plasma levels of chlorpromazine in psychiatric patients. *Agressologie 9:*115-121, 1968.

13. R. Whelpton and S. H. Curry, Gas-chromatographic separation of chlorpromazine, diazepam, and N-desmethyldiazepam. *J. Pharm. Pharmacol. 27:*970-971, 1975.
14. S. H. Curry and S. Evans, Assay of 7-hydroxychlorpromazine, and failure to detect more than small quantities, in plasma of responding schizophrenics. *Psychopharmacol. Commun. 1:*481-490, 1975.
15. R. Whelpton and S. H. Curry, Chromatographic properties of imines formed from dedimethylchlorpromazine and various aldehydes and ketones. *J. Chromatogr. 121::*88-92, 1976.
16. S. H. Curry and S. Evans, A note on the assay of chlorpromazine N-oxide and its sulphoxide in plasma and urine. *J. Pharm. Pharmacol. 28:*467-468, 1976.
17. S. H. Curry, Gas-chromatographic methods for the study of chlorpromazine and some of its metabolites in human plasma. *Psychopharmacol. Commun. 2:*1-15, 1976.
18. S. H. Curry and R. Whelpton, Hydrophobic character of 15 model chlorpromazine metabolites determined from partition ratios in mixed solvents. *Brit. J. Pharmacol. 51:*143P, 1974.
19. C. L. Huang and B. H. Ruskin, Determination of serum chlorpromazine metabolites in psychotic patients. *J. Nerv. Ment. Dis. 139:*381-386, 1964.
20. C. L. Huang and A. A. Kurland, Chlorpromazine blood levels in psychotic patients. *Arch. Gen. Psychiatry 5:*509-513, 1961.
21. C.-G. Hammar, B. Holmstedt, and R. Ryhage, Mass fragmentography-identification of chlorpromazine and its metabolites in human blood by a new method. *Anal. Biochem. 25:*532-548, 1968.
22. D. H. Efron, S. R. Harris, A. A. Manian, and L. E. Gaudette, Radioassay of chlorpromazine and its metabolites in plasma. *Psychopharmacologia 19:* 207-210, 1971.
23. D. R. Flint, C. R. Ferullo, P. Levandoski, and B. Hwang, More sensitive gas chromatographic measurement of chlorpromazine in plasma. *Clin. Chem. 17:*830-831, 1971.
24. G. W. Christoph, D. Schmidt, D. S. Janowsky, and J. M. Davis, A method for the determination of chlorpromazine in human blood serum. *Clin. Chim. Acta 38:*265-270, 1972.
25. K. Kawashima, R. Dixon, and S. Spector, Development of radioimmunoassay for chlorpromazine. *Eur. J. Pharmacol. 32:*195-202, 1975.
26. G. Alfredsson, B. Wode-Helgodt, and G. Sedvall, A mass fragmentographic method for the determination of chlorpromazine and two of its active metabolites in human plasma and CSF. *Psychopharmacology 48:*123-131, 1976.
27. P. Turano and W. J. Turner, Quantitation of chlorpromazine and its metabolites by two-dimensional thin-layer chromatography and direct scanning microdensity. *J. Chromatogr. 64:*347-354, 1972.
28. T. L. Chan, G. Sakalis, and S. Gershon, Quantitation of chlorpromazine and its metabolites in human plasma and urine by direct spectrodensitometry of thin-layer chromatograms. In *Phenothiazines and Structurally*

Related Compounds (I. S. Forrest, C. J. Carr, and E. Usdin, eds.). New York, Raven Press, 1974, pp. 323-333.
29. P. N. Kaul, L. R. Whitfield, and M. L. Clark, Chlorpromazine metabolism, VII: New quantitative fluorometric determination of chlorpromazine and its sulphoxide. *J. Pharm. Sci. 65:*689-694, 1976.
30. S. H. Curry, Chlorpromazine analysis by gas chromatography with an electron-capture detector. In *Phenothiazines and Structurally Related Compounds* (I. S. Forrest, C. J. Carr, and E. Usdin, eds.). New York, Raven Press, 1974, pp. 335-346.
31. S. H. Curry, Assay of chlorpromazine and some of its metabolites in biological fluids. In *Assay of Drugs and Other Trace Compounds in Biological Fluids* (E. Reid, ed.). Amsterdam, North Holland, 1976, pp. 185-192.
32. M. Spirtes, Artifactual contamination of control serum extracts in gas chromatographic analyses for chlorpromazine. *Clin. Chem. 18:*317-318, 1972.
33. L. Rivera-Calimlim, L. Castaneda, and L. Lasagna, Effects of mode of management on plasma chlorpromazine in psychiatric patients. *Clin. Pharmacol. Ther. 14:*978-986, 1973.
34. W. J. Turner, P. Turano, and S. Badzinski, An attempt to establish quality control in determination of plasma chlorpromazine by a multi-laboratory collaboration. In *Pharmacokinetics of Psychoactive Drugs.* (L. A. Gottschalk and S. Merlis, eds.). New York, Spectrum, 1976, pp. 33-44.
35. S. H. Curry and J. H. L. Marshall, Plasma levels of chlorpromazine and some of its relatively non-polar metabolites in psychiatric patients. *Life Sci. 7:*9-17, 1968.
36. S. H. Curry, Plasma protein binding of chlorpromazine. *J. Pharm. Pharmacol. 22:*193-197, 1970.
37. S. H. Curry, J. H. L. Marshall, J. M. Davis, and D. S. Janowsky, Factors affecting chlorpromazine plasma levels in psychiatric patients. *Arch. Gen. Psychiatry 22:*209-215, 1970.
38. S. H. Curry, J. H. L. Marshall, J. M. Davis, and D. S. Janowsky, Chlorpromazine plasma levels and effects. *Arch. Gen. Psychiatry 22:*289-296, 1970.
39. L. E. Hollister, S. H. Curry, J. E. Derr, and S. Kanter, Studies of delayed action medication, V: Plasma levels and urinary excretion of four different dosage forms of chlorpromazine. *Clin. Pharmacol. Ther. 11:*49-59, 1970.
40. L. E. Hollister and S. H. Curry, Urinary excretion of chlorpromazine metabolites following single doses in steady-state conditions. *Res. Comm. Chem. Path. Pharmacol. 2:*330-338, 1971.
41. S. H. Curry, A. D'Mello, and G. P. Mould, Destruction of chlorpromazine during absorption in the rat in vivo and in vitro. *Brit. J. Pharmacol. 42:* 403-411, 1971.
42. S. H. Curry, Relation between binding to plasma protein, apparent volume of distribution, and rate constants of disposition and elimination for chlorpromazine in three species. *J. Pharm. Pharmacol. 24:*818-819, 1972.

43. J. D. Maxwell, M. Carrella, J. D. Parkes, R. Williams, G. P. Mould, and S. H. Curry, Plasma disappearance and cerebral effects of chlorpromazine in cirrhosis. *Clin. Sci. 43:*143-151, 1972.
44. S. H. Curry, Plasma level studies in psychotropic drug evaluation. *Brit. J. Clin. Pharmacol., Suppl. (1) 3:*20-28, 1976.
45. S. H. Curry, Metabolism and kinetics of chlorpromazine in relation to effect. In *Antipsychotic Drugs: Pharmacodynamics and Pharmacokinetics* (G. Sedvall, B. Uvnas, and Y. Zotterman, eds.). Oxford, Pergamon, 1976, pp. 343-352.
46. L. Whitfield, P. N. Kaul, and M. L. Clark, Chlorpromazine metabolism, IX: Pharmacokinetics of chlorpromazine following oral administration in man. *J. Pharmacokinetics and Biopharmaceutics, 6:*187-196, 1978.
47. G. Sakalis, S. H. Curry, G. P. Mould, and M. H. Lader, Physiologic and clinical effects of chlorpromazine and their relationship to plasma level. *Clin. Pharmacol. Ther. 13:*931-946, 1972.
48. S. G. Dahl and R. E. Strandjord, Pharmacokinetics of chlorpromazine after single and chronic dosage. *Clin. Pharmacol. Ther. 21:*437-448, 1977.
49. O. Phillipson, J. Baker, F. Sebastianpillai, G. Sheppard, and P. Brook, Disappearance of chlorpromazine from plasma following drug withdrawal. *Psychol. Med. 8:*331-384, 1978.
50. S. H. Curry, J. E. Derr, and H. M. Maling, The physiological disposition of chlorpromazine in the rat and dog. *Proc. Soc. Exp. Biol. Med. 134:*314-318, 1970.
51. B. Wode-Helgodt, S. Borg, B. Fyrö, and G. Sedvall, Clinical effects and drug concentrations in plasma and cerebrospinal fluid in psychotic patients treated with fixed doses of chlorpromazine. *Acta Psychiat. Scand. 58:*149-173, 1978.
52. R. P. Maickel, M. C. Braunstein, M. McGlynn, W. R. Snodgrass, and R. W. Webb, Behavioural, biochemical, and pharmacological effects of chronic dosage of phenothiazine tranquillizers in rats. In *Phenothiazine and Structurally Related Compounds* (I. S. Forrest, C. J. Carr, and E. Usdin, eds.). New York, Raven Press, 1974, pp. 593-602.
53. G. Sakalis, T. L. Chan, S. Gershon, and S. Park, The possible role of metabolites in therapeutic response to chlorpromazine treatment. *Psychopharmacologia 32:*279-284, 1973.
54. A. V. P. Mackay, A. F. Healey, and J. Baker, The relationship of plasma chlorpromazine to its 7-hydroxy and sulphoxide metabolites in a large population of chronic schizophrenics. *Brit. J. Clin. Pharmacol. 1:*425-430, 1974.
55. P. Turano, J. March, W. J. Turner, and S. Merlis, Qualitative and quantitative report on chlorpromazine and metabolites in plasma, erythrocytes, and erythrocyte washings from chronically medicated schizophrenic patients. *J. Med. Exp. Clin. 3:*109-120, 1972.
56. J. E. March, D. Donato, P. Turano, and W. J. Turner, Interpatient variation and significance of plasma levels of chlorpromazine in psychotic patients. *J. Med. Exp. Clin. 3:*146-165, 1972.
57. A. A. Manian, D. H. Efron, and S. R. Harris, Appearance of monohydroxy-

lated chlorpromazine metabolites in the central nervous system. *Life Sci. 10:*679-684, 1971.
58. M. L. Clark, H. R. Ramsey, R. E. Raglund, D. K. Rah al, E. A. Serafetinides, and J. P. Costiloe, Chlorpromazine in chronic schizophrenia; behavioural dose-response relationships. *Psychopharmacologia 18:*260-270, 1970.
59. D. J. Kupfer, R. J. Wyatt, F. Snyder, G. P. Mouls, and S. H. Curry, Chlorpromazine plasma levels and sleep in psychiatric patients. *Commun. Behav. Biol. 6:*237-240, 1971.
60. S. H. Curry, Pharmacokinetics and psychotropic drugs. *Psychol. Med. 8:* 177-180, 1978.
61. N. R. Schooler, G. Sakalis, T. L. Chan, S. Gershon, S. C. Goldberg, and P. Collins, Chlorpromazine metabolism and clinical response in acute schizophrenia: A preliminary report. In *Pharmacokinetics of Psychoactive Drugs* (L. A. Gottschalk and S. Merlis, eds.). New York, Spectrum, 1976, pp. 199-220.
62. G. Sakalis, T. L. Chan, G. Sathananthan, N. Schooler, S. Goldberg, and S. Gershon, Relationships among clinical response, extrapyramidal syndrome, and plasma chlorpromazine and metabolite ratios. *Commun. Psychopharmacol. 1:*157-166, 1977.
63. O. T. Phillipson, J. M. McKeown, J. Baker, and A. F. Healey, Correlation between plasma chlorpromazine and its metabolites and clinical ratings in patients with acute relapse of schizophrenic and paranoid psychosis. *Brit. J. Psychiatry 131:*172-184, 1977.
64. D. J. Boullin, D. G. Grahame-Smith, R. P. J. Grimes, and H. F. Woods, Inhibition of human blood platelet aggregation by chlorpromazine and its metabolites. *Brit. J. Pharmacol. 53:*121-126, 1975.
65. D. J. Boullin, H. F. Woods, R. P. J. Grimes, D. G. Grahame-Smith, D. Wiles, M. G. Gelder, and T. Kolakowska, Increased platelet aggregation responses to 5-hydroxytryptamine in patients taking chlorpromazine. *Brit. J. Clin. Pharmacol. 2:*29-35, 1975.
66. T. Kolakowska, D. H. Wiles, A. S. McNeilly, and M. G. Gelder, Correlation between plasma levels of prolactin and chlorpromazine in psychiatric patients. *Psychol. Med. 5:*214-215, 1975.
67. D. H. Wiles, T. Kolakowska, A. S. McNeilly, B. M. Mandelbrote, and M. G. Gelder, Clinical significance of plasma chlorpromazine levels, I: Plasma levels of the drug, some of its metabolites, and prolactin during acute treatment. *Psychol. Med. 6:*407-415, 1976.
68. T. Kolakowska, D. H. Wiles, M. G. Gelder, and A. S. McNeilly, Clinical significance of plasma chlorpromazine levels, II: Plasma levels of the drug, some of its metabolites, and prolactin in patients receiving long-term phenothiazine treatment. *Psychopharmacology 49:*101-107, 1976.
69. P. N. Kaul and M. L. Clark, A novel approach to quantitative determination of subnanomoles of psychoactive drugs in blood. In *Pharmacokinetics of Psychoactive Drugs* (L. A. Gottschalk and S. Merlis, eds.). New York, Spectrum, 1976, pp. 3-14.
70. P. N. Kaul, L. R. Whitfield, and M. L. Clark, Chlorpromazine metabolism,

VIII: Blood levels of chlorpromazine and its sulphoxide in schizophrenic patients. *J. Pharm. Sci. 65:*694–697, 1976.
71. M. L. Clark and P. N. Kaul, A preliminary report on clinical response and blood levels of chlorpromazine and its sulphoxide during chlorpromazine therapy in chronic schizophrenic patients. In *Pharmacokinetics of Psychoactive Drugs* (L. A. Gottschalk and S. Merlis, eds.). New York, Spectrum, 1976, pp. 191-197.
72. M. L. Clark, P. N. Kaul, L. R. Whitfield, A. Paredes, J. P. Costiloe, and F. Wood, Chlorpromazine kinetics and clinical response. *Psychopharmacol. Bull. 14:*43-45, 1978.
73. Y. Sakurai, T. Nakahara, and R. Takahashi, Prediction of response to chlorpromazine treatment in schizophrenics. *Psychopharmacologia 44:*195-203, 1975.
74. V. F. Smolen, H. R. Murdock, W. P. Stoltman, J. W. Clevenger, L. W. Combs, and E. J. Williams, Pharmacological response data for comparative bioavailability studies of chlorpromazine oral dosage forms in humans, I: Pupilometry. *J. Clin. Pharmacol. 15:*734–751, 1975.
75. V. F. Smolen, E. J. Williams, and P. B. Keuhn, Bioavailability and pharmacokinetic analysis of chlorpromazine in humans and animals using pharmacological data. *Canad. J. Pharm. Sci. 10:*95-106, 1975.
76. V. F. Smolen, H. R. Murdock, and E. J. Williams, Bioavailability analysis of chlorpromazine in humans from pupilometric data. *J. Pharmacol. Exp. Ther. 195:*404–415, 1975.
77. V. F. Smolen, H. R. Murdock, W. P. Stoltman, J. W. Clevenger, L. W. Combs, and E. J. Williams, Pharmacological response data for comparative bioavailability studies of chlorpromazine dosage forms in humans, III: Heart rate and body temperature. 1978.
78. E. J. Williams, J. W. Clevenger, W. P. Stoltman, H. R. Murdock, and V. F. Smolen, Pharmacological response data for comparative bioavailability studies of chlorpromazine dosage forms in humans II: Tonometry, 1978.
79. W. J. Turner, P. A. Turano, J. E. March, and J. Kochnower, Excretion patterns of chlorpromazine metabolites by acutely medicated healthy control and by chronically medicated schizophrenic men. 1978.
80. J. Levine, M. L. Clark, and A. A. Manian, Chlorpromazine metabolism: Clinical-Chemical correlations in humans. In *The Present Status of Psychotropic Drugs* (A. Cerletti and F. J. Bové, eds.). Amsterdam, Excerpta Medica, 1969, p. 106.
81. N. C. Moran and W. M. Butler, The pharmacological properties of chlorpromazine sulfoxide, a major metabolite of chlorpromazine: A comparison with chlorpromazine. *J. Pharmacol. Exp. Ther. 118*:328-337, 1956.
82. J. D. Davidson, L. L. Terry, and A. Sjoerdsma, Action and metabolism of chlorpromazine sulfoxide in man. *J. Pharmacol. Exp. Ther. 121:*8-12, 1957.
83. A. R. Freeman and M. A. Spirtes, Effect of some phenothiazine derivatives

on the hemolysis of red blood cells in vitro. *Biochem. Pharmacol. 11:*161-163, 1962.
84. H. S. Posner, E. Hearst, W. L. Taylor, and G. J. Cosmides, Model metabolites of chlorpromazine and promazine: Relative activities in some pharmacological and behavioural tests. *J. Pharmacol. Exp. Ther. 137:*84-90, 1962.
85. G. G. Brune, H. H. Kohl, W. G. Steiner, and H. E. Himwich, Relevance of the N,N-dimethyl configuration to the pharmacological action of chlorpromazine. *Biochem. Pharmacol. 12:*679-685, 1963.
86. W. G. Steiner and H. E. Himwich, An electroencephalographic study of the blocking action of selected tranquillizers as a function of terminal methyl amine group. *Biochem. Pharmacol. 12:*687-691, 1963.
87. H. S. Posner and E. Hearst, Pharmacological activity of 1-, 2-, and 3-hydroxypromazine and 7-methoxychlorpromazine. *Int. J. Neuropharmacol. 3:*635-641, 1964.
88. H. H. Kohl, G. G. Brune, and H. E. Himwich, A comparative study of chlorpromazine and its demethylated derivatives: Potency and tissue distribution. *Biochem. Pharmacol. 13:*539-541, 1964.
89. T. L. Perry, C. F. A. Culling, K. Berry, and S. Hansen, 7-Hydroxychlorpromazine: Potential toxic drug metabolite in psychiatric patients. *Science 146:*81-83, 1964.
90. A. A. Manian, D. H. Efron, and M. E. Goldberg, A comparative pharmacological study of a series of monohydroxylated and methoxylated chlorpromazine derivatives. *Life Sci. 4:*2425-2438, 1965.
91. T. Mao and J. J. Noval, Some relationships concerning the chemical structure, hemolytic activity, and therapeutic potency of phenothiazines. *Biochem. Pharmacol. 15:*501-504, 1966.
92. N. Waltzman, A. A. Manian, H. Barry, and J. P. Buckley, Comparative effects of chlorpromazine hydrochloride and quaternary chlorpromazine hydrochloride on the central nervous systems of rats and mice. *J. Pharm Sci. 57:*2089-2093, 1968.
93. J. Nyback and G. Sedvall, Effect of chlorpromazine and some of its metabolites on synthesis and turnover of catecholamines formed from ^{14}C-tyrosine in mouse brain. *Psychopharmacologia 26:*155-160, 1972.
94. P. N. Kaul, P. R. Pabrai, and M. F Farmer, Chlorpromazine metabolism, VI: Adrenolytic and antiseratogenic activities of chlorpromazine and its various metabolites. *Arch. Int. Pharmacodyn. Ther. 206:*325-327, 1973.
95. J. P. Buckley, M. L. Steenberg, H. Barry, and A. A. Manian, Pharmacology of mono- and disubstituted chlorpromazine metabolites. *J. Pharm. Sci. 62:*715-722, 1973.
96. R. J. Miller and L. L. Iversen, Effect of chlorpromazine and some ot its metabolites on the dopamine-sensitive adenylate cyclase of rat brain striatum. *J. Pharm. Pharmacol. 26:*142-144, 1974.
97. P. Dally, *Chemotherapy of Psychiatric Disorders.* London, Logos Press, 1967.
98. S. H. Curry and L. Adamson, Double-blind trial of fluphenazine decanoate. *Lancer 2:*543-544, 1972.

99. L. Adamson, S. H. Curry, P. K. Bridges, A. F. Firestone, N. I. Lavin, D. M. Lewis, R. D. Watson, C. M. Xavier, and J. A. Anderson, Fluphenazine decanoate trial in chronic in-patient schizophrenics failing to absorb chlorpromazine. *Dis. Nerv. Syst. 34:*181-191, 1973.
100. S. H. Curry, D. M. Lewis, G. Samuel, and G. P. Mould, Fluphenazine decanoate in patients absorbing oral chlorpromazine ineffectively. In *The Future of Pharmacotherapy: New Drug Delivery Systems* (F. J. Ayd, ed.). Baltimore, International Drug Therapy Newsletter, 1973, pp. 53-60.
101. NIMH-PSC Collaborative Study Group, Phenothiazine treatment in acute schizophrenia: Effectiveness. *Arch. Gen. Psychiatry 10:*246-261, 1964.
102. S. Loga, S. H. Curry, and M. H. Lader, Interactions of orphenadrine and phenobarbitone with chlorpromazine: Plasma concentrations and effects in man. *Brit. J. Clin. Pharmacol. 2:*197-208, 1975.
103. A. G. Bolt, I. S. Forrest, and M. T. Serra, Quantitative studies of urinary excretion of chlorpromazine metabolites in chronically-dosed psychiatric patients. *J. Pharm. Sci. 55:*1205-1208, 1966.
104. S. H. Curry, Clinical significance of measuring plasma levels of psychotropic drugs: Phenothiazines. In *Neuro-Psychopharmacology* (P. Deriker, C. Radoues-Thomas, and A. Villeneuve, eds.). Oxford, Pergamon, 1978, pp. 865-869.
105. I. Creese and S. Snyder, A simple and sensitive radioreceptor assay for antischizophrenic drugs in blood. *Nature* (Lond.) *270:*180-182, 1977.
106. B. Meyers, L. E. Tune, and J. T. Coyle, Clinical response and serum neuroleptic levels in childhood schizophrenia. *Amer. J. Psychiat. 137:* 483-484, 1980.
107. L. E. Tune, I. Creese, J. R. Depaulo, P. R. Slavney, J. T. Coyle, and S. H. Snyder, Clinical state and serum neuroleptic levels measured by radioreceptor assay in schizophrenia. *Am. J. Psychiat. 137:*187-190, 1980.
108. S. H. Curry, Methodological pitfalls: the influence of experimental design on results. In *Drug Concentrations in Neuropsychiatry* (Ciba Foundation). Amsterdam: Elsevier/North-Holland and Excerpta Medica, 1980, pp. 35-49.
109. E. Usdin (ed.), *Clinical Pharmacology in Psychiatry.* Amsterdam, Elsevier, 1980 (in press).
110. A. Rosen and S. Y. Tham, The binding of chlorpromazine to some fractions of homogenized rat brain. *J. Pharm. Pharmacol. 32:*357-359 (1980).
111. R. Casper, D. L. Garver, H. Dekermenjian, S. Chang, and J. M. Davis, Phenothiazine levels in plasma and red blood cells—their relationship to clinical improvement in schizophrenia. *Arch. Gen. Psychiat. 37:*301-305, 1980.

9

Antipsychotic Agents *Fluphenazine*

George Sakalis and Louis Traficante* / *Department of Psychiatry, New York University Medical Center, New York, New York, United States*

I. INTRODUCTION

The failure of neuroleptic and antidepressant treatment to bring about rapid and complete relief of the features of schizophrenia and depressive illness with minimal unwanted drug effects has stimulated a growing interest in plasma concentration assays of these drugs over the past 10 years. The work was initiated mainly by Curry and coworkers [1,2] on chlorpromazine, and was encouraged by B. B. Brodie, who went further to suggest that even if the results of examining the plasma concentrations of the parent compounds were to prove inconclusive, i.e., if no clinical-chemical relationship were to be discovered, the researcher should go on to look at active metabolites. The assumption made is that a mathematical derivation of drug concentration at the target receptors involved in the "process" can be arrived at; and here one must keep in mind that not only does the concentration of these drugs vary in different parts of the brain, but also that no one area has been singled out as being the site of the lesion for either one of the two diseases.

Over the same period of time other researchers have elected to study the effect of these drugs on the computer-analyzed electroencephalogram [3,4] as

*Present affiliation: Department of Biobehavioral Sciences, Boston University Medical Center, Boston, Massachusetts, United States.

being a more direct measure. More recently, Raynaud [5] has investigated the uptake of isotopes of chlorpromazine and imipramine in humans by brain scan. Plasma levels of fluphenazine, which is the most widely used drug as a long-acting neuroleptic (intramuscularly in its decanoate or enanthate form) are of special interest. Often the psychiatric resident will call and ask for the corresponding dose of long-acting fluphenazine to that of the neuroleptic with which he or she has been treating the patient. The question is of course invalid, since metabolism in the gut and during first pass through the liver vary, not only from patient to patient (due to genetic factors, motility of gut, enzyme induction, etc.) but also in the same patient from time to time, though not as widely. It is therefore important to have a method which will make possible the assay of plasma fluphenazine over 1 to 2 weeks following a 25-mg intramuscular (i.m.) dose.

At this point the authors must stress their view that the assay of inactive metabolites of neuroleptic drugs is just as important, so that patients with high concentrations of such metabolites—for example, the sulfoxide of chlorpromazine—may be switched to an intramuscular preparation at an earlier point in treatment, thus bypassing the metabolism in the gut and by first pass through the liver. Alternatively, a substance that would diminish monooxygenase activity could be administered concurrently. The authors have had some success in thioridazine-chloroquine treatment in patients not responding to thioridazine alone [6]. We shall now examine certain methodological difficulties, which have led to reports from different laboratories of widely ranging values of fluphenazine blood concentration.

II. METHOD OF FLUPHENAZINE PLASMA LEVEL DETERMINATION

There are many difficulties associated with the determination of fluphenazine levels; indeed, attempts to assess plasma levels of this drug and its metabolites (Fig. 1) differ widely in methodology as well as in reported concentrations. Consequently, correlations of plasma levels to clinical response or the establishment of the concept of a "therapeutic window" have not yet been achieved.

In the past five years a number of analytical methods have been reported for determinations of fluphenazine in biological material; however, because of technical impracticalities, lack of reliability, and/or requisite nanogram sensitivity to measure the low concentrations of fluphenazine and metabolites in the plasma of patients undergoing treatment, these methods are not easily applicable in routine clinical determinations. Forrest et al. [7] devised a semiquantitative colorimetric spot test for total fluphenazine in urine. This test was based on the reaction of the phenothiazine with an acidic solution of ferric chloride. The method does not distinguish between parent compound and metabolites and

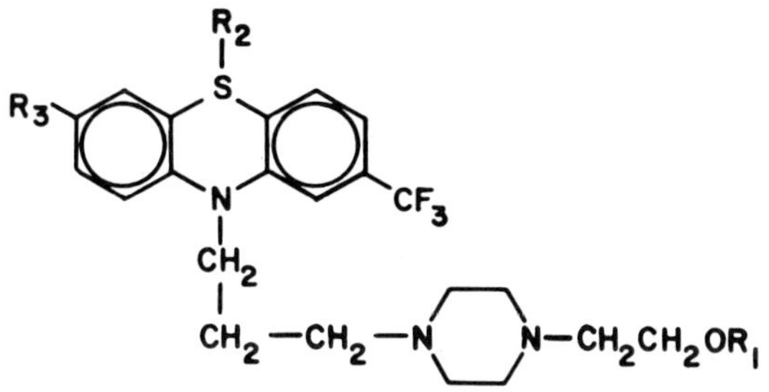

Compound	Pharmacological Activity	R_1	R_2	R_3
Fluphenazine	active	H	-	H
Fluphenazine enanthate	*	$-CO-(CH_2)_5-CH_3$	-	H
Fluphenazine decanoate	*	$-CO-(CH_2)_8-CH_3$	-	H
Fluphenazine sulfoxide	inactive	H	0	H
7-Hydroxyfluphenazine	active	H	-	OH
7-Hydroxyfluphenazine sulfoxide	---	H	0	OH

* Converted in blood to Fluphenazine.

Figure 1 Structure of fluphenazine and its major metabolites.

may yield inadequate color reaction when the daily drug dose is 20 mg or less. They did find, however, that peak levels of the total drug in urine occurred between 1½ to 3 hours after drug intake. This method provides a simple assay for total urinary phenothiazines, but is not applicable for plasma level determinations.

Schreiber and Grozier [8] reported on metabolic studies of various forms of fluphenazine (the short-acting hydrochloride tablets and injection and the long-acting fluphenazine enanthate and decanoate) in volunteer schizophrenic patients in remission. A single dose of one of the above forms containing up to 50 μCi of ^{14}C ring-labeled drug was administered, and these patients were then followed for a period of up to 30 days, with frequent sampling of blood, urine, and feces. While only measurement of total radioactivity (i.e., parent drug plus metabolites) was reported, a number of key observations were made. Their findings suggest that (1) fluphenazine and/or fluphenazine metabolites persist in detectable amount in blood for at least 3 days and are excreted for at least 7 days; (2) patients receiving an i.m. injection of the long-acting forms had detectable levels of radioactivity in plasma for up to 30 days. Although such studies using radioactive phenothiazines are very sensitive, they are not applicable for routine monitoring.

Kelsey et al. [9] described the gas-liquid chromatography (GLC) analysis of urinary fluphenazine and fluphenazine sulfoxide as their trimethylsilyl ethers from patients receiving a daily oral dose of fluphenazine hydrochloride (20 mg). The preliminary procedures involved to prepare a sample for GLC analysis include (1) filtration of urine and a volume adjustment with water; (2) ion-exchange chromatography on Amberlite XAD-2 resin; (3) treatment with ammonium hydroxide to remove urinary pigments; (4) evaporation under reduced pressure for concentration; and (5) silylation prior to chromatography. They found fluphenazine sulfoxide to be the major metabolite in urine, but did not apply their method for plasma level determinations. Although the separation of the parent compound from its sulfoxide was achieved, 7-hydroxyfluphenazine was not detected. This method is cumbersome when handling many samples and may not be applicable for determinations in plasma. Another GLC method was reported by Larsen and Naestoft [10] but was not applied to routine clinical determinations.

A number of other investigators, including Smulevitch et al. [11], used fluorescence measurements to determine parent drug and sulfoxide levels after selective extraction procedures. One-ml samples of plasma were subjected to alkaline hydrolysis at 100°C for 10 min and then fluphenazine was extracted by 2 ml of n-heptane containing 1.7% isoamyl alcohol. The fluphenazine sulfoxide and hydroxylated analogues were back-extracted into 0.1-M phosphate buffer solution (pH 5.0). Both preparations were oxidized with a mixture of acetic acid and H_2O_2 and fluorescence intensity was measured with a spectrofluorimeter at 405 mμ (excitation 350 mμ). Sensitivity was reported to be as low as 0.0002 μg of fluphenazine in the sample. In their study, fluphenazine decanoate (12.5 to 250 mg) was given intramuscularly to schizophrenic patients and periodic measurements were made in the blood. They suggest that a therapeutic effect is observed when the drug content in the blood remains at the level 0.8-1.5 μg/ml 6 to 7 days after injection of the decanoate. We have not been able to reproduce this method, since control plasma samples (after extraction and oxidation with H_2O_2) exhibited excessively high background fluorescence activity and no distinction could be made between control samples and those containing the phenothiazines.

Whelpton et al. [12] have recently reported a procedure to measure urinary excretion products in which they employ GLC after selective extraction of the parent drug and some metabolites. Since the method is not applicable for determinations in plasma, they suggest that the study of the urinary excretion pattern may prove useful to investigate the pharmacokinetics of fluphenazine until a satisfactory assay for fluphenazine in plasma is developed. We have applied the extraction method of these investigators on plasma from patients who received fluphenazine decanoate but were unable to detect or measure fluphenazine or any other metabolites. Essentially, after evaporation of solvents, we performed thin-layer chromatography on these samples. The thin-layer plate (silica gel G) was sprayed with a 0.4% solution of H_2O_2, heated at 100°C for 5 min, cooled, and scanned with a Schoeffel densitometer set for fluorescence measurement $_{ex}$300 mμ $_{fl}$420 mμ.

To study fluphenazine and metabolite concentrations in animal tissues, Gaertner et al. [13] employed thin-layer chromatography and quantitation by ultraviolet (UV) spectroscopy. After extraction of the drug from tissues with 1,2-dichloroethane, the extracts were applied to plates and developed with chloroform/isopropanol (10:1 v/v) and with isopropanol/chloroform/ammonia/water (32:16:2:1 v/v). Then, after detection with UV, the substances were isolated from the gel by distribution between NH_4OH and chloroform. The purified substances were finally dissolved in 0.1-N HCl or H_2SO_4 and molar absorbance determined. The experiments were designed to investigate kinetics during chronic treatment, and it is interesting to note that repeated oral treatment of male rats with fluphenazine, 25 mg/kg or more daily, led to an accumulation of metabolites containing an ethylenediamine group (with and without removal of the N-alkyl group) instead of the piperazine ring. These ring degradation products were found together with the parent drug and their N-dealkylated metabolites in liver, lung, kidney and spleen, as well as in brain when high doses were administered. Furthermore, after termination of treatment, the ethylenediamine derivatives were eliminated at a much slower rate than the intact piperazine ring congeners. Parallel observations were reported in dogs given fluphenazine in daily doses up to 40 mg/kg. To our knowledge, this analytical method has not been applied to human blood and no one has reported the presence of these ethylenediamine derivatives in humans.

Chien et al. [14] found a high ratio of fluphenazine to fluphenazine sulfoxide in schizophrenic patients with good clinical response to long-acting injectable preparations. They utilized thin-layer chromatography to measure plasma levels of depot fluphenazines and reported levels of parent drug up to 800 ng/ml and ring sulfoxide up to 400 ng/ml, which are in contrast to the very low levels found by other groups using radioisotope or GLC methods. Whereas the reported values of fluphenazine and its sulfoxide seem high, one would expect the ratios of parent compound to sulfoxide to be meaningful. Hopefully, the significance of these ratios to clinical response might be assessed in future studies.

A GLC method employing an OV-17 column and a ^{63}Ni electron capture detection was recently reported by Rivera-Calimlim and Siracusa [15] for the determination of fluphenazine in plasma. The plasma fluphenazine is first purified by solvent extraction and subsequent derivatization. This is accomplished by partitioning the crude product into isopropanol-heptane from alkalinized plasma. Then the heptane layer, after washing with phosphate buffer, is back-extracted into HCl. The acid layer is then made alkaline and extracted into toluene. This layer is then treated with NO-bis(trimethylsilyl)trifluoroacetamide for derivatization and analysis by GLC. They report the sensitivity of the assay to be 3 ng/ml plasma. Their preliminary results from six patients indicate that 7 to 14 days after a dose (presumably 50 mg of the dec. i.m.), plasma levels of fluphenazine range between 9 and 12 ng/ml. They do not, however, report detection of fluphenazine sulfoxide or other metabolites, which may indicate that their extraction procedure is more specific for parent drug. Factors affecting fluphenazine assays by GLC are: (1) long standing of blood samples in vacutainers before separation of plasma; (2) light sensitivity; (3) storage of samples for more than 2 months; (4) GLC temperatures above 200°C; and (5) standing of plasma extracts before injection into the column. Thus far they have not reported any correlations of fluphenazine concentrations to clinical response.

A sophisticated analytical method employing a special detector in combination with reversed-phase high-pressure liquid-chromatography was used by Tjaden et al. [16] to determine blood levels of fluphenazine in humans. The stationary phase was methyl silica, and buffered mixtures of methanol and water were used as the mobile phase. Extraction of phenothiazine was complex but basically involved an N-hexane extraction from an alkaline solution (recovery of each standard compound was reported to be 50% ± 5). Very low levels of the drug in blood (0-1.5 ng/ml) were detected with this method. The observed serum levels after i.m. doses of the decanoate were reported to be as little as 0.7 ng/ml of fluphenazine (detected 23 days after a 19-mg dose) and as high as 6.1 ng/ml (6 days after a 125-mg dose). No correlations were made with clinical response. These data support Schreiber and Grozier's original observation that after an intramuscular injection of fluphenazine decanoate, fluphenazine (and/or metabolites) can be detected for up to 30 days later. Further work on the selectivity of the measurement via anodic electrochemical oxidation, as applied to biological samples, is necessary.

Among other analytical techniques, competitive protein binding assays, and especially those that utilize specific antibodies, are being used currently to quantitate many different types of compounds [17]. Radioimmunoassay (RIA) depends upon the affinity of an antibody for an antigen (e.g., a drug or its metabolite). The sensitivity of these assays is made possible through the use of radioactive tracer molecules of high specific activity. The extraordinary specificity of antibodies permits them to bind their respective ligands even in the presence of myriad other compounds. The extent to which unlabeled ligand competes with radioactive ligand for a limited number of binding sites on the antibody molecules serves as a basis for quantitation. Often picogram amounts of a specific compound can be estimated, and the assays are relatively simple to perform once the proper antibodies and labeled ligand (drug or metabolites) are available [18]. Radioimmunoassays have been reported for several phenothiazine drugs [19,20]. At Brandeis University, a RIA for fluphenazine, which can be also used to assay chlorpromazine, has been developed recently (Van Vunakis, unpublished). It can detect picogram quantities of fluphenazine and some related metabolites in physiological fluids. Since the immunizing conjugate was prepared by linking the hemisuccinate of fluphenazine to protein by carbodiimide, the antibody can discriminate certain substitutions on the aromatic ring system. Thus, fluphenazine sulfoxide competes for the antibody only 1/150 as effectively as fluphenazine and would not be detected by the antibody unless it occurred in very large amounts. Compounds containing modification on the piperazine ring react significantly with the antibody; e.g., CF_3 phenothiazine propyl-N-methyl (ethylenediamine) is only slightly less effective than fluphenazine in inhibiting [^{3}H] antigen-antibody reaction. Because in addition to fluphenazine some metabolites with alterations in the aromatic ring may also contribute to the values obtained when using this RIA to determine blood levels of serologically reactive material in patients receiving fluphenazine, the results are expressed as *fluphenazine equivalents.*

III. CLINICAL STUDIES

In view of the wide discrepancies in reports from different laboratories cited above, it would be futile at the present time to attempt to draw any conclusions on the pharmacokinetics of fluphenazine or even to examine the relationship between plasma levels and clinical response. However, some general remarks on the available data would be appropriate, even if only to point out that they should be examined with caution.

In a preliminary communication, Curry [21] demonstrated by administering 25 mg radioactive fluphenazine to five patients in different forms (see Table 1) that urinary concentrations of fluphenazine equivalents reflect plasma concentrations. Table 1 summarizes the peak plasma concentrations and times at which they were observed as well as half-lives. The approach of urinary assays is advanced by the author for the study of fluphenazine kinetics, until a sensitive assay method for plasma fluphenazine becomes available.

It is significant that Itil et al. [22] also found the decanoate to have a longer-lasting effect than the enanthate on the computer-analyzed electroencephalogram. Thus, Curry estimates the interdose fluctuation in the plasma of a patient receiving weekly 50-mg injections of the decanoate to be 10-25 ng/ml with a half-life of 4-5 days. Interestingly, this figure is comparable to that given

Table 1 Fluphenazine Plasma Levels, Different Routes of Administration (Dose 25 mg)

Preparation	Peak in Plasma: Time	Peak in Plasma: Concentration (ng/ml)	$T_{1/2}$
Hydrochloride–i.m.[a]	1.5 h	26	15 h
Hydrochloride–oral	1 h	2	15 h
Enanthate	24 h	2	3.5 days
Decanoate	1 h	3.5	
	24 h	0.7	10 days
	Plateau (1-5 days)	0.6	

[a]Two patients with almost identical figures.
Source: Ref. 21.

by Rivera-Calimlim [15] who employed gas-liquid chromatography and found a plasma level of 19 ng/ml 4 days after injection in a patient receiving 50 mg of the decanoate every 2 weeks. However, Muusze (personal communication), reviewing available data from 20 patients, reports plasma levels of the order of 2 ng/ml following similar doses over the same period of time. This author has additionally observed interpatient variability in concentrations up to threefold. Although Rivera-Calimlim has listed a number of factors that may give rise to low concentrations, one must also take into account the fact that Muusze's method is more sophisticated [16]. Criticism must therefore be reserved at least until these studies are completed.

We presented a preliminary communication [23] on peak plasma levels after morning dose, in patients receiving orally either the standard or high dose of fluphenazine (i.e., 30 mg/day or 750 mg/day) at steady state. Assays were carried out by Van Vunakis' method of radioimmunoassay, and values reflect fluphenazine equivalents, i.e., parent plus metabolites, though the inactive sulfoxide competes for the antibody only 1/150 effectively as the parent and therefore its contribution to the figures is negligible.

This study was undertaken because of previous reports of uncontrolled studies made mainly by French workers in the 1960s [24] who claimed that a high oral dose (exceeding 1 g) is more effective in controlling psychotic symptomatology without increasing the incidence of unwanted effects with the exception of drowsiness. Briefly, the population of the ongoing study is drawn from newly admitted physically healthy patients, aged 20 to 45 years, with a diagnosis of acute schizophrenia established on independent clinical interviews by two psychiatrists on the basis of the criteria laid down in DSM II [25] and presenting, at least, one of Schneider's first-rank symptoms. Following 1 week's placebo washout the patients are randomly assigned to either high- or low-dose fluphenazine hydrochloride or chlorpromazine (CPZ) treatment in a double-blind procedure for a total period of 4 weeks. Since high fluphenazine dosage was expected to induce drowsiness in some patients the inclusion of a group of patients receiving CPZ, which would also encounter such effect, was decided upon to keep the study blind.

All drugs are given orally in liquid form to enhance absorption and according to a t.i.d. schedule. High-dose fluphenazine treatment is started with 75 mg on the first day, gradually increased to 750 mg daily by the end ot the second week, and kept fixed thereafter. Similarly, low-dose fluphenazine is increased from 3 to 30 mg daily and CPZ from 150 to 1,500 mg daily by the end of the second week and kept fixed thereafter. Psychiatric and nursing evaluations as well as routine laboratory tests are conducted at baseline and thereafter weekly. Physical and ophthalmological examinations and electrocardiogram (ECG) recordings are carred out at baseline and termination times.

Blood samples are drawn, if possible, both before and between 2 and 6 h after administration of the morning dose (peak) for plasma level determinations by RIA. Peak fluphenazine concentrations had occurred during such a period in samples from six male physically healthy inpatients who participated in a separate study on single-dose kinetics.

In 14 out of 24 patients that have completed the trial to date, plasma level determinations from samples obtained at either study termination or the end of the third treatment week are available. Of these 14 patients, 4 had been assigned to high-dose fluphenazine treatment, 3 to low-dose fluphenazine, and 7 to CPZ treatment. No abnormalities were noted in the laboratory tests or ECG recordings from these patients. RIA results of plasma level determinations as well as the scores obtained on the Clinical Global Impressions Scale at baseline and termination and occurrence of extrapyramidal side effects in each of the above patients are presented in Table 2. While no valid comparison of therapeutic efficacy and incidence of side effects can be made between treatment groups in this selected sample of patients, it is of interest to point out that a direct relationship between dose and plasma levels, but not between plasma levels and clinical response, is clearly apparent with regard to fluphenazine. Similarly, no relationship between increased plasma level and extrapyramidal side effects can be established since such symptoms developed both in the one patient with the lowest plasma concentration among those receiving high dosage and in one of the patients in the low-dose group. However, if no significant difference in efficacy between the two dosages is established, one must consider the possibility that schizophrenic

Table 2 Fluphenazine Plasma Levels, High versus Low Dose

Patient	Peak plasma total fluphenazine equivalents (μg/ml)		Clinical Global Impression Scale Scores		Extrapyramidal side effects
	Day 21	Termination	Baseline	Termination	
High Dose[a]					
1	6.3	–	5	5	–
2	15.2	–	4	4	–
3	4.9	–	4	1	Pseudo-Parkinsonism
4	–	5.6	4	2	–
Low Dose[b]					
1	0.086[c]	–	5	3	Pseudo-Parkinsonism
2	0.088	–	4	3	–
3	0.025	–	4	1	–

[a]Clinical assessment and plasma levels of fluphenazine by radioimmunoassay determination in acute schizophrenic patients receiving high dose (250 mg, t.i.d.) oral fluphenazine hydrochloride treatment. Blood samples were drawn between 2 and 6 h after morning dose administration.
[b]Clinical assessment and plasma levels of fluphenazine by radioimmunoassay determination in acute schizophrenic patients receiving low dose (10 mg, t.i.d.) oral fluphenazine hydrochloride treatment. Blood samples were drawn between 2 and 6 h after morning dose administration.
[c]Day 20.

subgroups respond differently as was demonstrated by Itil et al. [26]. In that study chronic, drug-resistant patients who showed increased slow-wave activity in the ECG did better on a high-dosage regimen. Though we do not include chronic patients in the ongoing study, a large proportion of our new admissions fall into the "subchronic" type as defined in the *Research Diagnostic Criteria* [27] and might correspond more closely to Itil's chronic subsample than to the acute and subacute types also represented in our population

A significant development is the availability at present of Snyder's [28] radio receptor method for the assays of total active neuroleptic equivalents. Patients entering the study will now have their blood fluphenazine concentration assayed by both radioimmunoassay and by radioreceptor assay. The latter, in which essentially fluphenazine in the patient's blood competes with [^{3}H] spiroperidol for striatal dopaminergic receptors in vitro, will enable us to determine both the total plasma concentration and the free fraction after dialysis, as well as red cell concentration.

Finally, mention should be made of the association of high concentrations of the inactive sulfoxidized metabolite with failure to respond. The values given by Chien and Chan [14] are, as discussed above, very high. Nevertheless, this does not necessarily invalidate the ratios of parent drug to sulfoxide. These authors reported that patients with higher plasma concentrations of parent drug showed a good clinical response, whereas patients with higher plasma concentrations of sulfoxide did not. These findings are in agreement with a similar trend observed in treatment with chlorpromazine [29-32] and thioridazine [33].

Traficante et al. [6] attempted to potentiate the antipsychotic effect of thioridazine by the concurrent administration of chloroquine with some success. This was attributed to partial inhibition of ring sulfoxidation by chloroquine, whereas the rate of side chain sulfoxidation resulting in the formation of mesoridazine, the active metabolite, was unaffected. It is of interest to note, however, that chloroquine also possesses an immunosuppressant effect, which would tend to support reports by Soviet psychiatrists that cyclophosphamide, by suppressing the immune response, makes it possible for nonresponding patients on phenothiazines to be converted to responders [34]. This combined treatment follows logically from the findings of Amkraut et al. [35] that patients with elevated immunoglobulins were resistant to treatment. What is the relationship of high immunoglobulins to increased sulfoxidation and why should the latter be related with poor response even in the presence of relatively high levels of the parent compound remains unclear at present. Stanley (personal communication) found that the increased concentration of 3,4-dihydroxyphenylacetic acid in rat striatum after acute chlorpromazine treatment was unaffected by concomitant treatment with sulfoxide. It may be that sulfoxide, being less bound to plasma protein [36], tends to decrease the free fraction of the parent drug. This mechanism might explain the high sulfoxide concentration found in the cerebrospinal fluid of a chlorpromazine nonresponder by Axelsson et al. [37]. Whatever the case may be, Van Kempen [38] demonstrated that the concentration of perphenazine sulfoxide in the urine decreased to a greater extent than did that of the parent compound after switching a group of patients from oral to long-acting i.m. preparation, presumably by avoiding first-pass metabolism. More recently Hansen et al. [39], who actually monitored plasma concentrations, also found a decrease in perphenazine sulfoxide after switching patients to the long-acting i.m. preparation. It may be relevant to note at this point that a number of patients out of a group of chlorpromazine nonresponders showed clinical improvement after being switched to i.m. fluphenazine [40], though these authors attributed this change to poor absorption of chlorpromazine from the gut. What then may be the explanation of failure to respond to the i.m. long-acting preparation in some cases? It seems to us that one of two possibilities may be the cause. Either the drug is rapidly sulfoxidized nonspecifically in the blood circulation, or the patient despite high concentration of the parent drug fails to respond because in his particular case the pathological process does not involve the dopaminergic system.

It is obvious from this brief exposition that there is an urgent need for the development of a sensitive method that will make it possible for fluphenazine and its metabolites, particularly the sulfoxide and the 7-hydroxy derivative to be assayed both in total plasma as well as the determination of their free fraction. The latter metabolite is of particular interest since it is probably pharmacologically active. We have reported an association between EPS and high plasma levels of 7-hydroxychlorpromazine [41]. On the other hand, Curry [42] failed to detect the presence of this metabolite in high concentrations. Even so, Snyder (personal communication) estimates the protein binding of 7-hydroxychlorpromazine to be much lower than that of the parent drug. What this may signify one can conjecture from the finding that the plasma concentration of mesoridazine, which is only about 85% bound to protein [36], and not that of the parent drug thioridazine (95% bound) is related to clinical response [33,43]. At this point it seems to us that only by taking all these factors into account can progress in this field be made.

REFERENCES

1. S. H. Curry, Determination of nanogram quantities of chlorpromazine and some of its metabolites using gas liquid chromatography with an electron capture detector. *Anal. Chem. 40:*1251-1255, 1968.
2. S. H. Curry and J. H. Marshall, Plasma levels of chlorpromazine and some of its relatively non-polar metabolites in psychiatric patients. *Life Sci. 7:* 9-17, 1968.

3. M. Fink, T. M. Itil, and D. M. Shapiro, Digital computer analysis of the human EEG in psychiatric research. *Comp. Psychiatry 8:*521-538, 1967.
4. T. M. Itil, in *Biological Mechanisms of Schizophrenia* (H. Mitsuda, ed.). Tokyo, Igaku-Shoin, 1974.
5. C. Raynaud and A. E. Todd-Pokropek, IAEA-SM-185/84; 45, 1974.
6. L. J. Traficante, B. Hine, S. Gershon, and G. Sakalis, Potentiation of thioridazine effects in rats and drug-resistant schizophrenic patients: A preliminary report. *Commun. Psychopharmacol. 1:*407, 1977.
7. F. M. Forrest, I. S. Forrest, and A. S. Mason, Review of rapid urine tests for phenothiazines and related drugs. *Amer. J. Psychiatry 118:*300-307, 1961.
8. E. C. Schreiber and M. L. Grozier, [Metabolic studies with long-acting compounds]. *Therapie 28:*441-458, 1973.
9. M. Kelsey, A. Keskiner, and E. A. Moscatelli, Gas-liquid chromatographic analysis of fluphenazine and fluphenazine sulfoxide in the urine of chronic schizophrenic patients. *J. Chromatogr. 75:*294-297, 1973.
10. N. E. Larsen and J. Naestoft, Determination of perphenazine and fluphenazine in whole blood by gas chromatography. *Med. Lab. Technol. 30:*129-132, 1973.
11. A. B. Smulevitch, E. I. Minsker, and N. A. Mazayewa, The problem of clinical activity of long-acting neuroleptics. *Comp. Psychiatry 14:*227-297, 1973.
12. R. Whelpton and S. H. Curry, Methods for study of fluphenazine kinetics in man. *J. Pharm. Pharmacol. 28:*869-873, 1976.
13. H. J. Gaertner, U. Breyer, and G. Liomin, Metabolism of trifluoperazine, fluphenazine, prochlorperazine, and perphenazine in rats: In vitro and urinary metabolites. *Biochem. Pharmacol. 23:*303-311, 1974.
14. C. P. Chien, T. L. Chan, and D. Damiano, *Abstracts of the Tenth Congress of the CINP, Quebec, 1976.*
15. L. Rivera-Calimlim and A. Siracusa, Plasma assay of fluphenazine. *Commun. Psychopharmacol. 1:*233-242, 1977.
16. U. R. Tjaden, J. Lankelma, H. Poppe, and R. G. Muusze, Anodic coulometric detection with a glassy carbon electrode in combination with reversed-phase high-performance liquid chromatography: Determination of blood levels of perphenazine and fluphenazine. *J. Chromatogr. 125:*275-286, 1976.
17. W. E. O'Dell and W. H. Daughaday, eds., *Principles of Competitive Protein Binding Assays.* Philadelphia, Lippincott, 1971.
18. S. A. Berson and R. Yallow, In *Immunobiology* (R. A. Good and A. W. Fisher, eds.). Stamford, Conn., Sinauer Associates, 1971, pp. 287-293.
19. M. Shostak, In *The Phenothiazines and Structurally Related Drugs* (I. S. Forrest, C. J. Carr, and E. Usdin, eds.). New York, Raven Press, 1974, pp. 365-377.
20. K. Kawashima, R. Dixon, and S. Spector, Development of radioimmunoassay for chlorpromazine. *Eur. J. Pharmacol. 32:*195-202, 1975.

21. S. H. Curry, Fluphenazin und Fluphenazindekanoat-Plasmaspiegel. Paper presented to the Alpenlandisches Psychiatrie-Symposion, Seefeld-Tirol, 1976, pp. 75-83.
22. T. Itil, A. Keskiner, H. Han, W. Hsu, and G. A. Ulett, EEG changes after fluphenazine enanthate and decanoate based on analog power spectra and digital computer period analysis. *Psychopharmacologia 20:*230-241, 1971.
23. G. Sakalis and A. Sudilovsky, In *Depot Fluphenazines* (F. Ayd, ed.). Baltimore, Ayd Medical Communications, in press.
24. 62eme Congres de Psychiatrie et de Neurologie de Langue Française, Marseille, September 1964.
25. DSM II; In *Diagnostic and Statistical Manual of Mental Disorders.* Washington, D.C., American Psychiatric Association, 1968.
26. T. Itil, B. Saletu, W. Hsu, N. Kireritci, and A. Keskiner, Clinical and quantitative EEG changes at different dosage levels of fluphenazine treatment. *Acta Psychiatr. Scand. 47:*440-451, 1971.
27. R. L. Spitzer, J. Endicott, and E. Robins, *Research Diagnostic Criteria.* New York, New York State Psychiatric Institute, 1977.
28. I. Creese and S. H. Snyder, A simple and sensitive radio-receptor assay for antischizophrenic drugs in blood. *Nature 270:*180-182, 1977.
29. G. Sakalis, T. L. Chan, S. Gershon, and S. Park, The possible role of metabolites in therapeutic response to chlorpromazine treatment. *Psychopharmacologia 32:*279-284, 1973.
30. A. V. MacKay, A. F. Healey, and J. Baker, The relationship of plasma chlorpromazine to its 7-hydroxy and sulfoxide metabolites in a large population of chronic schizophrenics. *Brit. J. Clin. Pharmacol. 1:*425-430, 1974.
31. Y. Sakurai, T. Nakahara, and R. Takahashi, Prediction of response to chlorpromazine treatment in schizophrenics. *Psychopharmacologia 44:*195-203, 1975.
32. D. H. Wiles, T. Kolakowska, A. S. McNeilly, B. M. Mandelbrote, and M. G. Gelder, Clinical significance of plasma chlorpromazine levels, I: Plasma levels of the drug, some of its metabolites, and prolactin during acute treatment. *Psychol. Med. 6:*407-415, 1976.
33. G. Sakalis, L. J. Traficante, and S. Gershon, Thioridazine metabolism and clinical response: A pilot study. *Curr. Ther. Res. 21:*720-724, 1977.
34. Z. P. Gurevich, In *Therapeutic Resistance in Schizophrenia and Affective Psychoses* (R. Y. Vovin, ed.). Leningrad, V. M. Bekhterev Psychoneurological Research Institute, 1975, pp. 69-74.
35. A. Amkraut, G. F. Solomon, M. Allansmith, B. McClellan, and M. Rappaport, Immunoglobulins and improvement in acute schizophrenic reactions. *Arch. Gen. Psychiatry 28:*673-677, 1973.
36. F. M. Belpaire, F. A. J. Vanderheeren, and M. G. Bogaert, Binding of thioridazine and some of its metabolites to human serum protein and human albumin. *Arzneim.-Forsch. 25:*1969-1971, 1975.

37. S. Axelsson, S. Jonsson, and L. Nordgren, Cerebrospinal fluid levels of chlorpromazine and its metabolites in schizophrenia. *Arch. Psychiatr. Nervenkr. 221:*167-170, 1975.
38. G. M. J. Van Kempen, Urinary excretion of perphenazine and its sulfoxide during administration of oral and long-acting injectable form. *Psychopharmacologia 21:*283-286, 1971.
39. C. E. Hansen, T. R. Christensen, J. Elley, L. B. Hansen, P. Kragh-Sorensen, N. E. Larsen, J. Naestoft, and E. F. Hvidberg, Clinical pharmacokinetic studies of perphenazine. *Brit. J. Clin. Pharmacol. 3:*915-923, 1976.
40. D. M. Lewis, S. H. Curry, and G. Samuel, Long-acting phenothiazines in schizophrenia. *Brit. Med. J. 1:*671-672, 1971.
41. G. Sakalis, T. L. Chan, G. Sathananthan, N. Schooler, S. Goldberg, and S. Gershon, Relationships among clinical response, extrapyramidal syndrome and plasma chlorpromazine and metabolite ratios. *Commun. Psychopharmacol. 1:*157-166, 1977.
42. S. H. Curry and S. Evans, A note on the assay of chlorpromazine N-oxide and its sulfoxide in plasma and urine. *J. Pharm. Pharmacol. 28:*467-468, 1976.
43. F. A. J. Vanderheeren and R. G. Muusze, Plasma levels and half lives of thioridazine and some of its metabolites, I: High doses in young acute schizophrenics. *Eur. J. Clin. Pharmacol. 11:*135-140, 1977.

10

Antipsychotic Agents
Thioridazine: Pharmacokinetics, Plasma Levels, and Clinical Response

John L. Crammer / *Institute of Psychiatry, University of London, London, England*

I. INTRODUCTION

Thioridazine is a phenothiazine drug with a range of clinical uses and doses very similar to those of chlorpromazine. It is perhaps the more effective of the two in suppressing worry and agitation and therefore in providing symptomatic relief in agitated depression or in Huntington's chorea, and it has been claimed also to be an antidepressant in its own right [1]. It is considerably less likely than chlorpromazine to release the neurological syndrome of parkinsonism, with its stiffness, lack of mobility, and tremor. On the other hand, in the higher-dose range it appears to be more cardiotoxic and sometimes to provoke retinal damage [2]. These clinical differences are paralleled by pharmacological differences in in vitro and in animal tests between the two drugs. Thioridazine has much more anticholinergic potency, and its antidopaminergic activity at different brain sites may differ somewhat from that of chlorpromazine. Closer analysis of these intriguing differences might help to clarify the mechanism of action of phenothiazines in the nervous system, and thereby also throw light on the physical disturbances at work in schizophrenic and manic-depressive psychoses.

A. Metabolism of Thioridazine and Chlorpromazine

Some of these clinical differences may be related to the general metabolism of the two drugs in man. Chlorpromazine is converted largely to 7-hydroxychlorpromazine metabolites (phenols) and their glucuronides [3], and the former may still have some pharmacological activity. The middle-ring sulfur, as in all phenothiazines, can also be oxidized (yielding ring sulfoxides which are for practical purposes inert), but for chlorpromazine sulfoxidation is less important than hydroxylation. In contrast, thioridazine is converted predominantly to ring sulfoxides, and hydroxy metabolites appear to play a very minor part [4,5]. Secondly, the metabolically inert chlorine atom in chlorpromazine at position 2 of the phenothiazine three-ring structure is replaced in thioridazine by a thiomethyl group, $-S.CH_3$, which undergoes rapid metabolic oxidation to mesoridazine (addition of one oxygen atom to make thioridazine side chain sulfoxide), and then more slowly to sulforidazine (addition of a second oxygen atom to form thioridazine side chain sulfone). Both of these metabolites have antipsychotic clinical potency, and both can be inactivated by further oxidation, this time of the phenothiazine ring sulfur, to form ring sulfoxides. These two different metabolic pathways are summarized in Fig. 1.

B. Application of Fluorimetry to Phenothiazine Studies

It was quite early observed that solutions of phenothiazines gave rise to red-, purple-, or blue-colored products when oxidized by concentrated sulfuric acid or

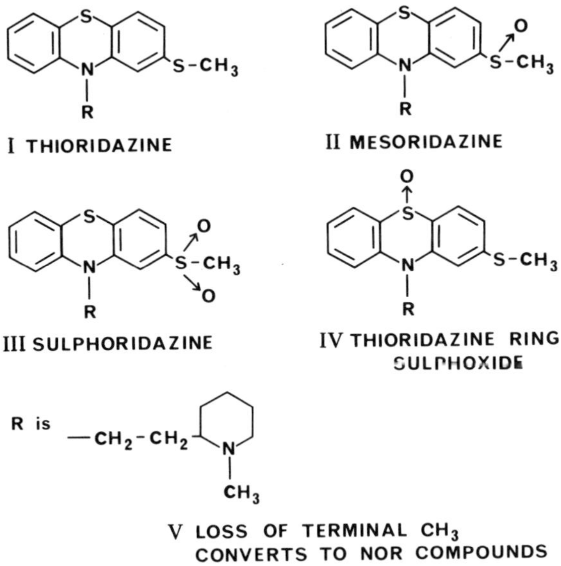

Figure 1 Thioridazine (1) is metabolized partly by oxidation in the thiomethyl group to active metabolites (2 and 3), partly by oxidation of the central-ring sulfur (4). Side chain demethylation also occurs (5), and other processes.

chromic acid or perchloric acid, particularly if a small amount of an iron salt was present. This was applied in the Forrest test [6] to make a simple ward or clinic test for phenothiazines in urine. Surveys of psychiatric patients with this test showed that a significant minority even of inpatients, particularly chronic schizophrenics, were not taking their prescribed phenothiazine. Some treatment failures could be ascribed to this fact, and nursing procedures had to be modified in an attempt to combat noncompliance [7]. This was the opening of a new field of effort for laboratory help to psychiatry, one where more still remains to be done. The physician would ideally like to know not just whether the patient has taken the prescribed drug or not, but whether he has taken the actual dose according to the intended time schedule. Some patients regularly take half whatever the doctor gives them, or are erratic in drug taking, and may not admit this. Some new type of plasma or urine test, perhaps the plasma concentration curve after a single dose, might prove useful in clinical assessment.

A second important step was the use of milder and more controllable oxidation methods to produce fluorescent substances. Thioridazine and many of its derivatives when treated with hydrogen peroxide underwent oxidation at both sulfur atoms of the molecule to form sulfones which give very bright blue solutions under ultraviolet light. The fluorescence could be measured in a fluorimeter, and the sensitivity was such that for the first time plasma levels of phenothiazine could be quantified reliably. The application of this measurement to urine and blood by Mellinger and others [8] resulted first in studies of drug bioavailability. It was possible to compare patients for the speed with which they excreted fluorigenic substances in the urine after standard oral doses of thioridazine, and to compare in the same patient the excretions after different oral and liquid formulations. It was also now possible to begin the study of the rate of rise and fall of these substances in plasma under a variety of conditions, particularly after Pacha [9] had published his particular method, in which the oxidation with hydrogen peroxide was carefully timed, and then stopped by the addition of just enough permanganate as shown by a persisting faint pink in the reaction solution. Of course all fluorimetric methods carry two basic flaws. Fluorescence may on occasion be partly or wholly quenched by some other substance in the biological sample or extract, a phenolic substance for instance; and fluorescence is a rather nonspecific property of many substances so that a sample may give a positive measurement even when thioridazine is certainly absent. However, these possibilities can to an extent be allowed for if one is aware of them.

From compliance and bioavailability interest moved on to two other clinical problems, metabolic differences between individuals and the prediction of success in therapy. As with other drugs, numerous studies confirmed that different people given the same thioridazine dose in milligrams per kilogram body weight per day by mouth developed quite different steady concentrations of phenothiazines in their plasmas. It was hoped that these measurements might prove useful in dose adjustment in therapy—for instance, that only those with high concentrations of phenothiazine in plasma would later recover from their schizophrenic psychosis [10,11] or their depressive illness [12,13]. This hope was not confirmed. Measurements by the Pacha method have not yielded clinically useful correlations of this sort.

Before rather too hastily concluding that therefore measurement of antipsychotic drugs in plasma has no practical utility, one should recognize both the flaws of the Pacha method and the dimensions of the clinical problem. Indeed, one should pause to consider the underlying philosophy, the theoretical assumptions, in the application of laboratory methods to the treatment of patients. We may not be asking the right questions, or at least putting them in the right way.

At least two metabolites of thioridazine, mesoridazine and sulforidazine, are believed to be clinically active, though not identically so, against psychosis [14]. Ring sulfoxide metabolites are thought to be inert. But the Pacha method makes no distinction between metabolites. Anything oxidizable to a sulfone is likely to fluoresce powerfully, and therefore the measurement is of a mixed group of active and inactive substances. It may be insufficiently specific to reveal a correlation which might be there.

But what is to be correlated on the clinical side? The measurement, if it can be called that, is even more imprecise, and usually has been little more than a physician's subjective impression that a patient has lost the bulk of his symptoms, or at least the most impressive ones. Clinical improvement from a psychosis may not be evident until after some weeks of drug treatment, and may of course be due to the spontaneous course of the illness or to supervening events and not the drug. If it is a result of drug action, is a drug plasma concentration an adequate correlate, or should some factor for duration of exposure to the drug be included?

The trouble is that a good many investigations have been of the hit-or-miss variety. One uses what is to hand, and hopes a correlation will turn up: the misses are unfortunately much commoner than the hits, and do not deepen understanding. It is better to clarify clinical and scientific purposes first, and then to choose the technical approaches most suitable to answering a particular general or practical question, and as far as possible to design the investigation so that the results always add something to the body of knowledge for future use.

II. PROBLEMS OF PREDICTION OF OUTCOME OF PHARMACOTHERAPY

The clinician wants laboratory help in coping now; and he wants help also predictively. In the coping situation, he finds his prescription has produced no response or, worse, new symptoms are appearing which might be drug related—side effects, toxic reaction, drug interaction—or might be quite unconnected with treatment. He wants the laboratory to help him act in changing the dose up or down, or altering the patient's drugs and general handling. Lithium carbonate treatment of manic-depressive disorders is a simple instance of this aid at work, since lithium can be measured easily and specifically in body fluids. Suitably timed plasma and urine collections with lithium measurement can tell a good deal about compliance, bioavailability, and the lithium concentrations to which the brain is exposed. If new symptoms of nausea and vomiting supervene during treatment a plasma concentration below 1.0 mmol/liter lithium may be a strong indication to look for another cause for the nausea. If the patient is not improving, a value below 0.7 mmol/liter lithium will suggest an increase in drug dose until the level lies in the range which experience has established as therapeutically most propitious. Thioridazine presents complexities of metabolism and measurement, but it might be possible to offer similar support in its use.

Under prediction, the clinician wants to know how much drug to prescribe for that individual patient, and how often, to produce particular clinical effects in future weeks or months. Three distinct types of factors come into this: (1)

individual metabolism; (2) individual susceptibility; (3) individual cerebral modifiability.

A. Individual Metabolism

It is now well established that different individuals present very different amounts of drug to the brain when treated with identical doses. This arises because of individual differences, in absorption from the gut, in liver metabolism, in renal function. Part of it is a constant, derived from genetic and constitutional factors, part a variable determined by previous nutritional, chemical, and other physical experience which influences the magnitude of blood flow or the activity of liver enzymes, for example. If the amount of drug delivered to the brain per hour or per day is a big enough factor in therapeutic effect, and if the size of this cerebral dose is fairly constant—determined mainly by constitutional factors—then an acute measure of the cerebral dose to be expected from any dosage schedule might have predictive value for the clinician. Taking the steady-state plasma level as a quantitative indicator of cerebral dose, one can predict the later actual steady-state level from a short series of plasma drug measurements following an initial acute dose of the drug in question, for lithium [15] and for nortriptyline [16]. However the clinician at present usually finds it simpler with these drugs to start the patient off on likely doses, and only seek laboratory help when treatment is not succeeding. Clinical response to lithium or nortriptyline in affective disorders tends to be quicker than it is to neuroleptics in schizophrenia.

One gets into difficulties with this approach where what is to be measured in the plasma is not one substance but several pharmacologically active metabolites. Even if analysis for each is complete and quick (as it may be for amitriptyline or imipramine) one is still left with the problem of how to total them up in a meaningful way, in terms of equivalent cerebral and clinical effect. This is why an alternative plasma measurement approach may be better. Instead of trying for quantitation with chemical specificity it may be better to use pharmacological specificity. Neuroleptics seem to act at least in part by blocking dopamine receptors. A test system has been devised which measures the plasma's power to compete with radioactive haloperidol in binding to a preparation containing partially purified dopamine receptors [17], and this measurement of dopamine blockade potency can be made on plasma samples at various times after each dose of many neuroleptics, separately or in mixture. It is too early to say whether this will be clinically useful, and whether similar assays for cholinergic, α-adrenergic, serotoninergic blockades and so on will need to be applied at the same time, but the potential is there.

B. Individual Susceptibility

There is already increasing evidence that different brains have different susceptibilities to the same cerebral dose of a drug. Some manic patients will respond readily to a basal lithium plasma level of 0.8 mmol/liter, whereas others are untouched by this but will respond at a level of 1.2 mmol/liter. The therapeutic range so often quoted is of course a statement about a population, whereas the individual has a much narrower requirement lying somewhere between the extremes. Later, we shall discuss evidence that thioridazine's acute effects in causing prolactin release and affecting psychophysiological measures [18] are different from individual to individual independently of plasma concentration. It is possible, therefore, that measures of cerebral susceptibility might have clinical predictive value in some way, but they have not yet been applied.

C. Individual Cerebral Modifiability

Whereas concepts of responsiveness, learning, behavioral modification, and psychodynamics are the very stuff of psychotherapy, pharmacotherapy has developed with a static model of the brain as a physically constant responding system. However, there is plenty of evidence that this is incorrect, and that biodynamics —the ways in which brain functions are reset in response to a variety of situations, such as exposure to drugs of dependence (alcohol or opiates), or sleep deprivation, or nutritional or endocrine experiences—are going to be important in predicting the effects of neuroleptic treatment and in the prophylaxis of mental disorders [19]. Later, the way in which the release of prolactin changes on chronic treatment with thioridazine will be discussed, with its use as a biodynamic indicator in mind.

Thus the laboratory's help to the psychiatrist is still at a primitive stage of development, and a narrow concentration on the measurement of specific chemical substances in plasma and on the pharmacokinetics of their dispersion into various quasi-theoretical body spaces is not going to take us very far. Some actual body spaces *have* latterly begun to receive attention—the red cell mass in particular—but urine is a body space sample freely available in quantity, and deserving of fuller study. Of course, renal blood flow determines urinary excretion, as liver blood flow determines liver metabolism, and blood flows in general, whether through fat, brain, or muscle, determine drug dispersion. Urine measurements can add an extra dimension to the indirect study of the drug dose being delivered to the brain. But the brain's responsiveness and the brain's adaptiveness or physical changeability remain uncharted.

In sum, the practical aims of plasma level measurements are to assess drug compliance and bioavailability, and to aid the clinician in coping with the difficult patient or in predicting the probable outcome of pharmacotherapy where response is likely to follow weeks after initiation of therapy. The scientific aims are wider and somewhat different. Some of them lie within chemical physiology —the mechanisms of membrane transport and of protein binding for a particular drug, the enzymatic equipment of various tissues which transform it, the possibilities of interaction with normal somatic functions or with other drugs administered, and so on.

Other scientific aims focus on responses. Drugs interact in a molecular way with receptors, and the problem is to link the altered receptors with the ultimate behavioral display. We are forced to think not only in terms of numbers of receptors, their spatial distribution, and variation in sensitivity and quality, but also of the interplay of other influences bearing on receptor qualities and on the forward transmission of their messages. Therapeutic benefits are too far and wide from receptor stimulation or blockade, and narrower cerebral effects must be sought, where quantitation is easier, objective, and can throw light on brain mechanisms and brain integration. Side effects such as parkinsonism, sedation, hypothermia, hormonal secretion, and electroencephalogram (EEG) change can be related to plasma concentrations of drugs. Or instead of examining human mammalian processes in general, one can use the fate of drugs and the responses to them as so many probes of the ways in which the individual human being changes from time to time, and the ways in which individuals differ from one another. This listing of aims may seem rather obvious. Its corollary, however, is that a particular aim is best served by a particular technical approach–in choice of biological samples and sampling times as well as in measurement techniques. At present the field shows a tendency to be constricted between the narrow walls of ritual measurements of plasma concentrations with calculations of routine pharmacodynamic parameters, and without more consideration of aims this is bound to prove infertile.

III. REVIEW OF ESTABLISHED KNOWLEDGE OF THIORIDAZINE METABOLISM AND CLINICAL RESPONSES

There are many gaps in our knowledge of thioridazine metabolism and clinical responses. A review of what is established, first with single (acute) doses and then with chronic regular treatment, may help to see where the next explorations should profitably go.

A. Metabolism

A single dose of thioridazine by mouth [5] or of mesoridazine by intramuscular injection [20] usually appears quickly in the plasma and almost as quickly gives rise to metabolites which appear in plasma and urine. With gas chromatographic measures 50 mg drug in oral syrup reliably produced a plasma peak in male volunteers about 1 to 2 h after swallowing, with a decline back to baseline in about 8 to 10 h thereafter. Mesoridazine began to be measurable in the plasma within an hour or two of the thioridazine dose, those subjects with the lowest plasma peaks of thioridazine having the most rapid conversion to mesoridazine. Examination of timed urine specimens showed that mesoridazine and sulforidazine were appearing there in detectable amount in an hour or two (by thin-layer chromatography as well as gas-liquid chromatography). This 50-mg dose caused only minimal subjective sensations and did not significantly affect blood pressure or pulse. Gottschalk et al. [20], giving 100-150 mg mesoridazine by intramuscular injection, produced marked sedation and hypotension, and the latter would be expected to delay drug absorption and metabolism. Nevertheless, the peak plasma levels of mesoridazine occurred mostly in 0.5-3 h, the half-lives were mostly 2-10 h, and sulforidazine as an important metabolite was observable in plasma 1 h after injection and reached its maximum about 3 h later. This rapidity of absorption and metabolism was originally established by the careful gas chromatographic work of the Swedish group [21-23], who showed that oral tablets gave lower and later peaks (were absorbed more slowly) than oral syrup, that there was a small influence of advancing age on the range of plasma levels to be expected from a standard dose, and that there was no sex difference in metabolism. Thioridazine 50 mg orally may give rise to peak plasma levels commonly of 100-200 ng/ml, occasionally much lower.

Apart from the clinically active metabolites mesoridazine and sulforidazine, the inert metabolite thioridazine ring sulfoxide was also rapidly formed: one alternative metabolic pathway. It can be measured in the plasma and urine provided chloroform rather than hexane extraction of the sample is used with sulfuric acid back-extraction (Papadopoulos, unpublished), and it occurs in the urine about as soon as and in comparable amounts to the two clinically active metabolites. Free thioridazine itself may be undetectable in urine samples, depending on their dilution and the number of hours of renal function they represent, or exist as a few micrograms in total: metabolic change of administered drug is clearly efficient.

If we try to assess the relative importance of these substances (Ng and Crammer [5]; Papadopoulos, unpublished) by balancing the oral dose against their 24-hour urinary excretion, the answer is illuminating. Only 1-2% of the dose is appearing as these metabolites in urine. Of course, it is highly likely that phenothiazine in quantity is disappearing through the liver-biliary system into the gut for eventual fecal excretion. Eiduson and Geller [4] long ago gave ^{35}S-labeled thioridazine to three patients and found that 50% of the radioactivity was in the stools and 30% in the urine. In other words, the stool is important, but even in urine a great amount of metabolite is being overlooked, and since we do not know what it is we cannot be sure that none of it might influence clinical response. We can only recognize metabolites if they have some characteristic color test or physical property—fluorescence, gas chromatographic retention time, radioactivity, or mass spectrum. On the other hand, to give ^{35}S compounds to patients is an unacceptable risk, and possibly, if it were available, thioridazine securely labeled with ^{14}C would be better. For the present all we can say is that thioridazine once absorbed is rapidly metabolized by at least three independent processes, largely to unknown substances, only a minority of which appear in the urine. It is therefore not surprising that attempts to correlate thioridazine plasma level with therapeutic effects have not met with much success.

This does not, however, exclude the possibility that individual differences in metabolic capacity might correlate with success or failure in therapy. Mackay et al. [24] suggested for chlorpromazine that the ratio of inactive ring sulfoxide to active metabolite in the individual's plasma or urine might predict future clinical effect, and this remains open for thioridazine also.

B. Clinical Effects

Apart from its slow action in the therapy of psychoses, thioridazine has acute cerebral effects such as sedation and production of fast activity in the EEG, systolic hypotension, and the release of prolactin from the pituitary into the circulation [25]. An attempt to correlate these clinical changes with thioridazine plasma levels after single doses in normal men failed [18]. The men were given different acute doses on different occasions and had a variety of plasma levels of thioridazine at different times. They showed cerebral changes of varying magnitude—drowsiness, fast EEG waves, increased finger tremor—and a variable plasma prolactin concentration, all of which correlated quite highly so that the timing and magnitude of the prolactin change was a good indicator for thioridazine response in general. Yet none of this correlated with plasma thioridazine or drug dose. Unlike lithium, or nortriptyline, therefore, thioridazine appeared to have no simple reactive relationship with human brain in these acute responses.

This conclusion emerged from the group of subjects as a whole. When, however, the subjects were examined individually an important further fact emerged. In an individual plasma prolactin and plasma thioridazine might be closely related, to an extent which was stable over months of testing, but individuals differed markedly in the quantitative aspect of this relationship. One might have a very big linear response to the drug, another a very small one (Fig. 2), and these individual responses canceled one another in the group and so hid a correlation which was there. In other words, individuals differed not only in thioridazine metabolism but also in cerebral responsiveness.

Prolactin release is under both positive and negative control: the pituitary secretes prolactin in response to a humoral stimulus released from the hypothalamus, but this secretion is held in check by a second hypothalamic substance, prolactin-inhibiting factor (PIF), which is either dopamine itself or something released by neural excitation across dopaminergic synapses. Phenothiazines as blockaders of dopamine receptors prevent the release of this PIF (and/or prevent the action of dopamine on the pituitary) and so allow prolactin to be secreted. This regulatory system differs in phenothiazine responsiveness from person to person. Does its state bear any relation to the sensitivity of other dopaminergic systems in the brain?

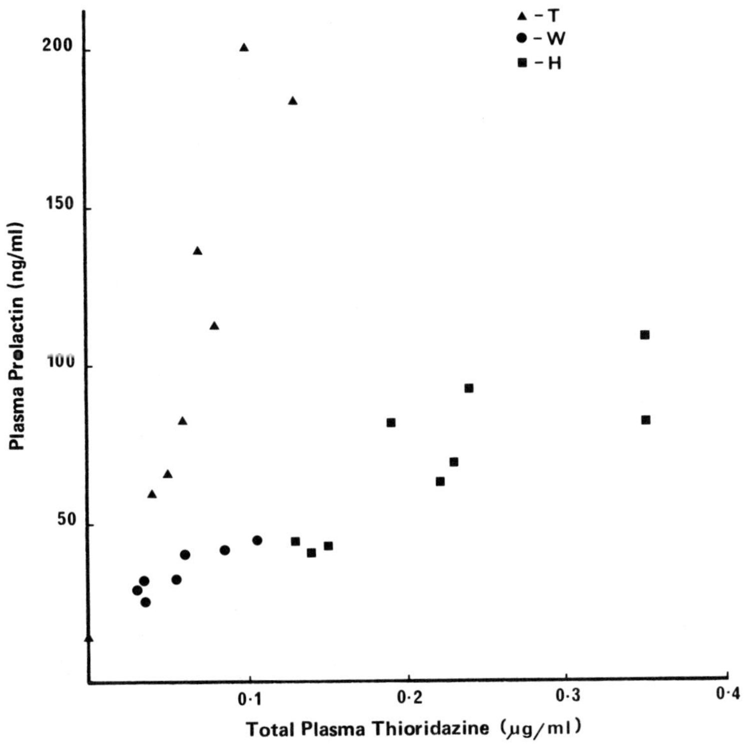

Figure 2 The relation between total plasma thioridazine and plasma prolactin in different individuals T, W, and H (sum of acute tests on various occasions). This variation between individuals could be due to differences in degree of plasma protein binding of the drug, or to differences in the receptor system. (From Ref. 31.)

Gottschalk et al. [20] has approached the acute effects of thioridazine differently, comparing the responses of drug-free acute schizophrenics and normal volunteers to single injections of saline or mesoridazine on a number of psychological tests. Three rating scales were used—Overall-Gorham brief psychiatric, Hamilton depression, and Wittenborn—and 5-min samples of speech taped for analysis by the author's own social alienation/personal disorganization method. Some individual items on the three rating scales declined in the patients given mesoridazine (depression, anxiety, anergy, apathy) 24 h after drug, and the social alienation/personal disorganization score was likewise significantly reduced. The anergy score appeared to be related to the measure of plasma mesoridazine plus sulforidazine, but otherwise plasma levels and clinical changes seemed independent. Unfortunately the methods were not ideal in this study, and the validity of even these results must be in doubt. The scoring of the three rating scales was not done blind, and the patients all received saline injections first, mesoridazine second (5 days later) instead of a random allocation of treatments. One would have liked to know also whether the psychological changes found could have been produced by any nonspecific sedation.

If a more exact study confirmed the findings and showed them specific, however, they would speak against the value of plasma measurements in clinical prediction but introduce two interesting ideas. The first is that an acute dose of drug may have a prolonged influence on the nervous system, extending even beyond the time when detectable drug has vanished from the body fluids; this would explain the poor correlation with drug plasma concentrations and suggest that something more than simple dopamine blockade was the mode of action. The second idea is that the clinical responses to a single dose might predict clinical outcome later on chronic treatment. However, there are reasons for thinking that this attractive thought will not work. It relates to a static model for drug action, whereas there is evidence that both drug metabolism and cerebral responsiveness change with continued drug treatment, and therefore a dynamic approach is necessary.

Chronic treatment with thioridazine appears to lead to higher persistent levels of mesoridazine and thioridazine in the plasma, while the thioridazine level itself appears to reach an equilibrium or steady state and then drop a little. Daily urine analysis shows that the amount of urinary ring sulfoxide increases severalfold in a few days and then stabilizes [5]. Experience with induction of liver hydroxylases by many drugs suggests that metabolic changes will continue for at least the first 2 weeks of treatment. Individual differences are evident in these changes [5], and therefore what happens clinically on the first day of treatment may not be the same on the 15th.

C. Cerebral Self-Modification under Phenothiazine Treatment

There are a number of hints also that the neuroleptic action of a phenothiazine involves the capacity for cerebral self-modification under prolonged treatment. The antipsychotic effect appears slowly, over a week or more, the parkinsonian side effects of the drug may be prominent at first but disappear on long-continued treatment (disappearance of the need for cotreatment with orphenadrine, etc.), the drug dose for suppression of symptoms may decline with time, and if the drug is stopped altogether the symptoms may not return for weeks or months. Sudden total cessation of treatment may lead to nausea and vomiting, suggestive of a state of dopamine receptor supersensitivity. In the case of thioridazine itself, unrest, tremor, fever, and incontinence suggestive of cholinergic supersensitivity have been reported [14]. It is surprising, therefore, that there has been so little study of thioridazine pharmacokinetics and cerebral responses at the end of treatment rather than at the beginning, during and after withdrawal.

IV. CONCLUSION

Hopes that the plasma prolactin level in relation to thioridazine might be an indicator of cerebral functional change have not so far been fulfilled. The limited data of Papadopoulos (unpublished) do not suggest any change in the individual's thioridazine-prolactin response curve over 14 days of treatment. Data of Meltzer and Fang [25] showed a steady raised prolactin over months of treatment of chronic schizophrenics with thioridazine, with a rapid return to basal values when the drug was stopped. But these changes occurred whether or not there was clinical change. At least two explanations have been offered for this. One supposes simply a different sensitivity of different dopaminergic systems; tuberoinfundibular prolactin release is very sensitive to thioridazine and is already complete at low plasma concentrations of thioridazine which are yet too low to affect the less sensitive caudate nucleus, for instance [26]. The other takes up the hypothesis that neuroleptics act by provoking slow cerebral modification; and clearly prolactin release is not modified with time and therefore is not comparable with other dopaminergic systems which are, as shown by changes in the liberation of the dopamine metabolite homovanillic acid into cerebrospinal fluid during prolonged phenothiazine treatment. Either way, prolactin release is out of step with long-term antipsychotic effects. There is no difference between normals and schizophrenics in its release by phenothiazines, nor between patients who improve on drug and those who do not.

Surveys of the plasma levels in groups of patients have been made often enough, whether by old [10-13] or by newer techniques, [5,22] to make it clear that such measurements are naive and uninformative. Thioridazine differs from lithium and nortriptyline in this respect. Neuropathological heterogenicity among clinically selected schizophrenics may be one factor, individual biological variability at the levels of cerebral responsiveness and cerebral modification another, but the complexities of drug metabolism may still be of prime importance. Since thioridazine is so rapidly metabolized, clinically active metabolites need more study. Axelsson [14] carried out a clinical trial on 10 chronic patients who would relapse when thioridazine was withdrawn and replaced this drug with mesoridazine or sulforidazine to produce renewed clinical remission. Sulforidazine appeared to have about half the potency of thioridazine itself, as judged by plasma levels at remission, while mesoridazine was intermediate. Although they were effective neuroleptics, after several weeks apathy, depression, and restlessness gradually appeared (and disappeared on return to thioridazine treatment later), so that these metabolites may produce signs of their own, and might even be responsible for a part of the picture usually thought of as a residuum of the psychosis. Electrocardiographic changes, principally T-wave changes, were also noted. However, it has recently been suggested [27] that these may be due to another metabolite–ring sulfoxide rather than side chain sulfoxide. A surprising finding in the plasmas of those on mesoridazine was the presence of thioridazine, implying that somewhere a chemical reduction of mesoridazine can take place, and showing that we have a great deal more yet to learn about thioridazine metabolism.

We still have to account chemically for over 95% of the thioridazine dose, and until the metabolite picture is clearer it seems premature to worry about the metabolites attached to or contained in erythrocytes [28]. Thioridazine itself is largely bound to plasma proteins [29], and it is still an open question whether the high plasma levels sometimes found in individuals on modest drug doses may not be due to exceptional binding power rather than low liver metabolism. It is not only laboratory workers who have much to do. Clinically there is a great need to refine the biological response to be observed, titrating against the presence of hallucinations or of thought disorder, or of insomnia or of neurological signs in parkinsonism or Huntington's chorea, or of neuroendocrine responses [30].

Somewhere, at some level, a quantity of drug is reacting with a quantity of receptors. It is the relation between receptor action and manifest behavioral function which is so totally obscure, and which can begin to be clarified once the actual substances acting on the receptors have been established.

REFERENCES

1. J. E. Overall, L. E. Hollister, F. Meyer, I. Kimbell, Jr., and J. Shelton, Imipramine and thioridazine in depressed and schizophrenic patients: Are there specific antidepressant drugs? *JAMA 189:*605-608, 1964.
2. S. L. Delong, Ocular reactions to psychopharmacologic drugs. In *Psychopharmacology: A Review of Progress, 1957-67* (D. H. Efron, J. O. Cole, J. Levine, and J. R. Wittenborn, eds.). PHS publication 1836. Washington, D.C., U.S. Government Printing Office, 1968.
3. T. L. Chan, G. Sakalis, and S. Gershon, Quantitation of chlorpromazine and its metabolites in human plasma and urine by direct spectrodensitometry of thin layer chromatograms. In *Phenothiazines and Structurally Related Drugs* (I. S. Forrest, C. J. Carr, and E. Usdin, eds.). New York, Raven Press, 1974.
4. S. Eiduson and E. Geller, The excretion and metabolism of ^{35}S-labelled thioridazine in urine, blood, bile, and feces. *Biochem. Pharmacol. 12:* 1429-1437, 1963.

5. T. H. Ng, and J. L. Crammer, Measurement of thioridazine in blood and urine. *Brit. J. Clin. Pharmacol. 4:*173-183, 1977.
6. F. M. Forrest, I. S. Forrest, and A. S. Mason, Review of rapid urine tests for phenothiazine and related drugs. *Amer. J. Psychiatry 118:*300-307, 1961.
7. B. Blackwell, Treatment adherence. *Brit. J. Psychiatry 129:*513-531, 1976.
8. T. J. Mellinger, E. M. Mellinger, and W. T. Smith, Thioridazine blood levels in patients receiving different oral forms. *Clin. Pharmacol. Ther. 6:*486-491, 1965.
9. W. L. Pacha, A method for the fluorimetric determination of thioridazine or mesoridazine in plasma. *Experientia* (Basel) *25:*103-104, 1969.
10. R. Bergling, T. Mjorndal, L. Oreland, W. Rapp, and S. Wold, Plasma levels and clinical effects of thioridazine and thiothixene. *J. Clin. Pharmacol. 15:* 178-186, 1975.
11. L. A. Gottschalk, R. Biener, E. P. Noble, H. Birch, D. E. Wilbert, and J. F. Heiser, Thioridazine plasma levels and clinical response. *Comp. Psychiatry 16:*323-337, 1975.
12. F. E. R. E. R. de Jonghe and H. J. van der Helm, Plasma concentrations of thioridazine in patients with depression. *Acta Psychiatr. Scand. 46:* 36-363, 1970.
13. F. E. R. E. R. de Johghe, H. J. van der Helm, H. F. Schalken, and J. H. Thiel, Therapeutic effect and plasma level of thioridazine. *Acta Psychiatr. Scand. 49:*535-545, 1973.
14. R. Axelsson, On the serum concentrations and antipsychotic effects of thioridazine, thioridazine side chain sulphoxide and thioridazine side chain sulphone in chronic psychotic patients. *Curr. Ther. Res. 21:*587-605, 1977.
15. P.-E. E. Bergner, K. Berniker, T. B. Cooper, J. R. Gradijan, and G. M. Simpson, Lithium kinetics in Man: Effect of variation in dosage pattern. *Brit. J. Pharmacol. 49:*328-339, 1973.
16. R. Braithwaite, S. Montgomery, and S. Dawling, Nortriptyline in depressed patients with high plasma levels, II. *Clin. Pharmacol. Ther. 23:*303-308, 1978.
17. I. Creese and S. H. Snyder, A simple and sensitive radioreceptor assay for antischizophrenic drugs in blood. *Nature 270:*180-182, 1977.
18. G. Nikitopolou, M. Thorner, J. Crammer, and M. Lader, Prolactin and psychophysiologic measures after single doses of thioridazine. *Clin. Pharmacol. Ther. 21:*422-429, 1977.
19. A. J. Mandell, *Neurobiological Mechanisms of Adaptation and Behaviour.* Advances in Biochemical Psychopharmacology series, vol. 13. New York, Raven Press, 1975.
20. L. A. Gottschalk, E. Dinovo, R. Biener, H. Birch, M. Syben, and E. P. Noble, Plasma levels of mesoridazine and its metabolites and clinical response in acute schizophrenia after a single intramuscular drug dose. In *Pharmacokinetics of Psychoactive Drugs: Blood Levels and Clinical Re-*

sponses (L. A. Gottschalk and S. Merlis, eds.). New York, Spectrum, 1976, pp. 171-189.
21. E. Martensson and B. E. Roos, Serum levels of thioridazine in psychiatric patients and healthy volunteers. *Eur. J. Clin. Pharmacol. 6:*181-186, 1973.
22. R. Axelsson and E. Martensson, Serum concentration and elimination from serum of thioridazine in psychiatric patients. *Curr. Ther. Res. 19:*242-265, 1976.
23. R. Axelsson, On the pharmacokinetics of thioridazine in psychiatric patients. In *Antipsychotic Drugs: Pharmacodynamics and Pharmacokinetics* (G. Sedvall, B. Uvnäs, and Y. Zotterman, eds.). Oxford, Pergamon, 1976, pp. 353-358.
24. A. V. P. Mackay, A. F. Healey, and J. Baker, The relationship of plasma chlorpromazine to its 7-hydroxy and sulphoxide metabolites in a large population of chronic schizophrenics. *Brit. J. Clin. Pharmacol. 1:*425-430, 1974.
25. H. Y. Meltzer and V. S. Fang, The effect of neuroleptics on serum prolactin in schizophrenic patients. *Arch. Gen. Psychiatry 33:*279-286, 1976.
26. E. J. Sachar, P. H. Gruen, T. B. Karasu, N. Altman, and A. G. Frantz, Thioridazine stimulates prolactin secretion in man. *Arch. Gen. Psychiatry 32:*885-886, 1975.
27. L. A. Gottschalk, E. Dinovo, R. Bremer, and B. R. Nandi, Plasma concentrations of thioridazine metabolites and electrocardiographic abnormalities. *J. Pharmac. Sci. 67:*155-157, 1978.
28. I. A. Zingales, Detection of chlorpromazine and thioridazine metabolites in human erythrocytes. *J. Chromatogr. 44:*547-562, 1969.
29. F. M. Belpaire, F. A. J. Vanderheeven, and M. G. Bogaert, Binding of thioridazine and some of its metabolites to human serum protein and human albumin. *Arzneim.-Forsch. 25:*1969-1971, 1975.
30. S. A. Checkley and J. L. Crammer, Hormone responses to methylamphetamine in depression: A new approach to the noradrenalin depletion hypothesis. *Brit. J. Psychiatry 131:*582-586, 1977.
31. A. S. Papadopoulos, M. Thorner, and J. L. Crammer. Unpublished.

11

Butyrophenones
Plasma Levels and Therapeutic Effect

Larry Evans / *Department of Psychiatry, University of Queensland, Brisbane, Queensland, Australia*

I. INTRODUCTION

The butyrophenones are a group of neuroleptic drugs which were first synthesized by Janssen in 1956, as he searched for a meperidine related drug with greater morphinelike potency than meperidine itself. Initially he studied a large series of 4-phenylpiperidines and eventually produced a propriophenone derivative which possessed the qualities of a morphinelike analgesic but which also appeared to have neuroleptic properties when studied in animals [1]. By the addition of fluorine in the para position of the ketonic phenyl ring and the substitution of a hydroxy group into the piperidine nucleus he produced the haloperidol molecule, (Fig. 1). This compound is completely devoid of morphinelike properties. Di Mascio [2] suggested its activity comes close to fitting Delay and Deniker's concept of neuroleptic action. He thought that this would also prove to be the case with other members of the butyrophenone group, many of which have

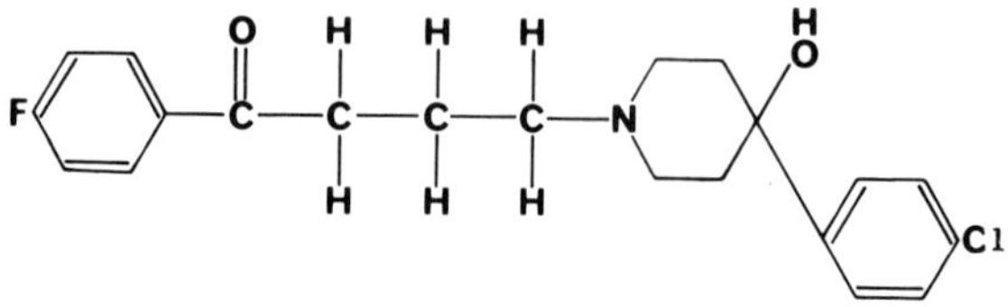

Figure 1 The haloperidol molecule.

been subsequently shown to be potent neuroleptics experimentally. Since haloperidol was the first of this group to have been introduced to clinical psychiatry as it was in 1958, it has also been the compound which has received most attention.

Early animal studies with haloperidol suggested that it would have potent antipsychotic activity, with less anticholinergic effects than most of the phenothiazines then available [3]. This potent neuroleptic activity can be explained by the physical characteristics of the butyrophenones. These characteristics are also present in some other neuroleptic drugs where they have been shown to be associated with high neuroleptic potency. Potent neuroleptic activity in these groups of drugs is probably related to a structural similarity of the molecules to γ-aminobutyric acid (GABA), resulting in the molecule occupying the GABA receptors easily and for prolonged periods of time. By this activity they prevent glutamic acid from polarizing the membrane and thus dopamine from reaching the appropriate receptors [4]. The physical properties accounting for this neuroleptic potency are a 6-membered basic heterocyclic ring with a straight chain of 3 carbon atoms linking the basic ring nitrogen with a carbon, nitrogen, or oxygen atom as shown in Fig. 2 [5]. As it is this configuration of the 3 carbon atoms with the nitrogen atom on the basic ring which attaches itself to the neurotransmitter site, it is thought that this part of the molecule is responsible for the neuroleptic activity. If this structure stays intact during the metabolism of neuroleptic molecules, the metabolites are likely to have some neuroleptic activity. In man, for example, the phenothiazines pass through a number of metabolic steps before this important part of the molecule is ruptured, resulting in the first metabolites of the phenothiazines being active [6].

The presence of active metabolites has made it difficult to interpret the results of studies of neuroleptic plasma levels and their relationship to therapeutic effect [7].

With the butyrophenones this appears less likely to be the case. Soudijn et al. [8] have shown the presence of flurophenyl carbonic acid in rats given tritiated haloperidol. This observation, coupled with the identification of flurophenyl acetylurenic acid as the major metabolite of haloperidol in the urine

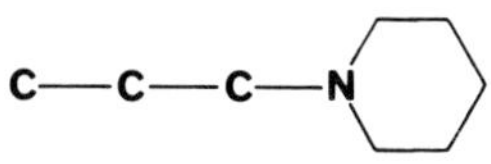

Figure 2 The active moiety of the neuroleptic molecule.

[9], led them to propose N-oxidative dealkylation as the major and general metabolic pathway of haloperidol in rats. In this metabolic pathway the C–C–C–N part of the haloperidol molecule is split during the first metabolic step. If this is the metabolic pathway of haloperidol and other similar butyrophenones in man, there would be few, if any, active metabolites making these compounds ideal for studies relating plasma level and therapeutic effect. Forsman and Ohman [10] have shown that N-oxidative dealkylation of haloperidol occurs in man by isolating both flurobenzoyl propionic acid and flurophenyl acetylurenic acid from the urine of patients treated with haloperidol. They concluded that haloperidol did not form active metabolites in man. Recently doubt has been cast on this by the identification of the hydrated metabolite in the serum and urine of patients on high doses of haloperidol. This compound is produced by hydroxylation of haloperidol and appears to be present in equal proportions to haloperidol. This could well be the first metabolic step in man before N-oxidative dealkylation occurs, and would produce a compound with the vital C–C–C–N fragment intact, which has been shown to have about a quarter of the neuroleptic potency of haloperidol in animals [11]. However, if this compound is in equilibrium with haloperidol in equal proportions, plasma haloperidol levels will still be a valid assessment of the active drug present in the body. Thus haloperidol would appear to be a most appropriate neuroleptic in which to seek a relationship between the plasma level and the therapeutic effect. Despite an apparent suitability, haloperidol has not been among the first neuroleptics to be studied for this relationship. This might be explained by the difficulties encountered in developing a method for estimating the plasma level and also by the initial insensitivity of such methods [12]. An accurate and sensitive method has now been developed using a gas chromatography electron capture technique [13,14]. Recently a radioimmunoassay (RIA) method has been developed, and this method also seems to be sensitive and accurate [15,16]. These developments led to a much greater interest in the clinical pharmacology and pharmacokinetics of haloperidol and the butyrophenones, and there have been a number of studies published over the past few years examining these drugs. An assay method has also been developed for penfluridol [17] which is a drug closely related to the butyrophenones.

II. DEVELOPMENTS OF CLINICAL USE OF HALOPERIDOL AND PENFLURIDOL

Haloperidol was first used routinely in clinical psychiatry in 1960, and within a few years Crane [18] wrote, "its value as a psychotropic agent has been documented by an impressive number of clinical studies." At that time he also commented that the best therapeutic dose for the average psychotic patient had not been established. Prior to this time there had been a tendency for haloperidol to be used in what would now be termed "low doses." At first it had been used in the treatment of chronic nonresponding schizophrenics who has been treated unsuccessfully with other drugs [19-21]. Later it was found to be more effective in treating acutely disturbed patients [22], and particularly schizophrenics and manics [23,24]. In his review Crane [18] surveyed 98 original articles describing the treatment of more than 5,300 patients. He found that the range of maximum dosage varied between 1 and 20 mg/day with one patient reported as having received 1,000 mg/day. There was obviously a preference for the lower doses, as the median was only 15 mg/day, with the largest number of studies utilizing dosages between 9 and 16 mg/day. The drug seemed to be most effective in treating overactivity, agitation, social withdrawal, and paranoia in schizophrenics. The mean improvement of patients on haloperidol based on 66 studies totaling 3,817 patients was 51%, with two-thirds of the studies reporting an improvement from 41 to 70%. Among the variables which Crane [18] considered might have influenced these responses were factors relating to dosage levels. He also commented that the margin between therapeutic doses and toxic doses was high.

These comments of Crane's [18] suggest that not all patients responded to the lower doses of haloperidol which were being prescribed at that time. This had already been noted in an unpublished report by Waelkens [25], who commented that the effective dose varied greatly from one patient to another and also within the same patient at different times during therapy. Since this time many other reports have shown that some patients need higher doses of haloperidol than others [26-33]. This led to the concept of adequate individualized dosages (AID) [34]. Patients were also treated with haloperidol for acute symptoms by titrating the dose against the changing clinical state, and it was suggested that this method could be used in much the same way that patients were digitalized in the past [35]. This method could be used parenterally or orally and has developed into the technique of rapid neuroleptization or rapid tranquilization which is now undertaken with those high-potency, low-dosage neuroleptic drugs available for parenteral use [36-41].

The other members of the butyrophenone group have as yet received little attention in clinical psychiatry. Droperidol has been used extensively in anesthetics in the procedure of neuroleptanalgesia.

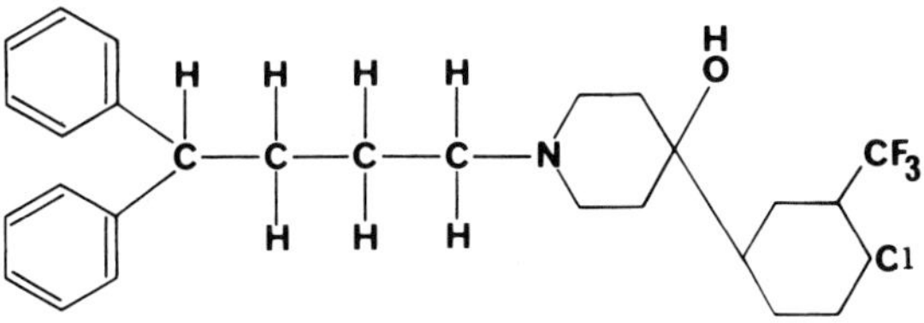

Figure 3 The penfluridol molecule. The active moiety of the neuroleptic molecule.

Closely related to the butyrophenones are the diphenylbutylpiperidine group of drugs, which have similar properties but are longer acting than the butyrophenones. Pimozide has been shown to be effective in treating schizophrenia [42].

Penfluridol is an even longer acting compound which has been shown to be effective in a single weekly oral dose in the treatment of acutely psychotic patients [43] and also in the treatment of the chronic schizophrenic syndrome [44]. Although these two drugs are strictly speaking not butyrophenones, their chemical structure is clearly derived from that family of compounds, as shown by the structure of penfluridol in Fig. 3.

III. HALOPERIDOL PLASMA LEVELS AND THERAPEUTIC EFFECT

Haloperidol is available in tablet, liquid concentrate, and injectible form, and can thus be used orally or parenterally. It is readily absorbed in whatever form it is given. When taken orally it will produce a peak plasma level within 2-6 h [45,46]. It is absorbed rapidly by normal subjects following intramuscular injection, with the maximum plasma level being reached within 20 min [47]. Protein binding is high, being about 92% for concentrations ranging between 0.5 and 20 ng/ml [10]. Forsman and Ohman [45] found the bioavailability to vary between 44 and 74% with a mean of 60% ± 11. They also discovered that the half-life of the drug varied depending on the route of administration. When given orally to 10 healthy volunteers, the half-life ranged from 12.0 to 36.3 h, with a mean of 24.1 h. When given by intravenous injection, the half-life ranged between 10.1 and 19 h, with a mean of 14.1 h. They suggested that the longer oral half-life was probably as a result of a substantial enterohepatic recirculation. It has been shown that about 15% of any given dose is excreted in the bile, with a further 40% being excreted by the kidney during the first 5 days after an oral dose [48].

Haloperidol appears to be concentrated in the liver and the brain [49].

The ratio between haloperidol concentration in the serum and erythrocytes was 1:1; thus the serum level is identical to the plasma level [45].

Forsman [10] showed a positive correlation between the serum level of haloperidol and the daily dose per kg body weight of the drug. This correlation has also been found by Penny et al. [50]. A fivefold variation in serum levels was found by Forsman and Ohman [10], which was not the case with the study of Penny et al., where a much smaller interpatient variation was reported. On the basis of their results Forsman and Ohman [10] suggested the need for adjusting the dose of haloperidol according to the serum level of the drug, though in this study they made no attempt to assess the clinical effect of the drug.

Shostak and Perel [15], using an RIA method of estimating serum haloperidol, obtained values comparable to those obtained by Forsman and Ohman [10]. Clarke et al. [16] also used an RIA method to estimate serum haloperidol in psychiatric patients receiving daily oral doses of 20-200 mg and found serum levels ranging between 5.8 and 245 ng/ml. Neither of these studies related the serum level to the therapeutic effect. There is some evidence to suggest that the neuroleptic effect of haloperidol correlates with the brain concentration of the drug [51].

It has been suggested in one study than antiparkinson medication can lower the plasma levels of haloperidol [52]. However, Forsman and Ohman [53] did not confirm this when they studied the effects of biperidine and orphenadrine. They did show that barbiturates and phenytoin lowered the plasma levels.

There have been few studies as yet published on the relationship between the therapeutic effect of haloperidol and its plasma level. Ericksen and colleagues [54] studied a group of 42 acutely decompensated schizophrenic patients who had been drug free for an average of 2 weeks. Patients were randomly assigned to one of two treatment groups. The first group were given haloperidol 60 mg intramuscularly (i.m.) daily in 6 divided doses for the first 5 days of the study plus placebo tablets. These patients were treated with oral haloperidol which was gradually reduced to 45 mg/day for 2 days, 30 mg/day for 2 days, 20 mg/day for 3 days, and then to 15 mg/day for the final week of the study. The other group of patients received a standard dose of 15 mg/day oral haloperidol throughout the study in addition to placebo injections. Patients were rated clinically using the Brief Psychiatric Rating Scale (BPRS) and a Clinical Global Impression Scale (CGIS). The patients receiving the higher dose of haloperidol showed much higher plasma levels at day 3 and day 11 than those patients who were taking the smaller dose. The mean values at day 3 for the loading dose group were 26.24 ng/ml versus 6.72 ng/ml for the standard-dose group. By day 11 this was 24.83 ng/ml as opposed to 9.86 ng/ml. By day 18 plasma levels had changed to 9.27 ng/ml for the loading-dose group and 9.72 ng/ml for the standard-dose group. The clinical ratings for the two treatment groups showed very little difference, as both groups showed considerable improvement, and the authors concluded that the patients with the higher plasma level of haloperidol held no advantage over those on a more conservative oral regime and lower plasma levels.

Evans and colleagues [55,56] studied a group of hospitalized schizophrenic patients who were treated with haloperidol at varying dosages. After a 2-week placebo period all patients were treated with a standard daily dose of 5 to 10. mg/day of haloperidol for the next 8 weeks. At the end of this period those patients who had shown a satisfactory clinical response as judged by the Inpatient Multidimensional Psychiatric Scale (IMPS) and by clinical assessment were withdrawn from the study. Ten patients remained and these patients were given escalating doses of haloperidol over the next 10 weeks up to a maximum dose of 80 mg/day. The dosages were changed at weekly intervals, and this adjustment was made after blood specimens had been taken for plasma haloperidol investigation. At the same time as blood was taken for the plasma haloperidol levels to be assessed, patients were rated on the IMPS and a side effect rating scale. During the latter 10-week part of the study, as patients showed a satisfactory response to their treatment, judged by a significant reduction in the IMPS and clinical assessment of the patient, these increments of dosage of haloperidol were ceased and the patient was continued on the study. A significant correlation was shown between the dose of haloperidol and the plasma level and also between the plasma level and the therapeutic effect. It is important to note in this study that the patients had their dose of haloperidol adjusted upward on the basis of their clinical response. This design avoided the situation where patients might be given increased doses of the drug after they have shown a satisfactory therapeutic response. While it is possible that this design might have produced a bias in the direction of a correlation, it has avoided a possible difficulty in studies of this type. When patients are given increasing doses of neuroleptic drug beyond their maximum therapeutic response, it is possible that developing behavioral toxicity might be registered on sensitive rating scales, thereby confusing the results.

IV. PENFLURIDOL PLASMA LEVELS AND THERAPEUTIC EFFECT

Penfluridol has only recently been made available for clinical use, and as yet there are not many studies showing its use in clinical practice. Cooper and colleagues [15] studied 22 hospitalized schizophrenic patients treated with varying doses of penfluridol ranging from 30 to 120 mg/week. They studied these patients for 13 weeks and found a good relationship between the mean steady-state plasma concentration and the dose expressed in mg of penfluridol per kg of body weight. A further study found a 10-fold variation in plasma levels of penfluridol but a significant correlation between dosage and plasma level and also between dosage and changes in psychopathology [44]. Chouinard et al. [57] claimed that the antiparkinsonism medication procyclidine decreased the steady-state plasma level of penfluridol.

REFERENCES

1. P. A. J. Janssen, C. Van de Westeringh, A. H. M. Jageneau, Chemistry and pharmacology of CNS depressants related to 4-(4-hydroxy-4-phenyl-piperidino)butyrophenone, I: Synthesis and screening data in mice. *J. Med. Pharmaceut. Chem. 1:*281, 1959.
2. A. Dimascio, The butyrophenones: An overview of their pharmacologic and metabolic properties. In *Butyrophenones in Psychiatry.* New York, Raven Press, 1972, p. 11.
3. P. A. J. Janssen, Chemical and pharmacological classification of neuroleptics. In *Modern Problems in Pharmaco-psychiatry.* New York, Karger, 1970, p. 33.
4. P. A. J. Janssen, The pharmacology of haloperidol. *Int. J. Neuropsychiatry 3(1):*10-18, 1967.
5. P. A. J. Janssen, The pharmacological and clinical mode of action of neuroleptic drugs. *Clin. Trials J. 3(1):*370-379, 1966.
6. D. H. Wiles, T. Kolakowska, A. S. McNeilly, Clinical significance of plasma chlorpromazine levels, I: Plasma levels of the drug, some of its metabolites, and of prolactin during acute treatment. *Psychol. Med. 6:*407-415, 1976.
7. T. B. Cooper, Plasma level monitoring of antipsychotic drugs. *Clin. Pharmacokinetics 3:*14-38, 1978.
8. W. Soudijn, I. Van Wijngaarden, and F. Allewijn, Distribution, excretion, and metabolism of neuroleptics of the butyrophenone type. *Eur. J. Pharmacol. 1:*47-57, 1967.
9. G. A. Braun, G. I. Poos, and W. Soudijn, Distribution, excretion, and metabolism of neuroleptics of the butyrophenone type. *Eur. J. Pharmacol. 1:*58-62, 1967.
10. A. Foraman and R. Ohman, On the pharmacokinetics of haloperidol. *Norsk. Psyk. Tidsskr. 28:*441-448, 1974.
11. A. Forsman and M. Larssen, Personal communication, 1978.
12. F. Marcucci, L. Airoldi, and E. Mussini, A method for the gas chromatographic determination of the butyrophenones. *J. Chromatogr. 59:*174-177, 1971.
13. I. A. Zingales, A gas chromatograph method for the determination of haloperidol in human plasma. *J. Chromatogr. 54:*15-24, 1971.

14. A. Forsman, E. Martensson, and G. Nyberg, A gas chromatographic method for determining haloperidol. *Naunyn-Schmiedebergs Arch. Pharmakol. Exp. Pathol. 286:*113-124, 1974.
15. M. Shostak and J. M. Perel, Radioimmunoassay for haloperidol. *Fed. Proc. 35:*531, 1976.
16. B. R. Clark, B. B. Tower, and R. T. Rubin, Radioimmunoassay of haloperidol in human serum. *Life Sci. 20:*319-326, 1977.
17. S. F. Cooper, R. Dugal, and M. J. Albert, Penfluridol steady-state kinetics in psychiatric patients. *Clin. Phar. Ther. 18:*325-329, 1975.
18. G. E. Crane, A review of clinical literature on haloperidol. *Int. J. Neuropsychiatry 3:*111, 1967.
19. M. D. Enoch and A. A. Robin, A controlled trial of haloperidol in chronic schizophrenics. *J. Ment. Sci. 106:*1459-1467, 1960.
20. E. Brandrup and P. Kristjansen, Controlled clinical test of a new psycholeptic drug (haloperidol). *J. Ment. Sci. 107:*778-782, 1961.
21. L. Prasad and M. C. Townley, Haloperidol and thioridazine in the treatment of chronic schizophrenics. *Dis. Nerv. Syst. 27:*722-726, 1966.
22. C. Entwistle, R. M. Taylor, and I. A. MacDonald, The treatment of mania with haloperidol (Serenace). *J. Ment. Sci. 108:*373-375, 1962.
23. P. E. Feldman, A. P. Bay, and A. N. Baser, Parenteral haloperidol in controlling patient behaviour during acute psychotic episodes. *Curr. Ther. Res. 11:*6, 362-366, 1969.
24. B. Shopsin, L. J. Hekimian, and S. Gershon, A controlled evaluation of haloperidol chlorpromazine and sodium amylobarbitone: Intramuscular short-term use in acute psychotic patients. *Curr. Ther. Res. 11:*9, 561, 1969.
25. J. Waelkens, Clinical report on R 1625. Unpublished paper, 1958.
26. A. J. Oldman and M. Bott, The management of excitement in a general hospital psychiatric ward by high dosage haloperidol. *Acta Psychiatr. Scand. 47:*369-376, 1971.
27. F. J. McLeod, Haloperidol. *Med. J. Aust. 2:*1040, 1971.
28. F. J. Ayd, Haloperidol: Fifteen years of clinical experience. *Dis. Nerv. Syst. 33:*459-469, 1972.
29. R. McMurdo, Haloperidol. *Med. J. Aust. 2:*1506, 1972.
30. F. Sangiovanni, M. A. Taylor, and R. Abrams, Rapid control of psychotic excitement states with intramuscular haloperidol. *Amer. J. Psychiatry 130(10):*1155-1156, 1973.
31. S. J. Dencker, High-dose treatment with neuroleptics in the acute phase of mental disease. *Proc. Roy. Soc. Med. 69(1):*32-34, 1976.
32. W. H. Anderson, Rapid treatment of acute psychosis. *Amer. J. Psychiatry 133:*9, 1976.
33. F. J. Ayd, Guidelines for using short-acting intramuscular neuroleptics for rapid neuroleptization. *Int. Drug Ther. Newsletter (12(2-3):*5-12, 1977.
34. J. C. Maerz, Adequate individualized dosages (A.I.D.) in perspective. *Proc. Roy. Soc. Med. 69(1):*35-39, 1976.

35. P. T. Donlon and J. Tupin, Rapid "digitalization" of decompensated schizophrenic patients with antipsychotic agents. *Amer. J. Psychiatry 131:*310–312, 1974.
36. W. H. Anderson and J. C. Kuehnle, Strategies for the treatment of acute psychosis. *JAMA 229(14):*1884–1889, 1974.
37. R. W. Reschke, Parenteral haloperidol for rapid control of severe, disruptive symptoms of acute schizophrenia. *Dis. Nerv. Syst. 35:*112-115, 1974.
38. N. L. Hoell, Technique of rapid tranquillization. *West. J. Med. 122:*5, 418, 1975.
39. A. S. Mason and R. P. Granacher, Basic principles of rapid neuroleptization. *Dis. Nerv. Syst. 37:*547-551, 1976.
40. R. G. Carter, Psychotolysis with haloperidol rapid control of the acutely disturbed psychotic patient. *Dis. Nerv. Syst. 38(4):*237-239, 1977.
41. F. J. Ayd, Intravenous haloperidol therapy. *Int. Drug. Ther. Newsletter 13:*6, 1978.
42. F. Baro, R. Van Lommel, and R. Dom, Pimozide treatment of chronic schizophrenics as compared with haloperidol and penfluridol maintenance treatment. *Acta Psychiatr. Belg.* 199-214, 1972.
43. H. M. Van Praag, T. Schut, and L. Dols, Controlled trial of penfluridol in acute psychosis. *Brit. Med. J. 4:*710–713, 1971.
44. L. Jacobsson, L. Von Knorring, and B. Mattsson, Penfluridol and thiothixene. *Int. Pharmaco-psychiatry 11:*206-214, 1976.
45. A. Forsman and R. Ohman, Pharmacokinetic studies on haloperidol in man. *Curr. Ther. Res. 20(3):*319–336, 1976.
46. T. A. Ban and J. C. Pecknold, Haloperidol and the butyrophenones. In *Drug Treatment in Mental Disorders.* New York, Raven Press, 1976.
47. W. A. Cressman, J. R. Bianchine, and V. B. Slotnick, Plasma level profile of haloperidol in man following intramuscular administration. *Eur. J. Clin. Pharmacol. 7:*99-103, 1974.
48. T. A. Ban, *The Butyrophenones in Psychopharmacology.* Baltimore, Williams and Wilkins, 1969.
49. P. J. Lewi, J. J. P. Heykants, and F. T. N. Allewijn, Distribution and metabolism of neuroleptic drugs (haloperidol). *Arzneim.-Forsch. 7:* 943, 1970.
50. J. Penny, L. Evans, and M. J. Eadie, Plasma levels of haloperidol with high dose therapy. Paper presented to the 11th A.S.C.E.P. meeting, Sydney, 1977.
51. P. A. J. Janssen and F. T. N. Allewijn, Chemistry and pharmacology of compounds related to 4-(4-hydroxy-4-phenyl-piperdino)butyrophenone. *Arzneim.-Forsch. 19:*199, 1969.
52. J. Gautier, A. Jus, and A. Villeneuve, Influence of the antiparkinsonian drugs on the plasma level of neuroleptics. *Biol. Psychiatry 12(3):*389-399, 1977.
53. A. Forsman and R. Ohman, Applied Pharmacokinetics of haloperidol in man. *Curr. Ther. Res. 21(3):*396–411, 1977.

54. S. E. Ericksen, S. W. Hurt, and S. Chang, Haloperidol dose, plasma levels, and clinical response. *Psychopharmacol. Bull. 14(2):*15-16, 1978.
55. L. Evans, M. J. Eadie, and J. Cox, Haloperidol: Plasma levels and therapeutic effect with low dose therapy. Paper presented to the 11th A.S. C.E.P. meeting, Sydney, 1977.
56. L. Evans, M. J. Eadie, and J. Penny, The relationship between the therapeutic effect and plasma level of high doses of haloperidol. Paper presented to the 11th International Congress C.I.N.P., Vienna, 1978.
57. C. Chouinard, L. Annable, and S. Cooper, Antiparkinsonian drug administration and plasma levels of penfluridol, a new long-acting neuroleptic. *Comm. Psychopharm. 1:*325-331, 1977.

12

Cerebrospinal Fluid and Plasma as Tools for Obtaining Biochemical and Pharmacokinetic Data in Neuroleptic Therapy

Göran Sedvall and Veronika E. Grimm* / *Department of Psychiatry, Karolinska Hospital, Stockholm, Sweden*

*Present affiliation: The Hebrew University of Jerusalem and The Weizmann Institute of Science, Rehovot, Israel.

I. INTRODUCTION

The present chapter summarizes results obtained in a series of studies performed in our laboratory over the past five years. In these studies clinical, biochemical, and pharmacokinetic variables were investigated in chlorpromazine (CPZ) treated patients, with the aim of establishing their predictive value for practical pharmacotherapy in the treatment of psychosis.

Ever since the introduction of neuroleptic drugs in 1952 [1,2] they have been extensively used in the treatment of psychotic patients. The way neuroleptics are used today, however, is the same as when they were introduced 25 years ago, i.e., dose levels are established pragmatically on the basis of patient response. Moreover, the clinical response to the drug varies extensively for reasons that are still not clearly understood. This relative standstill in clinical practice is in contrast with the progress made in the understanding of the mechanisms of action of these drugs on the brain of experimental animals.

The developments in analytical chemistry over the last decades have made it possible to measure plasma levels of the antipsychotic drugs and to initiate studies on the relationships between these concentrations and clinical effects in patients. Some authors found relationships to pharmacokinetic variables, others did not. This inconsistency in the findings may be partly due to the great variation in the biochemical and clinical response in the patient groups studied [3-6].

Simultaneous investigation of clinical, biochemical, and pharmacokinetic data may prove to be useful in the analysis of these observed discrepancies. It may also be useful for the selection of optimal drug dosage in psychotic patients, elucidate the problem of "nonresponders" and generally extend our understanding of the mechanism of action of these drugs in psychosis.

Most antipsychotic drugs block receptors for dopamine (DA) and norepinephrine (NE) in the animal brain [7-13]. The receptor blockade is reflected by an elevation in the brain concentrations of the major metabolites of DA and NE, i.e., homovanillic acid (HVA) and 3-methoxy-4-hydroxyphenylethylene-glycol (MOPEG) [14,15]. Treatment with neuroleptic drugs is also followed by a marked elevation of the HVA concentration in the cerebrospinal fluid (CSF) of psychotic patients [16-18]. The elevation of the concentrations of the monoamine metabolites is thought to result from feedback mechanisms activated by receptors blocked by the antipsychotic drugs [7].

Another reproducible biochemical effect of antipsychotic drugs is the elevation of prolactin levels in plasma [19]. This effect also is related to interference with dopaminergic mechanisms. DA neurons in the hypothalamus inhibit the release of prolactin from the pituitary gland [20]. When DA receptors are blocked by antipsychotic drugs the inhibitory influence ceases, resulting in elevation of prolactin in the plasma. Prolactinlike immunoreactive material has recently been demonstrated also in the CSF of animals and man [21-23]. Antipsychotic drugs but neither antidepressants nor lithium were found to elevate prolactin in the CSF, confirming the mediation of this effect by DA receptor blockade [22].

Thus it is possible to monitor at least some of the central biochemical effects of the antipsychotic drugs in clinical studies by measuring concentrations of monoamine metabolites and prolactin in CSF. If, as has been suggested, the antipsychotic effect of the neuroleptic drugs results from the blockade of DA receptors [24,25] there may be demonstrable relationships between these biochemical pharmacodynamic signs of DA receptor blockade caused by the drug and its clinical antipsychotic effects.

Previous animal data demonstrated that after CPZ treatment the elevation of brain HVA concentrations was highly correlated with the drug levels in brain and plasma [26]. It is therefore of interest to study whether similar relationships occur between central biochemical effects and drug concentrations in the body fluids of neuroleptic-treated patients.

As already pointed out, previous attempts to find relationships between plasma concentrations of neuroleptic drugs and clinical response have been ambiguous. This may be partly due to considerable pathophysiological variability within the groups of psychotic patients studied and/or the methodological difficulties involved in the measurement of clinical response and of drug levels. Of these variance factors the clinical and biochemical heterogeneity of the psychotic patient population is probably the major problem.

In an attempt to clarify the relationships between clinical response and drug levels it may be wise to proceed in a stepwise analysis. The objective measures of biochemical variables influenced by the drug may be more reliable than the subjective rating of degree of psychosis and therapeutic response. Analyzing first the relationships between drug levels and biochemical responses in patients may help to elucidate the reason for the unclear relationship to clinical response.

In all previous studies the plasma of patients was used to monitor drug concentrations in relation to treatment. This procedure is based on the assumption of a close correlation between drug concentrations at central receptor sites and in plasma. So far this relationship has not received too much attention in studies on experimental animals or man. The few results available indicate that the brain and plasma concentrations may differ very much and the size of the difference varies from drug to drug [26,27]. In the plasma of patients most neuroleptic drugs occur predominantly in protein-bound form [28,29]. Only the free fraction of the drug in plasma may be expected to be in equilibrium with the tissue concentration. The plasma protein binding of psychoactive drugs has been shown to vary considerably between patients [30]. For this reason the total plasma concentration of the drug cannot be expected to show as high a correlation with drug levels at central receptor sites as the free fraction should. Technical difficulties involved in measuring the free fraction in plasma, however, have prevented the detailed analysis of this problem in human subjects.

The CSF has direct connections to the cerebral extracellular space. In the CSF protein binding of drug is probably small due to the very low protein concentration in this medium. The drug concentration in CSF may be in more direct equilibrium with brain receptors than the free fraction in the plasma. It is therefore of interest to examine whether drug concentration in the CSF may be more highly correlated to central effects of psychoactive drugs than the total plasma concentration. The concentration of neuroleptic drugs in the CSF has not previously been analyzed. In this research project CSF was primarily sampled for the evaluation of the biochemical effects of CPZ. With the sensitive analytical tools available in this project drug concentrations could be established within the same samples. The relationships between these drug concentrations and the biochemical and clinical effects of drug treatment could accordingly be investigated. The present approach using drug concentrations in the CSF represents an extension of previously used research strategies that relied on plasma measurements.

CPZ was selected as the tool for this study for the following reasons. Since its introduction in 1952 it remains one of the most frequently used antipsychotic drugs. Its extensive use has given reasonable empirical bases for setting effective dose ranges [31]. The biochemical effects of CPZ in the central nervous system of animals have been more extensively studied than those for any other neuroleptic drug. Although the metabolism of the compound shows a remarkable complixity [32], it has been carefully studied in animals and men. All these facts make CPZ a highly interesting tool for research aiming at studying the complicated relationships between psychotherapeutic and biochemical drug effects and pharmacokinetic variables.

II. EXPERIMENTAL METHODS

A. Mass Spectrometric Determination of Chlorpromazine Concentrations in Plasma and Cerebrospinal Fluid

Neuroleptic drugs occur in very low concentrations in the plasma of drug-treated patients [33]. Therefore, the pharmacokinetic studies reviewed here called for the selection of a highly specific and sensitive method for drug level determination.

The use of gas chromatography in combination with mass spectrometry offers several advantages over previously used methods [34]. This technique, called mass fragmentography, makes possible the use of internal standards labeled with stable isotopes in the analytical procedure [35]. The deuterium-labeled standard has the same chemical properties as the authentic compound, but it can be distinguished from the latter in the mass spectrometer by the difference in mass. CPZ was labeled with three deuterium atoms in one of the side chain methyl groups. This compound was used as the internal standard in the mass fragmentographic procedure [36]. The method was shown to have high sensitivity and precision, allowing the determination of CPZ concentrations in plasma as well as in CSF of drug-treated patients. In the CSF, concentrations down to 0.1 ng/ml could be determined with satisfactory precision. A typical recording of a CPZ determination in plasma and CSF from a schizophrenic patient treated with 400 mg CPZ daily is shown in Fig. 1.

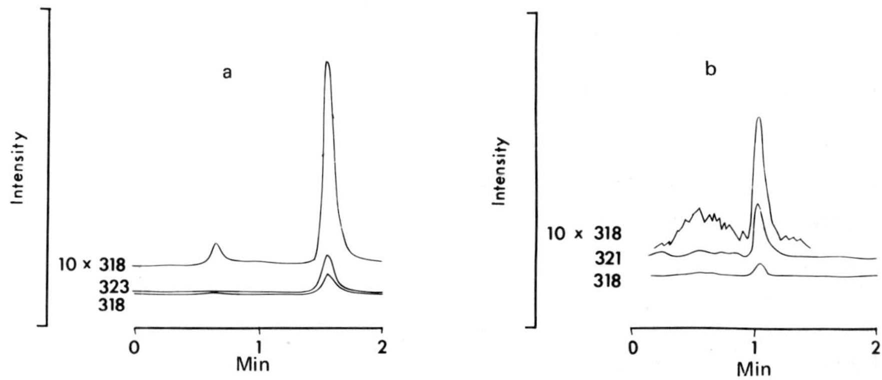

Figure 1 Mass fragmentographic analysis of CPZ in (A) plasma; (B) CSF of a psychotic patient treated for 2 weeks with 400 mg CPZ daily. Channel 318 represents the authentic compound and 321 the deuterium-labeled internal standard. (From Ref. 36.)

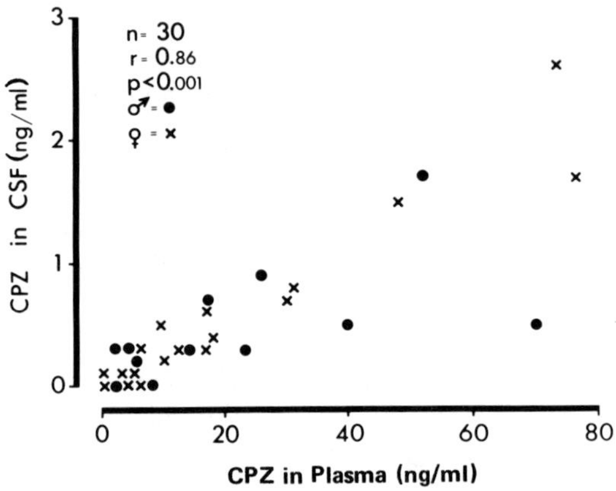

Figure 2 Relationship between CPZ concentrations in CSF and plasma of psychotic patients treated for 4 weeks with CPZ (200–600 mg). Samples were taken at 8:00 A.M. before morning dose. (From Ref. 37.)

In a series of CPZ-treated patients, plasma and CSF were sampled simultaneously and CPZ concentrations were determined in both fluids. There was a fairly high and significant correlation between plasma and CSF values. The average amount of CPZ in CSF was about 3% of the plasma level (Fig. 2). The range of CPZ values in plasma was 0-80 and in CSF 0-3 ng/ml.

The amount of CPZ in CSF is of similar magnitude to the concentration of free drug in plasma [29]. The marked interindividual variation in the CSF/plasma ratio of CPZ may be at least partially due to differences in plasma protein and possibly also CSF protein binding of CPZ. This problem is currently being analyzed in this laboratory.

B. Mass Spectrometric Determination of Chlorpromazine Metabolites in Plasma and Cerebrospinal Fluid

CPZ has a great number of metabolites [38]. Some of them have been shown to block DA receptors in rat brain [39-41]. The most potent of the metabolites in this respect are monodesmethyl-CPZ (nor_1-CPZ) and 7-hydroxy-CPZ (7-OH-CPZ). The CPZ sulfoxide has been shown to be inactive, whereas the above-mentioned two metabolites have been claimed to participate in the clinical effect of the drug [42,43]. However, strong evidence for this case has not yet been presented.

Using a similar methodological approach as with CPZ, we designed mass fragmentographic methods for the determination of nor_1-CPZ and 7-OH-CPZ in

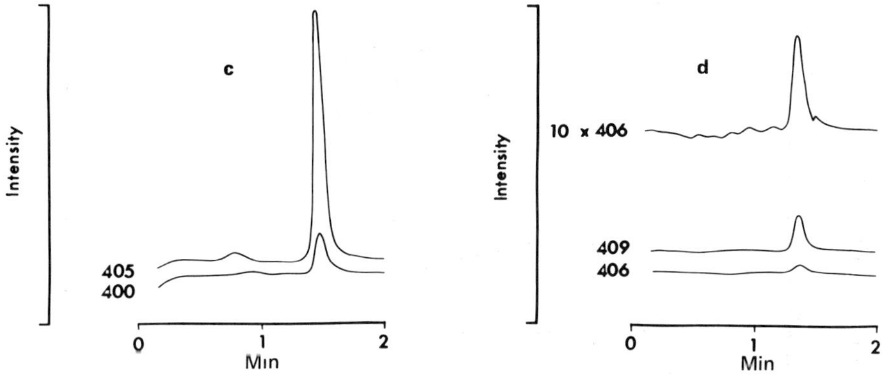

Figure 3 Mass fragmentographic analysis of (C) nor$_1$-CPZ in plasma and (D) 7-OH-CPZ in plasma of a psychotic patient treated for 2 weeks with 400 mg CPZ daily. The lower mass numbers reflect the authentic compounds. (From Ref. 36.)

body fluids [36] (Fig. 3). Confirming previous data by Curry and Marshall [42], the occurrence of both these metabolites could be demonstrated in the plasma of drug-treated patients [44]. Only occasionally did the concentration of the metabolites exceed the CPZ concentration in plasma. The average 7-OH-CPZ concentration was below 40% of the parent compound, and the average nor$_1$-CPZ concentration was generally less than 20% of CPZ (Figs. 4 and 5). None of the available animal data has shown or suggested any of the metabolites to have stronger effect on dopaminergic mechanisms than CPZ, the parent compound [45]. The drug level determinations in animals therefore indicated that generally the CPZ molecule itself is responsible for most of the effects of the compound on the DA system [45]. However, since the metabolites may have specific effects on other systems not yet elucidated by animal experiments, it should be of interest to analyze the relationship between these metabolite concentrations and different biochemical and clinical effects. Since CPZ and the two metabolites (nor$_1$-CPZ, 7-OH-CPZ) are all blocking DA receptors, the sum of their concentrations in the body fluids may be more closely related to DA receptor blockade than the concentration of each of them separately.

Naturally it was of great interest to analyze also levels of the active CPZ metabolites in CSF. But generally the concentrations of CPZ metabolites in CSF were too low to give a satisfactory precision for quantitative evaluation. Therefore, the evaluation of the very low CSF concentrations of active CPZ metabolites has to await future methodological advances.

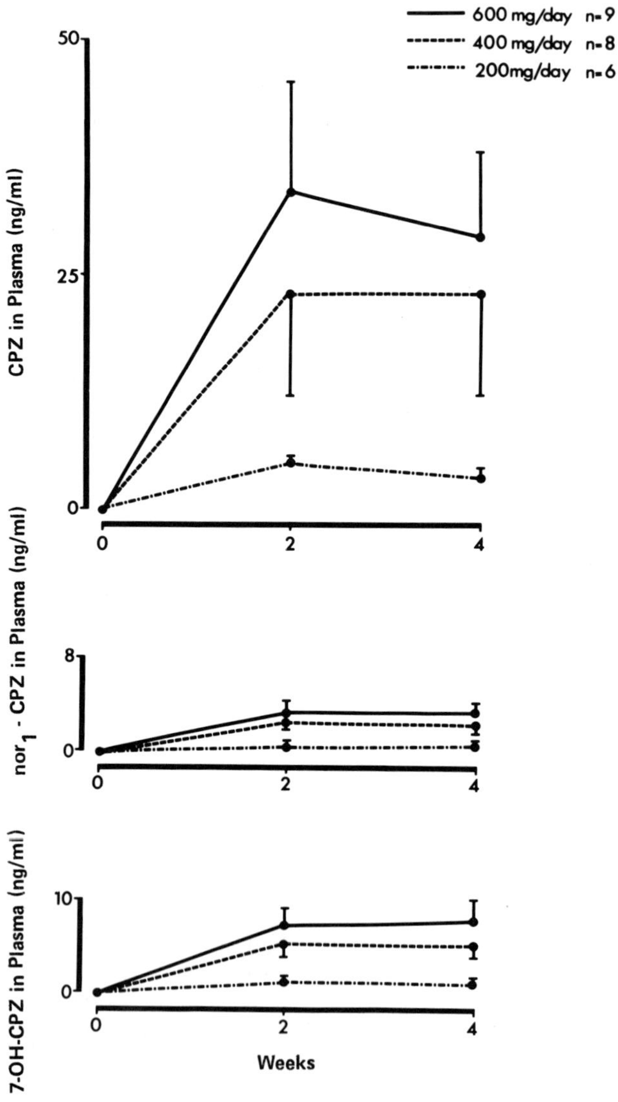

Figure 4 Concentrations of chlorpromazine and two of its active metabolites in plasma from patients treated with 3 different doses. Samples were obtained at 8:00 A.M. (From Ref. 44.)

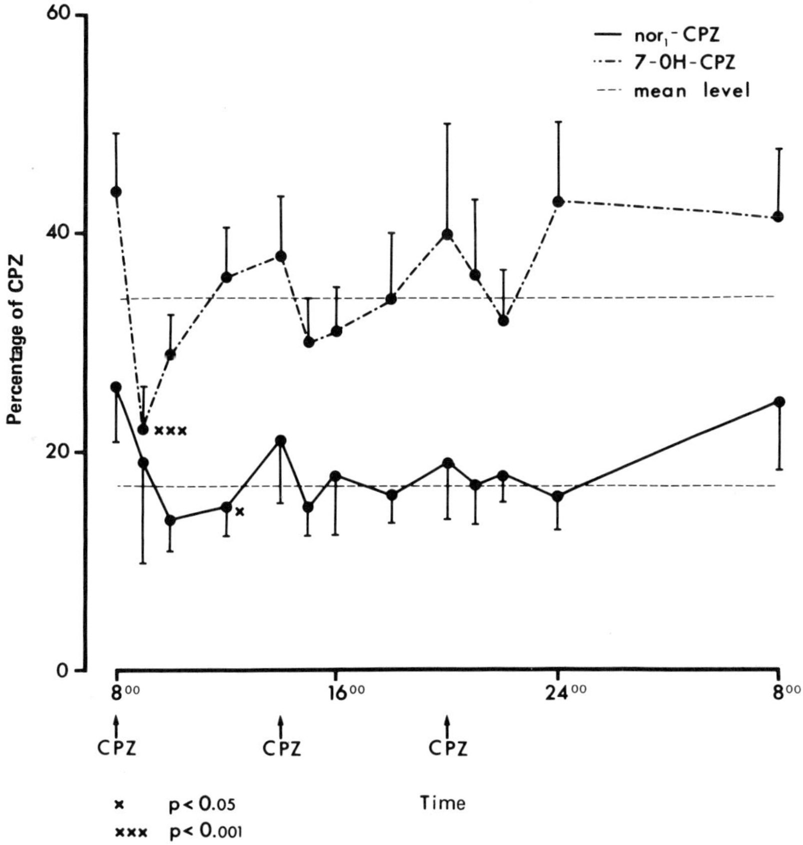

Figure 5 Concentrations of nor$_1$-CPZ and 7-OH-CPZ in percentage of the CPZ level of 10 patients treated with 200–400 mg CPZ per day. (From Ref. 44.)

C. Mass Spectrometric Determination of Monoamine Metabolites in Cerebrospinal Fluid

As mentioned above, changes in the concentrations of the major monoamine metabolites in the lumbar CSF can be used to monitor some biochemical effects of neuroleptic treatment in patients. For that purpose sensitive and reliable methods were required. Also here mass fragmentography was selected as the most appropriate methodology. A procedure allowing the simultaneous determination of the three major monoamine metabolites, i.e., HVA, MOPEG, and 5-HIAA, in 1 ml of CSF was developed [46] (Fig. 6). The specificity was proved

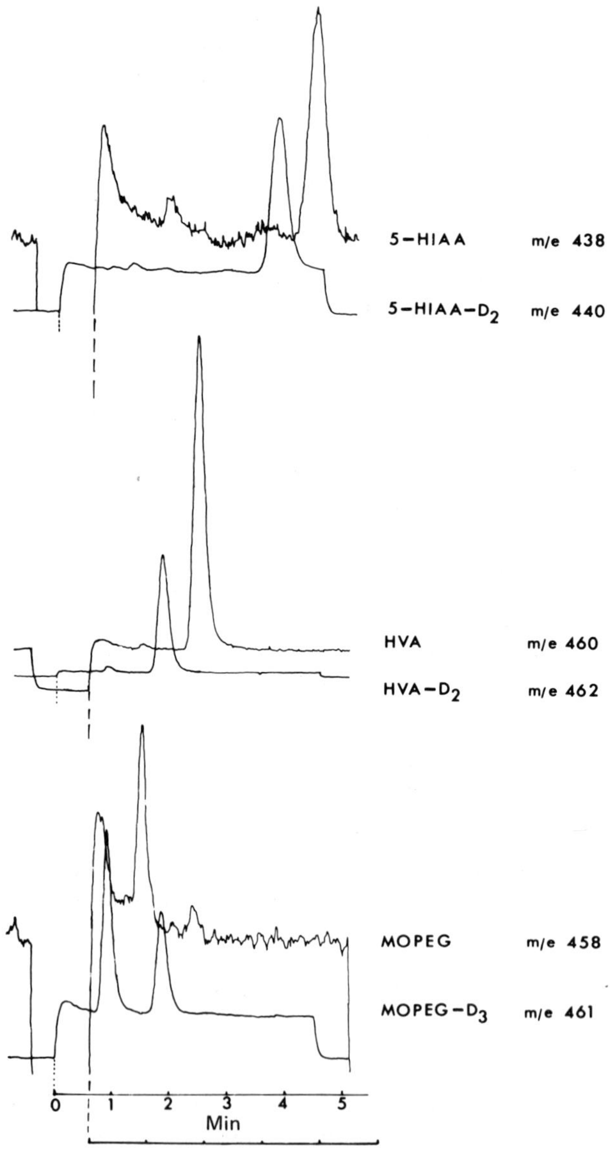

Figure 6 Mass fragmentograms demonstrating simultaneous determination of 5-HIAA and HVA as 1,1,1,2,2-pentafluoropropyl ester pentafluoropropionyl derivatives and MOPEG as trispentafluoropropionyl derivative in CSF. (From Ref. 46.)

by multiple ion analysis. The experimental error was below 7% when applied to the analysis of baseline concentrations of the metabolites in human lumbar CSF.

When CSF samples were analyzed independently for HVA and MOPEG by two different laboratories using mass fragmentography, the data showed high correlation. On the other hand, a comparison with a fluorimetric method gave a very unsatisfactory correlation. The low correlation obtained was due to a poor reliability of the fluorimetric method [47].

D. Radioimmunological Determination of Prolactin in Plasma and Cerebrospinal Fluid

To monitor the effect of CPZ treatment on DA receptors controlling prolactin release from the pituitary gland the hormone levels in plasma were measured by conventional radioimmunological technique. Prolactinlike immunoreactive material could also be demonstrated in the CSF of patients [22], confirming data previously obtained in animals [21]. Antipsychotic but not antidepressant drugs were found to elevate prolactin in CSF of patients [22]. In groups of neuroleptic-treated psychotic patients prolactin in CSF tended to be positively related to the plasma prolactin concentration. However, there were considerable interindividual differences in the CSF/plasma prolactin concentration ratio [48, 49]. Prolactin levels in the CSF as well as plasma of untreated patients tended to be higher in women than in men (Fig. 7).

E. Measurement of Psychotic Morbidity and Side Effects in Chlorpromazine-Treated Patients

The CPRS (Comprehensive Psychopathology Rating Scale [50]) was used for evaluation of changes in psychotic morbidity of patients. Various item combinations were selected that were thought to reflect severity of schizophrenic-type psychosis. Ratings were performed for each patient by two psychiatrists. The interrater reliability was satisfactory for ratings both before and during treatment [51].

The side effects were evaluated by an extended version of the Simpson and Angus rating scale for extrapyramidal symptoms [52,53].

F. Design of the Experimental Drug Trial with Chlorpromazine

The protocol for the study was approved by the Ethics Committee of the Karolinska Institute. Acutely admitted men and women with schizophrenic-type psychosis and age below 57 years were selected from the emergency ward. The inclusion and exclusion criteria used were in accordance with those described in *The International Pilot Study on Schizophrenia* [54].

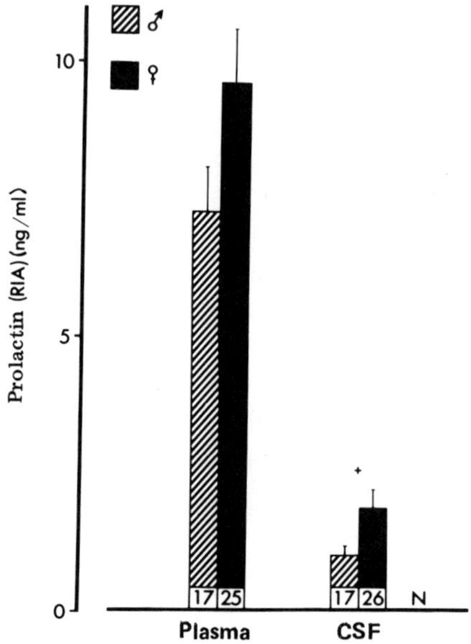

Figure 7 Pretreatment levels of PRL of psychotic patients. The blocks represent mean with standard error. Difference between sexes significant at $P < .05$. (From Ref. 48.)

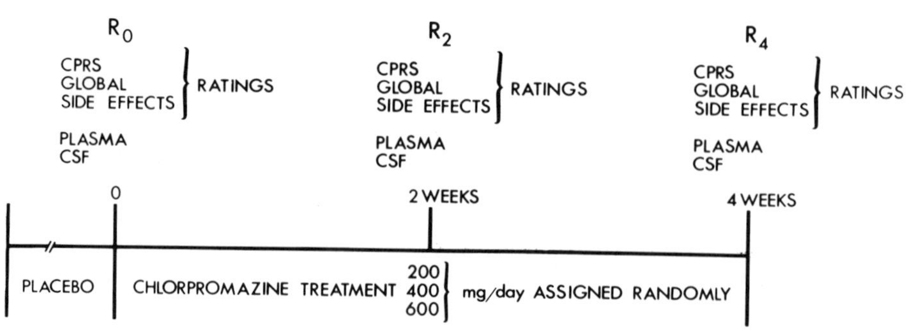

Figure 8 Protocol for chlorpromazine study. (From Ref. 37.)

The design of the experiment is shown in Fig. 8. The patients, not treated with any neuroleptic drug during the month preceding the study, were assigned on a double-blind basis to one of three doses of CPZ: 200, 400, or 600 mg/day. Each patient was examined before as well as 2 and 4 weeks after the initiation of drug administration. The selected dose range is empirically considered to be appropriate for schizophrenic patients [31]. This type of rigorous experimental approach has not been previously used with drug-treated psychotic patients. Such a double-blind dose response study should be the optimal design for the analysis of possible relationships between clinical, biochemical, and pharmacokinetic variables. The use of three fixed dose levels should result in great inter-individual variation in CPZ concentrations in the body fluids, thereby optimizing the possibility for disclosing realtionships between the drug concentrations and clinical and biochemical effects.

III. CLINICAL AND EXPERIMENTAL RESULTS

A. Effect of Chlorpromazine Treatment on Monoamine Metabolite Levels in Cerebrospinal Fluid of Psychotic Patients

CPZ treatment induced significant changes in the concentrations of all three monoamine metabolites measured in CSF (Fig. 9). The concentrations of HVA and MOPEG were most consistently altered [17].

The elevation of HVA was consistent with previous data in experimental animals and patients. This effect presumably reflects the blockade of DA receptors in the nigroneostriatal pathway. As seen in Table 1, CPZ dose showed no correlation with HVA concentrations. Inspection of the scatter diagrams relating the various CPZ measures (i.e., dose, dose mg/kg, concentration in plasma, and concentration in CSF) to concentration of HVA in CSF suggests a leveling off of HVA values at high CPZ values. An example of this can be seen in Fig. 10. Here, as in the other scatter plots, if one takes the whole range of CPZ values into account, then the relationship to HVA looks curvilinear. In the low ranges of CPZ values—where the larger number of patients are found (i.e., between 0 and 40 ng/ml in plasma)—the relationship between CPZ and HVA looks linear. Within this range a Pearson's r is significant ($r = .5, P < 0.01$). CPZ concentrations in plasma and CSF show significant correlation to HVA levels after 2 weeks of treatment despite this tendency for leveling off at the higher values of CPZ. At the 4-week testing, however, these correlations disappeared. The results indicate that the CPZ concentration directly influences the rate of DA metabolism in the central nervous system. Taking also into account the concentrations of the active CPZ metabolites, nor_1-CPZ and 7-OH-CPZ, did not result in higher

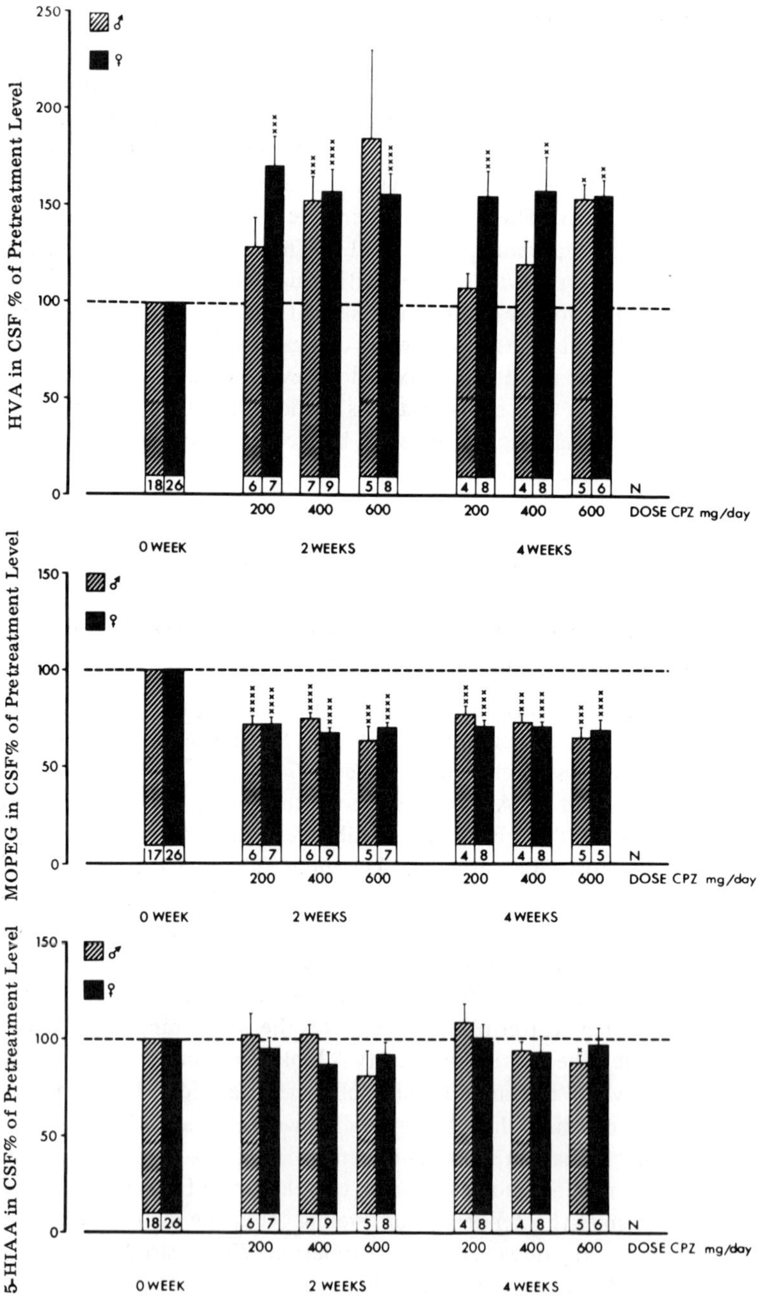

Figure 9 Effects of CPZ treatment on HVA, MOPEG, and 5-HIAA concentrations in the CSF of psychotic patients. The blocks represent means and standard errors. The asterisks mark significant differences from pretreatment levels. (From Ref. 17, by permission of Munksgaard International Publishers, Ltd., Copenhagen, Denmark.)

Table 1 Relationship between Pharmacokinetic Data and HVA Levels in CSF of CPZ-Treated Psychotic Patients

	2 weeks			4 weeks		
Sex:	M + F	M	F	M + F	M	F
n:	30	12	18	23	9	14
CPZ dose (mg)	.13	.33	.04	.16	.56	.06
CPZ dose (mg/kg)	.16	.51	−.08	.17	.66*	−.01
CPZ conc. in plasma	.44***	.48	.53**	.31	.49	.21
CPZ conc. in CSF	.52***	.41	.54**	.26	.27	.22

Note 1: n represents minimum number of patients.
Note 2: Pearson's product-moment correlation: $*P < .05$; $**P < .02$; $***P < .01$.
Source: Ref. 55.

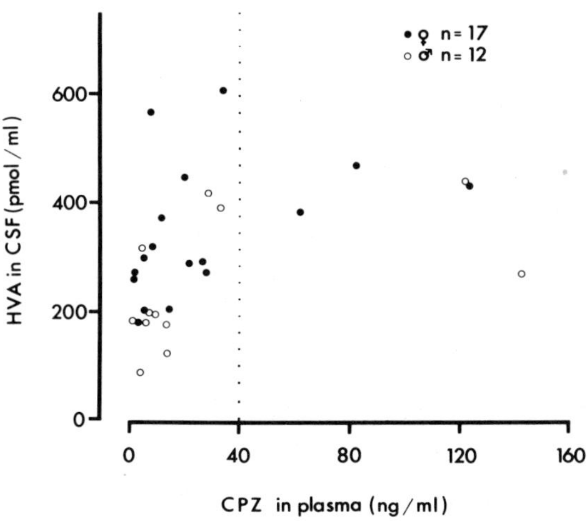

Figure 10 Scatter diagram showing relationship between CPZ concentration in plasma and HVA concentration in CSF from patients treated with CPZ for 2 weeks.

correlations, supporting the view that the unchanged CPZ molecule is the major determinant for the effect of drug treatment on the DA metabolism.

The MOPEG concentration declined (Fig. 9), which was opposite to what is usually found in animal experiments [15,36]. The lack of correlation between the CPZ concentrations and the MOPEG concentration (Table 2) contradicts the view that this effect is directly mediated by the CPZ molecule. Neither were the

Table 2 Relationship between Pharmacokinetic Data and Change in MOPEG Levels in CSF of CPZ-Treated Psychotic Patients

	2 weeks			4 weeks		
Sex:	M + F	M	F	M + F	M	F
n:	29	12	17	23	9	14
CPZ dose (mg)	.22	.40	.05	.33	.51	.20
CPZ dose (mg/kg)	.12	.21	.07	.21	.20	.24
CPZ conc. in plasma	.17	.11	.30	.06	-.04	.13
CPZ conc. in CSF	.22	.09	.38	.16	.15	.18

Note 1: n represents minimum number of patients.
Note 2: Pearson's product-moment correlation.
Source: Ref. 55.

active CPZ metabolites correlated to the MOPEG change. Thus the mechanism for the MOPEG change will have to be elucidated in future studies.

The concentration of 5-HIAA in CSF was reduced by CPZ treatment (Fig. 9). This effect also tended to be correlated to the CPZ concentrations in the body fluids. However, the correlation coefficients were generally lower than the correlations between HVA and CPZ. Since the concentrations of HVA and 5-HIAA both before and during CPZ treatment were significantly correlated [17], a correlation between 5-HIAA and CPZ was expected. The correlations between the concentrations of the two acid metabolites may be related to their common mechanism for transport out of the CSF.

B. Effect of Chlorpromazine Treatment on Prolactin Levels in Cerebrospinal Fluid and Plasma of Psychotic Patients

There was a marked elevation of the prolactin concentrations in both CSF and plasma during CPZ treatment. The prolactin elevation was related to the dose of CPZ administered. Women showed a significantly greater elevation than the men (Fig. 11).

The prolactin elevations were significantly correlated with both plasma and CSF concentrations of CPZ (Fig. 12). Taking into account the active CPZ metabolites did not increase the correlation with prolactin levels. In contrast to the HVA data, the prolactin elevation was highly correlated also to the dose of CPZ administered regardless whether this was expressed in mg/day or mg/body weight per day.

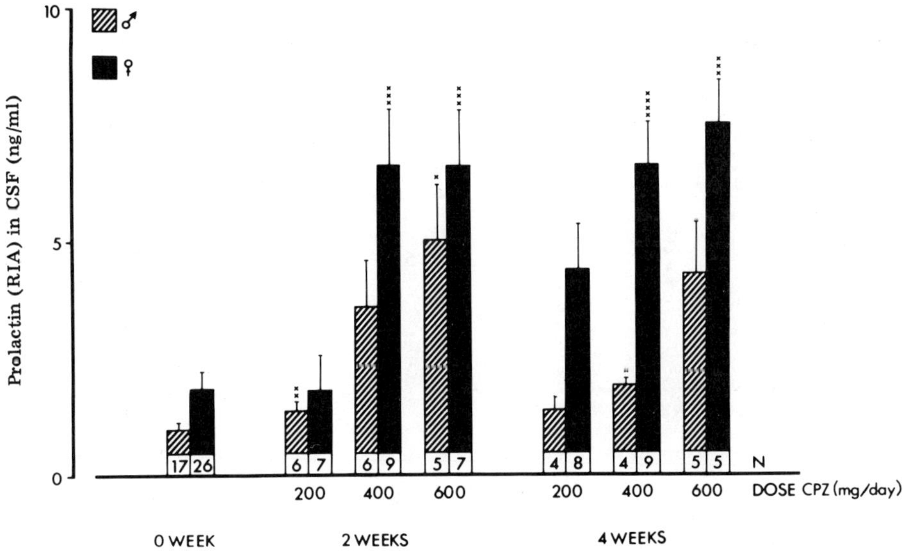

Figure 11 Effect of CPZ treatment on prolactin levels in CSF of psychotic patients. The blocks represent means and standard errors. The asterisks mark significant change from pretreatment levels. (From Ref. 48.)

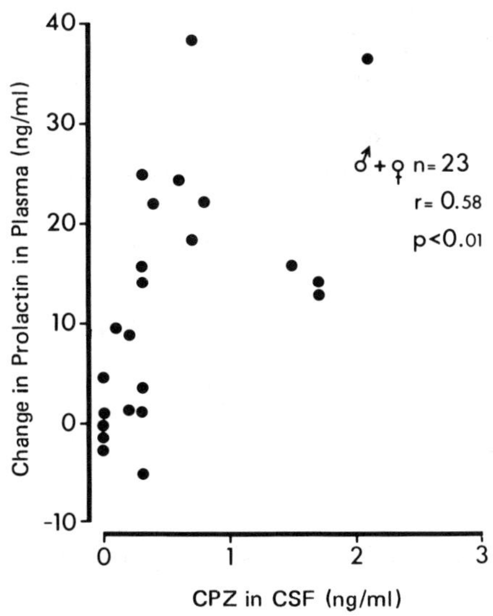

Figure 12 Relationships between change in prolactin in plasma and concentration of CPZ in CSF of psychotic patients after 4 weeks of treatment.

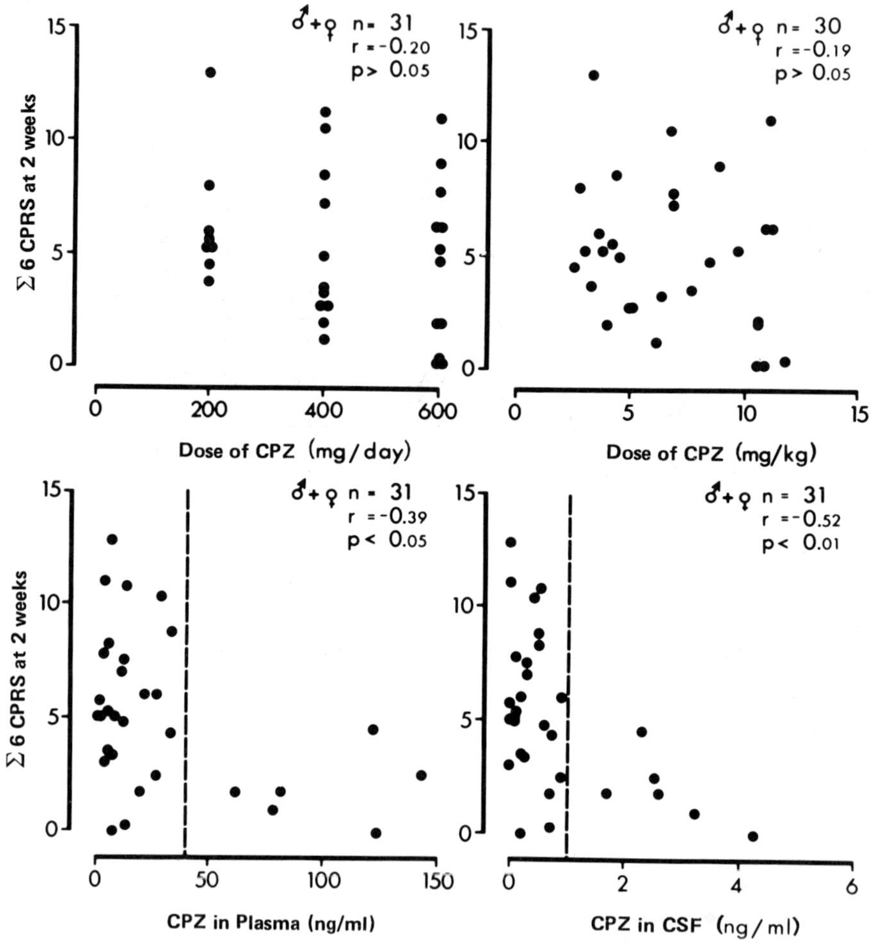

Figure 13 Relationships between pharmacokinetic data and final morbidity scores; r = Spearman's rank correlation. (From Ref. 51.)

C. Effect of Chlorpromazine Treatment on Psychotic Morbidity

There was a marked reduction of psychotic morbidity as measured by the CPRS scale in the CPZ-treated patients. The reduction in morbidity after 2 weeks of CPZ treatment was significantly related to both plasma and CSF concentration of CPZ (Fig. 13). At this time interval there were no significant correlations to the dosage of CPZ administered. After 4 weeks' treatment neither dose nor concentrations of CPZ were related to morbidity. This disappearance of the relationship may have been partly due to the dropout of some patients with high CPZ concentrations and excellent improvement between 2 and 4 weeks' treatment. However, the diagrams also indicated that a real change in the relationship between CPZ concentrations and final morbidity took place between 2 and 4 weeks' treatment. Thus a greater number of patients with low CPZ concentrations reached a high degree of improvement after 4 weeks' treatment. This finding may indicate that between 2 and 4 weeks of CPZ treatment additional factors besides the CPZ concentrations in the body fluids are responsible for the psychotic improvement in patients. Summation of the concentrations of CPZ and the active metabolites did not appreciably improve the correlations, indicating an only minor role, if any, of the active metabolites in the therapeutic response.

D. Side Effects in Chlorpromazine-Treated Psychotic Patients

A number of side effects, including extrapyramidal symptoms and sedation, were recorded in the patients during CPZ treatment [51]. Interestingly, the extrapyramidal symptoms were highly correlated to both the dose of CPZ administered as well as the concentrations of the unchanged drug in plasma and CSF (Table 3).

Sedation also was a fairly common side effect reported during the study. Sedation, while not related to the doses of CPZ, was significantly correlated to both CSF and plasma concentrations of the drug (Table 4).

Table 3 Relationships between Pharmacokinetic Data and Extrapyramidal Side Effects $\Sigma\ 6_{EP}$ in CPZ-Treated Psychotic Patients

	2 weeks			4 weeks		
Sex:	M + F	M	F	M + F	M	F
n:	31	12	19	28	12	16
CPZ dose (mg)	.51***	.39	.56***	.57****	.59*	.54*
CPZ dose (mg/kg)	.36* (n = 30)	.31	.39 (n = 18)	.44**	.49	.38
CPZ conc. in plasma	.50***	.12	.71****	.68**** (n = 26)	.53 (n = 11)	.73*** (n = 15)
CPZ conc. in CSF	.53***	.33	.62***	.71**** (n = 24)	.75** (n = 9)	.73*** (n = 15)

Note: Spearman's rank correlation: $*P < ,05$; $**P < .02$; $***P < .01$; $****P < .001$.
Source: Ref. 51

Table 4 Relationships between Pharmacokinetic Data and Somnolence in CPZ-Treated Psychotic Patients

	2 weeks			4 weeks		
Sex:	M + F	M	F	M + F	M	F
n:	31	12	19	28	12	16
CPZ dose (mg)	.27	.45	.16	.13	.13	.13
CPZ dose (mg/kg)	.15 (n = 30)	.24	.05 (n = 18)	.03	−.02	.11
CPZ conc. in plasma	.31	.20	.41	.46** (n = 26)	.40 (n = 11)	.47 (n = 15)
CPZ conc. in CSF	.44**	.32	.50*	.49** (n = 24)	.77*** (n = 9)	.38 (n = 15)

Note: Spearman's rank correlation: $^{*}P < .05$; $^{**}P < .02$; $^{***}P < .01$.
Source: Ref. 51.

E. Relationships between Biochemical and Clinical Variables in Chlorpromazine-Treated Psychotic Patients

As demonstrated in Fig. 14, there was a significant correlation between the HVA concentration in the CSF and reduction in morbidity after CPZ treatment for 2 weeks. However, the correlation coefficient was rather low. Moreover, such a correlation could not be found after CPZ treatment for 4 weeks. It is possible that the disappearance of the correlation between 2 and 4 weeks is related to the development of tolerance to the HVA-elevating effect of CPZ treatment [56,57]. The development of tolerance in some patients will probably increase the variability in the HVA data, which may explain the disappearance of the relationship between the HVA level and psychotic improvement after 4 weeks.

Similar to the HVA elevation, the 5-HIAA concentration also tended to be positively related to clinical improvement. However, the correlation coefficients were generally lower than those involving the HVA elevation.

Interestingly enough, the MOPEG change in CSF was the biochemical effect that was most consistently and highly correlated with clinical improvement. Thus, as shown in Table 5, there were high positive correlations between the reduction of the MOPEG concentration in CSF and several measures of psychotic morbidity [51]. The correlations occurred both in men and women, and they were apparent after both 2 and 4 weeks' treatment (Fig. 15).

As mentioned previously, the mechanism for the MOPEG reduction is so far not clear. The effect was not correlated to the CPZ concentration (Table 2) or to the sum of concentrations of CPZ and the active metabolites (Table 6).

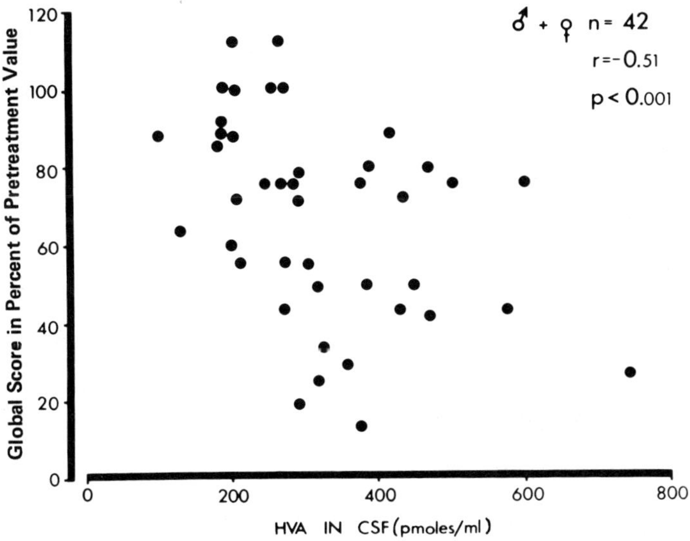

Figure 14 Relationship between HVA in CSF and global morbidity score after 2 weeks of CPZ treatment. (From Ref. 37.)

Table 5 Relationship between Reduction in MOPEG Level and Reduction in Morbidity Scores

		MOPEG in CSF					
		2 weeks			4 weeks		
	Sex:	M + F	M	F	M + F	M	F
Morbidity score	n:	40	17	23	34	13	21
Σ 10		.51****	.70	.31	.51***	.52	.43
Σ 7_R		.42***	.67***	.26	.41***	.73***	.23
Σ6		.43***	.51*	.24	.57****	.45	.62***
Global score		.23	.28	.16	.30	.04	.41

Note: Spearman's rank correlation: *$P < .05$; ***$P < .01$; ****$P < .001$.
Source: Ref. 37.

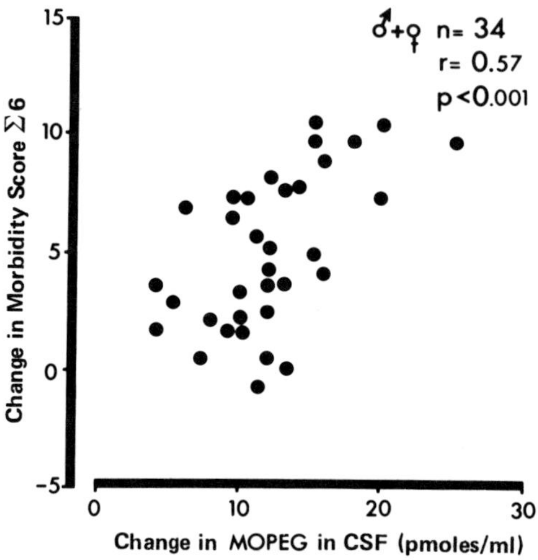

Figure 15 Correlation between change in MOPEG level in CSF and morbidity score Σ 6 (CPRS) after 4 weeks of CPZ treatment; r = Spearman's rank correlation. (From Ref. 37.)

However, the change in MOPEG appears to be a real pharmacological effect of CPZ treatment since the MOPEG concentrations at the end of treatment were significantly lower in the CPZ-treated patients than in a group of healthy volunteers examined (unpublished data). There was no correlation between reduction in motor activity and the reduction in MOPEG concentrations in CSF [37]. Therefore, the data may indicate that CPZ treatment results in a specific alteration of central NE metabolism, an effect which is fairly highly correlated to clinical improvement. The demonstration of this relationship may suggest that

Table 6 Relationship between MOPEG Levels in CSF and CPZ in Plasma and Sum-CPZ (CPZ + Nor_1–CPZ + 7-OH-CPZ) in Plasma of Psychotic Patients

	2 weeks			4 weeks		
Sex:	M + F	M	F	M + F	M	F
CPZ	.19 (n = 29)	.11 (n = 12)	.32 (n = 17)	.24 (n = 23)	.53 (n = 9)	.07 (n = 14)
Sum-CPZ	.12 (n = 24)	.01 (n = 12)	.33 (n = 12)	.14 (n = 25)	.51 (n = 9)	–.04 (n = 16)

Note: Pearson's product-moment correlation.

an alteration of central noradrenergic transmission is involved in the antipsychotic effect of CPZ treatment. The results may alternatively be interpreted as a reflection of an indirect normalization of an abberant noradrenergic transmission in psychotic patients treated with CPZ. In fact, several of the psychotic patients had supranormal MOPEG concentrations in the CSF at the beginning of treatment (unpublished data). Whatever the mechanism for the high correlation between the reduction in morbidity and the reduction of MOPEG concentrations in CSF, its high consistency recommends its further exploration.

F. Relationships between Prolactin Concentrations and Psychotic Morbidity in Chlorpromazine-Treated Patients

There were fairly high correlations between the prolactin concentrations in plasma and CSF and the reduction in psychotic morbidity in CPZ-treated men after treatment for both 2 and 4 weeks. The lack of such a relationship in the CPZ-treated women may be due to the high variability in estrogen secretion in the group of psychotic patients examined in this study. Prolactin secretion has been shown to be markedly influenced by estrogen secretion [58]. The relationship between prolactin concentrations and psychotic morbidity in men as demonstrated in Fig. 16 indicates that a prolactin elevation in plasma above 15 ng/ml is required for obtaining a satisfactory reduction of psychotic morbidity in CPZ-treated schizophrenic men.

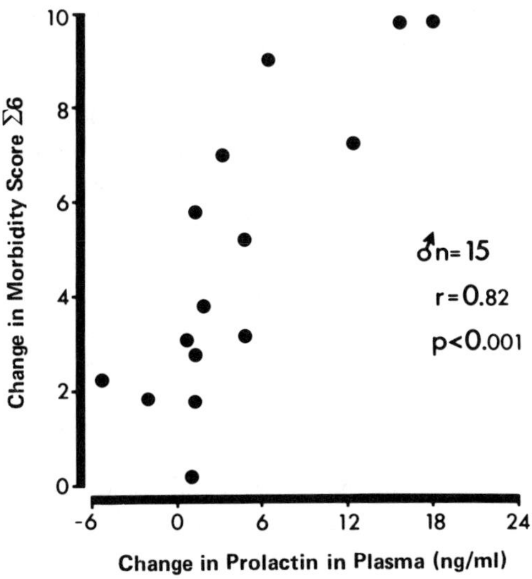

Figure 16 Correlation in men between change in prolactin in plasma and morbidity score Σ 6 (CPRS) after 4 weeks of CPZ treatment; r = Spearman's rank correlation. (From Ref. 37.)

IV. CONCLUDING REMARKS

A. Relationships between Biochemical Variables and Clinical Response

The present study demonstrated that several biochemical variables are reproducibly influenced in CPZ-treated patients. Thus the concentrations of HVA, 5-HIAA, and MOPEG in CSF are significantly altered by the treatment. Prolactin concentrations both in plasma and CSF are also consistently elevated during the treatment. In the earlier phase of treatment, i.e., after 2 weeks, the HVA concentration in CSF was significantly correlated to the CPZ concentration in the body fluids. The data indicated a curvilinear relationship. This supports the view that the CPZ molecule is directly influential in the alteration of central DA metabolism during CPZ treatment in man. The doses of CPZ administered were not significantly correlated to the HVA concentration. Accordingly, the results indicate that the CPZ concentrations in the body fluids are more useful predictors than the doses for the evaluation of the effect on central DA metabolism during CPZ treatment. Taking into account also the two active metabolites did not appreciably alter the results.

The prolactin elevations in plasma and CSF were significantly correlated both with doses and concentrations of CPZ in the body fluids. The prolactin elevation appears to be mediated by DA receptors located both in the hypothalamus and in the pituitary gland, which is situated outside the blood-brain barrier [59]. The high correlation between prolactin levels and both doses and levels of CPZ may support the view of a dominating role of the pituitary DA receptors for the prolactin elevation obtained.

The lack of correlation between the MOPEG change and the CPZ and CPZ-metabolite concentrations in the body fluids is noteworthy. The MOPEG reduction was the most consistent biochemical effect induced in the CPZ-treated patients. There tended to be positive correlations between this effect and the CPZ concentrations in the body fluids, but the correlation coefficients were low and nonsignificant. This lack of correlation indicates that the alteration of the MOPEG concentration may be a secondary effect of CPZ treatment, induced by other biochemical variables affected by the drug.

B. Predictive Value of Different Pharmacokinetic Variables

The present results demonstrated that some of the biochemical and clinical effects of CPZ treatment were more consistently correlated with CPZ concentrations in the body fluids than with the doses of CPZ administered. This held true for the HVA and 5-HIAA concentrations in the CSF. The prolactin concentrations were correlated with CPZ doses and concentrations to about the same extent.

Reduction in psychotic morbidity was not related to the doses of CPZ administered during any phase of the treatment. However, after 2 weeks the CPZ concentration in the plasma and to an even higher extent in the CSF were significantly correlated with improvement. Patients with CPZ concentrations in the CSF above 1 ng/ml showed a significantly greater reduction in morbidity than patients with a lower concentration. These results support the view that CPZ concentrations in the body fluids but not doses have a predictive value for therapeutic outcome, at least during the initial phases of treatment. The lack of correlation in the later phases of treatment may indicate that factors other than the CPZ concentration in the body fluids are influential in the therapeutic effect of CPZ treatment. Taking also the active CPZ metabolites into account did not increase the possibility to predict therapeutic outcome.

Central DA blockade may be just one of several factors in the mechanism of CPZ's antipsychotic effect. This factor may be most important in the early phases of treatment and is directly related to the concentration of the drug in both plasma and CSF. Later secondary phenomena may come into play that may be less directly related to the CPZ concentrations in the body fluids. These later mechanisms may be related to the demonstrated alteration of central noradrenergic metabolism. These may also be unrelated and hitherto unclarified effects of CPZ.

The present results thus demonstrated that some biochemical and clinical effects of CPZ treatment may be significantly related to CPZ concentrations in the body fluids. However, the relationships could only be demonstrated during the early phases of treatment, and the correlation coefficients were generally of a low order, explaining only 20-40% of the variance observed. These low correlation coefficients have little practical value for the treatment of the individual patient.

It should be noted that the pharmacokinetic variables studied were obtained at one predetermined time point (8:00 A.M.). Since CPZ has a fairly short half-life (on the order of 8-33 h), fairly marked shanges in the tissue concentration of the drug occurred during the day [44] (see also Chap. 10 of this volume). Ideally one should measure the area under the CPZ curve (AUC) during the day and study its relationship to the different biochemical and clinical effects. However, for practical purposes this will not be possible. Fairly low correlation coefficients were obtained here between effects and the plasma concentration of the drug at 8:00 A.M. We have demonstrated that the morning values for the CPZ concentrations in the plasma are highly correlated to the area under the curve for the CPZ concentration during the day [44]. Therefore it is unlikely that the AUC would have been better correlated to therapeutic outcome. It seems more probable that a great variation in interpatient biochemistry and/or pathophysiology explains the low correlation coefficients obtained.

Even if only fairly low correlations were found between different pharmacokinetic and biochemical variables and the clinical responses to CPZ treatment, the study demonstrated new and interesting relationships which have to be further explored. The data indicated that the relationships between drug concentrations and drug effects may vary with time. Moreover, they suggested the importance of noradrenergic mechanisms in addition to the alteration of central dopaminergic metabolism for the mechanism of action of CPZ treatment. The combined analysis of clinical, biochemical, and pharmacokinetic variables as performed here will turn out to be a fruitful approach for the analysis of the mechanism for the psychotherapeutic effect of CPZ treatment in schizophrenic patients.

REFERENCES

1. J. Delay, P. Deniker, and M. Harl, Traitement des états d'excitation et d'agitation par une methode medicamenteuse derivée de l'hibernotherapie. *Ann. Med. Psychol.* (Paris) *110:*267-273, 1952.
2. J. Hammon, J. Paraire, and J. Velluz, Remarques sur l'action du 4560 RP sur l'agitation maniaque. *Ann. Med. Psychol.* (Paris) *110:*331, 1952.
3. S. H. Curry, J. H. L. Marshall, J. M. Davis, and D. S. Janowsky, Factors affecting chlorpromazine plasma levels in psychiatric patients. *Arch. Gen. Psychiatry 22:*209–215, 1970.
4. L. Rivera-Calimlim, L. Castaneda, and L. Lasagna, Effects of mode of managements on plasma chlorpromazine in psychiatric patients. *Clin. Pharmacol. Ther. 14:*978, 1973.
5. B. Sakalis, S. H. Curry, G. P. Mould, and M. H. Lader, Physiologic and clinical effects of chlorpromazine and their relationship to plasma level. *Clin. Pharmacol. Ther. 13:*931, 1972.
6. T. Kolakowska, D. H. Wilcs, M. G. Gelder, and A. S. McNeilly, Clinical significance of plasma chlorpromazine levels, II: Plasma levels of the drug, some of its metabolites, and prolactin in patients receiving long-term phenothiazine treatment. *Psychopharmacology 49:*101, 1976.
7. A. Carlsson and M. Lindqvist, Effect of chlorpromazine or haloperidol on formation of 3-methoxytyramine and normetanephrine in mouse brain. *Acta Pharmacol. Toxicol. 20:*140–144, 1963.
8. J. M. van Rossum, The significance of dopamine-receptor blockade for the mechanism of action of neuroleptic drugs. *Arch. Int. Pharmacodyn. 160:*492, 1966.
9. H. Nybäck and G. Sedvall, Effect of chlorpromazine on accumulation and disappearance of catecholamines formed from C^{14}-tyrosine in the brain. *J. Pharmacol. Exp. Ther. 162:*294, 1968.
10. J. W. Kebabian, G. L. Petzold, and P. Greengard, Dopamine-sensitive adenylate cyclase in caudate nucleus of rat brain, and its similarity to the "dopamine receptor." *Proc. Nat. Acad. Sci. U.S. 69:*2145, 1972.

11. B. S. Bunney, J. R. Walters, R. H. Roth, and G. K. Aghajanian, Dopaminergic neurons: Effect of antipsychotic drugs and amphetamine on single cell activity. *J. Pharmacol. Exp. Ther. 185:*560-571, 1973.
12. P. Seeman, J. Chau-Wong, J. Tedesco, and K. Wong, Brain receptors for antipsychotic drugs and dopamine: Direct binding assays. *Proc. Nat. Acad. Sci. U.S. 72:*4376, 1975.
13. I. Creese, D. R. Burt, and S. H. Snyder, Dopamine receptor binding: Differentiation of agonist and antagonist states with ^{3}H-dopamine and ^{3}H-haloperidol. *Life Sci. 17:*993, 1975.
14. N. E. Andén, B. E. Roos, and B. Werdinius, Effects of chlorpromazine haloperidol and reserpine on the levels of phenolic acids in rabbit corpus striatum. *Life Sci. 3:*149-158, 1964.
15. H. H. Keller, G. Bartholini, and A. Pletscher, Increase of 3-methoxy-4-hydroxyphenylethylene glycol in rat brain by neuroleptic drugs. *Eur. J. Pharmacol. 23:*183, 1973.
16. G. Sedvall, B. Fyrö, H. Nybäck, F.-A. Wiesel, and B. Wode-Helgodt, Mass fragmentometric determination of homovanillic acid in lumbar cerebrospinal fluid of schizophrenic patients during treatment with antipsychotic drugs. *J. Psychiatr. Res. 11:*75-80, 1974.
17. B. Wode-Helgodt, B. Fyrö, B. Gullberg, and G. Sedvall, Effect of chlorpromazine treatment on monoamine metabolite levels in cerebrospinal fluid of psychotic patients. *Acta Psychiatr. Scand. 56:*129-142, 1977.
18. L. Bjerkenstedt, B. Gullberg, C. Härnryd, and G. Sedvall, Monoamine metabolite levels in cerebrospinal fluid of psychotic women treated with melperone or thiothixene. *Arch. Psychiatr. Nervenkr. 224:*107-118, 1977.
19. A. G. Frantz and D. L. Kleinberg, Prolactin: Evidence that it is separate from growth hormone in human blood. *Science 170:*745, 1970.
20. A. G. Frantz, Catecholamines and the control of prolactin secretion in humans. *Progr. Brain. Res. 39:*311, 1973.
21. J. A. Clemens, E. B. Smalstig, and B. D. Sawyer, Antipsychotic drugs stimulate prolactin release. *Psychopharmacologia* (Berlin) *40*:123-127, 1974.
22. G. Sedvall, G. Alfredsson, P. Eneroth, B. Fyrö, C. Härnryd, C.-G. Swahn, F.-A. Wiesel, and B. Wode-Helgodt, Selective effects of psychoactive drugs on levels of monoamine metabolites and prolactin in cerebrospinal fluid of psychiatric patients. In *Proceedings of the VI Int. Congr. Pharmacol. Helsinki,* vol. 3, 1975.
23. R. M. MacLeod and I. S. Login, Regulation of prolactin secretion through dopamine, serotonin, and the cerebrospinal fluid. *Adv. Biochem. Psychopharmacol. 16:*147-157, 1977.
24. S. H. Snyder, S. P. Banerjee, H. I. Yamamura, and D. Greenberg, Drugs, neurotransmitters, and schizophrenia. *Science 184:*1243, 1974.
25. A. Carlsson, Does dopamine have a role in schizophrenia? *Biol. Psychiatry 13:*3-21, 1978.
26. F. A. Wiesel, G. Alfredsson, V. Likwornik, and G. Sedvall, A relation between drug concentrations in brain and striatal homovanillic acid levels in chlorpromazine treated rats. *Life Sci. 16:*1145-1156, 1975.

27. R. Öhman, M. Larsson, I. M. Nilsson, J. Engel, and A. Carlsson, Neurometabolic and behavioral effects of haloperidol in relation to drug levels in serum and brain. *Naunyn-Schmiedeberg's Arch. Pharmakol. Exp. Pathol. 299:*105-114, 1977.
28. S. H. Curry, Plasma protein binding of chlorpromazine. *J. Pharm. Pharmacol. 22:*193-197, 1970.
29. S. H. Curry, Relation between binding to plasma protein, apparent volume of distribution, and rate constants of disposition and elimination for chlorpromazine in three species. *J. Pharm. Pharmacol. 24:*818-819, 1972.
30. B. Alexanderson and O. Borgå, Interindividual differences in plasma protein binding of nortriptyline in man: A twin study. *Eur. J. Clin. Pharmacol. 4:*196-200, 1972.
31. D. F. Klein and J. M. Davis, *Diagnosis and Drug Treatment of Psychiatric Disorders.* Baltimore, Williams and Wilkins, 1969.
32. I. S. Forrest, C. J. Carr, and E. Usdin, eds., Phenothiazine and structurally related drugs. *Adv. Biochem. Psychopharmacol. 9.* New York, Raven Press, 1974.
33. S. H. Curry, Chlorpromazine plasma levels and effects. *Arch. Gen. Psychiatry 22:*289, 1970.
34. G. Alfredsson and G. Sedvall, Mass fragmentographic analysis of chlorpromazine in human plasma. In *Wenner-Gren Center Int. Symp. Series 25:*367-372. Oxford, Pergamon Press, 1976.
35. B. Holmstedt and L. Palmer, Mass fragmentography: Principles, advantages, and future possibilities. *Adv. Biochem. Psychopharmacol. 7:*1, 1973.
36. G. Alfredsson, B. Wode-Helgodt, and G. Sedvall, A mass fragmentographic method for the determination of chlorpromazine and two of its active metabolites in human plasma and CSF. *Psychopharmacology 48:*123-131, 1976.
37. B. Wode-Helgodt, Clinical and biochemical effects of chlorpromazine in psychotic patients. Doctoral thesis, Karolinska Institutet, Stockholm, Sweden, 1977.
38. I. S. Forrest and D. E. Green, Phenothiazines: Metabolism and analytical detection. *J. Forensic Sci. 17:*592-617, 1972.
39. J. Dailey, G. Sedvall, and B. Sjöqvist, Effect of chlorpromazine and some of its metabolites on the accumulation of homovanillic acid in brain of mice. *J. Pharm. Pharmacol. 24:*580-581, 1972.
40. H. Nybäck and G. Sedvall, Effect of chlorpromazine and some of its metabolites on synthesis and turnover of catecholamines formed from ^{14}C-tyrosine in mouse brain. *Psychopharmacologia* (Berlin) *26:*155, 1972.
41. R. S. Miller and L. L. Iversen, Effect of chlorpromazine and some of its metabolites on the dopamine-sensitive adenylate cyclase of rat brain striatum. *J. Pharm. Pharmacol. 25:*142-144, 1974.
42. S. H. Curry and J. H. L. Marshall, Plasma levels of chlorpromazine and some of its relatively non-polar metabolites in psychiatric patients. *Life Sci. 7:*9-17, 1968.

43. O. T. Phillipson, J. M. McKeown, J. Baker, and A. F. Healey, Correlation between plasma chlorpromazine and its metabolites and clinical ratings in patients with acute relapse of schizophrenia and paranoid psychosis. *Brit. J. Psychiatry 131:*172, 1977.
44. B. Wode-Helgodt, G. Alfredsson, and G. Sedvall, Concentrations of chlorpromazine and two of its active metabolites in CSF and plasma of drug treated patients. To be submitted to *Psychopharmacology*, 1979.
45. G. Alfredsson, F. A. Wiesel, and P. Skett, Levels of chlorpromazine and its active metabolites in rat brain and the relationship to central monoamine metabolism and prolactin secretion. *Psychopharmacology 53:*13–18, 1977.
46. C. G. Swahn, B. Sandgärde, F. A. Wiesel, and G. Sedvall, Simultaneous determination of the three major monoamine metabolites in brain tissue and body fluids by a mass fragmentographic method. *Psychopharmacology 48:*147–152, 1976.
47. F. A. J. Muskiet, H. J. Jeuring, J. Korf, G. Sedvall, B. H. C. Westerink, A. W. Teelken, and B. G. Wolthers, Correlations between fluorimetric and mass fragmentographic methods for the determination of 3-methoxy-4-hydroxyphenylacetic acid and 3-methoxy-4-hydroxyphenylethylene glycol in cerebrospinal fluid. *Clin. Chem.*, in press, 1978.
48. B. Wode-Helgodt, P. Eneroth, B. Fyrö, B. Gullberg, and G. Sedvall, Effect of chlorpromazine treatment of prolactin levels in cerebrospinal fluid and plasma of psychotic patients. *Acta Psychiatr. Scand. 56:*280–293, 1977.
49. L. Bjerkenstedt, P. Eneroth, C. Härnryd, and G. Sedvall, Effects of melperone and thiothixene on prolactin levels in cerebrospinal fluid and plasma of psychotic women. *Arch. Psychiatr. Nervenkr. 224:*281–293, 1977.
50. M. Åsberg, S. A. Montgomery, C. Perris, D. Schalling, and G. Sedvall, A comprehensive psychopathological rating scale. *Acta Psychiatr. Scand., Suppl. 271*, 1978.
51. B. Wode-Helgodt, S. Borg, B. Fyrö, and G. Sedvall, Clinical effects and drug concentrations in plasma and cerebrospinal fluid in psychotic patients treated with fixed doses of chlorpromazine. *Acta Psychiatr. Scand. 58:*1978.
52. G. M. Simpson and J. W. S. Angus, A rating scale for extrapyramidal side effects. *Acta Psychiatr. Scand., Suppl. 212:*11, 1970.
53. L. Bjerkenstedt, C. Härnryd, V. Grimm, B. Gullberg, and G. Sedvall, A double-blind comparison of melperone and thiothixene in psychotic women using a new rating scale, the CPRS. *Arch. Psychiatr. Nervenkr.*, in press, 1978.
54. World Health Organization, *The International Pilot Study of Schizophrenia,* Geneva, 1973.
55. G. Sedvall, L. Bjerkenstedt, H. Nybäck, and B. Wode-Helgodt, The biochemical pharmacology of chlorpromazine treatment. In *Proceedings of the 7th Int. Congr. Pharmacol.*, Paris, Pergamon Press, 1978.
56. R. M. Post and F. K. Goodwin, Time-dependent effects of pheno-

thiazines on dopamine turnover in psychiatric patients. *Science 190:* 488-489, 1975.

57. I. Møller-Nielsen, A. V. Christensen, and B. Fjälland, Receptor blockade and receptor supersensitivity following neuroleptic treatment. In *Wenner-Gren Center Int. Symp. Series 25:*257-260. Oxford, Pergamon Press, 1976.

58. E. Wiedeman, E. Schwartz, and A. G. Frantz, Acute and chronic estrogen effects upon serum somatomedin activity, growth hormone, and prolactin in man. *J. Clin. Endocrinol. Metab. 42:*942, 1976.

59. G. M. Besser, J. A. H. Wass, T. Yeo, G. Delitala, A. Jones, W. A. Stubbs, and M. O. Thorner, Clinical neuroendocrine relationships in normal and disordered prolactin secretion. In *The Peptide Neuron,* New York, Plenum, 1978.

13

Benzodiazepine Pharamacokinetics, Plasma Levels, and Clinical Response

Ann Fulton, Kay P. Maguire, Trevor R. Norman, and Jeremy M. E. Wurm / *Department of Psychiatry, University of Melbourne, Parkville, Victoria, Australia*

I. INTRODUCTION

The benzodiazepines (see Fig. 1) have been widely accepted in clinical practice for the treatment of specific anxiety conditions. They have largely replaced older drugs, such as meprobamate, which were used as antianxiety agents. Some benzodiazepines, e.g., nitrazepam and flurazepam, are used as hypnotics.

Controlled clinical trials have demonstrated that, when given in adequate doses, each of the benzodiazepine antianxiety agents is consistently more effective than placebo in anxious nonpsychotic patients [1]. Clinically meaningful differences between the benzodiazepines have also been demonstrated, based on pharmacokinetic and plasma level measurements [2]. A review of the pharmacokinetics and metabolism of the more widely used benzodiazepines—chlordiazepoxide, diazepam, and chlorazepate—is presented here. The relationship between plasma levels of these drugs and clinical response, insofar as it is known, is also reviewed. Plasma level clinical response relationships for the psychotropic drugs have become an important area of research in recent years, as analytical techniques for drug measurement have become more refined.

II. CHLORDIAZEPOXIDE

A. Structure and Metabolism

Chlordiazepoxide chemically is 7-chloro-2-(methylamino)-5-phenyl-3H-1,4-benzodiazepine-4-oxide. The compound was introduced in 1960 [3] as an adjunct in the management of anxiety, and was the first of the benzodiazepine tranquilizers. Its acceptance by clinicians has resulted in the fact that 22.7 million prescriptions for the drug were filled by American retail pharmacies in 1973 [4].

Autoradiographic assay of intravenously injected [^{14}C] chlordiazepoxide in mice has revealed that the drug was rapidly concentrated in the brain, liver, kidney, myocardium, and skeletal muscles [5]. In the rat, chlordiazepoxide (CDX) was found to be distributed into all the tissues [6]. The metabolism of CDX in rats appeared to vary from the similar patterns observed in the dog and

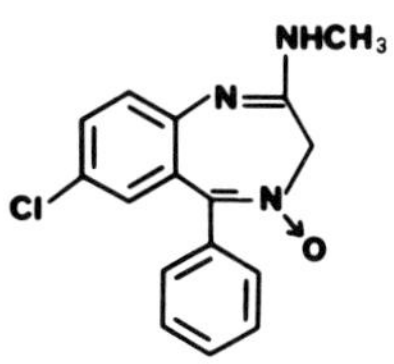

CHLORDIAZEPOXIDE

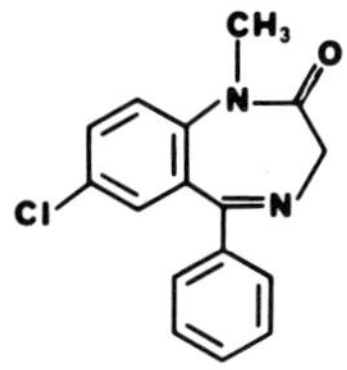

DIAZEPAM

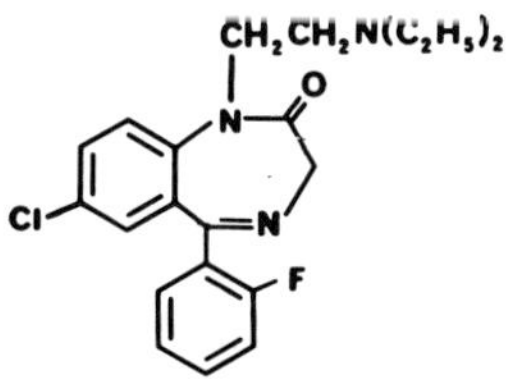

FLURAZEPAM

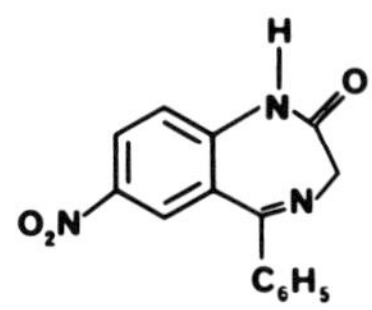

NITRAZEPAM

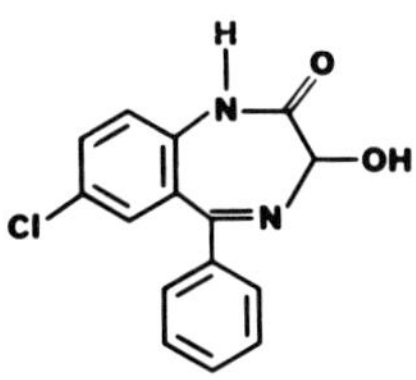

OXAZEPAM

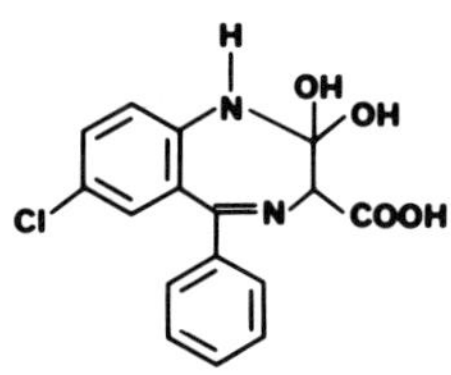

CHLORAZEPATE

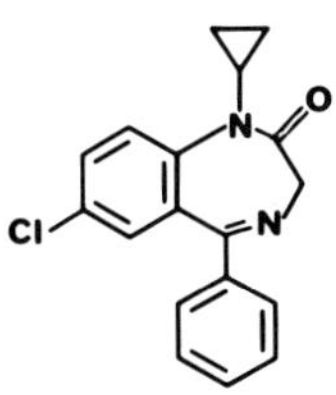

PRAZEPAM

Figure 1 Structures of some benzodiazepines

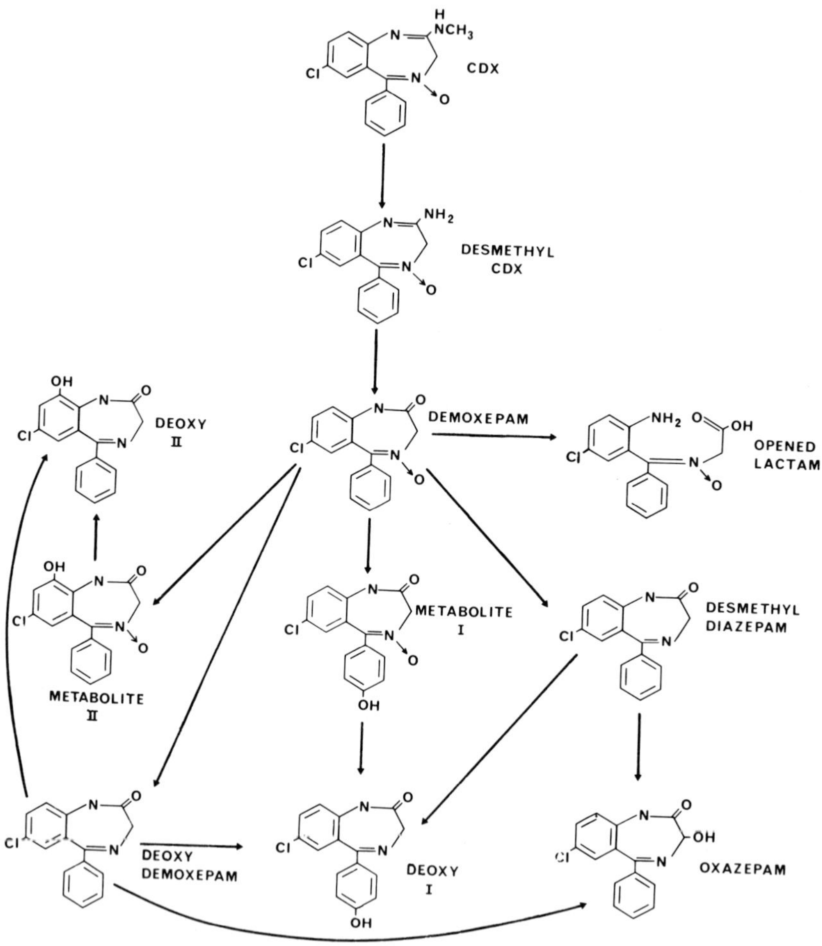

Figure 2 Metabolism of chlordiazepoxide.

in humans, since an unidentified metabolite was produced instead of N-desmethyl-chlordiazepoxide. Demethylation of CDX has been reported in the rat following in vitro and in vivo investigations [7], and the formation of N-desmethylchlor-diazepoxide has also been observed in the dog [7-12] and in humans [1,4,6-9, 11-23]. Other studies have postulated that demoxepam (7-chloro-1,3-dihydro-

5-phenyl-2H-1,4-benzodiazepine-2-one-4-oxide) is formed in dogs [9-12] and in man [1,6,8,9,11-14,19-22]. Demoxepam biotransformation may lead to the "opened lactam" amino acid N-(2-amino-5-chloro-phenylbenzylidene)glycine N-oxide [1,6,7,11,21,24], to N-desoxydemoxepam [8,11,13,24], or to desmethyldiazepam [1,19-22,25]. The conversion of N-desoxydemoxepam to oxazepam has been postulated in the dog [24] and in man [11,14], and oxazepam excretion was confirmed in the dog [10], while the formation of oxazepam from desmethyldiazepam has been described in humans [1,19,21]. Oxazepam may also give rise to 3-hydroxy metabolites, according to one study [13]. Demoxepam is also thought to give rise to metabolite I [7-chloro-1,3-dihydro-5-(4-hydroxyphenyl)-2H-1,4-benzodiazepin-2-one-4-oxide] in man [1,11,13] and dog [24], which may undergo cleavage to form the N-desoxyphenol known as desoxy I [1,11,24]. Metabolite II (7-chloro-1,3-dihydro-9-hydroxy-5-phenyl-2H-1,4-benzodiazepin-2-one-4-oxide) may similarly arise in the dog [24] and in humans [1,11,13], from which the corresponding N-desoxyphenol desoxy II may be formed [1,11,24]. It has been proposed that in the dog, N-desoxydemoxepam might be converted to deoxy I or deoxy II [24]. Deoxy I may also be metabolized from desmethyldiazepam [1].

The metabolic pathways proposed for the metabolites of CDX are depicted in Fig. 2.

B. Single-Dose Pharmacokinetics

1. Animal Studies

A six-compartment open-system pharmacokinetic model has been postulated [9] following a series of three separate intravenous administrations of chlordiazepoxide, N-desmethylchlordiazepoxide and demoxepam respectively to each of two dogs. The findings confirmed the pathways proposed in Fig. 1. Oral administration of [^{14}C] CDX to the dog produced a peak plasma level 7 h after ingestion of the labeled drug, with a half-life of 10-14 h, while plasma levels in rats reached maxima 2 h after administration, with half-lives in most tissues of about 4 h [6]. The half-life in rat brain was found to be shorter in this study.

The pharmacokinetics of the CDX metabolite demoxepam have been studied in the dog and a two-compartment model has been postulated [24]. The half-life of the fast disposition rate (α) ranged from 0.1 to 0.2 h, indicating a very rapid transfer of a portion of the drug to the peripheral compartment. The elimination rate (β) was markedly slower, with a half-life ranging from 11 to 16 h. This has also been expressed as 16 ± 2.0 (SE) h as a total half-life for demoxepam in the dog [11].

2. Human Studies

a. Oral Administration. It has been reported [26] that oral administration of 25 mg of CDX hydrochloride produced higher serum CDX levels than intramuscular administration, when serum levels were measured 1 to 2 h after ingestion of the drug. This apparent anomaly may be explicable by slow absorption of CDX from muscle or by the possibility of faster metabolism being associated with the intramuscular mode.

The elimination half-life of CDX has been given as 5-30 h [22], although the mode of administration was not specified, while an overall half-life of 22-24 h was reported after a single dose of 30 mg was orally administered to two healthy volunteers [6]. In a six-patient single-dose crossover study, 20 mg CDX and demoxepam were given orally with an interval of 7 days between the dose of each drug [12]. The half-life of plasma CDX ranged from 6.6 to 28 h, and the half-life of demoxepam had a range of 14 to 95 h, which was alternatively expressed as 45 ± 14 (SE) h [11]. This group believed that the figure of 20-24 h for the half-life of CDX in man was an overestimation [12]. They cited two possible causes, the first being that the assay used [27] was not specific and measured the total levels of CDX and its demethylated metabolite N-desmethylchlordiazepoxide, and the second factor being the increase in metabolite concentration with time.

Several other studies have estimated the absorption half-life ($T_{1/2a}$) of CDX, and the results from these investigations are summarized in Table 1, taken from Ref. 20. The mean CDX absorption half-life has also been estimated at 11 min in a 10-subject single-dose study, which indicated an apparent elimination half-life of 8.4 h after a 25-mg oral dose [17]. A mean bioavailability parameter encompassing the value of 1.0 indicated that chlordiazepoxide was approximately 100% systemically available after an oral dose [8]. The observation that total CDX clearance was consistently less than 1 ml/min/kg indicated that first-pass hepatic extraction was negligible following oral administration [21].

b. Intravenous Administration. The half-life of plasma CDX was reported to be about 16 h, following a study of two subjects who were each given a 100-mg intravenous dose of the drug [7]. A biexponential CDX disappearance curve found in a study of a single female subject revealed an elimination half-life of 13 h and an apparent volume of distribution (V_d) of 0.35 liter/kg [20]. These results were similar to those found in other studies (summarized in Table 2). Triexponential patterns of elimination of intravenously administered CDX have also been reported [4,14,20]. One study reported higher values under this disappearance mode than the elimination half-life of 5 to 36 h encountered with observed biexponential kinetics [4]. In a study of 11 healthy volunteers [14], 6 exhibited biexponential CDX elimination and 5 subjects had triexponential kinetics. Half-lives were 5 to 26 h in the biexponential instances, where the V_d values ranged from 0.2 to 0.45 liter/kg. Males with triexponential elimination had apparent distribution volumes of 0.4 to 0.7 liter/kg, and females had values of 1.4 to 1.5 liters/kg, while the half-life in these subjects ranged from 36 to 96 h. It has been stressed [14,20] that pharmacokinetic studies can underestimate V_d and $T_{1/2}$

Table 1 Absorption Kinetics of Oral Chlordiazepoxide[a]

Reference	Sex and no. of subjects	Age range (years)	Body fluid sampled	Dose (mg)	Peak concentration (μg/ml)	Time of peak concentration (h after dose)	$T_{1/2a}$ (min)
[12]	M,2; F,4	25-43	Plasma	20[b]	NA	NA	NA
[18]	M,4; F,5	18-38	Whole blood	25[c]	(0.76-2.05)	(1.0-12.0)	NA
[8]	M,6	25-29	Plasma	30[c]	NA	NA	32.3 (15.5-57.4)
[39]	M,28	21-30	Whole blood	25[c]	0.86 (0.48-1.25)	(0.5-2.0)	5.5[d]
	M,8	63-74	Whole blood	25[c]	0.69 (0.37-0.98)	3.3 (1.0-8.0)	19.6[d]
[45]	M,8; F,6	21-38	Whole blood	50[c]	1.65 (1.15-2.07)	2.3 (1.0-6.0)	42.6 (19.2-193)

[a]Mean and/or range (in parentheses) of kinetic variables given when appropriate; NA indicates values not available; $T_{1/2a}$ = absorption half-life.
[b]Given as free base
[c]Given as hydrochloride salt.
[d]Based upon across-subject mean data points.

Oral chlordiazepoxide was first assayed by Koechlin and D'Arconte [46].

Table 2 Pharmacokinetics of Intravenous Chlordiazepoxide in Healthy Young Volunteers[a]

Reference	No. of subjects	Age range (years)	Sex	Body fluid sampled	$T_{1/2\alpha}$ (h)	$T_{1/2\beta}$ (h)	V_d (liters/kg)	Clearance (ml/min)	Clearance (ml/min/kg)
[12]	1	NA	M	Plasma	0.06	14.2	0.26	14.5	0.21
[33]	1	23	M	Plasma	0.2	12.1	0.31	22.3	0.30
[8]	6	25-29	M	Plasma	0.25 (0.15-0.61)	9.4 (6.6-13.6)	0.31 (0.27-0.37)	30.2 (17.7-38.8)	0.37 (0.30-0.46)
[15]	7	21-38	M	Whole blood	0.77 (0.25-1.97)	18.4 (9.9-29.1)	0.45 (0.36-0.59)	23.9 (11.8-41.9)	0.32 (0.17-0.50)
	7	24-30	F	Whole blood	1.72 (0.75-3.36)	17.3 (9.1-34.1)	0.58 (0.49-0.67)	28.9 (11.0-49.8)	0.50 (0.19-0.81)
[29]	NA	Under 40	M	Plasma	NA	9.5	NA	27	NA
[47]	14	21-31	M	Plasma	NA	10.0 (4.1-16.4)	0.38 (0.22-0.75)	37.4 (19.8-127.8)	0.54 (0.26-2.16)

[a]Mean and/or range (in parentheses) of kinetic variables given; $T_{1/2\alpha}$ = distribution half-life; $T_{1/2\beta}$ = elimination half-life; V_d = apparent volume of distribution; NA indicates values were not available.

values if sampling periods are too short or assay techniques are not sufficiently sensitive to distinguish between CDX and its metabolites. The latter point is essentially valid since CDX metabolites are thought to have similar pharmacological activity to the parent drug [28].

CDX binding to plasma protein is extensive [19], with 94-97% of the drug being bound in plasma at any time [8,23,29], while the figure has been estimated at 87-88% in dogs [1]. Another study has cited a figure of 87% of CDX bound to human albumin [30], while an estimate of greater than 90% binding has also been suggested [15]. The uptake of CDX into erythrocytes has been shown to be limited [8,15], since values for the apparent volume of distribution based on whole blood are consistently greater than the V_d estimates taken from plasma levels.

c. Intramuscular Administration. The intramuscular mode of administration was found to lead to relatively slow absorption of chlordiazepoxide in man [4,8,19-22,31]. In addition, pain, muscle damage, and creatine phosphokinase level elevation were caused by intramuscular injection [2,4,31] and lower serum CDX levels were attained than through oral ingestion of the drug [26]. The acidity and high osmolarity of the solvent have been suggested as possible reasons for the pain and muscle damage experienced [2].

The slow absorption of intramuscular CDX is in keeping with its physicochemical profile [21,32]. The buffering of the drug and its vehicle in muscle tissue, which converts the water-soluble hydrochloride salt to the water-insoluble free base, can lead to the situation where only 30% of the injected dose remains in solution within the muscle tissue [8,21]. The solubilized drug had a half-life of about 13.4 min, while the precipitated drug's half-life was approximately 5 h [8], and a two-compartment model has been suggested to describe the absorption of an intramuscular dose of CDX [19,33].

In the light of the anomalous finding that CDX peak levels were lower and were reached later with intramuscular injection than with oral administration [4], it is interesting to note that after 72 h the completeness of absorption is, on the average, equivalent with both modes [31]. This is consistent with the bicompartmental model [8] in which rapid precipitation at the injection site is followed by slow redissolution of the drug [21,26].

C. Multiple-Dose Pharmacokinetics

Just as the blood levels of CDX varied considerably across different individuals after similar single oral or intramuscular doses [34], multiple-dose therapy led to the accumulation of active metabolites and parent drug at varying rates between and within individuals [21]. The steady-state drug concentrations for all psychoactive metabolites were generally reached 2 to 3 weeks after the commencement of therapy [21], although CDX itself achieved a steady-state level after 3 days [13]. It was found that average CDX steady-state plasma levels on a once-daily dosage scheme were not significantly different from the levels produced by a 3 times daily pattern of dosage [13].

A study in which volunteers were given 50 mg of CDX orally over a 14-day period indicated an accumulation half-life of CDX of up to 53 h [35]. The half-lives for N-desmethyl CDX and demoxepam ranged from 9.9 to 17.7 h and from 21.1 to 78.5 h, respectively, in the same study.

The results of other studies on multiple dosing with CDX are presented in Table 3. Another study found that in a single female volunteer given 50 mg CDX daily over 15 days, the CDX disappearance half-life was 9.0 h. CDX did not accumulate, although N-desmethyl CDX and demoxepam reached steady-state concentrations after the first 3 days. CDX disappeared rapidly following the cessation of therapy, and N-desmethyl CDX and demoxepam were detectable for 84 and 108 h, respectively, after the doses had ceased [20].

Clinically it may be advantageous to have an anxiolytic which is compatible with once-daily dosage and which gives rise to pharmacologically active metabolites for some time after the patient has stopped taking the drug.

D. Factors Influencing Pharmacokinetics

Individual differences in drug metabolism have been proposed as a possible cause for variation in CDX plasma levels, following a study in which 18 anxious individuals received 25 mg CDX orally [36,37]. The wide differences observed in CDX plasma levels were not held to be attributable to fluctuations in time lag between ingestion of the dose and venous sampling, nor to body weight, nor to sex.

Multiple regression analysis was applied to one study [38] in which three groups of males and females of diverse age were given 25, 100, or 200 mg CDX either as a single oral dose or in divided dose form. This group concluded that age, sex, body weight, and time of sampling were all factors worthy of investigation in relation to the pharmacokinetics of CDX. These and other influences will be discussed in turn.

1. Age

Increasing age was found to be associated with lower levels of N-desmethyl CDX following multiple regression analysis [38]. This is corroborated by another study [39], in which the impaired ability of elderly patients to convert CDX to its demethylated metabolite was noted. The findings of this group are included in Table 4, which compares the effects of age on CDX pharmacokinetics in two studies. The second study [29] found no significant difference between V_d values in young and old subjects, whereas the first group reported larger apparent

Table 3 Multiple-Dose Pharmacokinetics of Chlordiazepoxide[a]

Reference	No. of subjects or patients	Dose per day (mg)	Body fluid sampled	Mean steady-state concentration (μg/ml)		
				CDX	DMCDX	DMX
[13]	8	30[b]	Plasma	(0.38-1.31)	(0.31-0.85)	(0.24-0.46)
[44]	19	28 (10-15)	Plasma	1.78 (0.46-3.21)	1.74 (0.85-3.54)	1.82 (0.67-3.80)
[35]	3	50[b]	Whole blood	(0.32-0.39)	(0.58-0.86)	(0.49-0.56)
[48]	15	55.3 (41-60)	Plasma	2.25 (0-4.5)	1.41 (0.7-2.2)	0.67 (0.-1.3)

[a]Mean and/or range (in parentheses) given as appropriate; CDX = chlordiazepoxide, DMCDX = desmethylchlordiazepoxide, DMX = demoxepam.
[b]Fixed dosage.

Table 4 Effect of Age on Chlordiazepoxide Pharmacokinetics[a]

Reference	No of subjects	Age range	CDX dose and route	Body fluid sampled	$T_{1/2\beta}$ (h)	V_d (liters/kg)	Clearance
[39]	28	21-30	25 mg oral	Whole blood	10.1	0.42	0.61 ml/min/kg
[39]	8	63-74	25 mg oral	Whole blood	18.2	0.52	0.35 ml/min/kg
[29]	NA	24-40	0.6 mg/kg i.v.	Plasma	9.5	NA	27 ml/min
[29]	NA	60-86	0.6 mg/kg i.v.	Plasma	37.0	NA	13 ml/min

[a]Mean values are given for kinetic variables; $T_{1/2\beta}$ = elimination half-life; V_d = apparent volume of distribution; NA indicates values not available.

volumes of distribution in the elderly [39]. Both studies indicated extended elimination half-lives in older individuals; for example, the mean $T_{1/2\beta}$ was 9.5 h in young subjects but increased to 37 h in older people [29]. The extent of CDX binding to plasma protein was reported to be independent of age [29]. Reduced clearance of CDX has also been discussed [22], and the findings of this study, which evaluated the effects of a single 25-mg oral CDX dose on 8 volunteers over 65 years against 10 healthy subjects aged 30 or less, also indicated that the half-life increased with age and N-desmethyl CDX appeared later and in smaller concentrations with older subjects.

2. Sex

In a study of 11 healthy male and female subjects who each received 50 mg CDX by intravenous infusion [14], differences between apparent volumes of distribution for males and females were observed. In 5 of the subjects who exhibited triexponential clearance of CDX, V_d values for males ranged between 0.4 and 0.7 liter/kg, and for females between 1.4 and 1.5 liters/kg. A later study carried out by the same group on 7 male and 7 female volunteers similarly dosed with CDX gave a range of V_d values for males (0.36 to 0.59 liter/kg) and for females (0.49 to 0.67 liter/kg) [15]. This study found no significant difference between sexes for half-life and drug clearance. The use of multiple regression analysis in another study [38] revealed that females exhibited lower blood levels of CDX and N-desmethyl CDX than males, but the authors stressed that their results with small groups of subjects merely highlighted the need for more investigation in this area.

In a study of 14 anxious male and 4 anxious female patients, sex appeared to have no discernible effect on the blood level of CDX following a 25-mg oral dose [36,37].

3. Body Weight

Multivariate regression analysis of grouped data showed that CDX and N-desmethyl CDX blood levels were negatively correlated with body weight [38]. Few other references to the effects which weight may exert on pharmacokinetic parameters are available, possibly since most studies require their healthy volunteers to fall within the normal range of height and body weight.

In a study of nine healthy volunteers given 25 mg CDX as a single oral dose, an overall negative rank-order correlation ($r = -.48$) of peak CDX blood concentration with body weight was found, but this figure was only marginally significant from a statistical point of view. If the females were excluded from the analysis, the rank-order correlation figure became $-.80$ for the four male volunteers [18].

Another group concluded that the between-subject fluctuations in peak CDX concentrations were only partially attributable to variations in body weight (r = -.37) [14], while no appreciable influence of body weight on CDX blood levels was observed in a separate study [36,37].

4. Time of Sampling

The concentration of CDX decreased as the time between the single dose of 25, 100, or 200 mg and venous sampling increased, while the concentration of N-desmethyl CDX accumulated [38]. This finding is predictable in the knowledge that demethylation is the initial step in the metabolism of CDX in man (see Sec. II.A).

Following 25-mg oral doses of CDX to nine volunteers, peak levels of CDX were observed between 1 and 12 h after dosing [18]. The four male subjects all showed peak plasma CDX levels 3 h after the dose. Oral administration of 50 mg CDX to eight subjects gave peak levels when sampled 90 min after dosage in seven individuals, while the CDX level for the eighth healthy volunteer peaked 4 h after ingestion [31]. Maximum levels following intramuscular injection were detected at significantly later times after administration, ranging from 2½ to 12 h after dosage.

Six subjects were given 20 mg CDX orally in another study [12], after which peak CDX levels arose 2, 4, or 6 h after ingestion, while N-desmethyl CDX had maximum detectable concentrations between 8 and 24 h after the dose was taken.

Intravenous infusion of 50 mg CDX to 11 healthy male and female volunteers produced maximum N-desmethyl CDX levels between 8 and 36 h after dosing [14].

A study of intravenous injection of 100 mg of CDX to three surgical patients produced measurable CDX levels in the cerebrospinal fluid (CSF) within 15 min of injection, with the concentration increasing for 2 to 4 h. The demethylated metabolite was also measurable in two of the three patients, after 2.5 and 4 h, respectively [23].

The above findings are impossible to compare from a between-study pharmacokinetic point of view, since a common denominator of patient/ subject selection, mode of administration, sampling/detection method, or fluid measured is not present. Another study concluded that plasma level differences noted between the 18 anxious subjects who were each given 25 mg CDX orally were not due to differences in the time between ingestion of the drug and sampling of the blood.

It is agreed that pharmacokinetic parameters such as apparent volume of distribution and half-life can be underestimated if venous sampling is not carried out for a sufficiently long period after the drug was taken [14,20]. If the sampling time is truncated, triexponential elimination patterns may well be classified as examples of biexponential drug disposition.

5. Antacids

The first of the two reported studies on the effects of an antacid containing magnesium and aluminum hydroxides (Maalox) on the pharmacokinetics of CDX compared the administration of 25 mg of drug with either water or the antacid solution in a single-dose crossover study using 10 healthy male volunteers [17]. The rationale for looking into any possible interaction was that many anxious patients also suffer from gastrointestinal disorders, requiring the use of antacids with concurrent benzodiazepine therapy [40].

The mean CDX absorption half-life was extended significantly from 11 to 24 min by the antacid preparation, while the elimination half-life shortened marginally from 8.4 to 8.2 h. Six of the 10 individuals did not exhibit CDX levels until 3 h after the drug/antacid mixture was ingested, whereas with CDX alone the peak level was detected 30 min after oral administration. Metabolic conversion to N-desmethyl CDX was delayed by the antacid. It was concluded that coadministration of CDX with the antacid reduced the rate at which the drug was absorbed, but not the completeness of its absorption.

A second study involving antacid [16] served to confirm the authors' earlier contention that differences in the rate of drug absorption could influence the clinical response to antianxiety agents [18]. The later study [16] used a self-rating analogue scale to evaluate the effects of antacid in a four-way single-dose 25-mg CDX/placebo crossover trial on 10 male volunteers. Their findings indicated that the subjective effects of antianxiety agents may be dependent on the rate of drug absorption and may be ameliorated if the rate of absorption is reduced—for example, by the use of antacid preparations.

6. Ethanol

Coadministration of absolute ethanol with CDX was compared against the ingestion of placebo with drug [41]. The effect of the ethanol was to reduce the rate of CDX absorption more so than with placebo, although the study has been criticized [21] for sampling plasma only during the first 6 h after ingestion of the CDX.

7. Liver Disease

Patients suffering from liver cirrhosis exhibited longer elimination half-lives of CDX than normal subjects, and their total metabolic clearance was impaired by the disease. Metabolic conversion to N-desmethyl CDX was also reduced in cirrhotics [42].

The above results were supported in a separate investigation concerning liver malfunction [29]. The demethylated metabolite was not detected in three of the eight patients studied. The remaining five showed delayed appearance and elimination of N-desmethyl CDX from plasma.

8. *Disulfiram Therapy*

The effects of disulfiram on CDX pharmacokinetics have been reported in two studies [42,43]. The elimination half-life of CDX was significantly prolonged, and the total metabolic clearance was reduced in investigations conducted on healthy volunteers dosed with disulfiram 500 mg daily for 2 weeks.

E. Plasma Levels and Clinical Response

Little information concerning the relationship which may exist between plasma levels of CDX and clinical responses is available [36,37].

Attempts at correlation of these two variables have been made difficult by the fact that considerable interindividual variation exists in the blood concentrations of CDX [34].

A study of 18 anxious individuals dosed with 25 mg CDX orally strongly suggested that the blood level of CDX needed to exceed a threshold concentration in order for an anxiolytic effect to be experienced in most individuals [36, 37]. The figure of 0.7 μg/ml was cited as a possible demarcation zone, since patients whose blood concentrations did not achieve this level show no significant decrease in anxiety score, according to the rating scale employed.

A study of 20 anxious patients receiving a mean dose of 28 mg CDX daily was carried out in double-blind placebo-controlled crossover trial but was unable to discern a correlation between the concentration of CDX (or its metabolites) and clinical response [44]. A separate study of volunteers dosed for 2 weeks with CDX, on the other hand, enabled correlations between steady-state plasma levels of N-desmethyl CDX and demoxepam and clinical effect to be drawn, but such a correlation was unable to be reported for the parent drug CDX.

Chlordiazepoxide is a drug which is widely prescribed, but whose mode of action and relationship of blood level to anxiolytic effect are still obscure. Further research in the area is required.

III. DIAZEPAM

A. Structure and Metabolism

Diazepam, synthesized in 1959, was marketed as Valium 4 years later, after it was discovered to be a potent anticonvulsant with muscle-relaxing, antiaggressive, anxiolytic, and sedating properties. By labeling with [^{3}H] diazepam, the site of benzodiazepine action was located in the human cerebral cortex [49]. The mechanism of action of diazepam is unknown Evidence suggests that in some way γ aminobutyric acid or neurons regulated by this transmitter are involved [50].

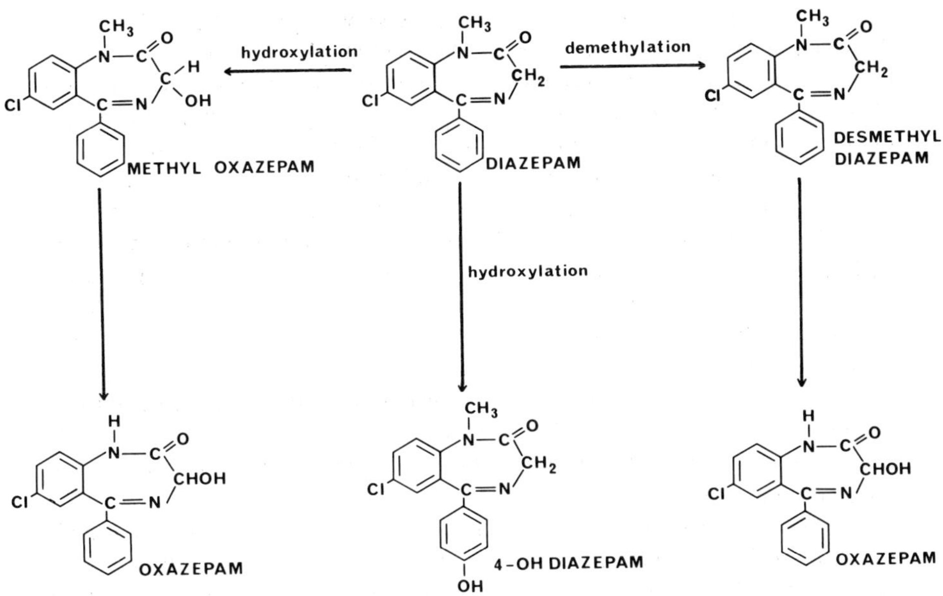

Figure 3 Metabolism of diazepam.

Diazepam is a weak acid, with pK_a 3.3 [51]. It is lipid soluble and water insoluble. The latter property causes precipitation when the usual solution in 40% propylene glycol, 10% ethanol, and aqueous sodium benzoate/benzoic acid is diluted for intravenous infusions. The comparatively frequent occurrence of thrombophlebitis after intravenous administration has been attributed to precipitated diazepam penetrating the wall of a vein [52]. The search for better solvents led to the use of Cremaphor-EI and soya bean oil/water emulsions in which media dilution may be readily carried out without untoward effects [53, 54]. Diazepam is also available as tablets, as syrupy suspensions, and as suppositories.

Metabolism is carried out in the liver via three main pathways (see Fig. 3). Diazepam is N-demethylated, yielding the major metabolite desmethyldiazepam or nordiazepam; diazepam is also hydroxylated in position 3 to give N-methyloxazepam and oxazepam; and diazepam may also hydroxylate onto the phenyl ring in the 4 position [55-57]. Desmethyldiazepam, N-methyloxazepam, and oxazepam all possess to some extent the clinical characteristics of their common parent compound.

The main metabolites have been identified in human blood, bile, and urine, most of the hydroxylated derivatives being excreted in the urine as the glucuronides. From a study on five patients who were given 40-50 μCi of [^{14}C]-diazepam in a single intravenous bolus, Mahon et al. [58] concluded that the chief metabolite in blood was desmethyldiazepam. In urine the average recovery of activity was 48.9% of the dose and consisted of 3-hydroxy- and 4-hydroxy-diazepam and oxazepam. The average recovery from bile was 5.4% and was composed of the same metabolites that appeared in urine.

Less than 5% of diazepam and desmethyldiazepam in plasma is free [59, 60]. The amounts of drug and metabolite that were protein bound did not vary with food intake, nor with the nature of the meal [61,62], but did appear to decrease in patients with renal disease to 92-95% [63]. A reanalysis of the data of Kangas et al. [64] suggested that the difference in protein binding may be due to sex differences.

Larger free-drug fractions can be measured in cirrhotic patients and hypoalbuminemic patients [60,62,65] and a higher incidence of diazepam side effects has been noted in patients with hypoalbuminemia than in patients with normal serum protein composition [66].

Diazepam and desmethyldiazepam have been found to be present in body fat, cerebrospinal fluid (CSF), brain tissues, liver, and saliva. As well they have been identified in the milk of lactating females and in the placenta, the umbilical cord, and various organs of the fetus.. That diazepam is stored in adipose tissue has been demonstrated in humans from whom serial samples of subscapular fat were taken during surgery [67]. The lipophilic nature of diazepam and its metabolite favors their storage in other lipid-rich depots such as the tissues of the brain. The maximum drug concentration in animals initially appears in the grey matter, thereby correlating with the rapid hypnotic and anticonvulsant effects, followed by accumulation into the white matter [68,69].

Free (unbound) diazepam and desmethyldiazepam readily leave the plasma to equilibrate with CSF [70] and saliva [71,72]. Although long-term dosage regimen does not produce any alteration in CSF diazepam level, the ratio of desmethyldiazepam in CSF versus plasma is higher in patients after treatment of several months than after acute treatment [73].

The rate of movement of diazepam across the placenta depends on the placental and uterine circulation [74,75], and measurable quantities of diazepam were found in fetal liver, lung, and brain [76]. A single intramuscular or intravenous dose of diazepam given to the mother in the first stage of labor resulted in marked uptake by the fetus [77]. Since the diazepam-free fraction in the umbilical cord plasma may be higher than in the maternal plasma [77], muscular relaxation and limpness in neonates born to mothers given intravenous diazepam during labor is understandable and contraindicates its use as a parturitive analgesic [78]. The safety limit to the newborn, in cases where diazepam is for various reasons the drug of choice, is 20 mg, administered intramuscularly [78].

Levels of diazepam in human breast milk are of the order of one-tenth of that in plasma; and both diazepam and desmethyldiazepam can be found in the plasma of babies breast-fed by mothers who are on a course of diazepam therapy [79]. An infant fed by his mother who had taken 30 mg diazepam orally for 3 days reportedly lost weight and became lethargic, with electroencephalographic evidence of sedative medication [80]. Oxazepam was found in the urine of the infant. These studies indicate that breast-feeding should be discontinued by mothers taking more than 10 mg of diazepam in a daily dose [81].

Chronic medication of diazepam may result in absorption of the drug and its main metabolite by erythrocytes. In a study of patients receiving 4 mg to 60 mg of diazepam, absorption into red blood cells occurred after 11 or more weeks of treatment. Upon discontinuation of drug administration, the disappearance from the erythrocytes was slower than from the plasma [82].

B. Single-Dose Pharmacokinetics

The pharmacokinetics of diazepam after a single dose is characterized by a rapid absorptive phase, followed by a phase of rapid decline in plasma level and a much slower elimination phase.

Diazepam can be administered via various routes: orally, rectally, by intramuscular and intravenous injections. Absorption after oral administration is rapid and nearly complete, peak plasma levels being reached within 30 to 90 min [83], and similar intraindividual plasma levels result from different tablet formulations [84]. A major factor which influenced the rate of oral absorption is the nature of drugs coadministered. Alcohol, [85], morphine, pethidine, and atropine [86, 87] were found to lower absorption rates, whereas aluminum hydroxide, sodium citrate [88], and metoclopramide [87] displayed the opposite effect. Age is another factor: peak plasma levels appearing earlier in children than in the elderly [67].

The use of diazepam suppositories gave peak plasma times which differed with the nature of the suppository base [84]. The plasma levels reached after the use of certain brands of suppository can be higher than after the intramuscular injection of an equivalent dose [89].

Absorption is complete 15 min after an intravenous injection [86], but 90 min is required before plasma peaks appear after an intramuscular administration [90,91]. The peak heights after intramuscular injections are smaller than that following oral or intravenous administration of an equivalent dose, and depend on injection technique as well as injection site [92]. Exercise has reportedly shortened the time interval between injection and peak plasma level [86].

Peak serum concentrations of diazepam in normal healthy subjects were 1.6 μg/ml, 0.5 μg/ml, and 0.3 μg/ml after a single dose of 20 mg administered intravenously, orally, and intramuscularly [90]. A second peak appearing about

6 h after dosage has been reported by various groups [91,93,94] and was attributed initially to an enterohepatic recycling of diazepam, which was demonstrated in the metabolism by animals [59] and later to the release of diazepam from some storage compartment [61]. Mineral water ingested 5 h after intravenous diazepam was not followed by elevated serum drug levels 1 h later, as was the case when a light fatty meal was taken [95]. Furthermore, in a controlled food intake trial, it was shown that the secondary peaks all occurred after food intake [96]. The hypothesis of enterohepatic recycling was both supported [97,98] and contradicted [58,99] by later work. Using [^{14}C] diazepam given as intravenous bolus to five patients with T-tube biliary drainage, Mahon et al. [58] showed that the appearance of only 5% radioactivity in the bile over a period of 5 to 14 days was incompatible with the existence of an enterohepatic cycle. The rise in serum diazepam after food intake may be caused by the increased circulation in the gut mobilizing stored diazepam from storage sites in the gut wall [61,100].

The pharmacokinetics of diazepam have been fitted to a three-compartment [101] and also to a two-compartment open model [102]. There is rapid distribution between the central compartment and a "shallow" peripheral compartment, according to Kaplan et al. [101], and there is also slow movement between the central compartment and a "deep" peripheral compartment.

Elimination of diazepam from the central compartment is slow, the half-life of elimination $T_{1/2}$ being typically of the order of 30 h after a single intravenous dose of 10 mg, $T_{1/2}$ is affected by age, diseases of the liver and kidneys, halothane anesthesia, and microsomal enzyme induction.

The prolongation of $T_{1/2}$ with increasing age is dependent primarily on an increase in the apparent volume of distribution. From 20 h in 20-year-olds, $T_{1/2}$ rose to nearly 90 h in 30-year-olds [62]. In young children $T_{1/2}$ was found to be 18 h, in newborns 31 h, and in 38-34-week-old premature neonates 75 h [81].

Patients with alcoholic cirrhosis and with hepatitis showed a markedly lower-than-normal efficiency in clearance of diazepam. Klotz et al. [62], following the elimination of diazepam in such patients, found the $T_{1/2}$ doubled; while Andreasen [103] found $T_{1/2}$ increased fivefold in patients with similar diseases. The metabolic clearance rate was significantly impaired in patients with chronic liver disease, but there was no difference from paired controls in the degree and duration of sedation [104].

Protein binding of diazepam is decreased from 98 to 92% in patients with renal insufficiency [63], but the decrease is not associated with any drop in albumin concentration [103] in patients with acute renal failure. The decrease in plasma protein binding of diazepam may result in a bigger apparent volume of distribution and other changes in the dynamics of drug distribution. Very little data exists on this point.

Halothane anesthesia reduced the rate of disappearance of diazepam from the plasma without any concomitant rise in metabolite concentrations [105]. The induction of liver microsomal enzymes was thereby ruled out in this instance. Various drugs are suspected of inducing the metabolism of diazepam. Indeed, diazepam itself is suspected of being an autoinducer [106] because the rate of disappearance of diazepam from the plasma together with a more rapid increase of plasma desmethyldiazepam of patients on continuous diazepam therapy was faster than normal volunteers. That the steady-state plasma level of diazepam has been found to be lower in patients on long-term diazepam therapy by some workers [107,108] further supports the theory of self-induction.

Other inducers cited are cigarette smoke—the effect of central nervous system depression by diazepam being less marked in smokers compared to nonsmokers [109,110]—phenobarbital [69,111], and phenytoin [111], the steady state level of diazepam being lower than controls in patients on anticonvulsant treatment.

Two h after a single intravenous injection of diazepam, desmethyldiazepam was detected in plasma, rising to a peak at about 30 h and from there on declining slowly [108]. Multiple administration of diazepam was followed by serum accumulation of the metabolite. Administration of 15 mg diazepam daily for 2 weeks gave rise to plateau levels of plasma metabolite which exceeded that of diazepam, to decay with $T_{1/2}$ of 92 h when diazepam was discontinued [90].

C. Multiple-Dose Pharmacokinetics

The slow rates of elimination and the lipophilic nature of diazepam and desmethyldiazepam are the main reasons for their accumulation in the system after multiple doses. Steady-state plasma levels of each were reached after 1 and 2 weeks of regular dosage [59,112], a balance being formed between elimination and accumulation.

The plateau concentrations of desmethyldiazepam were in many cases higher than that of diazepam [44,82]. The interindividual variations of metabolism after chronic and subchronic dosage were wide [59,82,87,113]. Genetic factors having been concluded to play little part [114], the lipophilic nature of diazepam and its metabolite was thought to be a contributory cause.

The plasma levels of plasma diazepam and desmethyldiazepam after multiple doses were reportedly higher, in some cases, than after single administrations, and various reasons were given in explanation. The accumulation of desmethyldiazepam may inhibit the metabolism of diazepam by some sort of feedback mechanism [102,108], or tissues may become so saturated with the metabolite that further doses caused a spillover into plasma, resulting in elevated plasma levels [115]. In contrast, treatment periods of 1 to 6 weeks, and longer, were found by some workers to yield plasma diazepam and desmethyldiazepam levels lower than those after single doses [75,105]. The explanations given in these instances were enzyme induction [75,106] or removal of drugs for storage in sites such as adipose tissues and erythrocytes.

Upon discontinuation of drug therapy, both diazepam and its main metabolite dropped slowly in concentration, the latter with an apparent half-life of 4 to 8 days [86,116] and diazepam with an apparent half-life of 2 to 4 days.

D. Plasma Levels and Clinical Response

There does not appear to be any simple relationship between clinical response and plasma levels of diazepam and the main metabolite, desmethyldiazepam, either separately or together. Dasberg et al. [117] found in a trial with patients with acute anxiety that the minimum effective steady-state concentration was 400 ng/ml of diazepam and that the degree of the clinical effect was directly proportional to plasma concentrations and reciprocal clearance values of both diazepam and desmethyldiazepam. Hillestad et al. [90] reported a close relationship between serum levels of diazepam and effects such as sleepiness, mental alertness, coordination, vision, and amnesia, but that desmethyldiazepam was inactive. They also noticed that continuous administration developed tolerance and less response. While a serum concentration of 400 ng/ml diazepam after a single dose gave rise to impaired mental and physical functions, higher serum levels in controls after continuous administration of diazepam had less effect.

The sedative effect of diazepam was related only to the fast distributary phase of diazepam, according to Kanto [89], and when the plasma level of the drug had no further rapid changes, the sedative effect was over. During the distribution phase sedation originated from diazepam entry into the central nervous system. This movement ceased when equilibrium was established between drug concentrations in the plasma and other tissues.

A partial correlation between clinical effects and plasma levels was noted by Ghoneim et al. [113]. No correlation was found of plasma levels with tranquilizing effects and feelings of happiness, boredom, aggressiveness, and withdrawal, but there was a significant correlation between plasma levels of diazepam and moods like drowsiness, fuzziness, mental slowness, weakness, clumsiness, and laziness.

The clinical effects of desmethyldiazepam were concluded to be slightly different from those of diazepam. A study of the plasma levels of six subjects who had taken diazepam or desmethyldiazepam and their mood ratings showed desmethyldiazepam to be the more powerful hypnosedative and mood-lowering drug of the two [116]. Tansella et al. [118] could find no relationship connecting plasma levels of desmethyldiazepam and clinical ratings of hypnotic effect, although they detected a significant correlation of performance ability with plasma concentrations. An anxiolytic concentration/effect relationship had been noted before by Curry [119].

The results of recent work indicated that no simple relationship between diazepam plasma concentration and clinical effect existed. The effects of diazepam on anxiety, sedation, and mood change were not linearly related to peak blood levels, fall in blood level, or half-life of diazepam in plasma or red cells [120]. Similar conclusions were reached by bond[44] and Tansella et al. [121].

IV. CHLORAZEPATE

A. Structure and Metabolism

Chlorazepate is a 1,4-benzodiazepine (see Fig. 1), with a pharmacological profile similar to diazepam [122,123]. Clinical comparisons with diazepam and chlordiazepoxide indicate that chlorazepate is equal to or superior as an anxiolytic, and side effects are often less frequent [124-127].

Chlorazepate is essentially a "prodrug" for nordiazepam, the N-desmethyl metabolite of diazepam. Administration of chlorazepate to healthy individuals results in a complete and rapid hydrolysis and decarboxylation reaction in the gut, to form desmethyldiazepam [126]. The extent of hydrolysis appears to be dependent on gastric acidity, although the exact role of gastric acid is not established [128,129]. After conversion to nordiazepam, the metabolic pathways of chlorazepate are the same as those found for nordiazepam and described above. Nordiazepam is the major compound found in blood after chlorazepate ingestion. Only small amounts of unchanged chlorazepate are detected in blood, and these do not persist for more than a few hours [129].

B. Single-Dose Pharmacokinetics

After attainment of peak desmethyldiazepam levels, rapid distribution occurs, followed by a slow elimination phase. With equimolar oral doses, desmethyldiazepam appears more rapidly in plasma and reaches higher levels with chlorazepate than with diazepam [126].

Plasma levels of desmethyldiazepam were determined by electron capture gas chromatography after oral administration of 10 mg of chlorazepate with 100 ml of water to seven healthy volunteers [83]. Drug concentrations were determined up to 72 h after the dose. The mean plasma half-life was 62 h with a range of 32-146 h. Peak concentrations of desmethyldiazepam were in the range 191-384 ng/ml with a mean of 260 ng/ml and were achieved about 80 min after the dose. Data were fitted to a two-compartment open model from which the absorption rate constant was calculated as 3.3 h^{-1} and the half-life as 57 h. The discrepancy between the pharmacokinetic model and the raw data may be because the investigation was not carried out for a long enough period compared to the half-life.

Greenblatt [130] has described an electron capture gas chromatographic method for determining desmethyldiazepam and its application to the study of chlorazepate pharmacokinetics. In this limited study one healthy female volunteer received 15 mg of chlorazepate dipotassium with 100 ml of water. Plasma samples were drawn up to 144 h after the dose. The data were consistent with a two-compartment open model, with first-order absorption from the gastrointestinal tract. A peak plasma concentration of 380 ng/ml was found after 45 min. The apparent half-life of absorption was 10 min and of elimination 27 h. These values are within the range of values by Wretlind et al. [83].

Single oral doses of 0.3 mg/kg (15-30 mg) chlorazepate were administered to six epileptic patients and blood samples were drawn up to 36 h after the dose [131]. A biexponential decline from peak levels was observed and the data was fitted to a two-compartment open model. The mean time to reach peak serum level was 50 min (range 30-90 min). The half-life of elimination was 39.2 h with a distribution half-life of 1.28 h. The range of values observed for the elimination half-life of 28.3 to 67.3 h agree with the range observed by Wretlind et al. [83]. This points to a lack of drug interaction between chlorazepate and the anticonvulsants phenobarbital, phenytoin, and carbamazepine. Clearance rates in the epileptic patients averaged 35 ± 7.2 ml/min compared with 22.1 ml/min observed by others [132]. These workers also observed $T_{1/2\beta}$ of 46.8 h, not significantly different from that of the epileptic patients. Exposure to microsomal enzyme inducers significantly alters clearance rates without a significant effect on half-life of elimination.

C. Multiple-Dose Pharmacokinetics

Chlorazepate pharmacokinetics were determined in 12 volunteers who received 20 mg of the drug once a day at night for 14 days [133]. Blood samples were drawn daily during the medication period and for 5 days after cessation of drug treatment. Steady-state desmethyldiazepam levels were observed within 8-11 days with a mean concentration of 884 ng/ml (range 540-1347 ng/ml). The biological half-life of desmethyldiazepam was in the range 31-97 h (mean 53 h). A sex difference was observed in the apparent volume of distribution, with females exhibiting a higher value than males (1.40 and 0.97 liters/kg, respectively). This may be due to difference in water-body fat distribution. Results obtained in this study are similar to those observed for the administration of desmethyldiazepam alone [134].

A similar study has been carried in treated epileptics [132]. In this study all the patients received 0.3 mg/kg (7.5-15 mg) of chlorazepate every 12 hours for 6 days, in addition to their normal anticonvulsant medication (phenytoin or phenobarbital). The average serum half-life observed was 40.4 h. This was slightly shorter but within the range of values observed by Post et al. [133]. Total body clearance averaged 34.6 ml/min and the volume of distribution 1.63 liters/kg. No sex effect was observed on the volume of distribution, but epileptics tended to have a higher value than found in normal individuals (as by Post et al. [133], for example).

D. Factors Influencing Pharmacokinetics

Little data has been gathered on the effect of age and disease states on the pharmacokinetics of chlorazepate, and this is a subject where more research is required. The effect of antacid preparations on chlorazepate kinetics has been documented in two studies [129,135].

In the first study [129], 15 normal male volunteers were divided into three groups. One group received 15 mg of chlorazepate, another 15 mg of chlorazepate with 20 ml of antacid suspension, and the third group antacid suspension 2 h and 1 h before chlorazepate and 1 h and 2 h after chlorazepate. Each individual was crossed over to another treatment group after 2 weeks until all subjects received each treatment regimen. Plasma and urine samples were collected up to 96 h after the dose. Both nordiazepam and chlorazepate plasma levels were determined. Peak chlorazepate levels of 106, 113, and 99 ng/ml occurred at 1 h for groups 1, 2, and 3, respectively, and chlorazepate levels were not detectable after 6 h. For nordiazepam C_{max} was 257, 206, and 219 ng/ml for groups 1, 2, and 3, respectively. Significant differences in plasma levels occurring at the earlier sampling time indicated a slower absorption of nordiazepam with the antacid treatments. The time to reach maximum concentration was fastest for the nonantacid group (1 h) and slowest (2.2 h) for the group 2 (antacid with medication). Group 3 had a T_{max} of 1.4 h. Elimination half-life of nordiazepam did not change significantly (64.8, 67.3, and 70 h) for the three groups. For chlorazepate T_{max} was not significantly different, but $T_{1/2\beta}$ was 1.96, 2.66, and 1.65 h, respectively, for the three treatments. The urinary excretion pattern was comparable for the three treatment regimens.

A second study [135] investigated chlorazepate kinetics in a group of 10 volunteers, who ingested 15 mg of the drug with 60 ml of water, or with 60 ml of magnesium aluminum hydroxide on two occasions in a randomized crossover study. Plasma levels of desmethyldiazepam were measured up to 48 h after the dose. Peak plasma levels of desmethyldiazepam were lower (273 vs. 188 ng/ml) and reached later (1.8 vs. 2.8 h) when chlorazepate was administered with the antacid than with water. The absorption half-life was also longer (14.8 vs. 30.7 min) in the antacid group. The lag time before the start of the absorption did not significantly differ between the two groups. Administration of chlorazepate with magnesium aluminum hydroxide reduces the rate of appearance of desmethyldiazepam in the blood, but does not delay the start of absorption.

Chlorazepate is suitable for once-a-day antianxiety therapy, and multiple dosing with this drug leads to the accumulation of desmethyldiazepam, the substance responsible for its antianxiety effect.

V. OTHER BENZODIAZEPINES

A. Lorazepam

1. Metabolism

The major metabolic pathway for lorazepam is via direct conjugation with glucuronic acid. This metabolite accounts for 75% of the dose found in urine after oral administration. Three minor metabolites have also been found in urine: hydroxylorazepam, a quinazoline derivative, and a quinazoline carboxylic acid [136].

2. Single-Dose Pharmacokinetics

Single oral doses of 2 mg were given to eight healthy male volunteers [135]. A mean peak level of 17 ng/ml was observed 2 h after the dose. Complete absorption was indicated by recovery of 95% of the dose in urine (88%) and feces (7%) largely as the glucuronide metabolite. The mean half-life of elimination was 12 h.

A single dose of 4 mg was injected intramuscularly into six healthy male volunteers [137]. Lorazepam was rapidly absorbed, reaching a mean peak level of 57 ng/ml within 3 h. The mean apparent absorption half-life was 21.2 min, elimination half-life 13.6 h, volume of distribution 0.9 liter/kg, and total clearance 58.2 ml/min. Lorazepam glucuronide reached peak levels within 12 h then declined parallel to the parent drug.

Four male volunteers were given bolus intravenous injections of 5 mg lorazepam [138]. Mean pharmacokinetic parameters were determined as half-life 13.2 h, volume of distribution 0.84 liter/kg, and total clearance 55.3 ml/min. Peak levels of lorazepam glucuronide appeared 6 h after the dose and again declined similarly to its parent compound,

3. Multiple Dosing

Fifteen male volunteers received multiple doses of lorazepam ranging from 4 to 10 mg/day over a period of 26 weeks [139]. On a dose of 6 mg/day, steady-state concentrations of lorazepam were 88 ng/ml while its glucuronide reached 170 ng/ml (n = 15). Steady-state concentrations of lorazepam and its metabolite were 164 ng/ml and 266 ng/ml, respectively, on a daily dose of 10 mg/day (n = 7).

Concentrations fluctuated from week to week but not in any systematic fashion. Lorazepam did not appear to stimulate or inhibit its own metabolism. Mean steady-state lorazepam levels were highly correlated with daily-dose in mg/kg but were not related to age.

4. *Effects of Age and Liver Disease*

The disposition of lorazepam after intravenous administration of 2 mg was investigated in patients with alcoholic cirrhosis and viral hepatitis and compared to normal volunteers [140]. No statistically significant age-dependent relationships in the pharmacokinetic parameters measured were observed over the age range 15-73 years. The values obtained for the control group were higher than in the previously reported studies [136-138]; for example, half-lives in this study averaged 22 h. Volumes of distribution and total plasma clearances were also higher, and the authors suggested that differences in populations might account for the values found.

Cirrhosis was associated with a 70% increase in the elimination half-life and was due to an increase in the volume of distribution. No significant changes were observed in the patients with hepatitis. Comparison of systematic plasma clearance in patients in whom studies with other drugs had also been performed indicated that the degree of impairment, if any, in the metabolism of lorazepam was considerably less than for the other drugs.

B. Oxazepam

1. *Metabolism*

Oxazepam is metabolized to only one major metabolite, a glucuronide which is inactive [141].

2. *Single-Dose Studies*

In a preliminary study, 15 mg was given orally to four healthy volunteers [142]. About 85% of the dose was accounted for in urine and feces, largely as the glucuronide, indicating almost complete absorption. Peak levels of oxazepam ranged from 119 to 190 ng/ml occurring 2 to 4 h after the dose. Peak levels of the glucuronide were 60 to 357 ng/ml and occurred between 4 to 8 h postdose. The half-life of elimination of oxazepam was 12 to 20 h. Half-lives were measured in a further eight volunteers and were found to range from 9 to 21 h. Plasma clearances varied between 0.028 and 0.191 liter/h/kg.

Single oral doses of 15 mg were given to nine healthy volunteers [143]. Peak levels of oxazepam occurred between 1 and 4 h. Plasma clearance ranged from 0.05 to 0.17 liter/g/hr and half-lives from 6 to 25 h. Volume of distribution varied from 0.61 to 5.4 liters/kg. The total recovery of oxazepam conjugate was 79% of dose in urine (67%) and feces.

Seven healthy volunteers were given single oral doses of 15 mg oxazepam [83]. Peak levels of 301-399 ng/ml were reached in 1 to 4 h after the dose. Half-lives ranged from 8 to 18 h, plasma clearance from 0.0358 to 0.0919 liter/kg/h, and volume of distribution from 0.52 to 2.35 liters/kg.

3. *Multiple-Dose Studies*

Oxazepam was given 5 mg t.i.d. to the same volunteers who participated in the single-dose study [143]. Stable steady-state concentrations of oxazepam and its glucuronide were achieved within 2-3 days. Oxazepam ranged from 23 to 202 ng/ml with a mean of 61 ng/ml, while the conjugate varied from 27 to 130 ng/ml. Recovery of the conjugate in urine was 86% of the dose over a 24-h period during steady state.

4. *Effects of Renal Disease*

The pharmacokinetics of oxazepam were investigated in 13 patients with renal failure [144]. Plasma half-lives were increased ranging 24-91 h. Plasma concentrations showed secondary peaks about 24 h, but plasma clearance was normal. Conjugated oxazepam accumulated to 5-50 times the level of oxazepam after single doses and 14-50 times higher after multiple dosing. Steady-state levels of oxazepam itself were similar to those obtained in normal subjects (30-160 ng/ml). In some patients substantial fecal excretion was observed.

5. *Effects of Liver Disease*

Single oral doses of 45 mg were given to patients with acute viral hepatitis, cirrhosis, and age-matched controls [145]. Elimination half-life, plasma clearance, apparent volume of distribution, plasma binding, and urinary excretion were comparable in both groups to their controls. Oxazepam appears to be normally eliminated in patients with parenchymal liver disease.

C. Nitrazepam

1. *Structure and Metabolism*

Nitrazepam is a member of the 1,4-benzodiazepines which has been widely introduced into clinical practice as a hypnotic. Its principle advantage in comparison with other hypnotics is a wider margin of safety and an absence of drug interactions [146].

The metabolism of nitrazepam has been studied [147,148]. In both man and rats the major metabolic pathway is by reduction of the nitro group to the corresponding amine. Further metabolism by acetylation leads to the major metabolite, the 7-acetamido derivative. Hydroxylation in the 3 position also occurs, yielding both the hydroxylated amide and acetamido compounds. These are minor metabolites. Cleavage of the benzodiazepine ring also occurs to form 2-amino-3-hydroxy-5-nitrobenzophenone. The pharmacological profile of these compounds has been investigated by Randall and Kappell [28]. Only the parent compound nitrazepam rather than its metabolites exerted any pharmacological activity.

2. Single-Dose Pharmacokinetics

Despite the widespread use of nitrazepam, there is relatively little known about its pharmacokinetics. This may be in part due to the lack of sensitive analytical techniques for measuring the drug. The pharmacokinetics of nitrazepam were studied in six volunteers after a single oral dose and a single intravenous (i.v.) dose of 10 mg [149]. The half-life of elimination after i.v. infusion was 18-24 h (mean 21 h), and after oral administration was 21-28 h (mean 25 h). Absorption rates and distribution were not evaluated due to lack of plasma data in the first hour. Maximum plasma concentrations, reached after 2 h, were 68-108 ng/ml.

The bioavailability of two oral forms of nitrazepam were compared in 15 volunteers after single 5-mg oral doses [150]. Elimination half-lives were 28 and 25 h for the two brands. Peak levels were obtained at 2 h and ranged from 25 to 50 ng/ml. This data is consistent with that obtained by Rieder [149]. In a similar study, 7 volunteers received two nitrazepam-containing preparations as a single 5-mg oral dose [151]. Plasma levels were determined up to 80 h after the dose. The mean elimination half-life of nitrazepam was 27 h. The time to peak plasma concentrations varied between the two brands from 45 min in one to 2 h in the other. Bioavailability of both formulations was the same.

From these single-dose studies it is apparent that nitrazepam has a rather long half-life in comparison to its intended short duration of action. Accumulation of the drug would be expected to occur on repeated oral dosing.

3. Multiple-Dose Pharmacokinetics

Four healthy subjects received doses of 5 mg of nitrazepam at different intervals over a 29-day period [147]. Plasma levels of the drug and its metabolites were measured each day. A steady-state level of the drug was reached after 4 days. The average minimum concentration of nitrazepam during steady state was 38.6 ng/ml and did not show much interindividual variation (range 35.2-44.4 ng/ml). Half-lives determined after the first dose and at the end of the dosing period remained the same (mean 25.9 vs. 25.2 h), showing that nitrazepam did not induce its own metabolism.

Little information is available on the effects of age, disease states, and other factors on nitrazepam pharmacokinetics.

D. Prazepam

Like chlorazepate, prazepam may be considered as a "prodrug" for desmethyldiazepam. After oral administration the cyclopropylmethyl side chain is almost completely removed by the first-pass effect in the liver [152]. Prazepam is almost undetectable in blood, whereas desmethyldiazepam is the major component. Prazepam may be considered a long-acting benzodiazepine.

E. Flurazepam

Only trace amounts of flurazepam were detectable after daily 30-mg doses [153]. The hydroxyethyl metabolite was measurable for several hours, while the N-1-desalkyl metabolite had an elimination half-life of 47 to 100 h in four volunteers. Peak plasma levels following single doses were 10-22 ng/ml, and after continuous dosing rose to 49-142 ng/ml during 2 weeks. The desalkylated metabolite of flurazepam is probably responsible for the hypnotic activity of the drug.

REFERENCES

1. D. J. Greenblatt and R. I. Shader, *Benzodiazepines in Clinical Practice.* New York, Raven Press, 1974, pp. 19-42.
2. D. J. Greenblatt, R. I. Shader, and J. Koch-Weser, Serum creatine phosphokinase concentrations after intramuscular chlordiazepoxide and its solvent. *J. Clin. Pharmacol. 16:*118-121, 1976.
3. L. H. Sternbach, The discovery of Librium. *Agents and Actions 2:*193-196, 1972.
4. D. J. Greenblatt, R. I. Shader, J. Koch-Weser, and K. Franke, Clinical pharmacokinetics of chlordiazepoxide. *Psychopharmacol. Bull. 11:*34-35, 1975.
5. G. F. Placidi and G. B. Cassano, Distribution and metabolism of ^{14}C-labelled-chlordiazepoxide in mice. *Int. J. Neuropharmacol. 7:*383-389, 1968.
6. B. A. Koechlin, M. A. Schwartz, G. Krol, and W. Oberhansli, The metabolic fate of ^{14}C-labelled-chlordiazepoxide in man, in the dog, and in the rat. *J. Pharmacol. Exp. Ther. 148:*399-411, 1965.
7. M. A. Schwartz and E. Postma, Metabolic N-demethylation of chlordiazepoxide. *J. Pharm. Sci. 55:*1358-1362, 1966.
8. H. G. Boxenbaum, K. A. Geitner, M. L. Jack, W. R. Dixon, H. E. Spiegel, J. Symington, R. Christian, J. D. Moore, L. Weissman, and S. A. Kaplan, Pharmacokinetic and biopharmaceutic profile of chlordiazepoxide HCl in healthy subjects: Single dose studies by the intravenous, intramuscular, and oral routes. *J. Pharmacokinetics and Biopharmaceutics 5:*3-23, 1977.
9. S. A. Kaplan, M. Lewis, M. A. Schwartz, E. Postma, S. Cotler, C. W. Abruzzo, T. L. Lee, and R. E. Weinfeld, Pharmacokinetic model for chlordiazepoxide HCl in the dog. *J. Pharm. Sci. 59:*1569-1574, 1970.
10. H. B. Kimmel and S. S. Walkenstein, Oxazepam excretion by chlordiazepoxide-^{14}C-dosed dogs. *J. Pharm. Sci. 56:*538-539, 1967.
11. M. A. Schwartz and E. Postma, Metabolites of demoxepam, a chlordiazepoxide metabolite, in man. *J. Pharm. Sci. 61:*123-125, 1972.
12. M. A. Schwartz, E. Postma, and Z. Gaut, Biological half-life of chlordiazepoxide and its metabolite, demoxepam, in man. *J. Pharm. Sci. 60:*1500-1503, 1971.

13. H. G. Boxenbaum, K. A. Geitner, M. L. Jack, W. R. Dixon, and S. A. Kaplan, Pharmacokinetic and biopharmaceutic profile of chlordiazepoxide HCl in healthy subjects: Multiple-dose oral administration. *J. Pharmacokinetics and Biopharmaceutics 5:*25-39, 1977.
14. D. J. Greenblatt, R. I. Shader, K. Franke, and J. Koch-Weser, Pharmacokinetics of intravenous chlordiazepoxide. *Clin. Pharm. Ther. 17:*235, 1975.
15. D. J. Greenblatt, R. I. Shader, K. Franke, D. S. MacLaughlin, B. J. Ransil, and J. Koch-Weser, Kinetics of intravenous chlordiazepoxide: Sex differences in drug distribution. *Clin. Pharm. Ther. 22:*893-903, 1977.
16. D. J. Greenblatt, R. I. Shader, J. S. Harmatz, K. Franke, and J. Koch-Weser, Absorption rate, blood concentrations, and early response to oral chlordiazepoxide. *Amer. J. Psychiatry 134:*559-562, 1977.
17. D. J. Greenblatt, R. I. Shader, J. S. Harmatz, K. Franke, and J. Koch-Weser, Influence of magnesium and aluminum hydroxide mixture on chlordiazepoxide absorption. *Clin. Pharmacol. Ther. 19:*234-239, 1974.
18. D. J. Greenblatt, R. I. Shader, and J. Koch-Weser, Pharmacokinetic determinants of the response to single doses of chlordiazepoxide. *Amer. J. Psychiatry 131:*1395-1397, 1974.
19. D. J. Greenblatt, R. I. Shader, and J. Koch-Weser, Pharmacokinetics in clinical medicine: Oxazepam versus other benzodiazepines. *Dis. Nerv. Syst. 36:*6-13, 1975.
20. D. J. Greenblatt, R. I. Shader, J. Koch-Weser, and K. Franke, Blood levels and clinical response. In *Pharmacokinetics of Psychoactive Drugs* (L. A. Gottschalk and S. Merlis, eds.). New York, Spectrum, 1976, pp. 127-129.
21. D. J. Greenblatt, R. I. Shader, S. M. MacLeod, and E. M. Sellers, Clinical pharmacokinetics of chlordiazepoxide. *Clin. Pharmacokinetics 3:*381-394, 1978.
22. R. I. Shader and D. J. Greenblatt, Clinical implications of benzodiazepine pharmacokinetics. *Amer. J. Psychiatry 134(6):*652-655, 1977.
23. D. R. Stanski, D. J. Greenblatt, A. Selwyn, R. I. Shader, K. Franke, and J. Koch-Weser, Plasma and cerebrospinal fluid concentrations of chlordiazepoxide and its metabolites in surgical patients. *Clin. Pharmacol. Ther. 20:*571-578, 1976.
24. M. A. Schwartz, E. Postma, and S. J. Kolis, Metabolism of demoxepam, a chlordiazepoxide metabolite in the dog. *J. Pharm. Sci. 60:*438-444, 1971.
25. W. R. Dixon, M. A. Brooks, E. Postma, M. R. Hackman, and M. A. Schwartz, Identification and determination of N-desmethyl-diazepam in plasma following chronic administration of chlordiazepoxide hydrochloride (Librium) to man. *Fed. Proc. 33:*472, 1974.
26. L. A. Gottschalk, R. Biener, and E. C. Dinovo, Effect of oral and intramuscular routes of administration on serum chlordiazepoxide levels and the prediction of these levels from predrug fasting serum glucose concentrations. *Res. Commun. Chem. Pathol. Pharmacol. 8:*697-702, 1974.

27. D. Smyth and G. W. Pennington, The detection and excretion of chlordiazepoxide ("Librium") in human plasma and urine. *Arch. Int. Pharmacodyn. 145:*154-165, 1963.
28. L. O. Randall and B. Kappell, Pharmacological activity of some benzodiazepines and their metabolites. In *The Benzodiazepines* (S. Garattini, E. Mussini, and L. O. Randall, eds.). New York, Raven Press, 1973, pp. 27-51.
29. R. K. Roberts, G. R. Wilkinson, R. A. Branch, and S. Schenker, Effect of age and cirrhosis on the disposition and elimination of chlordiazepoxide (Librium). *Gastroenterology 73:*A45/1243, 1977.
30. W. Müller and V. Wollert, Characterization of the binding of benzodiazepines to human serum albumin. *Naunyn-Schmiedebergs Arch. Pharmacol. Exp. Pathol. 280:*229-237, 1973.
31. D. J. Greenblatt, R. I. Shader, and J. Koch-Weser, Slow absorption of intramuscular chlordiazepoxide. *N. Engl. J. Med. 291:*1116-1118, 1974.
32. K. Florey (ed.), *Analytical Profiles of Drug Substances,* vol. 1. New York, Academic Press, 1972, pp. 15-37.
33. D. J. Greenblatt and J. Koch-Weser, Clinical Pharmacokinetics. *N. Engl. J. Med. 293:*702-705, 964-970, 1975.
34. L. A. Gottschalk, E. Noble, and H. Elliott, Blood levels and dose response. *Psychopharm. Bull. 9:*40-43, 1973.
35. D. J. Greenblatt, R. I. Shader, K. Franke, and J. S. Harmatz, Pharmacokinetics of chlordiazepoxide and metabolites following single and multiple oral doses. *Int. J. Clin. Pharmacol. Biopharm. 16:*486-493, 1978.
36. L. A. Gottschalk and S. A. Kaplan, Chlordiazepoxide plasma levels and clinical responses. *Compr. Psychiatry 13:*519-527, 1972.
37. L. A. Gottschalk, E. P. Noble, G. E. Stolzoff, D. E. Bates, C. G. Cable, R. L. Uliana, H. Birch, and E. W. Fleming, Relationships of chlordiazepoxide blood levels to psychological and biochemical responses. In *The Benzodiazepines* (S. Garattini, E. Mussini, and L. O. Randall, eds.). New York, Raven Press, 1973, pp. 257-278.
38. D. J. Greenblatt, J. S. Harmatz, D. R. Stanski, R. I. Shader, K. Franke, and J. Koch-Weser, Factors influencing blood concentrations of chlordiazepoxide: A use of multiple regression analysis. *Pharmacology 54:*277-282, 1977.
39. R. I. Shader, D. J. Greenblatt, J. S. Harmatz, K. Franke, and J. Koch-Weser, Absorption and disposition of chlordiazepoxide in young and elderly male volunteers. *J. Clin. Pharmacol. 17:*709-718-1977.
40. D. J. Greenblatt and R. I. Shader, Psychotropic drugs, medical disease, and other medical therapies. In *Drugs in Combination with Other Therapies* (M. Greenblatt, ed.). New York, Grune & Stratton, 1975, pp. 83-99.
41. M. Linnoila, S. Otterstrom, and M. Anttila, Serum chlordiazepoxide, diazepam, and thioridazine concentrations after the simultaneous ingestion of alcohol or placebo drink. *Ann. Clin. Res. 6:*4-6, 1974.
42. E. M. Sellers, S. M. MacLeod, D. J. Greenblatt, and H. G. Giles, Influence of disulfiram and disease on benzodiazepine disposition. *Clin. Pharmacol. Ther. 21:*117, 1977.

43. E. M. Sellers, S. M. MacLeod, D. J. Greenblatt, and H. G. Giles, Inhibition of chlordiazepoxide biotransformation by disulfiram. *Clin. Res. 24:*652A, 1976.
44. A. J. Bond, D. M. Hailey, and M. H. Lader, Plasma concentrations of benzodiazepines. *Brit. J. Clin. Pharmacol. 4:*51-56, 1977.
45. D. J. Greenblatt, R. I. Shader, S. M. MacLeod, E. M. Sellers, K. Franke, and H. G. Giles, Absorption of oral and intramuscular chlordiazepoxide. *Eur. J. Clin. Pharmacol. 13:*267-274, 1978.
46. B. A. Koechlin and L. D'Arconte, Determination of chlordiazepoxide (Librium) and of a metabolite of lactam character in plasma of humans, dogs, and rats by a specific spectrofluorometric micro method. *Anal. Biochem. 5:*195-207, 1963.
47. S. M. MacLeod, D. J. Greenblatt, and E. M. Sellers, Determination of intravenous chlordiazepoxide pharmacokinetics: Plasma versus blood. *Clin. Res. 25:*273A, 1977.
48. K-M. Lin and R. O. Friedel, Relationship of plasma levels of chlordiazepoxide and metabolites to clinical response. *Amer. J. Psychiatry 136:*18-23, 1979.
49. H. Möhler, T. Okado, P. H. Heitz, and J. Ulrich, Biochemical identification of the site of action of benzodiazepines in human brain by ^{3}H-diazepam binding. *Life Sci. 22:*985-996, 1978.
50. E. Costa, A. Guidotti, C. C. Mao, and A. Suria, New concepts on the mechanism of action of benzodiazepines. *Life Sci. 17:*167-186, 1975.
51. J. M. Clifford and W. F. Smyth, The determination of some 1,4-benzodiazepines and their metabolites in body fluids: A review. *Analyst 99:* 241-272, 1974.
52. O. Lingjaerde and K. Nordbø, Thromboflebitt efter intravenøs injeksjon av diazepam. *Tidskrift der Norske Laegeforening 94:*455-456, 1974.
53. J. W. Dundee and G. M. Wyant, Tranquilizers. In *Intravenous Anesthesia* (J. W. Dundee and G. M. Wyant, eds.). Edinburgh, Churchill Livingstone, 1974, pp. 248-273.
54. O. von Dardel, C. Mebius, and T. Mossberg, Diazepam in emulsion form for intravenous usage. *Acta Anaesth. Scand. 20:*221-224, 1976.
55. J. A. De Silva, B. A. Koechlin, and G. Bader, Blood level distribution patterns of diazepam and its major metabolite in man. *J. Pharm. Sci. 55:* 692-702, 1966.
56. J. A. De Silva and C. V. Puglisi, Determination of medazepam (Nobrium), diazepam (Valium), and their major transformation products in blood and urine by electron capture gas-liquid chromatography. *Anal. Chem. 42:* 1725-1736, 1970.
57. M. A. Schwartz, B. A. Koechlin, E. Postma, S. Palmer, and G. Krol, Metabolism of diazepam in rat, dog, and man. *J. Pharm. Exp. Ther. 149:*423-435, 1965.
58. W. A. Mahon, T. Inaba, T. Umeda, E. Tsutsumi, and R. Stone, Biliary elimination of diazepam in man. *Clin. Pharmacol. Ther. 19:*443-450, 1976.

59. E. van der Kleijn, J. M. van Rossum, E. T. J. M. Muskens, and N. Rijntjes, Pharmacokinetics of diazepam in dogs, mice, and humans. *Acta Pharmacol. Toxicol., Suppl.* (3) *29:*109-127, 1971.
60. J. J. Thiessen, E. M. Sellers, P. Denbeigh, and L. Dolman, Plasma protein binding of diazepam and tolbutamide in chronic alcoholics. *J. Clin. Pharmacol. 16:*345-351, 1976.
61. K. Kortilla, M. J. Mattila, and M. Linnoila, Prolonged recovery after diazepam sedation: The influence of food, charcoal ingestion, and injection rate on the effects of intravenous diazepam. *Brit. J. Anaesth. 48:*333-340, 1976.
62. U. Klotz, G. R. Avant, A. Hoyumpa, S. Schenker, and G. R. Wilkinson, The effects of age and liver disease on the disposition and elimination of diazepam in adult man. *J. Clin. Invest. 55:*347-359, 1975.
63. L. Kangas, J. Kanto, J. Forsstrom, and E. Iisalo, The protein binding of diazepam and N-demethyldiazepam in patients with poor renal function. *Clin. Nephrol. 5:*114-118, 1976.
64. D. J. Greenblatt, J. S. Harmatz, and R. I. Shader, Sex differences in diazepam protein binding in patients with renal insufficiency. *Pharmacology 16:* 26-29, 1978.
65. P. B. Andreasen, J. Hendel, G. Greisen, and E. F. Hvidberg, Pharmacokinetics of diazepam in disordered liver function. *Eur. J. Clin. Pharmacol. 10:*115-120, 1976.
66. D. J. Greenblatt and J. Koch-Weser, Clinical toxicity of chlordiazepoxide and diazepam in relation to serum albumin concentrations: A report from the Boston Collaborative Drug Surveillance Program. *Eur. J. Clin. Pharmacol. 7:*259-262, 1974.
67. S. Garattini, Metabolism of diazepam in animals and man. In *The Benzodiazepines.* (S. Garattini, E. Mussini, and L. O. Randall, eds.). New York, Raven Press, 1973, pp. 84-89.
68. S. Garattini, F. Marcucci, P. L. Morselli, and E. Mussini, The significance of measuring blood levels of benzodiazepines. In *Biological Effects of Drugs in Relation to Their Plasma Concentrations* (D. S. Davies and B. N. C. Pritchard, eds.). London, Macmillan, 1973, pp. 211-225.
69. P. L. Morselli, G. B. Cassano, G. F. Placidi, G. B. Muscettola, and M. Rizzo, Kinetics of the distribution of ^{14}C-diazepam and its metabolites in various areas of cat brain. In *The Benzodiazepines.* S. Garattini, E. Mussini, and L. O. Randall, eds.), New York, Raven Press, 1973, pp. 129-143.
70. J. Kanto, L. Kangas, and T. Siirtola, Cerebrospinal-fluid concentrations of diazepam and its metabolites in man. *Acta Pharmacol. Toxicol. 36:* 328-334, 1975.
71. H. G. Giles, D. H. Zilm, R. C. Frecker, S. M. MacLeod, and E. M. Sellers, Saliva and plasma concentrations of diazepam after a single oral dose. *Brit. J. Clin. Pharmacol. 4:*711-712, 1977.
72. K. Feller and G. Le Petit, On the distribution of drugs in saliva and blood plasma. *Int. J. Clin. Pharmacol. Biopharm. 15:*468-469, 1977.

73. J. Hendell, Cumulation in cerebrospinal fluid of the N-desmethyl metabolite after long term treatment with diazepam in man. *Acta Pharmacol. Toxicol. 37:*17-22, 1975.
74. R. Erkkola, L. Kangas, and A. Pekkarinen, The transfer of diazepam across the placenta during labour. *Acta Obstet. Gynaecol. Scand. 52:*167-170, 1973.
75. J. Kanto and R. Erkkola, The feto-maternal distribution of diazepam in early human pregnancy. *Ann. Chir. Gynaecol. Fenn. 63:*489-491, 1974.
76. M. Mandelli, P. L. Morselli, S. Nordio, G. Pardi, N. Principi, F. Sereni, and G. Tognoni, Placental transfer of diazepam and its disposition in the newborn. *Clin. Pharmacol. Ther. 17:*564-572, 1975.
77. J. Kanto, R. Erkkola, and R. Sellman, Accumulation of diazepam and N-demethyldiazepam in the fetal blood during labour. *Ann. Clin. Res. 5:* 375-379, 1973.
78. J. Kanto, Studies of diazepam: Human and animal experiments with special reference to its pharmacokinetics. Master's thesis, University of Turku, Finland, 1976.
79. A. P. Cole and D. M. Hailey, Diazepam and active metabolite in breast milk and their transfer to the neonate. *Arch. Dis. Child. 50:*741-742, 1975.
80. M. J. Patrick, W. J. Wilstone, and P. Reavey, Diazepam and breast feeding. *Lancet 1:*542-543, 1972.
81. M. Mandelli, G. Tognoni, and S. Garattini, Clinical pharmacokinetics of diazepam. *Clin. Pharmacokin. 3:*72-91, 1978.
82. I. A. Zingales, Diazepam metabolism during chronic medication. Unbound fraction in plasma, erythrocytes, and urine. *J. Chromatogr. 75:*55-78, 1973.
83. M. Wretlind, A. Pilbrant, A. Sundwall, and J. Vessman, Disposition of three benzodiazepines after single oral administration in man. *Acta Pharmacol. Toxicol.* (Copenhagen), *Suppl. (1) 40:*28-39, 1977.
84. E. Arnold, A simple method for determining diazepam and its major metabolites in biological fluids: Application in bioavailability studies. *Acta Pharmacol. Toxicol. 36:*335-352, 1975.
85. D. J. Greenblatt, J. I. Shader, D. R. Weinberger, and M. D. Allen, Effect of a cocktail on diazepam absorption. *Clin. Pharmacol. Ther. 23:*114-115, 1978.
86. J. A. S. Gamble, Some factors influencing the absorption of diazepam. *Proc. Roy. Soc. Med. 68:*22, 1975.
87. J. A. S. Gamble, J. H. Gaston, S. G. Nair, and J. W. Dundee, Some pharmacological factors influencing the abosrption of diazepam following oral administration. *Brit. J. Anaesth. 48:*1181-1185, 1976.
88. S. G. Nair, J. A. S. Gamble, J. W. Dundee, and P. J. Howard, The influence of three antacids on the absorption and clinical action of oral diazepam. *Brit. J. Anaesth. 48:*1175-1180, 1976.
89. J. Kanto, Plasma concentrations of diazepam and its metabolites after peroral, intramuscular, and rectal administration. *Int. J. Clin. Pharmacol. 12:*427-432, 1975.

90. L. Hillestad, T. Hansen, H. Melsom, and A. Drivens, Diazepam metabolism in normal man. *Clin. Pharmacol. Ther. 16:*479-484, 485-489, 1974.
91. E. S. Baird and D. M. Hailey, Delayed recovery from a sedative: Correlation of the plasma levels of diazepam with clinical effects after oral and intravenous administration. *Brit. J. Anaesth. 44:*803-808, 1972.
92. R. A. E. Assaf, J. W. Dundee, and J. A. S. Gamble, The influence of the route of administration on the clinical action of diazepam. *Anaesthesia 30:*152-158, 1975.
93. E. S. Baird and D. M. Hailey, Plasma levels of diazepam and its major metabolite following intramuscular administration. *Brit. J. Anaesth. 45:* 546-548, 1973.
94. K. Kortilla and M. Linnoila, Skills related to driving after intravenous diazepam, flunitrazepam, or droperidol. *Brit. J. Anaesth. 46:*961-969, 1974.
95. M. Linnoila, K. Kortilla, and M. J. Mattila, Effect of food and repeated injections on serum diazepam levels. *Acta Pharmacol. Toxicol. 36:*181-186, 1975.
96. K. Kortilla and M. Linnoila, Recovery and skills related to driving after intravenous sedation: Dose-response relationship with diazepam. *Brit. J. Anaesth. 47:*457-463, 1975.
97. R. Sellman, J. Kanto, and A. Pekkarinen, Biliary excretion of diazepam and its metabolites in man. *Acta Pharmacol. Toxicol. 37:*242-249, 1975.
98. R. Sellman, J. Kanto, E. Raijola, and A. Pekkarinen, Human and animal study on elimination from plasma and metabolism of diazepam after chronic alcohol intake. *Acta Pharmacol. Toxicol. 36:*33-38, 1975.
99. P. W. Eustace, D. M. Hailey, A. G. Cox, and E. S. Baird, Biliary excretion of diazepam in man. *Brit. J. Anaesth. 47:*983-985, 1975.
100. K. Kortilla and L. Kangas, Unchanged protein binding and the increase of serum diazepam levels after food intake. *Acta Pharmacol. Toxicol. 40:* 241-246, 1977.
101. S. A. Kaplan, M. L. Jack, K. Alexander, and R. E. Weinfeld, Pharmacokinetic profile of diazepam in man following single intravenous and oral and chronic oral administrations. *J. Pharm. Sci. 62:*1789-1796, 1973.
102. U. Klotz, K. H. Antonin, and P. R. Bieck, Pharmacokinetics and plasma binding of diazepam in man, dog, rabbit, guinea pig, and rat. *J. Pharmacol. Exp. Ther. 199:*67-73, 1976.
103. F. Andreasen, The effects of dialysis on the protein binding of drugs in patients with renal failure. *Acta Pharmacol. Toxicol. 34:*284-294, 1974.
104. J. B. McConnell, M. Davis, S. Curry, and R. Williams, Diazepam kinetics and sedation in chronic liver disease. *Gut 18:*A988, 1977.
105. J. Kanot and E. U. M. Iisalo, Diazepam as an inductive agent in two kinds of combination anaesthesia: The disappearance of diazepam and its metabolites from the plasma. *Ann. Chir. Cynaecol. Fenn. 62:*251-255, 1973.
106. R. Sellman, J. Kanto, E. Raijola, and A. Pekkarinen, Induction effect of

diazepam on its own metabolism. *Acta Pharmacol. Toxicol. 37:*345-351, 1975.

107. J. Kanto, E. Iisalo, V. Lehtinen, and J. Salminen, The concentrations of diazepam and its metabolites in the plasma after an acute and chronic administration. *Psychopharmacologia* (Berlin) *36:*123-131, 1974.
108. U. Klotz, K. H. Antonin, and P. R. Bieck, Comparison of the pharmacokinetics of diazepam after single and subchronic doses. *Eur. J. Clin. Pharmacol. 10:*121-126, 1976.
109. M. S. Koppelman, Metabolism of benzodiazepines. *N. Engl. J. Med. 288:* 917, 1973.
110. Boston Collaborative Drug Surveillance Program, Clinical depression of the central nervous system due to diazepam and chlordiazepoxide in relation to cigarette smoking and age. *N. Engl. J. Med. 288:*277-280, 1973.
111. G. W. Hepner, E. Vesell, A. Lipton, H. Harvey, G. Wilkinson, and S. Schenker, Disposition of aminopyrine, antipyrine, diazepam, and indocyanine green in patients with liver disease or on anticonvulsant drug therapy: Diazepam breath test and correlations in drug elimination. *J. Lab. Clin. Med. 90:*440-456, 1977.
112. A. B. Berlin, B. Siwers, S. Agurell, A. Hiort, F. Sjöqvist, and S. Ström, Determination of bioavailability of diazepam in various formulations from steady-state plasma concentration data. *Clin. Pharmacol. Ther. 13:* 733-744, 1972.
113. M. M. Ghoneim, S. P. Mewaldt, and J. Ambre, Plasma levels of diazepam and mood ratings. *Anaesth. Analg. Cur. Res. 54:*173-177, 1975.
114. S. Eriksen, E. Dorus, H. Dekirmenjian, N. Segal, and J. M. Davis, Interindividual variability in diazepam metabolism: Preliminary evidence of an absence of genetic control. *Clin. Pharmacol. Ther. 21:*102, 1977.
115. K. Kortilla, M. J. Mattila, and M. Linnoila, Saturation of tissues with N-desmethyldiazepam as a cause for elevated serum levels of this metabolite after repeated administration of diazepam. *Acta Pharmacol. Toxicol. 36:*190-192, 1975.
116. H. H. Dasberg, Effects and plasma levels of N-desmethyldiazepam after oral administration in normal volunteers. *Psychopharmacologia* (Berlin) *43:*191-198, 1975.
117. H. H. Dasberg, E. van der Kleijn, P. Guelen, and H. van Praag, Plasma concentration of diazepam and of its metabolite N-desmethyldiazepam in relation to anxiolytic effect. *Clin. Pharmacol. Ther. 15:*473-483, 1974.
118. M. Tansella, O. Siciliani, L. Burti, M. Schiavon, C. H. Tansella, C. H. Zimmerman, M. Gerna, G. Tognoni, and P. L. Morselli, N-desmethyldiazepam and amylobarbitone sodium as hypnotics in anxious patients: Plasma levels, clinical efficacy, and residual effects. *Psychopharmacologia* (Berlin) *41:*81-85, 1975.
119. S. H. Curry, Concentration effect relationships with major and minor tranquillizers. *Clin. Pharmacol. Ther. 16:*192-197, 1974.
120. R. C. Smith, H. Dekirmenjian, J. Davis, R. Caspar, L. Gosenfeld, and

C. Tsai, Blood level, mood, and MHPG responses to diazepam in man. In *Pharmacokinetics of Psychoactive Drugs* (L. A. Gottschalk and S. Merlis, eds.). New York, Spectrum, 1976, pp. 141-154.

121. M. Tansella, C. H. Zimmermann, L. Tansella, L. Ferrario, L. Preziati, G. Tognoni, and M. Lader, Plasma concentrations of diazepam, nordiazepam, and amylobarbitone after short-term treatment in anxious patients. *Pharmakopsychiatrie Neuropsychopharmakol. 11*(2):68-72, 1978.

122. G. Holmberg and B. Livstedt, Clinical evaluation of a new benzodiazepine derivative, chlorazepate. *Arzneim.-Forsch. 22:*916, 1972.

123. K. D. Charalampous, W. Tooley, and C. Yates, Chlorazepate dipotassium: A new benzodiazepine antianxiety agent. *J. Clin. Pharmacol. 13:*114, (1973).

124. A. J. Cooper, R. V. Magnus, and M. Rose, Controlled trial of dipotassium chlorazepate ("Tranxene") in anxiety. *Brit. J. Psychiatry 123:*475, 1973.

125. S. I. Feurst, Clorazepate dipotassium, diazepam, and placebo in chronic anxiety. *Curr. Ther. Res. 15:*499, 1973.

126. A. Robin, S. H. Curry, and R. Whelpton, Clinical and biochemical comparison of clorazepate and diazepam. *Psychol. Med. 4:*388, 1974.

127. G. Burrows, P. Dumovic, J. A. Smith, T. Norman, and K. Maguire, A controlled comparative trial of clorazepate (Tranxene) and diazepam (Valium) for anxiety. *Med. J. Aust. 2:*525-528, 1977.

128. C. W. Abruzzo, T. Macasieb, R. Weinfeld, J. A. Rider, and S. Kaplan, Changes in oral absorption characteristics in man of dipotassium chlorazepate at normal and elevated gastric pH. *J. Pharmacokin. Biopharm. 5:* 377-390, 1977.

129. A. H. C. Chun, P. J. Carrigan, D. J. Hoffmann, M. S. Kershner, and J. D. Stuart, Effect of antacids on abosrption of clorazepate. *Clin. Pharmacol. Ther. 22:*329-335, 1977.

130. D. J. Greenblatt, Determination of desmethyldiazepam in plasma by electron capture GLC: Application to pharmacokinetic studies of clorazepate. *J. Pharm. Sci. 67:*427-429, 1978.

131. A. J. Wilensky, R. H. Levy, A. S. Troupin, L. Moretti-Ojemann, and P. Friel, Clorazepate kinetics in treated epileptics. *Clin. Pharmacol. Ther. 24:*22-30, 1978.

132. P. J. Carrigan, G. G. Chao, W. M. Barker, D. J. Hoffmann, and A. H. C. Chun, Steady-state bioavailability of two clorazepate dipotassium dosage forms. *J. Clin. Pharmacol. 17:*18-28, 1977.

133. C. Post, S. Lingren, A. Bertler, and H. Malmgren, Pharmacokinetics of N-desmethyldiazepam in healthy volunteers after single daily doses of dipotassium chlorazepate. *Psychopharmacology 53:*105-109, 1977.

134. G. Tognoni, R. Gomeni, D. De Maio, G. G. Alberti, P. Franciosi, and G. Scieghi, Pharmacokinetics of N-desmethyldiazepam in patients suffering from insomnia and treated with nortriptyline. *Brit. J. Clin. Pharmacol. 2:*227-232, 1975.

135. R. I. Shader, A. Georgotas, D. J. Greenblatt, J. S. Harmatz, and M. D.

Allen, Impaired absorption of desmethyldiazepam from clorazepate by magnesium aluminum hydroxide. *Clin. Pharmacol. Ther. 24:*308–315, 1978.

136. D. J. Greenblatt, R. T. Schillings, A. A. Kyriakopoulos, and R. I. Shader, Clinical pharmacokinetics of lorazepam, I: Absorption and disposition of oral ^{14}C-Lorazepam. *Clin. Pharmacol. Ther. 20:*329–341, 1976.

137. D. J. Greenblatt, T. H. Joyce, W. H. Comer, J. A. Knowles, R. I. Shader, A. A. Kyriakopoulos, D. S. MacLaughlin, and H. W. Ruelius, Clinical pharmacokinetics of lorazepam, II: Intramuscular injection. *Clin. Pharmacol. Ther. 21:*222–230, 1977.

138. D. J. Greenblatt, W. H. Comer, A. W. Elliott, R. I. Shader, J. S. Knowles, and H. W. Ruelius, Clinical pharmacokinetics of lorazepam, III: Intravenous injection. *J. Clin. Pharmacol. 17:*490–494, 1977.

139. D. J. Greenblatt, J. S. Knowles, W. H. Comer, R. I. Shader, J. S. Harmatz, and H. W. Ruelius, Clinical pharmacokinetics of lorazepam, IV: Long term oral administration. *J. Clin. Pharmacol. 17:*495–500, 1977.

140. J. W. Kraus, P. V. Desmond, J. P. Marshall, R. F. Johnson, S. Schenker, and G. R. Wilkinson, Effects of ageing and liver disease on disposition of lorazepam. *Clin. Pharmacol. Ther. 24:*411–419, 1978.

141. S. S. Walkenstein, R. Wiser, C. H. Gudmundsen, H. B. Kimmel, and R. A. Corradino, Absorption, metabolism, and excretion of oxazepam and its succinate half-ester. *J. Pharm. Sci. 53:*1181–1186, 1964.

142. J. Vessman, B. Alexanderson, F. Sjoqvist, B. Strindberg, and A. Sundwall, Comparative pharmacokinetics of oxazepam and nortriptyline after single oral doses in man. In *The Benzodiazepines* (S. Garattini, E. Mussini, and L. O. Randall, eds.), New York, Raven Press, 1973, pp. 165–173.

143. G. Alvan, B. Siwers, and J. Vessman, Pharmacokinetics of oxazepam in healthy volunteers. *Acta Pharmacol. Toxicol., Suppl. (1) 40:*40–51, 1977.

144. I. Oder-Cederlöf, J. Vessman, G. Alvan, and F. Sjöqvist, Oxazepam disposition in uremic patients. *Acta Pharmacol. Toxicol., Suppl. (1) 40:*52–62, 1977.

145. H. J. Shull, G. R. Wilkinson, R. Johnson, and S. Schenker, Normal disposition of oxazepam in acute viral hepatitis and cirrhosis. *Ann. Int. Med. 84:*420–425, 1976.

146. D. J. Greenblatt and R. I. Shader, The clinical choice of sedative-hypnotics. *Ann. Int. Med. 77:*91–100, 1972.

147. J. Rieder and G. Wendt, Pharmacokinetics and metabolism of the hypnotic nitrazepam. In *The Benzodiazepines* (S. Garattini, E. Mussini, and L. O. Randall, New York, Raven Press, 1973, pp. 99–127.

148. J. Rieder, Methoden zur Bestimmung von 1,3-dihydro-7-nitro-5-phenyl-2H-1,4-benzodiazepin-2-on und seinen Hauptmetaboliten in biologischen Proben und Ergebnisse von Versuchen uber die Pharmacokinetik und den Metabolismus dieser Substanz bei Mensch und Ratte. *Arzneim.-Forsch. 15:*1134–1148, 1965.

149. J. Rieder, Plasma levels and derived pharmacokinetic characteristics of unchanged nitrazepam in man. *Arzneim.-Forsch. 23:*212–218, 1973.

150. K. Moeller-Jensen, Determination of nitrazepam in serum by gas-liquid chromatography: Application in bioavailability studies. *J. Chromatogr. 111:*389-396, 1975.
151. A. G. De Boer, J. Rost-Kaiser, H. Bracht, and D. D. Breimer, Assay of underivatised nitrazepam and clonazepam in plasma by capillary gas chromatography applied to pharmacokinetic and bioavailability studies in humans. *J. Chromatogr. 145:*105-114, 1978.
152. D. J. Greenblatt, and R. I. Shader, Pharmacokinetic understanding of antianxiety drug therapy. *South. Med. J. Suppl. (2) 71:*2-9, 1978.
153. S. A. Kaplan, J. A. F. De Silva, M. L. Jack, K. Alexander, N. Strojny, R. E. Weinfeld, C. V. Puglisi, and L. Weissman, Blood level profile in man following chronic oral administration of flurazepam hydrochloride. *J. Pharm. Sci. 62:*1932-1935, 1973.

14

Sedatives and Hypnotics

Denis N. Wade / *Department of Clinical Pharmacology, University of New South Wales, and Department of Clinical Pharmacology, St. Vincent's Hospital, Sydney, New South Wales, Australia*

I. INTRODUCTION

The hypnosedatives are a group of chemically diverse drugs which are commonly grouped together because they possess to a varying degree common properties and because they are not readily classified with other psychoactive drugs, many of which are also sedatives. The properties shared by this class of compound include sedation at low dose, hypnosis at higher dosage, skeletal muscle relaxation, anxiolysis, and, in most cases, anticonvulsant action. Not all the hypnosedatives in clinical use possess all these actions at dosages used clinically but some, especially the benzodiazepines, find clinical use for all these properties. The use of hypnosedatives as antianxiety agents and as anticonvulsants has been discussed in Chaps. 13 and 15. This discussion is limited to their use as sedative and hypnotic agents.

Hypnotics are among the most widely used of all drugs. Surveys in most Western societies indicate a high level of usage, particularly by women [1-5]. The consumption appears to be remarkably similar in different countries [6] and varies little with socioeconomic status [1]. The use of hypnosedatives is a matter of concern both because of the number of people who become dependent on or habituated to hypnotics and because hypnotics are the agents most commonly used to attempt suicide. The economic cost has also been a major topic or debate, especially in countries where the government has assumed responsibility for the payment of all or part of the national drug bill.

Some of the most commonly used hypnotics and some of their important clinical and pharmacokinetic properties are shown in Table 1. The ideal properties for a hypnosedative depend very much on the indication for its use. A long half-life of action may be ideal for a drug being used as an antianxiety agent, but is clearly a disadvantage if the compound is to be used simply as a nighttime hypnotic. Residual effects the next day may not only be unpleasant but in many situations may be frankly dangerous. Furthermore, it must be remembered that the sedatives listed in Table 1 have different mechanisms of action and the quality of the sedation they produce varies considerably.

II. THE RELATIONSHIP BETWEEN PLASMA LEVEL AND CLINICAL RESPONSE

Plasma concentrations of hypnosedatives correlate poorly with their effects both at doses used clinically and in overdosage. The very large variations in the response of individuals to hypnosedatives is probably the major reason, although several other factors are involved.

The poor correlation between plasma concentration and the clinical picture seen with overdosage is surprising and applies to most hypnosedatives in common use. Some of the discrepancies are partly explained by poor analytical techniques and poor reporting systems used by some forensic toxicologists and coroner's courts. Toxicity has all too frequently been ascribed to a single substance in cases involving overdosage with multiple drugs, and failure to consider the importance of coincidental ingestion of alcohol has been common. It is unfortunate that much important clinical data has been lost because so many court reports are of limited value and some grossly incorrect. A death ascribed to diazepam in one such report occurred after a man drowned in a small puddle of water beside a footpath. A high blood alcohol concentration and a plasma concentration of diazepam often associated with normal dosage were reported in the court proceedings!

Table 1 Pharmacokinetic Features of Several Commonly Used Hypnosedatives[a]

	Pentobarbitone	Glutethimide	Diazepam	Flurazepam	Nitrazepam	Oxazepam	Chloral hydrate	Methaqualone
Hypnotic dose (mg)	100-200	500-1,000	5-15	15-30	5-10	30-45	500-1,500	300
V_d (liters/kg)	1	1.4	0.7-2.6	–	2.1	1.6	0.95	6
$T_{1/2}$ (h)	20-60	5-22	15-20	b	21-28	10-14	8.2	20-40
Active metabolites	No	No	Yes	Yes	No	No	Yes	No
$T_{1/2}$ of active metabolites	–	–	40	100	–	–	11 and 80	–

[a]Figures are from several sources and should be regarded as only approximate. V_d = volume of distribution; $T_{1/2}$ = half-life of elimination.
[b]Relative extensive first-pass metabolism of the parent drug.

Values of "toxic" and "lethal" plasma or blood concentrations quoted in many toxicology texts are based on such poor data and should be regarded at best as only very rough guides to the severity of intoxication. Measurement of the plasma concentration should never replace clinical judgment in dictating the management of the patient with an overdosage of a sedative drug.

Studies of patients with single overdosages of barbiturates other than phenobarbitone and barbitone have repeatedly failed to show any close correlation between the plasma concentration and the level of consciousness or the duration of coma [7-11]. Furthermore, various studies have reported a very wide range of plasma concentration associated with recovery of consciousness after barbiturate-induced coma. Some patients have coma with marked central nervous system (CNS) depression at plasma concentrations of barbiturate below that associated with the return of consciousness in others [11,12]. There is some evidence that there is a better correlation between the plasma concentrations of phenobarbitone and barbitone and the degree of CNS depression.

Similarly, poor correlations have been noted between plasma or "blood" concentrations of glutethimide and the clinical features of poisoning [13-15]. Although there is some correlation between mean blood concentration of glutethimide and degree of intoxication, the variation is so large as to be of no value in the management of the individual case. Some patients with mild intoxication and no coma have blood glutethimide concentrations less than those with severe intoxication manifest by coma and hypotension.

Methaqualone is another sedative frequently involved in serious suicidal overdosages, usually in combination with diphenhydramine. A study of 102 patients with overdosage of this combination showed little correlation between plasma concentration of methaqualone (diphenhydramine was not measured) and the degree of duration of coma [16].

Acute intoxication with chloral hydrate is often associated with respiratory depression and cardiac complications, including ventricular and supraventricular arrhythmias. Additionally, there is the risk of damage to the mucosa of the gastrointestinal tract, especially the stomach. It is not clear how much of the toxicity is associated with the parent molecule and how much is due to its metabolites, trichloroethanol and trichloroacetic acid. Chloral hydrate is normally rapidly metabolized to trichloroethanol, which is pharmacologically active, but there is some evidence that this conversion is slower with overdosage [17]. Measurement of the plasma level of trichloroethanol can be used to estimate the quantity of chloral hydrate ingested [17,18] and to follow the rate of spontaneous or dialysis-induced removal from the body, but there is no clear demonstration of a close correlation between the plasma level of trichloroethanol and the risk of serious toxicity. The clinical condition of the patient, especially the presence of shock and cardiac arrhythmias, should be the main factor indicating treatment, including dialysis [19-21]. The correlations between the blood concentration of ethanol and the level of intoxication appear to be much more precise than for other sedatives.

There are similarly poor correlations between plasma concentrations of hypnosedatives and their sedative effects when used at clinical dosages. The reasons are variable and relate to the complex pharmacokinetics and pharmacodynamics of many hypnotics and to the very many factors, including the large placebo effects, that influence arousal in man. Additionally, the rapid development of tolerance to the hypnotic effects of most hypnosedatives [21] indicates that any relationship between plasma concentration and effect may not be independent of time of exposure to the drug. The complexity of the problem is best illustrated by considering the relationship between the plasma concentration of a commonly used benzodiazepine and the sedation it produces.

Diazepam is one of the most commonly used sedatives, and there is marked intersubject variation in the plasma concentrations achieved after single or multiple doses of the drug. This variation reflects differences in the rates of metabolism and in the distribution of the drug. Furthermore, N-desmethyldiazepam, a major metabolite of diazepam, has a longer half-life than the parent drug and accumulates with chronic usage. The desmethyl metabolite also has sedative and anticonvulsant effects [22] but doesn't have the muscle relaxant effects of diazepam. Similarly, oxazepam, a further metabolite of diazepam, also has sedative and anticonvulsant activities, although less potent than diazepam. Oxazepam has little or no action as a skeletal muscle relaxant. Thus the various pharmacologic effects of the benzodiazepines are related not to a single compound but to a number of compounds, each with quite separate pharmacodynamics, pharmacokinetics, and variable distribution within the brain. Furthermore, it is clear that individual pharmacological effects may relate to different fractions of the total benzodiazepine concentration. Thus the muscle relaxant effect relates most closely to the level of diazepam, whereas the anticonvulsant and sedative effects are related to a complex function of the concentrations of diazepam, N-desmethyldiazepam, and oxazepam. The situation is a little less complicated with the first administration of benzodiazepine hyponotics. In this case, the degree of sedation in adult subjects does correlate with the blood level achieved (Table 2), but apparent recovery from the sedative effects can take place without any fall in the blood concentration or indeed while the concentration is still rising!

Flurazepam is another widely used hypnotic, particularly in the United States. A similarly complex metabolic and pharmacokinetic pattern complicates the relationship between concentrations of flurazepam and its effects. The hypnotic effect of this drug increases over 3 or 4 nights' administration [24], although the drug itself does not appear to accumulate [25] and hangover does

Table 2 Relationship between Blood Levels of Diazepam and Drowsiness[a]

	Adults		Children	
Blood level (ng/ml)	No. of subjects	No. of subjects with drowsiness	No. of subjects	No. of subjects with drowsiness
<100	11	2 (18%)	3	1 (33%)
100-180	15	5 (33%)	8	4 (50%)
>180	16	14 (87%)	4	0 (0%)

[a] $\chi^2 < 180/>180 = P < .001$.

Source: Ref. 23.

not seem to be a problem [26]. Two of the metabolites of flurazepam, the N-desalkyl and the N-hydroxymethyl derivatives, are more active than the parent drug [27], and there is considerable "first-pass" metabolism both in the small bowel mucosa as well as the liver [28]. These data indicate that the hypnotic effect of flurazepam does not reside in a single chemical substance, and that the "active" drug is the sum of the concentration of parent drug and active metabolites. The parent drug and active metabolites are known to have different potencies, and their relative proportion in the plasma changes with time after a single dose and with long-term administration. Thus it should not be surprising that there are no simple correlations between the blood levels of benzodiazepines and their sedative properties.

The subject is made even more difficult to study by the nature of the sedation produced by benzodiazepines, which largely results from attenuation of sensory stimulation rather than direct and relatively nonspecific depression of the CNS which characterizes sedation produced by drugs such as barbiturates, glutethimide, and chloral hydrate. Benzodiazepine-induced sedation is therefore very dependent on the level of sensory stimulation at the time.

While blood or plasma concentrations of a drug can be measured with some precision, it is much more difficult to obtain meaningful quantitative data of the degree of sedation produced by a drug. The reasons for this are readily understood by considering our knowledge of normal sleep and drug-induced sedation.

III. SLEEP AND HYPNOTIC DRUGS

A. Normal Sleep

Tir'd Nature's sweet restorer, balmy sleep!

Sleep is clearly an important part of our lives, yet it is surprising that we understand so little about its restorative powers and even less about disorders of sleep, including the very common problem of insomnia. The basic physiological mechanisms operating in normal sleep are ill understood, and it is only in the last 15 years that much effort has been directed at defining the effects of sleep deprivation and other abnormal patterns of sleep.

The time spent in sleep varies enormously between individuals and throughout life in the same individual. Young children and the elderly sleep longer and sleep more during daylight hours. Although it is clear that the time spent sleeping is partly determined by habit and influenced by opportunity and environment, there are obvious differences in the need for sleep. Some individuals function indefinitely with only a few hours of sleep, while others seem to need 8 to 10 hours of sleep to avoid decreasing performance, irritability, and malaise which characterize the individual deprived of sleep. Not only is the time spent in sleep ill understood, but there appear to be qualitative differences in the way people sleep. Many patients who complain bitterly of insomnia sleep for much the same total time as subjects who do not complain of insomnia [29]. Thus although objective signs of insomnia such as increased sleep latency (time to fall asleep), number of awakenings, and total length of sleep may be demonstrable, it is clear that a major component of the quality of sleep is not measured by the various physiological parameters which are commonly assessed.

Studies in sleep laboratories in the last 10 to 15 years have defined some of the physiological characteristics of normal sleep. It has been possible to divide arousal into three stages: (1) alert wakefulness; (2) non-rapid-eye-movement sleep (NREM or non-REM sleep); and (3) rapid-eye-movement sleep (REM sleep). The injection of physostigmine during periods of NREM sleep will induce REM sleep, suggesting that cholinergic mechanisms are involved in the induction of REM sleep [30]. The location of the REM-sleep-promoting area may be in the pons. Serotonergic mechanisms operate in the promotion of NREM sleep, while dopaminergic and noradrenergic pathways appear to be involved in maintaining the alert wakeful state. The overall level of arousal appears to be governed by the interplay of sleep-promoting mechanisms and wakefulness-promoting mechanisms, on which is superimposed an intrinsic circadian rhythm.

Falling asleep is associated with a fairly characteristic pattern of events in normal individuals. The early period of sleep is characterized by the deepest sleep. During the night sleep progressively becomes lighter so that for the 2 or 3 hours before awakening, the subject is in very light sleep and readily aroused. The depth of sleep is associated with a characteristic pattern of changes in the electroencephalogram (EEG) which are designated stages 1 to 4 in order of increasing depth of sleep (Fig. 1).

After an initial period of about 60 to 90 min of deep sleep (stage 3 and 4), most subjects experience a period of REM sleep during which rapid eye movements occur and the frequency of the EEG increases, although the average amplitude decreases. Several such periods of REM sleep occur at about 90-min intervals during a normal night's sleep, and somewhere on the order of 20 to 25% of the night is spent in REM sleep. It is believed that dreaming occurs during periods of REM sleep, and subjects awakened at this time often remember the content of the dream, but rarely do if awakened during periods of non-REM sleep. Modern physiologists owe much to the poet Shelley (1792-1822), who clearly understood much about sleep:

> I arise from dreams of thee
> In the first sweet sleep of night.
>
> —*Indian Serenade*

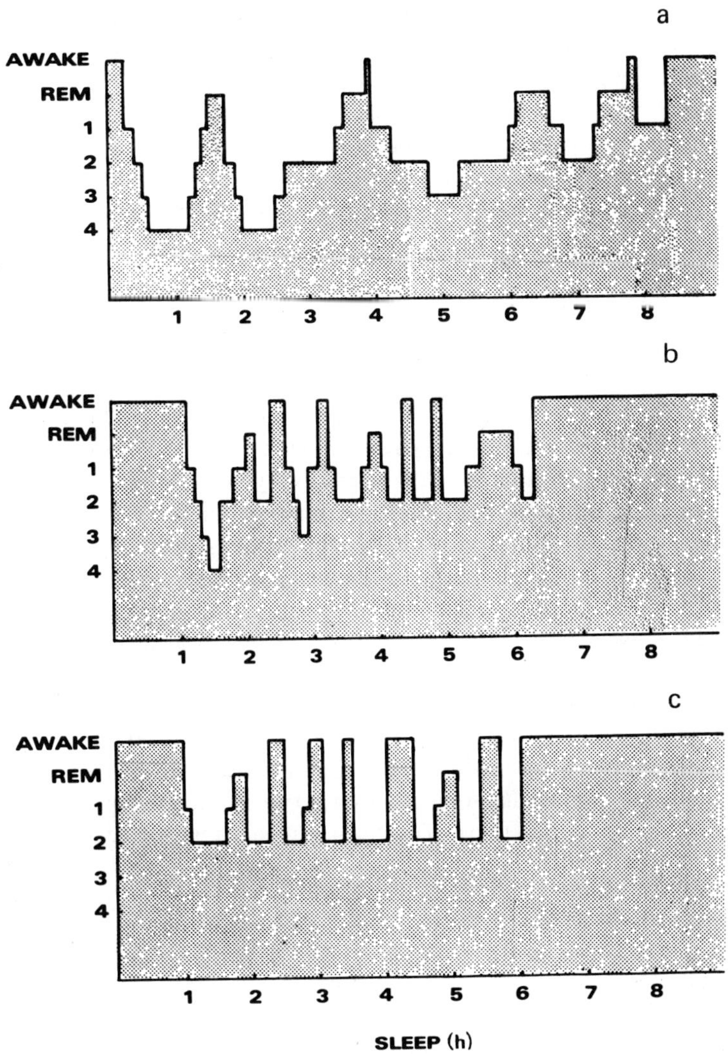

Figure 1 Schematic representations of the pattern of sleep in a normal subject (top), a subject with insomnia (middle), and a subject with insomnia who has taken barbiturates for some time (lower diagram). The stages of sleep are shown on the left (1 to 4). REM = rapid eye movement sleep.

With advancing age, less of the sleep period is spent in stage-3 and stage-4 sleep, and the number of awakenings during the night increases progressively, but the relative proportion of REM sleep remains fairly constant. Sleep during daylight hours, especially "catnaps," usually reflects reduced sensory input. True inversion of the sleep rhythm is most likely to be associated with organic illness such as cerebral arteriosclerosis or cardiac, respiratory, or hepatic failure.

Sleep is an important part of normal physiology and is certainly not a period of inactivity. Circulatory, hormonal, and metabolic events, including the output of growth hormone and the adrenal steroids, are known to be linked to the sleep-wakefulness cycle. There is evidence that sleep is an important component of synthetic processes, including those involved in normal growth and in the repair and replacement of tissues [31,32].

B. Insomnia

Insomnia is one of the most common symptoms encountered in medical practice and accounts for the major use of hypnosedatives. In the United Kingdom alone, it has been established that 22 million prescriptions for hypnosedatives are prescribed per annum [33], indicating that about 1 night's sleep in every 10 is influenced by a hypnotic drug. Indications are that this figure is not unrepresentative of most Western societies. Despite this enormous drug usage, little is known about the symptom of insomnia, and there remains considerable dispute about the existence of insomnia as a separate entity. It is, however, clear that most patients complaining of insomnia are suffering primarily from anxiety, depression, a drug effect, or other readily identifiable cause.

One of the most common causes of insomnia is the consumption of caffeine-containing beverages, especially coffee. A dose-related impairment of sleep can be demonstrated in normal subjects given between 1 and 4 cups of coffee or an equivalent dose of caffeine. The changes induced by coffee and caffeine resemble the pattern seen in many insomniacs. Sleep latency is increased with more frequent wakenings. REM sleep is not suppressed but is more frequent in the early hours of sleep, while stage-3 and stage-4 sleep shift to the later part of the sleep period [34]. The incidence of insomnia as a primary disorder of arousal is unknown. Of 48 patients complaining of insomnia and evaluated at the Stanford University Sleep Disorders Clinic, 18 (38.4%) were thought to have "true" insomnia, while 9 (19.1%) were thought to have a psychiatric disorder and 20 (42.5%) were thought to have drug-related insomnia [29].

Sleep laboratory studies have defined quantitative and qualitative abnormalities in the sleep of some insomniacs. Some subjects with difficulty going to sleep have clearly measured increases in the sleep latency period. Other insomniacs have sleep patterns characterized by more frequent awakenings, early awakening, or simply a decreased total sleep time. A further study by the Stanford group measured the sleep characteristics of 26 patients with presumed primary insomnia. These patients were selected on the basis of detailed inquiries, including sleep diaries, interviews, and other reports, and were all judged to be suffering from severe chronic insomnia. The mean sleep times without medication ranged continuously from a little over 4 hours to nearly 9 hours [29]! These studies and others [35-37] have clearly indicated that most patients complaining of insomnia give extremely inaccurate estimates of their sleep time. The objective measurements of sleep time in insomniacs have clearly shown that only those insomniacs with a sleep time of less than about 6 hours are likely to have an increased sleep time with hypnotics used in customary dosage.

The "quality" of sleep remains largely unmeasurable, although sleep characterized by an increased amount of REM (REM rebound) is often of poor quality, being nonrestful, often with an unpleasant dream content. This is seen particularly during periods following the withdrawal of some hypnosedatives. Changes in the REM content of sleep, however, do not relate directly to qualitative changes in sleep.

C. The Effect of Hypnosedatives on Sleep Patterns

There are many hypnosedatives capable of inducing sleep in normal individuals and in insomniacs, but there is no available sedative that induces sleep that is physiologically normal and none has an ideal pharmacodynamic or pharmacokinetic profile. Most sedatives used clinically are effective hypnotics when used for short periods but lose their effectiveness if used for more than a week or two. Kales et al. [21] studied the efficacy of chloral hydrate 1,000 mg, flurazepam 30 mg, glutethimide 500 mg, methaqualone 150 and 300 mg, and secobarbitone 100 mg, and while all were initially effective in inducing or maintaining sleep, all except flurazepam were ineffective when studied again at the end of 2 weeks' administration.

The characteristics of sleep induced by hypnosedatives vary somewhat, but most reduce the content of stage-3 and stage-4 sleep and most cause a reduction in REM sleep. Following the withdrawal of hypnosedatives, the quantity of stage-3 and stage-4 sleep returns to normal, but in most cases there is a rebound increase in the content of REM sleep and this period is often associated with unpleasant dream content and nonrestful sleep and is believed to be a major reason for continuation of the hypnotic habit in many patients. The features of some commonly used hypnosedatives are shown in Table 3.

1. Barbiturates

The barbiturates include a large number of derivatives of barbituric acid which have been widely used in clinical medicine for 70 years. Many barbiturates are undoubtedly effective as sedatives, hypnotics, and anxiolytics, and some as anti-

Table 3 Some Important Features Associated with the Use of Commonly Used Hypnotics[a]

	Pentobarbitone	Glutethimide	Flurazepam	Nitrazepam	Oxazepam	Chloral hydrate	Methaqualone
Effective hypnotic							
Under 2 weeks	++	++	++	++	+	++	++
Long-term	–	–	++	+	+	–	–
Hangover potential	++	++	±	++	+	++	++
REM suppression	++	++	–	±	±	±	++
REM rebound	++	++	–	±	±	±	++
Inhibition of Stage 4 sleep	±	±	++	+	+	–	±
Danger with overdosage	++	++	±	±	±	++	++
Risk of habituation	++	++	±	±	±	++	++
Drug interactions (pharmacokinetic)	++	++	–	–	–	++	++

[a]++ = marked effect; + = mild to moderate effect; ± = mild or doubtful effect; – = no effect. It should be remembered that any combination of CNS depressants will produce at least additive CNS depression. This type of interaction is not included in the table.

convulsants, but a low therapeutic index and other problems associated with long-term use now limits their clinical indications in situations other than epilepsy.

Barbiturates reversibly depress the CNS in a dose-dependent manner, probably by inhibiting transmembrane ion fluxes. Their actions are complex, but inhibition of synaptic transmission, particularly affecting pathways involved with repetitive discharges, is likely to be important. High doses of barbiturates depress respiratory drive, and this is the main cause of death with overdosage. The therapeutic index is low, the lethal dose only being about twice the anesthetic dose.

The anticonvulsant action of the barbiturates is not directly related to their potency as sedatives. Phenobarbitone and some very closely related compounds are much more potent anticonvulsants than other barbiturates which have significant anticonvulsant activity only at anesthetic doses. The relationship between plasma concentration of phenobarbitone and anticonvulsant or toxic effect is sufficiently precise to make plasma level measurement of phenobarbitone an important part of the safe and effective use of this anticonvulsant and other closely related compounds (see Chap. 15).

The major uses of barbiturates are as anticonvulsants and general anesthetics. The lipid-soluble compounds of the series are more potent hypnotics and are useful as induction agents in anesthesia. They have a rapid onset and short duration of action because of redistribution into tissues. Metabolism and elimination of the more lipid-soluble compounds is also more rapid. Barbiturates are potent inducers of oxidative drug metabolism and are involved in a number of clinically important interactions with drugs, including the coumarin anticoagulants and several corticosteroids.

Barbiturate-induced sleep differs from normal sleep in a number of ways. There is initially a marked reduction in the time spent in REM sleep [12], and on withdrawal there is an increase in the time spent in REM sleep. This "REM rebound" is associated with nonrestful sleep, often with an unpleasant dream content. The unpleasant nature of the withdrawal period is undoubtedly an important reason for the development of habituation. Prolonged use of barbiturates for periods longer than about 2 weeks is associated with a loss of hypnotic effect and increased restlessness during the late stages of sleep. Hormonal changes involving growth hormone and adrenocorticosteroids have been documented, but their significance is unknown.

Impaired performance, particularly in matters involving judgment, fast reactions, and skilled motor function, may be present for at least 24 h after a single dose of a barbiturate. This is an important risk in dangerous or demanding occupations. Additionally, subtle changes in mood are often present after waking from barbiturate-induced sleep. Subjects commonly display a "brittle" affect, and irritability, elation, depression, or excessive sensitivity may be provoked by minor situations.

Several factors contribute to the development of chronic states of intoxication which are unfortunately common among users of barbiturates. Loss of hypnotic potency after only a few nights' use follows from the rapid development of tolerance to the sedative effect together with accelerated metabolism of the drugs due to enzyme induction. Patients often take larger doses in an attempt to regain the hypnotic effect and to avoid the unpleasant and nonrestful sleep that is associated with withdrawal of barbiturates. Remarkable tolerance may develop, the patient being confused and tremulous with grossly altered affect but still unable to obtain a restful night's sleep. Convulsions may follow attempts to reduce the dosage especially if the drugs are withdrawn abruptly.

The lack of long-term efficacy, together with the numerous disadvantages and risks of long-term use, precludes the use of barbiturates for the treatment of chronic insomnia. Although effective hypnotics short term, their acute toxicity, particularly the risks of overdosage, together with the frequent "hangover" effect, indicates that they should no longer be used.

There is evidence from animal studies that barbiturates in high dosage can reduce the brain damage resulting from trauma and/or anoxia [38]. The efficacy of this treatment in reducing brain damage after cardiopulmonary arrest is not yet clear, but studies are now in progress in several centers.

2. *Glutethimide and Methyprylon*

Glutethimide, like methyprylon, is a piperidinedione whose pharmacology is similar to the medium-acting barbiturates. Hypnotic doses of 0.5 to 1.0 g are associated with the rapid development of tolerance and the risk of dependence and addiction. The drug is erratically absorbed and has a low therapeutic ratio, being particularly likely to cause coma with cardiac depression and arrhythmias. The lethal dose is in the order of 10 to 20 g. Long-lasting antimuscarinic effects, including paralytic ileus and bladder atony, may complicate recovery from only moderate overdosage. The drug is a potent inducer of the microsomal mixed-function oxidase, and interactions with coumarin anticoagulants, vitamin D_3, and cortisol metabolism have been documented.

The drug suppresses REM sleep even at doses that do not decrease awakenings in insomniacs [39]. The hypnotic effect of glutethimide is not sustained. There appears to be no clinical indication for the continued use of this drug.

Not a great deal is known of the pharmacology of methyprylon, but it appears to resemble the barbiturates and glutethimide. Its effect on sleep is similar to the barbiturates [39], and the drug has the same risks with overdosage and long-term use. Again, there would seem to be no indication for its continued use.

3. *Chloral Hydrate*

Chloral hydrate and the related compounds chloral betaine and triclofos sodium are widely used hypnotic agents, although chloral hydrate has now been in use for over a century. Like the barbiturates and many other hypnotics, they are effective short-term hypnotics but associated with the rapid development of tolerance and loss of efficacy after a few nights' use.

There is some dispute about the effect of chloral hydrate on sleep physiology. Doses of 0.5 and 1.0 g are associated with little suppression of REM sleep [40], but larger doses of 1,500-2,000 mg are not infrequently needed [41]. It is likely that chloral hydrate would suppress REM sleep at these doses, as it has been reported with a dose as low as 800 mg [42].

Chloral hydrate has a therapeutic ratio similar to the barbiturates, and acute intoxication is similar with the addition of gastric irritation.

Rapid tolerance, dependence, and addiction are all problems with long-term use, and chloral hydrate interacts significantly with coumarin anticoagulants [43,44] and should never be used at the same time.

Although the half-life of chloral hydrate and its major active metabolite trichloroethanol is shorter than most other hypnotics (8-11 h), a minor metabolite, trichloroacetic acid, accumulates with a much longer half-life and may be responsible for the interaction between chloral hydrate and the coumarin anticoagulants.

4. Benzodiazepines

Several components from this chemically distinct group of sedatives are now widely used as sedatives, hypnotics, anxiolytics, anticonvulsants, and skeletal muscle relaxants. The drugs are much safer in overdosage than any other hyposedatives, even enormous overdosages rarely if ever being fatal if taken as a single compound. The antianxiety and anticonvulsant actions of this class of compound have been discussed in Chaps. 13 and 15, and many of the features of their hypnotic effects have been mentioned.

Flurazepam is the most completely studied hypnotic compound from the series. It is the only hypnotic drug with proven long-term efficacy [21], and despite the relatively long half-life of some of its active metabolites, it does not appear to be associated with a problem of morning "hangover" [29]. In doses of 15-30 mg flurazepam is not associated with REM suppression or rebound, although like diazepam and most other hypnosedatives, δ-wave sleep is reduced. Diazepam is an effective hypnotic, and although associated with REM suppression and rebound it has an important place in the treatment of insomnia associated with anxiety.

Other benzodiazepine hypnotics have been less extensively studied. Nitrazepam is widely used in several countries, and data from several sleep laboratory studies are available. The drug is an effective hypnotic, but unlike flurazepam, nitrazepam reduces the content of REM sleep and is associated with REM rebound and an increased incidence of "bizarre" dreams on withdrawal. Chlordiazepoxide is a less potent hypnotic, and the more potent flunidiazepam has not yet been fully evaluated.

The effects of a number of benzodiazepine hypnotics on sleep have been reviewed by Kales and Scharf [45] and by Oswald et al. [46]. Doses of benzodiazepines used clinically are not associated with enzyme induction, and this class of hypnotic can safely be used in patients taking oral anticoagulants. The benzodiazepines have a low potential for abuse.

IV. THE PLACE OF DRUG THERAPY IN THE MANAGEMENT OF INSOMNIA

The available evidence indicates that hypnosedative drugs have much less to offer than the level of their consumption would suggest. Careful screening of patients presenting with chronic insomnia will disclose many that have an anxiety state or depression as the underlying cause, and this should determine the therapeutic approach. Hypnosedatives should be avoided in the depressed patient because of the suicide risk. The sedative effects of the tricyclic antidepressants can be used to provide useful nighttime sedation.

Many patients have insomnia that is itself drug related. Caffeine usually in the form of excessive consumption of coffee is a common cause of difficulty going to sleep, and alcohol is a common cause of disturbed sleep with frequent and early awakenings. A careful history followed by careful explanation and reassurance often results in a dramatic end to this type of insomnia.

The most difficult problems of drug-related insomnia are seen in patients habituated to hypnosedatives, especially barbiturates, chloral hydrate, or methaqualone. Full explanation is important, and these patients often need considerable encouragement and support to overcome their dependence on these drugs. Sudden withdrawal of sedatives may not be possible without the risk of precipitating epilepsy, particularly when very large doses of barbiturates are being taken. Gradual withdrawal in hospital is then the most appropriate method of management.

There remains a number of patients whose insomnia appears to be "primary." Every effort should be made to avoid the long-term use of hypnotics, particularly as up to half of these patients will have little or no objective evidence of decreased sleep time, and very little increase of sleep time if hypnotics are used [29]. If long-term usage of a hypnotic is indicated, then flurazepam appears to be the agent of choice.

REFERENCES

1. J. Carmody, R. Boyle, P. Butler, P. Douglas, and D. Dwyer, Patterns of use of benzodiazpeines in Australia. *Med. J. Aust. 2*:666–668, 1977.

2. J. S. Berkeley and I. M. Richardson, Drug usage in general practice. *J. R. Coll. Gen. Pract. 23:*155-161, 1973.
3. O. L. Wade and H. E. Hood, An analysis of prescribing of an hypnotic in the community. *Brit. J. Prev. Soc. Med. 26:*121-128, 1972.
4. G. G. Jenner, Prescriptions in general practice, *N. Z. Med. J. 78:*296-299 1973.
5. P. D. Stolley, M. H. Becker, J. D. McEvilla, L. Lasagna, M. Gainor, and L. M. Sloane, Drug prescribing and use in an American community. *Ann. Intern. Med. 76:*537-540, 1972.
6. F. M. Berger, Drugs and suicide in the United States. *Clin. Pharmacol. Ther. 8:*219-223, 1967.
7. H. Matthew and A. A. M. Lawson, Acute barbiturate poisoning: A review of 2 years' experience. *Q. J. Med. 35:*539-552, 1966.
8. L. W. Henderson and J. P. Merrill, Treatment of barbiturate intoxication. *Ann. Intern. Med. 64:*876-891, 1966.
9. J. G. Setter, J. F. Maher, and G. E. Schneiner, Barbiturate intoxication. *Arch. Intern. Med. 117:*224-236, 1966.
10. J. Hadden, K. Johnson, S. Smith, L. Price, and E. Gardina, Acute barbiturate intoxication. *JAMA 209:*893-900, 1969.
11. L. F. Prescott, P. Roscoe, and J. A. Forrest, Plasma concentrations and drug toxicity in man. In *Biological Effects of Drugs in Relation to Their Plasma Concentrations* (D. S. Davies and B. N. C. Prichard, eds.). London, Macmillan, 1973, pp. 51-81.
12. I. Haider and I. Oswald, Effects of amylobarbitone and nitrazepam on the electrodermogram and other features of sleep. *Brit. J. Psychiatry 118:* 519-522, 1971.
13. J. A. Chazen and J. J. Cohen, Clinical spectrum of glutethimide intoxication. *JAMA 208:*837-839, 1969.
14. N. Wright and P. Roscoe, Acute glutethimide poisoning: Conservative management of 31 patients. *JAMA 214:*1704-1706, 1970.
15. J. A. Chazen and S. Garella, Glutethimide intoxication: A prospective study of 70 patients treated conservatively without hemodialysis. *Arch. Intern. Med. 128:*215-219, 1971.
16. H. Matthew, A. T. Proudfoot, S. S. Brown, and A. C. A. Smith, Mandrax poisoning: Conservative management of 116 patients. *Brit. Med. J. 2:* 101-102, 1968.
17. N. E. Stalker, J. G. Gambertoglio, C. J. Fukumitsu, J. L. Naughton, and L. Z. Benet, Acute massive chloral hydrate intoxication treated with hemodialysis: A clinical pharmacokinetic analysis. *J. Clin. Pharmacol. 18:*136-142, 1978.
18. D. J. Berry, Determination of trichloroethanol at therapeutic and overdose levels in blood and urine by electron capture gas chromatography. *J. Chromatogr. 107:*107, 1975.
19. W. D. Loeser, C. J. Fisher, and G. Boulis, Forty-three dialyses in a community hospital. *JAMA 192:*809, 1965.
20. S. Locket, Hemodialysis in the treatment of acute poisoning. *Proc. Roy. Soc. Med. 63:*427, 1970.

21. A. Kales, W. C. Allen, M. B. Scharf, and J. D. Kales, Hypnotic drugs and their effectiveness: All-night EEG studies of insomniac subjects. *Arch. Gen. Psychiatry 23:*226-232, 1970.
22. F. Marcucci, E. Mussini, A. Guaitaini, R. Fanelli, and S. Garattini, Anticonvultant activity and brain levels of diazepam and its metabolites in mice. *Eur. J. Pharmacol. 16:*311-314, 1971.
23. S. Garattini, F. Marcucci, P. L. Morselli, and E. Mussini, The significance of measuring blood levels of benzodiazepines. In *Biological Effects of Drugs in Relation to Their Plasma Concentrations* (D. S. Davies and B. N. C. Prichard, eds.). London, Macmillan, 1973, pp. 211-225.
24. A. Kales, E. O. Bixler, M. Scharf, and J. D. Kales, Sleep laboratory studies of flurazepam: A model for evaluating hypnotic drugs. *Clin. Pharmacol Ther. 19:*576-583, 1976.
25. S. A. Kaplan, J. A. F. deSilva, M. L. Jack, J. K. Alexander, N. Strojny, R. E. Weinfeld, C. V. Puglisi, and L. Weissman, Blood level profiles in man following chronic oral administration of flurazepam hydrochloride. *J. Pharm. Sci. 62:*1932-1935, 1973.
26. J. D. Kales, A. Kales, E. O. Bixler, and E. S. Slye, Effect of placebo and flurazepam on sleep patterns in insomniac subjects. *Clin. Pharmacol. Ther. 12:*691-697, 1971.
27. L. O. Randall and B. Kappell, Pharmacological activity of some benzodiazepines and their metabolites. In *The Benzodiazepines* (S. Garattini, E. Mussini, and L. O. Randall, eds.). New York, Raven Press, 1973, pp. 27-51.
28. W. A. Mahon, T. Inaba, and R. M. Stone, Metabolism of flurazepam by the small intestine. *Clin. Pharmacol. Ther. 22:*228-233, 1977.
29. W. C. Dement, V. P. Zarcone, E. Hoddes, H. Smythe, and M. Carskadon, Sleep laboratory and clinical studies with flurazepam. In *The Benzodiazepines* (S. Garattini, E. Mussini, and L. O. Randall, eds.). New York, Raven Press, 1973, pp. 599-612.
30. R. J. Wyatt, S. Dawson, and J. C. Gillin, REM sleep induction by physostigmine infusion during sleep. *Science 191:*1281-1283, 1976.
31. I. Oswald, Human brain protein, drugs, and dreams. *Nature 223:*893-897, 1969.
32. I. Oswald, *Sleep.* Harmondsworth, Penguin Books, 1970.
33. D. D. Breimer, Pharmacokinetic and biopharmaceutical aspects of hypnotic drug therapy. In *Clinical Pharmacy and Clinical Pharmacology* (W. A. Gouveia, G. Tognoni, and P. P. O. Van der Kleijn, eds.). Amsterdam, Elsevier/North-Holland Biomedical Press, 1976, pp. 17-42.
34. I. Karacan, J. L. Thornby, A. M. Anch, G. H. Booth, R. L. Williams, and P. J. Salis, Dose related sleep disturbances induced by coffee and caffeine. *Clin. Pharmacol. Ther. 20:*682-689, 1976.
35. L. J. Monroe, Psychological and physiological differences between good and poor sleepers. *J. Abnorm. Psychol. 72:*255-264, 1967.
36. S. A. Lewis, Subjective estimates of sleep. *Brit. J. Psychol. 60:*203-208, 1969.

37. W. W. K. Zung, Insomnia and disordered sleep. *Int. Psychiatry Clin. 1:* 123-146, 1970.
38. E. M. Nemoto, W. A. Kofke, P. K. K-A. Mossman, S. W. Stezoski, and P. Safar, Studies on the pathogenesis of ischaemic brain damage and the mechanism of its amelioration by thiopental. *Acta Neurol. Scand. Suppl. (64) 56:* 142, 1977.
39. A. Kales, T. A. Preston, T-L. Tan, and C. Allen, Hypnotics and altered sleep-dream patterns, I: All night EEG studies of glutethimide, methyprylon, and pentobarbital. *Arch. Gen. Psychiatry 23:*211-218, 1970.
40. A. Kales, J. D. Kales, M. B. Scharf, and T-L. Tan, Hypnotics and altered sleep dream patterns, II: All night EEG studies of chloral hydrate, flurazepam, and methaqualone. *Arch. Gen. Psychiatry 23:*219-225, 1970.
41. K. Rickels and H. Bass, A comparative, controlled clinical trial of seven hypnotic agents in medical and psychiatric in-patients. *Amer. J. Med. Sci. 245:*142-152, 1963.
42. J. I. Evans and O. Ogunremi, Sleep and hypnotics. *Brit. Med. J. 3:*310-313, 1970.
43. E. M. Sellers and J. Koch-Weser, Potentiation of warfarin-induced hypoprothrombinaemia by chloral hydrate. *N. Engl. J. Med. 283:*827-831, 1970.
44. E. Sellers and J. Koch-Weser, Kinetics and clinical importance of displacement of warfarin from albumin by acidic drugs. *Ann. N.Y. Acad. Sci. 179:* 213-225, 1971.
45. A. Kales and M. B. Scharf, Sleep laboratory and clinical studies of the effects of benzodiazepines on sleep: Flurazepam, diazepam, chlordiazepoxide, and Ro 5-4200. In *The Benzodiazepines* (S. Garattini, E. Mussini, and L. O. Randall, eds.). New York, Raven Press, 1973, pp. 577-598.
46. I. Oswald, S. A. Lewis, H. Tagney, H. Firth, and I. Haider, Benzodiazepines and human sleep. In *The Benzodiazepines* (S. Garattini, E. Mussini, and L. O. Randall, eds.). New York, Raven Press, 1973, pp. 613-625.

15

Clinical Correlations of Anticonvulsant Drug Plasma Levels

Mervyn J. Eadie / *Department of Medicine, University of Queensland, Brisbane, Queensland, Australia*

I. INTRODUCTION

In the early 1970s the measurement of plasma anticonvulsant levels in epileptic patients was still a research tool. At that time the practical applications of the measurements were being explored by several groups of workers in different countries. Within a relatively short period, in many places measurement of plasma anticonvulsant levels has come to be regarded as little more than a routine aspect of the management of the patient with epilepsy. This rapid acceptance of the practice of monitoring plasma anticonvulsant levels attests to its clinical usefulness. However, the practice of monitoring the levels has come into widespread use before there has been time for the clinical correlations of the plasma level data to be thoroughly worked out. In addition, many of the generation of clinicians who are now using these measurements have received little formal education in clinical pharmacology. Because of these two circumstances, optimal use may sometimes not be made of the information provided by the drug levels. Moreover, the limitations of the measurement themselves may at times not be appreciated.

II. RATIONALE FOR THE MEASUREMENTS

The rationale for measuring plasma anticonvulsant concentration lies in the knowledge that the action of many drugs is proportional to the concentration of drug molecules in the biological fluid (the "biophase") around the receptors at which drug action is initiated. Drug molecules in the biophase are in dynamic equilibrium with drug molecules in plasma water. These molecules, in turn, are in dynamic equilibrium with any drug molecules which happen to be bound to plasma protein. Through these equilibria, drug concentration in whole plasma can provide a measure of drug concentration in the biophase. Therefore, for many drugs, drug concentrations in whole plasma provide a measure of the extent of drug action. There is now a tendency to assume that drug action will be proportional to plasma drug concentration for any new drug which comes into use. This assumption is generally born out in practice, but it is not always valid. For some of the newer anticonvulsants, and for certain older anticonvulsants which are not in common use, it has not yet been established that plasma drug levels are directly related to antiepileptic effect. However, for the well-established anticonvulsants, plasma drug level has been found related to capacity to prevent epileptic seizures (see Fig. 1).

The quantitative relation between drug concentrations in plasma and in the biophase that applies in the postdistributional state (when enough time has elapsed for the drug to have achieved its definitive distribution throughout the body) may not necessarily apply shortly after a dose of drug is given. In the immediate postdosage situation the ratio between drug levels in plasma and in the biophase may differ from the ratio found when postdistributional equilibria apply. Anticonvulsants are nearly always used in long-term therapy. Therefore, plasma anticonvulsant levels are almost always measured in the postdistributional state. However, if anticonvulsants are given in an acute situation and plasma drug levels are measured shortly after drug administration, the usual postdistributional relation between plasma drug level and anticonvulsant effect may not necessarily apply.

III. ANALYTICAL METHODS

Plasma anticonvulsant levels have been measured by a variety of methods. The clinician would probably regard detailed knowledge of these methods as un-

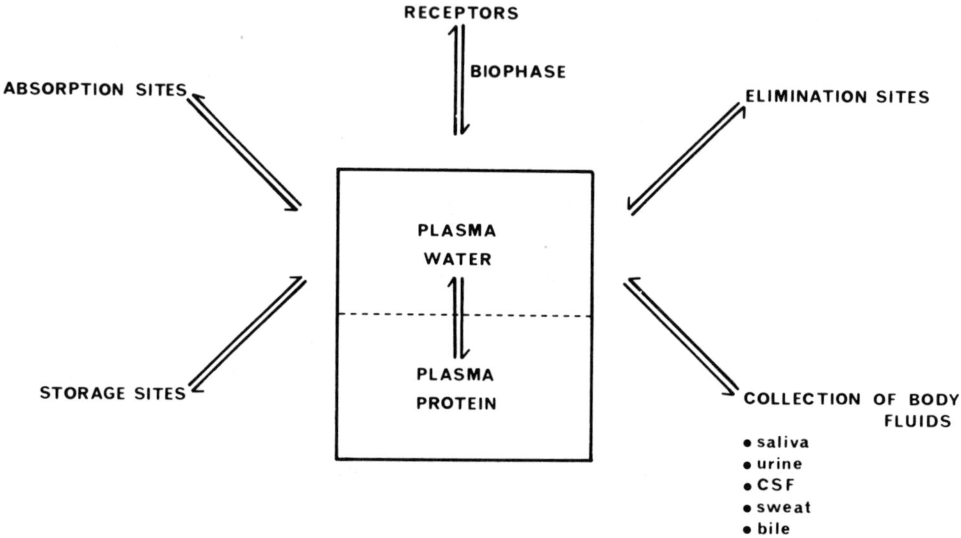

Figure 1 Scheme of drug distribution.

necessary for his purposes. However, he may find it useful to have some appreciation of the sensitivity and specificity of the assay method used to measure the plasma anticonvulsant drug levels which help influence his therapeutic decisions.

A. Spectrophotometric Techniques

Colorimetric or ultraviolet spectrophotometric techniques have been used to measure plasma anticonvulsant levels. In general, these methods are not very specific unless complicated partitioning techniques are introduced into the method. Such assays are usually of only marginally adequate sensitivity for drug given in doses of a few hundred mg daily.

Spectrofluorimetry offers enhanced sensitivity and possibly increased specificity for at least certain anticonvulsant drugs. However, the method is not widely used, largely because it is more demanding technically.

B. Immunoassay Techniques

Radioimmunoassay and enzyme multiplied immune test (EMIT) assays are highly sensitive and often are of adequate specificity for plasma anticonvulsant measurements. For those possessing the necessary apparatus the assays are relatively simple technically.

The major limiting factor in the use of immunoassays is that, to achieve simplicity, preliminary solvent partitioning steps are not carried out. Specificity of the method thus depends on the selectivity of the antibody used for the drug in question. Antibodies to particular drugs have not always proved completely specific. Thus in one EMIT system the assay for phenobarbitone also measures methylphenobarbitone, and another immunoassay for phenobarbitone also measures its weakly active metabolite p-hydroxyphenobarbitone [1]. Even when immunoassays distinguish between active drug and all known metabolites there is still the risk that the assay may not differentiate between the drug and an as-yet-unknown metabolite. This risk is reduced with other types of assay technique in which initial solvent partitioning steps are likely to separate the drug from any more polar metabolites [2].

C. Chromatographic Techniques

The separation capacity of the various chromatographic techniques, with the preceding solvent-partitioning stages often carried out before the drug is introduced into the chromatographic system, generally render such methods sufficiently specific for analytical purposes. Quantitative thin-layer chromatography may not always be sufficiently sensitive for measurement of plasma anticonvulsant concentrations. However, with suitable detectors gas-liquid chromatography and high-pressure liquid chromatography offer adequate sensitivity and specificity for the measurements. In general, high-pressure liquid chromatography is not quite as sensitive as gas chromatography, though it may offer advantages for the separation of thermolabile or polar substances. The use of a gas chromatograph-mass spectrometer operated in the specific ion detection mode offers the ultimate in assay specificity together with a sensitivity at least comparable to that of immunoassay. Unfortunately, the necessary apparatus is expensive to purchase and to maintain.

IV. PHARMACOKINETIC BACKGROUND

A knowledge of the pharmacokinetics of the individual anticonvulsant drug provides a desirable background for an interpretation of their plasma levels. There are several major sources of pharmacokinetic information available regarding these drugs (see Refs. 3-6). In the present section some of the more important of the available human pharmacokinetic data will be outlined.

A. Phenytoin

1. Absorption

After oral administration, phenytoin appears to absorb rather slowly but reasonably completely. Peak plasma levels occur 2 to 8 h from dosage [7]. The bioavailability of the drug in currently available preparations seems reasonably complete, though in the past a preparation with an approximate 75% bioavailability (due to an interaction between an excipient component and the drug) was marketed in Australia [8]. Despite its relatively full bioavailability, phenytoin from different preparations may exhibit different rates of entry into the circulation in the same subject [9]. Phenytoin is poorly soluble in water, particularly at acid pH. It seems likely that slow dissolution of the drug explains its rather slow absorption.

When given by intramuscular injection phenytoin absorbs slowly and unpredictably [10], so that it is difficult to give large enough doses of the drug to achieve satisfactory plasma levels. Wilder and Ramsay [11] have shown that a 50% increase in phenytoin dose is needed to maintain plasma phenytoin levels when intramuscular injection of phenytoin replaces oral therapy with the drug. Phenytoin crystals may deposit at sites of intramuscular injection of the drug, and remain in situ for many weeks [12].

2. Distribution

The apparent volume of distribution of phenytoin is approximately 0.6 liters/kg [13]. The great majority of the drug in plasma is bound to plasma protein. Figures for the plasma protein binding of the drug have usually been in the range 90-93% [7,14-16]. Protein binding capacity is reduced in the neonate [17] and in adult life decreases with age [18]. Protein binding of phenytoin is reduced in patients with uremia [19] or hepatic failure [18]. Phenytoin concentrations in cerebrospinal fluid (CSF) [7] and in saliva [20] are similar to those in plasma water. Phenytoin enters milk, where its concentration is about 25-30% of the simultaneous phenytoin concentration in plasma [21]. Phenytoin concentrations in human epileptic brain are generally similar to simultaneous phenytoin concentrations is plasma [22,23].

3. Elimination

Only about 5% of a phenytoin dose is excreted unchanged in urine [24]. A similar percentage of an oral phenytoin dose is excreted unaltered in the feces [8]. The remainder of an oral dose (approximately 90%) is eliminated by biotransformation. The drug molecule undergoes a variety of oxidative reactions on its aromatic rings, forming a number of hydroxylated metabolites of which 5-p-hydroxyphenyl-5-phenylhydantoin is generally accepted as the chief. For the most part, p-hydroxyphenytoin undergoes glucuronide conjugation prior to its excretion in urine. There is evidence that the capacity for the biotransformation of phenytoin to p-hydroxyphenytoin can become saturated at plasma phenytoin concentrations which are encountered during the course of antiepilepsy therapy in man [25]. However, there is also evidence [26] that formation of p-hydroxyphenytoin may play a decreasing role in the overall elimination of phenytoin as plasma phenytoin level increases. Despite this, the saturability of the enzymatic mechanism mediating p-hydroxyphenytoin formation at therapeutic plasma phenytoin levels ensures that the overall elimination of the drug is not adequately described by first-order kinetics. The elimination process is better described in terms of Michaelis-Menten kinetics [27]. Nevertheless, values for the half-life of phenytoin have been published, e.g., 22.0 ± 9.0 h [28]. A collection of half-life values for the drug was provided by Suzuki et al. [29]. Calculated values for the Michaelis-Menten parameters of phenytoin elimination are set out in Table 1.

The elimination of phenytoin is dose dependent, as is implicit in the fact that its elimination is better described by Michaelis-Menten than by first-order kinetics. As indicated by the V_{max} data shown in Table 1, and as was suggested by data on the relation between steady-state plasma phenytoin level and drug dose [33-36], phenytoin is eliminated more rapidly in children than in adults [37]. Sex appears to have little influence on elimination rate of the drug [38, 39], though it is possible that pregnancy enhances phenytoin elimination [40].

Phenytoin is known to be involved in a number of pharmacokinetic interactions with other drugs (see Ref. 4). It is likely that many of these interactions involve altered phenytoin elimination.

B. Methoin (Mephenytoin)

No accurate pharmacokinetic data are available for mephenytoin in man. Its demethylated derivative, Nirvanol, which is formed by biotransformation in man, is an anticonvulsant [41].

Table 1 Calculated Values for Phenytoin Elimination

Reference	K_m (μg/ml)	V_{max} (mg/kg/day)
[27]	6.77	6.1
[30]	16.3	14.4[a]
[31]	3.8	6.2
[32]	4.0	–
[26]	5.8 (adults)	8.1
	5.3 (children)	12.5

[a]This value was expressed in terms of mg/liter/day.

C. Phenobarbitone

1. Absorption

It has been suggested that phenobarbitone is absorbed slowly, since peak plasma levels may not occur till 6-18 h after oral dosage [42]. One's experience is that peak levels of the drug usually occur earlier than this after oral administration. According to Maynert [43], phenobarbitone is thought to be completely absorbed after oral administration. While there do not appear to be published data for the time course of plasma phenobarbitone levels after intramuscular administration of the drug, personal investigation has shown that peak plasma levels occur within 4 h of injection.

2. Distribution

The apparent volume of distribution of the drug is 0.7 liters/kg [13]. Some 50% of the drug in plasma is protein bound [44]. CSF levels of phenobarbitone are 40% of simultaneous levels of the drug in whole plasma [45]. If allowance is made for pH differences between plasma and saliva, phenobarbitone concentrations in saliva correspond reasonably well with concentrations of unbound phenobarbitone in plasma [46]. Phenobarbitone concentrations in brain and serum are said to be similar [47]. Melchior et al. [48] found that simultaneous concentrations of the drug in maternal serum and umbilical cord serum were similar.

3. Elimination

An average of 21% of a phenobarbitone dose is excreted unchanged in urine [42]. The major metabolite is p-hydroxyphenobarbitone [49], which is excreted in urine partly as conjugates (glucuronide and possibly sulfate). Little detailed quantitative work on the pattern of phenobarbitone excretion in human urine appears to have been published.

It seems generally accepted that the elimination of phenobarbitone follows first-order kinetics. However, the data of Eadie et al. [50], who studied the relation between steady-state plasma phenobarbitone level and different drug doses in individual patients, raised the possibility that the elimination kinetics of the drug may be more complex. Values for the half-life of phenobarbitone are 3-4 days [51], 4 days [52], and 4.3-6.7 days [42]. In children the half-life is shorter, e.g., 1.5-3.1 days [53].

D. Methylphenobarbitone

1. Absorption

On both a weight and a molar basis, roughly twice as much methylphenobarbitone as compared with phenobarbitone is required to produce similar plasma phenobarbitone levels. This discrepancy has raised the possibility that methylphenobarbitone is incompletely absorbed after oral administration [43]. Personal data suggest that the drug is fairly rapidly absorbed (T_{max} less than 7 h in seven of eight subjects). Therefore, one is reluctant to accept that methylphenobarbitone has a poor bioavailability. The answer to the dose discrepancy between phenobarbitone and methylphenobarbitone may lie in the pattern of elimination of the latter.

2. *Distribution*

Little information is available. In four subjects studied personally the apparent volume of distribution averaged 1.9 liter/kg. The extent of the plasma protein binding of methylphenobarbitone is unknown.

3. *Elimination*

Personal studies have shown that less than 5% of a methylphenobarbitone dose is excreted in urine unchanged. In one subject in whom appropriate data were collected, approximately 50% of a methylphenobarbitone dose was biotransformed to phenobarbitone. The pattern of elimination of the remainder of his dose was not determined.

In eight subjects the half-life of methylphenobarbitone averaged 32 h (range 17-76 h).

E. Primidone

1. *Absorption*

After oral administration primidone is thought to absorb reasonably rapidly. Peak plasma levels occur an average of 3 h after dosage [54,55]. Information on bioavailability of the drug is lacking.

2. *Distribution*

The apparent volume of distribution of primidone is 0.6 liter/kg [13]. The drug does not appear to be selectively concentrated in any region of the body [13]. Primidone is not bound to plasma protein [55,56] so that its simultaneous levels in whole plasma and CSF are similar [57].

3. *Elimination*

The extent of urinary excretion of unchanged primidone is unknown. It has been calculated that, in the steady state, 15% [58] or 24.5% [59] of a dose of primidone is biotransformed to phenobarbitone. Part of the primidone dose is converted to phenylethylmalonamide.

Primidone has a half-life of 6.5 ± 1.0 h [55] or 10-12 h [54]. There is no clear evidence that the elimination of the drug is influenced by age or sex. Pharmacokinetic interactions between primidone and phenytoin [60] or carbamazepine [55], both of which increase plasma phenobarbitone levels relative to primidone dose, probably do so by increasing the rate of elimination of primidone.

F. Carbamazepine

1. Absorption

Carbamazepine is poorly soluble in water. When given by mouth in tablet form its absorption is relatively slow, and there are intimations that the drug may not always be completely bioavailable [61,62]. No parenteral preparation of the drug is available.

2. Distribution

Carbamazepine has an apparent volume of distribution of approximately 1 liter/kg [62,63]. In man, brain/plasma concentration ratios for the drug range from 2.25:1 to 1.1:1 [64]. Some 70-75% of the drug in plasma is protein bound [65, 66]. The drug's simultaneous concentrations in plasma water and in CSF [67] or saliva [68] are similar.

3. Elimination

Less than 2% of a carbamazepine dose is excreted unchanged in urine [69]. Elimination occurs chiefly through biotransformation. Epoxide formation, with subsequent opening of the epoxide ring to form hydroxyl derivatives, occurs at the adjacent carbon atoms in the intermediate ring of the tricyclic carbamazepine molecule. Phenolic derivatives are formed if one of the benzene rings in the molecule undergoes oxidation. The initial product of epoxidation, carbamazepine-10,11-epoxide, is an anticonvulsant with a half-life of 6-14 h [64].

Carbamazepine in plasma has a half-life of 30 to 50 h after initial dosage [63,70,71]. With repeated administration of the drug the half-life shortens [71, 72]. In single-dose studies the half-life also appears to shorten in the individual as higher carbamazepine doses are given [63,71]. Concurrent intake of phenytoin or phenobarbitone may increase the elimination of carbamazepine [73].

G. Ethosuximide

1. Absorption

Ethosuximide appears to be fairly rapidly absorbed after oral administration. Peak plasma levels occur 3 to 7 h after intake [6]. The bioavailability of the drug has not been studied in detail, though it is probably reasonably complete. The drug absorbs faster from syrup than from capsules [74].

2. Distribution

The drug appears to be distributed through body water, its apparent volume of distribution being about 0.7 liter/kg [6]. Ethosuximide is not bound to plasma protein, and its simultaneous concentrations in whole plasma and in CSF [75] and in saliva [76] are similar. Ethosuximide concentrations in brain and in plasma also are similar [77].

3. *Elimination*

Between 17 and 38% of an ethosuximide dose is excreted unchanged in urine [78]. The remainder is biotransformed by alkyl side chain oxidation. In children the half-life is around 30 h [74]; in adults the half-life is about 60 h [79].

H. Troxidone

1. *Absorption*

After oral administration peak plasma levels of troxidone occur 30 min from intake [80]. Bioavailability data are lacking.

2. *Distribution*

The drug appears to be distributed throughout body water. It is not bound to plasma protein.

3. *Elimination*

Troxidone is biotransformed to an active anticonvulsant metabolite, dimethadione, which is excreted as such in urine. Troxidone has a half-life of about 16 h [80], but dimethadione has a much slower pattern of elimination, with a half-life of some 10 days [81].

I. Diazepam

1. *Absorption*

After oral administration diazepam absorbs rapidly with a T_{max} of about 1 h [82]. Bioavailability is probably in excess of 90% [83]. Given rectally, diazepam in solution absorbs rapidly (T_{max} 10-20 min), but if given in a suppository the drug absorbs less rapidly, then having a T_{max} of 60 min [84]. Diazepam absorbs more rapidly if given by mouth than if injected intramuscularly [85].

2. *Distribution*

It seems likely that diazepam undergoes substantial tissue binding, in view of its apparent volume of distribution of 1.75 liters/kg [13]. Diazepam in plasma is 97% bound to proteins [86,87]. CSF levels of the drug are 2-3% of simultaneous plasma levels [87]. Total brain diazepam levels are a good deal higher than simultaneous plasma levels of the drug [88].

3. *Elimination*

Less than 1% of a diazepam dose is excreted unchanged in urine [89]. Biotransformation is the chief route of elimination of the drug. N-demethylation leads to the formation of an anticonvulsant metabolite N-desmethyldiazepam (nordiazepam). This may be oxidized to a 3-hydroxy derivative, oxazepam, which also has some anticonvulsant properties.

The half-life of diazepam is 32 h [13] or 0.83-1.75 days [90]. Nordiazepam is more slowly eliminated, with a half-life of 60-95 h [90].

J. Nitrazepam

1. Absorption

Nitrazepam is fairly rapidly absorbed after oral administration, with a T_{max} of 2 h. Bioavailability is 53-94% [91].

2. Distribution

Nitrazepam has an apparent volume of distribution of 2.1 liters/kg [13]. Some 90% of the drug in plasma is protein bound [13]. Nitrazepam is found in human milk at 50% of its simultaneous plasma concentration [92].

3. Elimination

Nitrazepam is eliminated almost entirely by biotransformation, less than 1% of a dose of the drug appearing unchanged in urine. The main biotransformation products are 7-amino and 7-acetamido derivatives. The half-life of nitrazepam averaged 25.1 h [91].

K. Clonazepam

1. Absorption

Clonazepam appears to absorb fairly rapidly after oral administration, with a T_{max} of 2-4 h [93]. Bioavailability is about 90%. The efficiency of intramuscular administration has not been studied.

2. Distribution

Clonazepam has an apparent volume of distribution of 2.6 liters/kg [93]. Some 47% [94] or 82% [13] of the drug in plasma is protein bound.

3. Elimination

About 2% of a clonazepam dose is excreted unchanged in urine. Elimination is chiefly by means of biotransformation, with the formation of 7-amino, 7-acetamido, and various ring hydroxylated metabolites and their glucuronide conjugates. The half-life of the drug is 19-60 h [93,95,96].

L. Valproic Acid (Dipropylacetic Acid)

1. Absorption

Valproic acid (and its sodium salt) are water-soluble substances, which absorb rapidly after oral administration. Peak plasma levels often occur within 1 h of dosage [97]. Bioavailability data for the drug are not available.

2. Distribution

The apparent volume of distribution of valproate is 0.15-0.40 liters/kg [98]. These values suggest that the drug is distributed mainly in extracellular water. Figures for plasma protein binding of the drug are 84% [99] or 90% [100].

3. Elimination

Some 7% of a valproate dose is excreted unchanged in urine [97]. Biotransformation apparently accounts for the elimination of the remainder of the dose, various fatty acid derivatives being formed. The half-life of the drug is 10.3 ± 2.6 h [97] or 9.00 ± 1.01 h [98] in normal adults. However, the latter authors found that the drug was more rapidly eliminated in epileptic patients (half-life 5.88 ± 0.47), perhaps because previous anticonvulsant therapy had induced the hepatic microsomal mixed oxidase system in such patients.

V. PRACTICAL ASPECTS OF THE MEASUREMENTS

A. Fluids in Which the Anticonvulsant Measurements May Be Carried Out

The dynamic equilibria schematized in Fig. 1 suggest that drug concentrations in plasma water are likely to provide the best readily available measure of drug concentrations in the biophase. It is comparatively easy to separate blood cells from plasma by centrifuging. However, the further process of separating plasma water from plasma proteins (without displacing drug bound to plasma proteins) involves rather tedious technical procedures, e.g., ultrafiltration, dialysis. Further, if appreciable amounts of the drug are bound to plasma proteins, separating plasma water from plasma proteins reduces the amount of drug available for measurement. Consequently the separation imposes an increased demand on the sensitivity of the assay method used. Because of these considerations anticonvulsant levels are usually measured in whole plasma, as a matter of convenience, even though it has been shown that anticonvulsant levels in plasma water may correlate better with clinical effects of the drugs than do anticonvulsant levels in whole plasma [101].

The equilibria schematized in Fig. 1 also raise the possibility that anticonvulsant levels measured in biological fluids other than plasma might provide a reasonable measure of anticonvulsant effect. CSF, with its almost negligible protein content relative to that of plasma, is virtually equivalent to an ultrafiltrate of plasma. Concentrations of phenytoin, phenobarbitone, carbamazepine, and diazepam in CSF have proved very similar to concentrations of these drugs in plasma water, measured simultaneously (see above). However, it is not practicable to use CSF for routine anticonvulsant measurements. There has therefore been interest in using saliva for measurement of anticonvulsant concentrations. The protein concentration of saliva, though higher than that of CSF, is still only a small percentage of that of whole plasma. Unfortunately, the pH of saliva differs from that of plasma, and salivary pH may vary from time to time in the individual. This pH difference may cause a difference in the proportion of drug molecules ionized in plasma and saliva. Only nonionized drug molecules come into equilibrium across the cell membranes separating saliva and plasma water. Therefore, drug concentrations may alter between saliva and plasma water as salivary pH changes. This alteration would be of little magnitude for drugs which have pK_a values well away from the pH values of saliva and plasma, but could have major effects for drugs with pK_a values between the pH values of saliva and plasma. A correlation has been established between plasma water and salivary levels of phenytoin [20,46,68] and carbamazepine [46,68]. Levels of ethosuximide (which does not bind to plasma protein) are similar in saliva and in whole plasma [76]. If the pH of saliva is measured at the time of its collection and the pK_a value for the anticonvulsant in question is known, a correction can be applied for the effects of any pH discrepancy between saliva and plasma. If this is done, corrected salivary levels of phenytoin, phenobarbitone, carbamazepine, and ethosuximide correlate very well with simultaneous plasma water levels of these drugs [46]. The convenience of using saliva, rather than plasma water, to provide a reliable indication of the extent of potential anticonvulsant action suggests that increasing use may be made of salivary anticonvulsant assays in the future.

B. Measurement of Active Metabolites

Some anticonvulsant biotransformation products are known to possess antiepilepsy activity, as has been indicated above. In other instances it is not known whether anticonvulsant metabolites are pharmacologically active. Sometimes the active metabolites are more slowly eliminated than the parent drugs, e.g., phenobarbitone formed from methylphenobarbitone or from primidone. In such cases the parent drug serves in a sense as a "prodrug" for its metabolite. It may then be more useful clinically to measure plasma levels of the metabolite than of the drug itself. In such cases the situation would be more fully interpreted by measuring drug and metabolite simultaneously. However, data are not yet available correlating simultaneous plasma levels of drug and metabolite with therapeutic or toxic effects. Table 2 shows the major known metabolites of anticonvulsants and where possible indicates whether or not these metabolites have anticonvulsant activity.

Table 2 Major Known Metabolites and Half-Lives of Anticonvulsant Drugs

Drug	Metabolite(s)	Anticonvulsant activity	Half-life (h)
Phenytoin			22 ± 9
	p-Hydroxyphenytoin	0	?
Methoin (mephenytoin)			?
	Nirvanol	+	?
Phenobarbitone			96
	p-Hydroxyphenobarbitone	Weak	?
Methylphenobarbitone			32
	Phenobarbitone	+	96
Primidone			10–12
	Phenobarbitone	+	96
	Phenylethylmalonamide	+	29–36
Carbamazepine			30–50
	Carbamazepine epoxide	+	6–40
Ethosuximide			30–60
Troxidone			16
	Dimethadione	+	240
Diazepam			32
	Nordiazepam	+	60–95
	Oxazepam	+	9–22
Nitrazepam			25
	7-Aminonitrazepam	?	?
Clonazepam			19–60
	7-Aminoclonazepam	?	?
Valproic acid			9–10

C. Timing of Plasma Anticonvulsant Measurements

When a constant dose of a drug is given regularly, it requires the passing of 5 half-lives of the drug before plasma drug concentrations achieve 97% of their ultimate steady-state values. (In the steady state the amount of drug absorbed equals the amount eliminated over each dosage interval.) If the delay in achieving a steady state after dosage change is not appreciated, plasma anticonvulsant levels may be measured before a steady state applies. This may cause misleading correlations between the plasma drug level and the patient's subsequent clinical response. The half-lives of the anticonvulsants (or of their metabolites with known antiepilepsy actions) are also set out in Table 2. These values may serve as a basis for deciding when steady-state conditions are likely to apply. In general, bearing in mind that there is often a ±5-10% error in measuring drug concentration, it is realistic to anticipate that a reasonable approximation to the steady state will apply after 4 half-lives have elapsed. When therapy with a drug is begun, the drug may induce its own biotransformation, and also the biotransformation of other drugs taken concurrently. This effect, should it apply, will shorten drug half-life and speed the occurrence of steady-state conditions. However, should the dose be reduced for one of a number of drugs given concurrently, deinduction of the biotransformation of the other drugs may occur. Relatively little information is available about the speed of such deinduction in man, but one's impression is that the process may occur over several weeks. If so, it may take a long time for a new steady state to apply after dosage reduction. This point may not always be appreciated when plasma drug levels are measured.

In the steady state, plasma drug level may not be constant across the dosage interval, though the mean plasma level, over consecutive dosage intervals, is constant. After each dose, plasma drug level rises as absorption exceeds elimination, reaches a peak when absorption and elimination become equal, and then declines as elimination preponderates. For many of the anticonvulsants (e.g., Fig. 2) absorption of the drug after oral dosage and elimination of the drug are sufficiently slow processes for fluctuations in plasma level across an 8- or 12- or even a 24-h dosage interval to be negligible for practical purposes. For such drugs it matters little when steady-state levels are measured in relation to the time of dosage. However, for more rapidly eliminated anticonvulsants, e.g., valproate, steady-state plasma drug levels can show appreciable change within a dosage interval. For such drugs the timing of the measurements in relation to dosage becomes important. Usually only a single measurement is practicable. The time of peak plasma level in the individual is difficult to predict, and may change from dose to dose if rate of gastric emptying varies. Therefore, the most reproducible measurement is the plasma level immediately before the next dose is taken (the minimum steady-state plasma level). Uncertainty in the literature as to whether such minimum valproate levels have been measured makes some data about the drug difficult to assess.

D. Use of Appropriate Anticonvulsants

Empirically it has been found that certain types of epilepsy respond best to particular anticonvulsants and respond poorly to other anticonvulsants. If an anticonvulsant inappropriate to the patient's type of epilepsy is used, the therapeutic response is unlikely to be satisfactory no matter how well drug doses are adjusted.

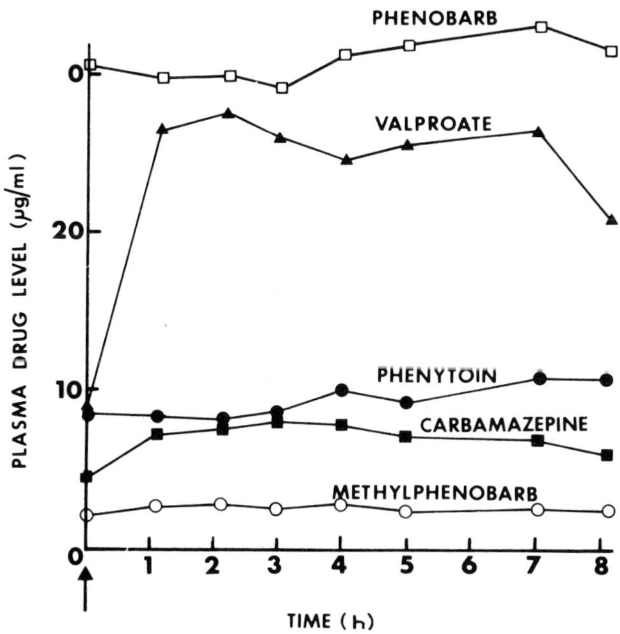

VALPROATE	400 mg
PHENYTOIN	230 mg
CARBAMAZEPINE	600 mg
METHYLPHENOBARB	100 mg

Figure 2 Variation in steady-state plasma level of valproate across a dosage interval compared with the relatively unchanged plasma levels of the other anticonvulsants. At the commencement of the study the patient took valproate 400 mg, phenytoin 230 mg, carbamazepine 600 mg, and methylphenobarbitone 100 mg, all by mouth. (From Ref. 76.)

Correct diagnosis of the patient's type of epilepsy is a prerequisite for successful anticonvulsant therapy.

The types of anticonvulsant most likely to be useful in particular varieties of epilepsy are set out in Table 3.

E. Problems of Compliance

Clinicians who treat epileptic patients become aware that these patients often fail to take their prescribed doses of anticonvulsant drugs. There have been several published reports describing this imperfect compliance [102-105]. Fail-

Table 3 Correlation of Types of Epilepsy with Drugs Useful in Their Treatment

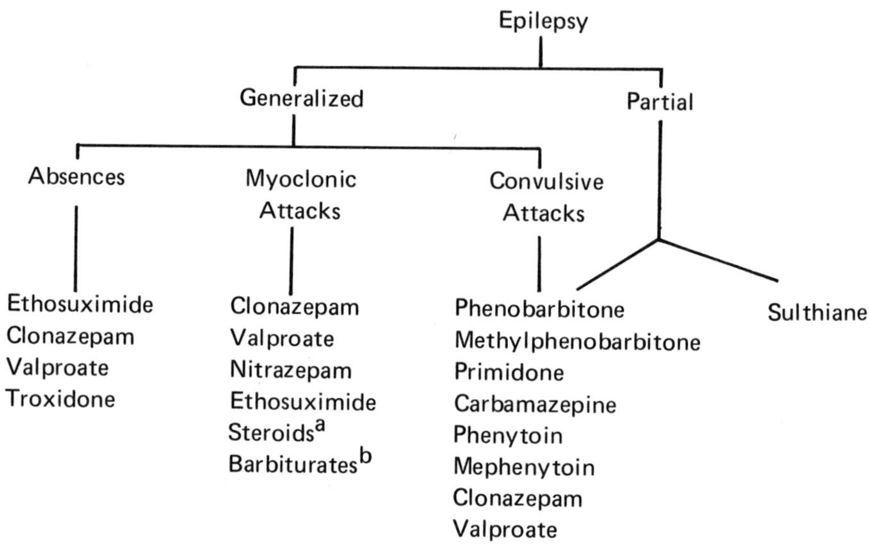

[a]For hypsarrhythmia.
[b]For adolescents.

ure to take therapy as prescribed may be due to a deliberate decision on the part of the patient. He may, for example, reject the diagnosis of epilepsy, reject the need to treat his epilepsy, or simply adopt the view that any drug intake is best avoided. Failure of compliance may also be due to the patient not understanding what is required of him, or be due to simple forgetfulness on his part.

However caused, imperfect compliance produces problems for the clinician who uses plasma anticonvulsant levels as a guide to the treatment of epilepsy. If drug dosage is adjusted to achieve a desired plasma drug level and the clinician believes that the patient is taking one drug dose when in reality he is taking a different dose, therapeutic misadventure may result. Whenever plasma drug levels deviate too widely from what the clinician's experience indicates is the expected level for the nominal drug dose being taken, the clinician should be suspicious of imperfect compliance. He should bear this in mind if he has to adjust drug dosages.

F. The Idea of a Therapeutic Range

Anticonvulsants are usually given with the aim of completely controlling the patient's epilepsy without producing any adverse effects on the patient's health.

The presence of adverse effects often becomes obvious soon after therapy is commenced or after drug dosage is increased. When the patient has infrequent seizures, or when treatment has been commenced before the natural history of his epilepsy has had time to declare itself, it is useful to know whether the patient has been given a sufficient drug dose for it to be likely to produce a reasonable anticonvulsant effect. In these circumstances, so long as the patient is taking drugs appropriate for his type of epilepsy, achieving a plasma anticonvulsant level in the "therapeutic range" is likely to offer the patient his best chance of epilepsy control without an undue risk of side effects of the type regarded as due to excessive drug dosage. It offers no protection against the occurrence of idiosyncratic-type unwanted drug effects.

In general, therapeutic ranges of plasma anticonvulsant levels appear to have been determined by clinicians setting the lower limit of the range at the plasma drug level at which a moderate number of patients' epilepsies come under control. The upper limit appears to be determined by the levels above which a significant number of patients begin to experience unwanted effects of the type usually regarded as due to drug overdosage. No more exact statistical correlation between plasma drug levels and success rates in controlling epilepsy or risks of producing unwanted effects are yet available for the majority of the anticonvulsants. For some of the newer anticonvulsants, or for the less widely used drugs, details of the therapeutic ranges are often tentative. Whether the therapeutic range of plasma concentrations of the one anticonvulsant drug is the same for different types of epilepsy for which it is appropriate therapy, whether the range changes as the patient's epilepsy becomes less active, and whether the range is the same if a second (or third) appropriate drug is added to therapy are as yet unanswered questions.

It should be recognized that achieving a plasma anticonvulsant level in the therapeutic range neither ensures that a patient's epilepsy will be fully controlled nor guarantees that he will not experience unwanted effects. Some patients may have their epilepsy controlled with plasma drug levels below, or above, the therapeutic range. In the latter case, some such patients may not be unduly troubled by drug side effects. On the other hand, certain patients may experience conventional overdosage-type toxicity with plasma drug levels in, or even below, the therapeutic range.

A detailed statistical analysis of the correlation between plasma anticonvulsant levels and biological effects of therapy in different types of epilepsy, carried out on a substantial body of data, could provide a very much better basis for determining appropriate anticonvulsant dose than that provided by the presently available, rather arbitrarily determined, values for the therapeutic ranges.

VI. CORRELATIONS OF CLINICAL EFFECTS AND PLASMA LEVELS FOR INDIVIDUAL DRUGS

A. Phenytoin

1. Anticonvulsant Effect

There is evidence that, at least up to the threshold of toxicity, increasing plasma phenytoin levels correlate with improved control of epilepsy (if the epilepsy is of a type normally responsive to the drug). Thus Lund [106] followed a group of 32 epileptic patients over a 3-year period. He showed that epileptic seizures in the group became less frequent (the mean annual grand mal rate falling from 5.8 to 1.6 attacks) as mean plasma phenytoin level was increased from 6.1 ± 2.9 to 15.0 ± 2.5 μg/ml, drug doses being adjusted on clinical grounds. Rowan et al. [107] found that epileptiform activity in the telemetered electroencephalogram (EEG) decreased as plasma phenytoin level was increased by dose adjustment. Terrence et al. [108] studied the question of unexpected inexplicable death in 37 epileptic patients. Only 3 had anticonvulsant levels in the therapeutic range, and almost 50% had no measurable drug in their plasmas. This finding raises the possibility that inadequate plasma anticonvulsant levels in epileptics are associated with an increased risk of death (perhaps death in epileptic seizures).

It seems fairly widely accepted that the therapeutic range of plasma phenytoin concentration is 10-20 μg/ml [109-111] or 12-25 μg/ml [112]. The earliest attempt to define the range was that of Buchthal and Svensmark [47], who found that phenytoin levels above 10 μg/ml were needed to control severe epilepsy, that no unwanted effects occurred at levels below 14 μg/ml, and that levels above 30 μg/ml tended to produce severe side effects. Subsequently Buchthal and Lennox-Buchthal [52] quoted a therapeutic range of 15-25 μg/ml for phenytoin. They based this opinion on Buchthal's earlier work which had shown that only 25% of epileptic patients had their seizures controlled with phenytoin levels below 10 μg/ml. At levels between 11 and 15 μg/ml, 67% of patients were controlled; and at levels above 15 μg/ml, 86% of patients had their seizures controlled. The figure of Norell et al. [112] of 12-25 μg/ml was based on their finding that phenytoin levels above 13 μg/ml always controlled mild epilepsy, that levels above 19 μg/ml were required to control severe epilepsy, that more severe epilepsy would not be controlled regardless of levels, and that the threshold for toxicity was 29 μg/ml. Some authors have quoted narrower ranges, e.g., van der Kleijn et al. [13], who set the range at 12-15 μg/ml, while others have accepted wider ranges, e.g., Winek [113] at 5-22 μg/ml. The general utility of the 10-20-μg/ml figure for the therapeutic range is reflected in the study of Reynolds et al. [114]. These workers treated with phenytoin as the sole anticonvulsant 31 previously untreated patients who had types of epilepsy which were likely to respond to the drug. By achieving phenytoin levels in the range

10-20 μg/ml they were able to achieve satisfactory seizure control in 90% of patients

It is well recognized that some patients do achieve seizure control with plasma phenytoin levels below the therapeutic range [111].

There have been several reports that epilepsy may be made worse if so much phenytoin is given that plasma drug levels are above the therapeutic range [115,116]. Paradoxically, in these circumstances, reduced plasma phenytoin levels may be associated with improved control of epilepsy.

2. Other Therapeutic Effects

Phenytoin is not invariably used as an anticonvulsant. Bigger et al. [117] found that plasma phenytoin levels up to 18 μg/ml would control 90% of cardiac arrythmias that were responsive to the drug. This finding suggests that the therapeutic range for phenytoin in cardiac arrhythmia may be similar to the range for epilepsy. In contrast, plasma phenytoin levels in excess of 4 μg/ml appeared sufficient to control pain in eight cases of Fabry's disease [118]. Personal experience in using phenytoin to prevent "hemiparesthetic" and "basilar artery" migraine has indicated that plasma drug levels as low as 2 μg/ml can be associated with complete prevention of previously frequent attacks, and that the majority of such cases do not appear to need plasma phenytoin levels as high as 10 μg/ml.

3. Unwanted Effects

Some information is available correlating plasma phenytoin level with the presence of a number of undesirable effects of the drug. The effects that have been studied involve (1) the nervous system at several levels and (2) the gums. The correlation does not appear to have been investigated at any length for other extraneural unwanted effects of the drug. Of course, the severity of idiosyncratic toxic effects will not necessarily be proportional to plasma drug concentration.

4. Neurotoxicity

The most simple and readily remembered correlation between plasma phenytoin level and neurotoxicity is that given by Kutt et al. [119] and Kutt and McDowell [109], viz., that plasma phenytoin levels of 20 μg/ml are associated with the onset of nystagmus, levels of 30 μg/ml with ataxia of gait, and 40 μg/ml with lethargy. These conclusions are in general agreement with the earlier findings of Buchthal and Svensmark [47] that severe side effects occurred once plasma phenytoin levels exceeded 30 μg/ml. Livingstone et al. [110] considered that most patients tolerated plasma phenytoin levels below 25 μg/ml, that levels of 30 μg/ml were associated with ataxia, nystagmus, and diplopia, that levels above 30 μg/ml produced drowsiness and lethargy, while levels above 50 μg/ml caused extreme lethargy and coma. These correlations are also in agreement with the findings of Wilder et al. [120], who studied plasma phenytoin levels in drug-intoxicated patients and noted that depression of consciousness cleared once the plasma drug level fell below 40 μg/ml. Winek [113] suggested that plasma phenytoin concentrations of 100 μg/ml and above might be lethal. Booker and Darcey [101] were interested in the relation between concentration and unbound phenytoin in plasma, and side effects. They established the following correlations: plasma-unbound phenytoin concentrations below 1.5 μg/ml were not associated with toxicity; mild toxicity occurred at levels of 1.5 to 3.0 μg/ml, and definite intoxication above this concentration of free (i.e., unbound) plasma phenytoin.

It should be recognized that toxicity does not always occur immediately when plasma phenytoin levels exceed the upper limit of the population therapeutic range. Conversely, occasional patients experience typical manifestations of phenytoin toxicity with plasma drug levels in or below the therapeutic range. Thus Eadie and Tyrer [121] referred to a ballet dancer who became too ataxic to carry out pirouettes when her plasma phenytoin level was only 5 μg/ml, though she was not ataxic in other circumstances. They also mentioned a patient with probable brainstem damage whose gait became ataxic at plasma phenytoin levels of 6 μg/ml. It seems likely that phenytoin accumulation progressively affects brain function, and does not suddenly disturb it at a critical drug concentration. The threshold for clinically apparent intoxication appears to be determined not only by drug concentration but also by the functional integrity of the cerebral mechanisms that are altered by the drug, and by the demands made on their functional capacity by the patient. The view that anticonvulsant toxicity is a progressive phenomenon is supported by the finding that there is a statistical correlation between increasing plasma phenytoin levels (in the therapeutic range) and psychomotor slowing, intellectual deterioration, psychiatric illness, and personality change [122].

Sometimes phenytoin neurotoxicity takes an unusual form. Phenytoin overdosage may affect basal ganglia dopamine mechanisms to cause choreoathetosis. Kooiker and Sumi [123] noticed this phenomenon in two cases with plasma phenytoin levels of 40 and 65 μg/mg. McLellan and Swash [124] encountered another two instances, with plasma phenytoin levels above 30 μg/ml. The phenomenon was also described in four cases with plasma phenytoin levels of 51, 42.5, 30, and 26.5 μg/ml, respectively [125].

One's experience has been that occasional patients with plasma phenytoin levels above 30 μg/ml experience depression rather than exhibit nystagmus, diplopia, and ataxia. Spector et al. [126] found total external ophthalmoplegia without depression of consciousness in one patient with a plasma phenytoin level of 36 μg/ml.

Clinical peripheral neuropathy due to phenytoin is rare, though a case has been described in the presence of a nontoxic serum phenytoin level [127]. The neuropathy recovered after phenytoin was withdrawn. Subclinical peripheral neuropathy is more common. Birket-Smith and Krogh [128] found that plasma phenytoin levels above 30 μg/ml were associated with slowed motor conduction in the deep peroneal nerve of man. Chokroverty and Rubino [129] and Chokroverty and Sayeed [130] confirmed that motor nerve conduction was slowed in patients who took phenytoin for over 10 years, or who had plasma phenytoin levels above 20 μg/ml. This neuropathy was not due to drug-induced folate deficiency.

Direkze and Fernanco [131] noted fasciculation in one patient with plasma phenytoin levels of 12-14 μg/ml. The involuntary movements ceased when drug intake was stopped.

6. Gingival Hypertrophy

There were earlier statements that phenytoin-induced gum hypertrophy was unrelated to plasma phenytoin level [109]. However, several authors have stated that gum hypertrophy increased with increasing plasma phenytoin levels [132-134]. The first group of authors found that 93.2% of a group of oligophrenic epileptics aged between 6 and 49 years, and with a plasma phenytoin level between 10 and 20 μg/ml, had gum hypertrophy.

B. Methoin (Mephenytoin)

Aird and Woodbury [135] quoted a therapeutic range for methoin of 5-16 μg/ml. One does not know how this figure was derived. Troupin et al [136] cited an impression that the therapeutic range for the drug was 25-40 μg/ml, but they used a nonspecific assay which measured the sum of the concentrations of methoin and its active anticonvulsant metabolite Nirvanol.

C. Phenobarbitone

1. Anticonvulsant Effects

The lower therapeutic limit of plasma phenobarbitone level is probably about 10 μg/ml [4,52,135]. Buchthal et al. [137] had noted that a plasma phenobarbital level of 10 μg/ml was associated with a 90% reduction in EEG paroxysmal activity in epileptic patients. Earlier Buchthal and Svensmark [47] had found that plasma phenobarbitone levels above 20 μg/ml were necessary to control severe epilepsy. Several groups of workers have investigated the question of the plasma phenobarbitone level necessary to prevent febrile convulsions in infancy. Faero et al. [138] found that a plasma phenobarbitone level of 15 μg/ml was required. This was confirmed by Thorn [139], who found that recurrent febrile convulsions occurred in 13% of children treated with phenobarbitone, but in 26% of untreated control children. However he also found that when plasma phenobarbitone level was measured at the time of further febrile convulsing, in only 4 of 23 treated subjects was the plasma drug level above 15 μg/ml. Heckmatt et al.

[140] encountered children in whom this plasma phenobarbitone level did not protect against febrile convulsions. However, the consensus appears to be that 15 μg/ml represents the lower therapeutic limit for treating febrile convulsions. Without specifying that it was the therapeutic range, Pippenger and Rosen [141] stated that neonates with epilepsy did well with plasma phenobarbitone levels of 15-30 μg/ml.

There is difficulty in assigning an upper limit to the therapeutic range of plasma phenobarbitone levels. Toxicity from the drug tends to begin gradually and at times an element of tolerance to the sedative effects of the drug appears to occur. A reasonable figure for the upper limit might be that set by Livingstone et al. [110], viz., 30 μg/ml, but some patients will tolerate much higher plasma levels of the drug without noticeable distress. Thus Feldman et al. [111] quoted a therapeutic range of 15-40 μg/ml.

2. *Unwanted Effects*

The chief dose-related unwanted effects of phenobarbitone are drowsiness and stupor. As indicated above, the threshold plasma level for the onset of these symptoms varies from individual to individual, and within the one individual may vary, depending on whether or not drug levels have been increased so rapidly that there has not been time for tolerance to develop. Livingstone et al. [110] associated plasma phenobarbitone levels of 30-50 μg/ml with the occurrence of definite drowsiness, and said that levels above 70 μg/ml were associated with marked drowsiness and perhaps coma. Winek [113] regarded plasma phenobarbitone levels of 40-60 μg/ml as toxic, and levels of 80-150 μg/ml as lethal.

D. Methylphenobarbitone

No information is available correlating plasma methylphenobarbitone level with therapeutic or toxic effect. Levels of phenobarbitone, derived from biotransformation of methylphenobarbitone, have their expected pharmacological correlations.

E. Primidone

In man primidone is biotransformed to phenobarbitone and phenylethylmalonamide. Both of these metabolites are anticonvulsants. Booker et al. [54] commented that plasma primidone levels above 10 μg/ml did not improve the control of epilepsy, and were likely to be associated with an increasing incidence of side effects. (On these authors' figures, the simultaneous plasma phenobarbitone level would have been above 30 μg/ml, sufficient for both an anticonvulsant and a toxic effect.) Winek [113] quoted 10 μg/ml as a therapeutic level of plasma primidone concentration, 50-80 μg/ml as toxic levels, and 100 μg/ml as a lethal level. Certain authors propose therapeutic ranges for primidone, e.g., 8-12 μg/ml

[13]. One wonders how useful this policy is when the simultaneous presence of phenobarbitone is apparently ignored.

F. Carbamazepine

1. Anticonvulsant Effects

Møller [142] stated that plasma carbamazepine levels above 6 μg/ml were needed to control epilepsy. Monaco et al. [143] found that plasma carbamazepine levels in the range 4-10 μg/ml tended to control epilepsy and suggested a therapeutic range for the drug of 4-12 μg/ml. Simonsen et al. [144] had put the therapeutic range at 6-10 μg/ml, and Perchalski and Wilder [145] suggested that, for most cases, plasma carbamazepine levels below 10 μg/ml were therapeutic. In patients with psychomotor epilepsy (i.e., complex partial seizures), Schneider [146] found 50-99% control of attacks with plasma carbamazepine levels of 4.6 ± 2.2 μg/ml and full control at levels of 5.9 ± 2.7 μg/ml. On the basis of these data he suggested that the therapeutic range was 6.5 ± 3.0 μg/ml. It would thus appear that contemporary opinion would set the therapeutic range of plasma carbamazepine concentrations at 4-12 μg/ml. However, the therapeutic ranges have often been determined on the basis of the response of patients taking other anticonvulsants with carbamazepine. As mentioned earlier, there is a very consistent pharmacokinetic interaction between phenytoin and carbamazepine which reduces plasma carbamazepine levels. Dam et al. [147] claimed that concurrent therapy with phenytoin increased the amount of carbamazepine-10,11-epoxide in plasma relative to the amount of carbamazepine. Personal unpublished data are in keeping with this finding. If the finding is correct, since epoxycarbamazepine is an anticonvulsant in animals [148], the lower limit for the therapeutic range of plasma carbamazepine level may be above 4 μg/ml when carbamazepine is used as the sole anticonvulsant. One's practice has been to work to a therapeutic range of 6-12 μg/ml in managing patients taking carbamazepine alone, but to accept that some patients tolerate higher plasma levels of the drug with benefit and without troublesome side effects.

No therapeutic range for epoxycarbamazepine has yet been established.

Troupin and Ojemann [116] suggested that plasma carbamazepine levels of 20 μg/ml, or levels above this, could be associated with a worsening of epilepsy.

2. Effect in Tic Douloureux

Personal experience has been that minimum plasma carbamazepine levels of 5 μg/ml are needed to control tic douloureux. Levels as high as 19 μg/ml have at times been necessary, and have been tolerated without unacceptable side effects.

Unwanted Effects

Meinardi [149] found that some patients taking carbamazepine developed nystagmus once the plasma level of the drug exceeded 1.5 μg/ml. At levels of 8.5-10 μg/ml about 50% of patients had other side effects, e.g., headache, dysequilibrium, disturbance of vision. Winek [113] regarded plasma carbamazepine levels of 8-10 μg/ml as "toxic." Schneider [146] had set 8 to 9 μg/ml as the threshold for the appearance of serious unwanted effects. The lowest plasma carbamazepine level he saw associated with side effects was 5.9 μg/ml, and the highest level without side effects was 16.9 μg/ml.

One's experience with carbamazepine side effects has been similar to one's experience with the unwanted effects of phenobarbitone. Excluding idiosyncratic reactions, for both drugs the major unwanted effects are sedative (drowsiness, mental dulling, minor dysequilibrium). A degree of pharmacological tolerance to such sedative side effects seems to occur. Therefore, if carbamazepine or phenobarbitone doses are adjusted to increase plasma levels of the respective drugs gradually, plasma levels may be tolerated quite readily which would have been associated with unacceptably severe side effects if these levels had been attained soon after therapy began. This fact may help explain some of the scatter of figures for the toxicity threshold of carbamazepine.

In a single-dose study Levy et al. [69] found no correlation between plasma carbamazepine levels and the time course of drug side effects, but in this study there may not have been time for definitive steady-state equilibria to occur.

G. Ethosuximide

1. Anticonvulsant Effect

Therapeutic resonse in petit mal "absence" epilepsy can nearly always be determined readily on clinical grounds. Therefore, one might expect that the therapeutic range of plasma levels for ethosuximide would be clearly defined. In fact, Penry et al. [150] stated that plasma ethosuximide levels of 40-60 μg/ml gave complete control of absence epilepsy, while Sherwin and Robb [75] set the therapeutic range for the drug at 40-120 μg/ml. Browne et al. [151] found that 79% of a series of 39 previously untreated cases of absence epilepsy derived a greater than 75% reduction in seizure frequency from plasma ethosuximide levels of 41-99 μg/ml. They therefore suggested that the therapeutic range for the drug was 40-100 μg/ml. Winek [113] set the therapeutic range of the drug at the rather lower figures of 25-75 μg/ml.

While accepting the general applicability of the 40-μg/ml lower limit to the therapeutic range for ethosuximide, one has seen a patient whose absence seizures were completely controlled at a plasma ethosuximide level of 26 μg/ml. One has also seen absence epilepsy not controlled till ethosuximide levels have reached a value of 180 μg/ml, and these levels were not associated with clinical toxicity.

2. Unwanted Effects

Little has been published on the correlation between ethosuximide toxicity and plasma levels of the drug. On a number of occasions one has increased ethosuximide dose to raise plasma ethosuximide levels above 100 μg/ml in an attempt to control absence epilepsy. In the majority of such cases control has been achieved at levels between 100 and 150 μg/ml, but at levels above 150 μg/ml some patients have begun to develop nausea and mental dullness. As mentioned above, one patient tolerated a plasma ethosuximide level of 180 μg/ml.

H. Troxidone

Troxidone is a largely outmoded drug, and little information is available on the clinical correlations of its plasma levels. In fact, the drug is biotransformed to an anticonvulsant substance, dimethadione, which is much more slowly eliminated than troxidone. Apparently plasma dimethadione levels of "700 μg/ml, or higher" provide the best chance of controlling absence epilepsy [80,152,153].

I. Diazepam

1. Anticonvulsant Effect

Agurell et al. [84] suggested that the anticonvulsant threshold plasma concentration of diazepam was 150-200 ng/ml, an opinion apparently based on clinical impression only. Booker and Celesia [154] found that serum diazepam levels in excess of 600 ng/ml were required to suppress spontaneous paroxysmal discharges in the human epileptic EEG. However, these workers administered diazepam intravenously, and the plasma levels they measured may not have necessarily reflected the brain diazepam levels which would have been present when post-distribution equilibria applied. There appears to be little adequate information on the correlation between plasma diazepam levels and anticonvulsant effects.

2. Other Therapeutic Effects

Fink et al. [155] found that plasma diazepam levels above 100 ng/ml were associated with increased β-activity in the surface EEG. Dasberg et al. [156] stated that the minimal plasma diazepam concentration to relieve anxiety was 400 ng/ml, and that plasma nordiazepam levels above 300 ng/ml were also capable of altering certain psychiatric symptoms. However Bond et al. [157] claimed that no relation had been shown to exist between plasma levels of any benzodiazepine and the measured response of anxiety.

3. Unwanted Effects

No information is available correlating unwanted effects of diazepam with plasma levels of the drug, possibly because a great deal of tolerance may occur to the sedative-type toxic effects of the drug. Winek [113] quoted plasma diazepam levels of 5-10 μg/ml as toxic, and levels above 50 μg/ml as lethal.

J. Nitrazepam

No data are available correlating plasma levels and pharmacological effects of nitrazepam.

K. Clonazepam

1. Anticonvulsant Effect

Huang et al. [158] in some preliminary work suggested that plasma clonazepam levels above 15 μg/ml correlated with protection against myoclonic epilepsy, and levels above 30 ng/ml with an anticonvulsant effect against other types of epilepsy. Subsequently they stated that the usually effective anticonvulsant dose of clonazepam was 6 mg/day, which gave an average plasma clonazepam concentration of 25-30 ng/ml [159]. Dreifuss et al. [160] improved the control of absence seizures in 8 of 10 children with plasma clonazepam levels in the range 13-72 ng/ml. However, Naestoft et al. [161] found no correlation between plasma clonazepam level and anticonvulsant effect.

Clonazepam is a comparatively recently introduced drug, and has not yet been in use long enough for sufficient experience to accumulate to allow its therapeutic range to be defined. It has often been used in very resistant epileptics who may already be taking multiple anticonvulsants. In these circumstances its success rate may not be high. It may be difficult to define a valid therapeutic range till the drug has a period of use as an initial anticonvulsant. One has seen clonazepam control absence epilepsy at plasma levels of 20-30 ng/ml, but has also seen it fail to control temporal lobe epilepsy at levels of 200 ng/ml.

2. Unwanted Effects

Hvidberg and Sjo [162] could not correlate plasma clonazepam levels with side effects of the drug, and Sjo et al. [96] could not define a threshold of toxicity for the drug. The main unwanted effects of clonazepam are sedative. Tolerance to these effects occurs, particularly if doses are increased gradually. Plasma clonazepam levels of 20-30 ng/ml may be associated with a prohibitive degree of drowsiness in some subjects, yet if doses are increased slowly, a patient may tolerate a plasma clonazepam level of 200 ng/ml without appreciable sedation.

L. Valproic Acid

There has not yet been any extensive study of the correlation between therapeutic effect and plasma levels of valproate. Further, certain workers appear not to have recognized that plasma valproate levels fluctuate more over a dosage interval than do plasma levels of the other anticonvulsants in common use. In order to obtain reproducible correlations for valproate, if these exist, plasma levels should always be measured at the same stage of the dose interval (with the immediate predose level being perhaps the most appropriate single measurement). A tentative lower limit to the therapeutic plasma range of valproate concentrations has been suggested as 50 μg/ml [163], and a therapeutic range of 60-80 μg/ml has been proposed [13]. It is not clear whether these suggestions refer to minimal plasma level values in the steady state.

2. Unwanted Effect

The only information so far available is Meinardi's [164] statement that plasma valproate levels above 110 μg/ml are usually associated with muscular weakness and tremor.

VII. CORRELATION OF CLINICAL EFFECTS WITH PLASMA LEVELS FOR DRUG COMBINATIONS

Two or more anticonvulsants are sometimes combined in the treatment of epilepsy, either because the patient has two types of epilepsy, each of which will respond best to a different drug, or because a single drug has failed to control the patient's seizures. When two anticonvulsants are combined there may be pharmacokinetic interactions which alter the plasma levels, and hence the pharmacological effects of one, or other, or both of the drugs involved. It is harder to establish whether there are also pharmacodynamic interactions which alter the relation between plasma level of each drug and its pharmacological effect. When two drugs are combined to treat one type of epilepsy it is hoped that there will be an additive or synergistic pharmacodynamic interaction between the two drugs to improve seizure control. Clinical experience suggests that this expectation is sometimes realized, though it is not certain whether additive or synergistic effects are involved. There does not appear to be any clear evidence that the relation between unwanted effects of anticonvulsants and drug plasma level is altered when anticonvulsants are combined. However, the whole question of clinical effect/plasma level correlations in the presence of multiple anticonvulsant drugs deserves much detailed study before one will be entitled to draw any firm conclusions.

VIII. CONCLUSION

Although a moderate amount of information is available regarding the clinical correlations of plasma anticonvulsant levels, there are still many unanswered questions. It is often much easier to measure the plasma concentrations of an anticonvulsant drug than it is to quantitate the individual clinical situation with which the plasma level measurement should be correlated. To some extent, as a consequence of this, one has seen in the treatment of epilepsy a growing tendency to regard the achieving of satisfactory plasma anticonvulsant drug levels as almost the final aim of anticonvulsant therapy. The levels are being regarded not merely as a guide to therapy, but as a goal of therapy. The patient's clinical state should always be the final criterion in management, and measurement of plasma anticonvulsant levels should be seen only as a means to an end.

REFERENCES

1. C. T. Viswanathan, H. E. Booker, and P. G. Welling, Interference by p-hydroxyphenobarbital in the ^{125}I-radioimmunoassay of serum and urinary phenobarbital. *Clin. Chem. 23:*873–876, 1977.
2. B. B. Brodie, S. Udenfriend, and J. E. Baer, The estimation of basic organic compounds in biological material, I: General principles. *J. Biol. Chem. 168:*299–309, 1947.
3. D. M. Woodbury, J. K. Penry, and R. Schmidt, *Antiepileptic Drugs.* New York, Raven Press, 1972.
4. M. J. Eadie and J. H. Tyrer, *Anticonvulsant Therapy: Pharmacological Basis and Practice.* Edinburgh and London, Churchill-Livingstone, 2nd. ed. 1980.
5. A. Richens, *Drug Treatment of Epilepsy.* London, Henry Kimpton, 1976.
6. E. F. Hvidberg and M. Dam, Clinical pharmacokinetics of anticonvulsants. *Clin. Pharmacokinetics 1:*161–188, 1976.
7. H. M. Triedman, R. A. Fishman, and M. D. Yahr, Determination of plasma and cerebrospinal fluid levels of Dilantin in the human. *Trans. Am. Neurol. Assoc. 85:*166–170, 1960.
8. F. Bochner, W. D. Hooper, J. H. Tyrer, and M. J. Eadie, Factors involved in an outbreak of phenytoin intoxication. *J. Neurol. Sci. 16:*481-487, 1972.
9. K. Arnold, N. Gerber, and G. Levy, Absorption and dissolution studies on sodium diphenylhydantoin capsules. *Canad. J. Pharm. Sci. 5:*89-92, 1970.
10. W. Wallis, H. Kutt, and F. McDowell, Intravenous diphenylhydantoin in treatment of acute repetitive seizures. *Neurology 18:*513–525, 1968.
11. B. J. Wilder and R. E. Ramsay, Oral and intramuscular phenytoin. *Clin. Pharmacol. Ther. 19:*360-364, 1976.
12. E. E. Serrano and B. J. Wilder, Intramuscular administration of diphenylhydantoin: Histologic follow-up study. *Arch. Neurol. 31:*276–278, 1974.
13. E. van der Kleijn, P. J. M. Guelen, C. van Wijk, and I. Baars, Clinical pharmacokinetics in monitoring chronic medication with anti-epileptic drugs. In *Clinical Pharmacology of Antiepileptic Drugs* (H. Schneider, D. Janz, C. Gardner-Thorpe, H. Meinardi, and A. L. Sherwin, eds.). Berlin, Springer, 1975, pp. 11-33.

14. P. K. M. Lunde, A. Rane, S. J. Yaffe, L. Lund, and F. Sjöqvist, Plasma protein binding of diphenylhydantoin in man: Interaction with other drugs and the effect of temperature and plasma dilution. *Clin. Pharmacol. Ther. 11:*846-855, 1970.
15. L. Lund, P. K. Lunde, A. Rane, O. Borgå, and F. Sjöquist, Plasma protein binding, plasma concentrations, and effects of diphenylhydantoin in man. *Ann. N.Y. Acad. Sci. 179:*723-728, 1971.
16. L. Lund, A. Berlin, and P. K. M. Lunde, Plasma protein binding of diphenylhydantoin in patients with epilepsy: Agreement between the unbound fraction in plasma and the concentration in the cerebrospinal fluid. *Clin. Pharmacol. Ther. 13:*196-200, 1972.
17 M. Ehrnebo, S. Agurell, B. Jalling, and L. O. Boreus, Age differences in drug binding by plasma proteins: Studies on human foetuses, neonates and adults. *Eur. J. Clin. Pharmacol. 3:*189-193, 1971.
18. W. D. Hooper, F. Bochner, M. J. Eadie, and J. H. Tyrer, Plasma protein binding of diphenylhydantoin. *Clin. Pharmacol. Ther. 15:*276-282, 1974.
19. D. W. Shoeman, D. M. Benjamin, and D. L. Azarnoff, The alteration of plasma proteins in uraemia as reflected in the ability to bind diphenylhydantoin. *Ann. N.Y. Acad. Sci. 226:*127-130, 1973.
20. F. Bochner, W. D. Hooper, J. M. Sutherland, M. J. Eadie, and J. H. Tyrer, Diphenylhydantoin concentrations in saliva. *Arch. Neurol. 31:*57-59, 1974.
21. B. L. Mirkin, Diphenylhydantoin: Placental transport, fetal localization, neonatal metabolism, and possible teratogenic effects. *J. Pediat. 78:*329-337, 1971.
22. F. Vajda, F. M. Williams, S. Davidson, M. A. Falconer, and A. Breckenridge, Human brain, cerebrospinal fluid, and plasma concentrations of diphenylhydantoin and phenobarbital. *Clin. Pharmacol. Ther. 15:*597-603, 1974.
23. G. W. Houghton, A. Richens, P. A. Toseland, S. Davidson, and M. A. Falconer, Brain concentrations of phenytoin, phenobarbitone, and primidone in epileptic patients. *Eur. J. Clin. Pharmacol. 9:*73-78, 1975.
24. A. J. Glazko, T. Chang, J. Baukema, W. A. Dill, J. R. Goulet, and R. A. Buchanan, Metabolic disposition of diphenylhydantoin in normal human subjects following intravenous administration. *Clin. Pharmacol. Ther. 10:* 498-504, 1969.
25. F. Bochner, W. D. Hooper, J. H. Tyrer, and M. J. Eadie, The effect of dosage increments on blood phenytoin concentrations. *J. Neurol. Neurosurg. Psychiatry 35:*873-876, 1972.
26. M. J. Eadie, J. H. Tyrer, F. Bochner, and W. D. Hooper, The elimination of phenytoin in man. *Clin. Exp. Pharmacol. Physiol. 3:*217-224, 1976.
27. N. Gerber and J. G. Wagner, Explanation of the dose-dependent decline of diphenylhydantoin plasma levels by fitting to the integrated form of the Michaelis-Menten equation. *Res. Com. Chem. Pathol. Pharmacol. 3:* 455-466, 1972.
28. K. Arnold and N. Gerber, The rate of decline of diphenylhydantoin in human plasma. *Clin. Pharmacol. Ther. 11:*121-134, 1970.

29. T. Suzuki, Y. Saitoh, and K. Nishihara, Kinetics of diphenylhydantoin disposition in man. *Chem. Pharm. Bull. 18:*405-411, 1970.
30. A. J. Atkinson and J. M. Shaw, Pharmacokinetic study of a patient with diphenylhydantoin toxicity. *Clin. Pharmacol. Ther. 14:*521-528, 1973.
31. G. E. Mawer, P. W. Mullen, M. Rodgers, A. J. Robins, and S. B. Lucas, Phenytoin dose adjustment in epileptic patients. *Brit. J. Clin. Pharmacol. 1:*163-168, 1974.
32. A. Richens, A study of the pharmacokinetics of phenytoin (diphenylhydantoin) in epileptic patients, and the development of a nomogram for making dose increments. *Epilepsia 16:*627-646, 1975.
33. O. Svensmark and F. Buchthal, Diphenylhydantoin and phenobarbital: Serum levels in children. *Amer. J. Dis. Child. 108:*82-87, 1964.
34. B. Jalling, L. O. Boreus, A. Rane, and F. Sjöquist, Plasma concentrations of diphenylhydantoin in young infants. *Pharmacologica Clinica 2:*200-202, 1970.
35. L. G. Borofsky, S. Louis, H. Kutt, and M. Roginsky, Diphenylhydantoin: Efficacy, toxicity, and dose-serum level relationship in children. *J. Pediat. 81:*995-1002, 1972.
36. W. D. Hooper, M. J. Eadie, and J. H. Tyrer, Plasma diphenylhydantoin levels in Australian children. *Aust. N.Z. J. Med. 4:*456-461, 1973.
37. P. J. M. Guelen, Discussion. In *Clinical Pharmacology of Antiepileptic Drugs* (H. Schneider, D. Janz, C. Gardner-Thorpe, H. Meinardi, and A. L. Sherwin, eds.). Berlin, Springer, 1975, pp. 45-46.
38. W. D. Hooper, J. H. Tyrer, and M. J. Eadie, Plasma diphenylhydantoin levels in Australian adults. *Aust. N.Z. J. Med. 4:*449-455, 1973.
39. G. W. Houghton, A. Richens, and M. Leighton, Effect of age, height, weight, and sex on serum phenytoin concentration in epileptic patients. *Brit. J. Clin. Pharmacol. 2:*251-256, 1975.
40. C. M. Lander, V. E. Edwards, M. J. Eadie, and J. H. Tyrer, Plasma anticonvulsant concentrations during pregnancy. *Neurology 27:*128-131, 1977.
41. H. J. Kupferberg and W. Yonekawa, The metabolism of 3 methyl 5 ethyl 5 phenylhydantoin (mephenytoin) to 5 ethyl 5 phenylhydantoin (Nirvanol) in mice in relation to anticonvulsant activity. *Metab. Disposition 3:*26-29, 1975.
42. P. Lous, Blood serum and cerebrospinal fluid levels and renal clearance of Phenemal in treated epileptics. *Acta Pharmacol. Toxicol. 10:*166-177, 1954.
43. E. W. Maynert, Phenobarbital, Mephobarbital, and Metharbital: Absorption, distribution, and excretion. In *Antiepileptic Drugs* (D. M. Woodbury, J. K. Penry, and R. P. Schmidt, eds.). New York, Raven Press, 1972, pp. 303-310.
44. L. R. Goldbaum and P. K. Smith, The interaction of barbiturates with serum albumin and its possible relation to their disposition and pharma cological actions. *J. Pharmacol. Exp. Ther. 111:*197-209, 1954.
45. I. P. Baumel, B. B. Gallagher, and R. H. Mattson, Phenylethylmalonamide

(PEMA): An important metabolite of primidone. *Arch. Neurol. 27:*34-41, 1972.
46. J. J. McAuliffe, A. L. Sherwin, I. E. Leppik, S. A. Fayle, and C. E. Pippenger, Salivary levels of anticonvulsants: A practical approach to drug monitoring. *Neurology 27:*409-413, 1977.
47. F. Buchthal and O. Svensmark, Aspects of the pharmacology of phenytoin (Dilantin) and phenobarbital relevant to their dosage in treatment of epilepsy. *Epilepsia 1:*373-384, 1959.
48. J. C. Melchior, O. Svensmark, and D. Trolle, Placental transfer of phenobarbitone in epileptic women, and elimination in newborns. *Brit. Med. J. 2:*860-861, 1967.
49. T. C. Butler, The metabolic hydroxylation of phenobarbital. *J. Pharmacol. Exp. Ther. 116:*326-336, 1956.
50. M. J. Eadie, C. M. Lander, W. D. Hooper, and J. H. Tyrer, Factors influencing plasma phenobarbitone levels in epileptic patients. *Brit. J. Clin. Pharmacol. 4:*541-547, 1977.
51. L. C. Mark, Metabolism of barbiturates in man. *Clin. Pharmacol. Ther. 4:* 504-530, 1963.
52. F. Buchthal and M. A. Lennox-Buchthal, Phenobarbital: Relation of serum concentration to control of seizures. In *Antiepileptic Drugs* (D. M. Woodbury, J. K. Penry, and R. P. Schmidt, eds.). New York, Raven Press, 1972, pp. 335-343.
53. L. K. Garrettson and P. G. Dayton, Disappearance of phenobarbital and diphenylhydantoin from serum of children. *Clin. Pharmacol. Ther. 11:* 674-679, 1970.
54. H. E. Booker, K. Hosokowa, R. D. Burdette, and B. Darcey, A clinical study of serum primidone levels. *Epilepsia 11:*395-402, 1970.
55. B. B. Gallagher and I. P. Baumel, Primidone: Absorption, distribution, and excretion. In *Antiepileptic Drugs* (D. M. Woodbury, J. K. Penry, and R. P. Schmidt, eds.). New York, Raven Press, 1972, pp. 357-359.
56. S. I. Johannessen, and R. E. Strandjord, Abosrption and protein binding in serum of several anti-epileptic drugs. In *Clinical Pharmacology of Antiepileptic Drugs* (H. Schneider, D. Janz, C. Gardner-Thorpe, H. Meinardi, and A. L. Sherwin, eds.). Berlin, Springer, 1975, pp. 262-273.
57. A. L. Sherwin, General discussion. In *Clinical Pharmacology of Antiepileptic Drugs* (H. Schneider, D. Janz, C. Gardner-Thorpe, H. Meinardi, and A. L. Sherwin, eds.). Berlin, Springer, 1975, p. 145.
58. T. C. Butler and W. J. Waddell, Metabolic conversion of primidone (Mysoline) to phenobarbital. *Proc. Soc. Exp. Biol. Med. 93:*544-546, 1956.
59. O. V. Olesen and M. Dam. The metabolic conversion of primidone (Mysoline) to phenobarbitone in patients under long-term treatment. *Acta Neurol. Scand. 43:*348-356, 1967.
60. E. H. Reynolds, G. Fenton, P. Fenwick, A. L. Johnson, and M. Laundy, Interaction of phenytoin and primidone. *Brit. Med. J. 2:*594-595, 1975.
61. K. Kauro and P. Tammisto, Comparison of two generically equivalent

carbamazepine preparations. *Ann. Clin. Res. Suppl. (11) 6:*21-25, 1974.

62. L. M. Cotter, M. J. Eadie, W. D. Hooper, C. M. Lander, G. A. Smith, and J. H. Tyrer, The pharmacokinetics of carbamazepine. *Eur. J. Clin. Pharmacol., 12:*451-456, 1977.
63. M. D. Rawlins, P. Collste, L. Bertilsson, and L. Palmer, Distribution and elimination kinetics of carbamazepine in man. *Eur. J. Clin. Pharmacol. 8:*91-96, 1975.
64. P. L. Morselli, L. Bossi, and M. Gerna, Pharmacokinetic studies with carbamazepine in epileptic patients. In *International Symposium on Epileptic Seizures-Behaviour-Pain* (W. Birkmayer, ed.). Berne, Huber, 1975, pp. 141-150.
65. P. L. Morselli, M. Gerna, D. De Maio, G. Zanda, F. Viani, and S. Garattini, Pharmacokinetic studies on carbamazepine in volunteers and in epileptic patients. In *Clinical Pharmacology of Antiepileptic Drugs* (H. Schneider, D. Janz, C. Gardner-Thorpe, H. Meinardi, and A. L. Sherwin, eds.). Berlin, Springer, 1975, pp. 166-179.
66. W. D. Hooper, D. K. Dubetz, F. Bochner, L. M. Cotter, G. A. Smith, M. J' Eadie, and J. H. Tyrer, Plasma protein binding of carbamazepine. *Clin. Pharmacol. Ther. 17:*433-440, 1975.
67. S. I. Johannessen and R. E. Strandjord, The concentration of carbamazepine (Tegretol) in serum and in cerebrospinal fluid in patients with epilepsy. *Acta Neurol. Scand., Suppl. (51) 48:*445-446, 1972.
68. A. S. Troupin and P. Friel, Anticonvulsant level in saliva, serum, and cerebrospinal fluid. *Epilepsia 16:*223-227, 1975.
69. R. H. Levy, W. H. Pitlick, A. S. Troupin, J. R. Green, and J. M. Neal, Pharmacokinetics of carbamazepine in normal man. *Clin. Pharmacol. Ther. 17:*657-668, 1975.
70. L. Palmer, L. Bertilsson, P. Collste, and M. Rawlins, Quantitative determination of carbamazepine in plasma by mass fragmentography. *Clin. Pharmacol. Ther. 14:*827-832, 1973.
71. A. P. Gerardin, F. V. Abadie, J. A. Campestrini, and W. Theobald, Pharmacokinetics of carbamazepine in normal humans after single and repeated oral doses. *J. Pharmacokinetics Biopharmaceutics 4:*521-535, 1976.
72. M. Eichelbaum, K. Ekbom, L. Bertilsson, V. A. Ringberger, and A. Rane, Plasma kinetics of carbamazepine and its epoxide metabolite in man after single and multiple doses. *Eur. J. Clin. Pharmacol. 8:*337-341, 1975.
73. J. Christiansen and M. Dam, Influence of phenobarbital and diphenylhydantoin on plasma carbamazepine levels in patients with epilepsy. *Acta Neurol. Scand. 49:*543-546, 1973.
74. R. A. Buchanan, L. Fernandez, and A. W. Kinkel, Absorption and elimination of ethosuximide in children. *Clin. Pharmacol. 9:*393-398, 1969.
75. A. L. Sherwin and J. P. Robb, Ethosuximide: Relation of plasma level to clinical control. In *Antiepileptic Drugs* (D. M. Woodbury, J. K. Penry, R. P. Schmidt, eds.). New York, Raven Press, 1972, pp. 443-448.

76. M. J. Eadie, J. H. Tyrer, G. A. Smith, and L. McKauge, Pharmacokinetics of drugs used for petit mal absence epilepsy. *Clin. Exp. Neurol., 14:*172-183, 1977.
77. W. A. Dill, L. Peterson, T. Chang, and A. J. Glazko, Physiologic disposition of α-methyl-α-ethyl succinimide (ethosuximide; Zarontin) in animals and man. *Amer. Chem. Soc. Abstracts,* 149th Annual Meeting, 1965, p. 30.
78. A. J. Glazko, Antiepileptic drugs: Biotransformation, metabolism, and serum half-life. *Epilepsia 16:*367-391, 1975.
79. T. Chang, W. A. Dill, and A. J. Glazko, Ethosuximide: Absorption, distribution, and excretion. In *Antiepileptic Drugs* (D. M. Woodbury, J. K. Penry, and R. P. Schmidt, eds.). New York, Raven Press, 1972, pp. 417-423.
80. H. E. Booker, Trimethadione and other oxazolidinediones: Relation of plasma levels to clinical control. In *Antieplieptic Drugs* (D. M. Woodbury, J. K. Penry, and R. P. Schmidt, eds.). New York, Raven Press, 1972, pp. 403-407.
81. T. C. Butler and W. J. Waddell, N-methylated derivatives of barbituric acids, hydantoin, and oxazolidine used in the treatment of epilepsy. *Neurology, Suppl. (1) 8:*106-112, 1958.
82. J. A. F. De Silva, B. A. Koechlin and G. Bader, Blood level distribution patterns of diazepam and its major metabolite in man. *J. Pharm. Sci. 55:*692-702, 1966.
83. D. E. Schwartz, B. A. Koechlin, E. Postma, S. Palmer, and G. Krol, Metabolites of diazepam in rat, dog, and man. *J. Pharmacol. Exp. Ther. 149:*432-435, 1965.
84. S. Agurell, A. Berlin, H. Ferngren, and B. Hellstrom, Plasma levels of diazepam after parenteral and rectal administration in children. *Epilepsia 16:* 277-283, 1975.
85. L. Hillestad, T. Hansen, H. Melsom, and A. Drivenes, Diazepam metabolism in normal man: Serum concentrations and clinical effects after intravenous, intramuscular, and oral administration. *Clin. Pharmacol. Ther. 16:*479-484, 1974.
86. U. Klotz, K.-H. Antonin, and P. R. Bieck, Pharmacokinetics and plasma binding of diazepam in man, dog, rabbit, guinea pig, and rat. *J. Pharmacol. Exp. Ther. 199:*67-73, 1976.
87. J. Kanto, L. Kangas, and T. Siirtola, Cerebrospinal fluid concentrations of diazepam and its metabolites in man. *Acta Pharmacol. 36:*328-334, 1975.
88. E. van der Kleijn, Kinetics of distribution and metabolism of diazepam in animals and humans. *Arch. Int. Pharmacodyn. 182:*433-436, 1969.
89. S. A. Kaplan, M. L. Jack, K. Alexander, and R. E. Weinfeld, Pharmacokinetic profile of diazepam in man following single intravenous and oral and chronic oral administrations. *J. Pharm. Sci. 62:*1789-1796, 1973.
90. E. van der Kleijn, J. M. van Rossum, E. T. J. M. Muskens, and N. V. M. Rijntjes, Pharmacokinetics of diazepam in dogs, mice, and humans. *Acta Pharmacol. Toxicol., Suppl. (3) 29:*109-127, 1971.
91. J. Rieder, Plasma levels and derived pharmacokinetic parameters of unchanged nitrazepam in man. *Arzneim.-Forsch. 23:*212-218, 1973.

92. J. Rieder and G. Wendt, Pharmacokinetics and metabolism of the hypnotic nitrazepam. Paper presented to the Symposium on Benzodiazepines, Milan, 1-4 Nov. 1971.
93. A. Berlin and H. Dahlström, Pharmacokinetics of the anticonvulsant drug clonazepam evaluated from single oral and intravenous doses and by repeated oral administration. *Eur. J. Clin. Pharmacol. 9:*155-159, 1975.
94. W. Müller and U. Wollert, Characterization of the binding of benzodiazepines to human serum albumin. *Naunyn-Schmiedebergs Arch. Pharmacol. Exp. Pathol. 280:*229-237, 1973.
95. S. A. Kaplan, K. Alexander, M. L. Jack, C. V. Puglisi, J. A. F. De Silva, T. L. Lee, and R. E. Weinfeld, Pharmacokinetic profiles of clonazepam in dog and humans and of flunitrazepam in dog. *J. Pharm. Sci. 63:*527-532, 1974.
96. O. Sjo, E. F. Hvidberg, J. Naestoft, and M. Lund, Pharmacokinetics and side-effects of clonazepam and its 7-amino-metabolite in man. *Eur. J. Clin. Pharmacol. 8:*249-254, 1975.
97. E. Schobben, E. van der Kleijn, and F. J. M. Gabreels, Pharmacokinetics of di-n-propylacetate in epileptic patients. *Eur. J. Clin. Pharmacol. 8:* 97-105, 1975.
98. A. Richens, I. T. Scoular, S. Ahmad, and B. J. Jordan, Pharmacokinetics and efficacy of Epilim in patients receiving long-term therapy with other anticonvulsants. In *Clinical and Pharmacological Aspects of Sodium Valproate (Epilim) in the Treatment of Epilepsy* (N. J. Legg, ed.). Turnbridge Wells, MCS Consultants, 1975, pp. 78-88.
99. H. Meinardi, E. van der Kleijn, J. W. A. Meijer, and H. van Rees, Absorption and distribution of antiepileptic drugs. *Epilepsia 16:*353-365, 1975.
100. B. J. Jordan, J. S. Shillingford, and K. P. Steed, Preliminary observations on the protein-binding and enzyme-inducing properties of sodium valproate (Epilim). In *Clinical and Pharmacological Aspects of Sodium Valproate (Epilim) in the Treatment of Epilepsy* (N. J. Legg, ed.). Turnbridge Wells, MCS Consultants, 1975, pp. 112-116.
101. H. E. Booker and B. Darcey, Serum concentrations of free diphenylhydantoin and their relationship to clinical intoxication. *Epilepsia 14:*177-184, 1973.
102. M. Lund, R. S. Jorgensen, and V. Kühl, Serum diphenylhydantoin (phenytoin) in ambulant patients with epilepsy. *Epilepsia 5:*51-58, 1964.
103. S. M. Wolf, A. C. Carr, R. A. Hanson, E. P. Dale, D. C. Davis, E. D. Goldenberg, G. A. Lulejian, K. S. Sharpe, P. Trietman, and A. W. Weinstein, Parental compliance in the continuous administration of phenobarbital for the prevention of febrile seizures. *J. Pediat. 83:*1085-1086, 1973.
104. J. Eisler and R. H. Mattson, Compliance in anticonvulsant drug therapy. *Epilepsia 16:*203, 1975.
105. O. Driessen and R. Höppner, Plasma levels of phenobarbital and phenytoin in epileptic outpatients. *Eur. Neurol. 15:*135-142, 1977.
106. L. Lund, Anticonvulsant effect of diphenylhydantoin relative to plasma

levels: A prospective three-year study in ambulant patients with generalized epileptic seizures. *Arch. Neurol. 31:*289–294, 1974.

107. A. J. Rowan, C. E. Pippenger, P. A. McGregor, and J. H. French, Seizure activity and anticonvulsant drug concentration. *Arch. Neurol. 32:*281-288, 1975.

108. C. F. Terrence, Jr., H. M. Wisotzkey, and J. A. Perper, Unexpected, unexplained death in epileptic patients. *Neurology 25:*594–598, 1975.

109. H. Kutt and F. McDowell, Management of epilepsy with diphenylhydantoin sodium. *JAMA 203:*969-972, 1968.

110. S. Livingstone, W. Berman, and L. L. Pauli, Anticonvulsant drug blood levels: Practical applications based on 12 years' experience. *JAMA 232:* 60-62, 1975.

111. R. G. Feldman, C. E. Pippinger, and M. L. Florence, The relation of anticonvulsant drug levels to complete seizure control. *Epilepsia 16:*203-204, 1975.

112. E. Norell, G. Lilienberg, and I. Gamstorp, Systematic determination of the serum phenytoin level as an aid in the management of children with epilepsy. *Eur. Neurol. 13:*232-244, 1975.

113. C. L. Winek, Tabulation of therapeutic, toxic, and lethal concentrations of drugs and chemicals in blood. *Clin. Chem. 22:*832-836, 1976.

114. E. H. Reynolds, D. Chadwick, and A. W. Galbraith, One drug (phenytoin) in the treatment of epilepsy. *Lancet 1:*923-926, 1976.

115. P. T. Lascelles, R. S. Kocen, and E. H. Reynolds, The distribution of plasma phenytoin levels in epileptic patients. *J. Neurol. Neurosurg. Psychiatry 33:*501-505, 1970.

116. A. S. Troupin and L. M. Ojemann, Paradoxical intoxication: A complication of anticonvulsant intoxication. *Epilepsia 16:*753-758, 1976.

117. J. T. Bigger, Jr., D. H. Schmidt, and H. Kutt, Relationship between the plasma level of diphenylhydantoin sodium and its cardiac antiarrhythmic effect. *Circulation 38:*363-374, 1968.

118. L. A. Lockman, D. B. Hunninghake, W. Krivit, and R. J. Desnick, Relief of pain of Fabry's disease by diphenylhydantoin. *Neurology 23:*871-875, 1973.

119. H. Kutt, W. Winters, R. Kokenge, and F. McDowell, Diphenylhydantoin metabolism, blood levels, and toxicity. *Arch. Neurol. 11:*642–648, 1964.

120. B. J. Wilder, R. A. Buchanan, and E. E. Serrano, Correlation of acute diphenylhydantoin intoxication with plasma levels and metabolite excretion. *Neurology 23:*1329–1332, 1973.

121. M. J. Eadie and J. H. Tyrer, The therapeutic range of plasma anticonvulsant levels. *La Clinica Therapeutica 83:*121-133, 1977.

122. E. H. Reynolds and R. D. Travers, Serum anticonvulsant concentrations in epileptic patients with mental symptoms: A preliminary report. *Brit. J. Psychiatry 124:*440-445, 1974.

123. J. C. Kooiker and S. M. Sumi, Movement disorder as a manifestation of diphenylhydantoin intoxication. *Neurology 24:*68-71, 1974.

124. D. L. McLellan and M. Swash, Choreo-athetosis and encephalopathy induced by phenytoin. *Brit. Med. J. 2:*204-205, 1974.
125. S. Ahmad, J. Laidlaw, G. W. Houghton, and A. Richens, Involuntary movements caused by phenytoin intoxication in epileptic patients. *J. Neurol. Neurosurg. Psychiatry 38:*225-231, 1975.
126. R. H. Spector, R. A. Davidoff, and R. J. Schwartzman, Phenytoin-induced ophthalmoplegia. *Neurology 26:*1031-1034, 1976.
127. B. H. Dobkin, Reversible subacute peripheral neuropathy induced by phenytoin. *Arch. Neurol. 34:*189-190, 1977.
128. E. Birket-Smith and E. Krogh, Motor nerve conduction velocity during diphenylhydantoin intoxication. *Acta Neurol. Scand. 47:*265-271, 1971.
129. S. Chokroverty and F. A. Rubino, Motor nerve conduction study in patients on long term diphenylhydantoin therapy: Correlation with clinical states and serum levels of diphenylhydantoin, folate, and cyanocobalamine. *Electromyography Clin. Neurophysiol. 13:*139-140, 1973.
130. S. Chokroverty and Z. A. Sayeed, Motor nerve conduction study in patients on diphenylhydantoin therapy. *J. Neurol. Neurosurg. Psychiatry 38:*1235-1239, 1975.
131. M. Direkze and P. S. L. Fernanco, Transient anterior horn cell dysfunction in diphenylhydantoin therapy. *Eur. Neurol. 15:*131-134, 1977.
132. R. N. Kapur, S. Girgis, T. M. Little, and R. E. Masotti, Diphenylhydantoin-induced gingival hyperplasia: Its relationship to dose and serum level. *Develop. Med. Child, Neurol. 15:*483-487, 1973.
133. G. J. Conard, H. Jeffay, L. Boshes, and A. D. Steinberg, Levels of 5,5-diphenylhydantoin and its major metabolite in human serum, saliva, and hyperplastic gingiva. *J. Dent. Res. 53:*1323-1329, 1974.
134. T. M. Little, S. S. Girgis, and R. E. Masotti, Diphenylhydantoin induced gingival hyperplasia: Its response to changes in drug dosage. *Develop. Med. Child, Neurol. 17:*421-424, 1975.
135. R. B. Aird and D. M. Woodbury, *The Management of Epilepsy.* Springfield, Ill., Charles C. Thomas, 1974.
136. A. S. Troupin, L. M. Ojemann, and C. B. Dodrill, Mephenytoin: A reappraisal. *Epilepsia 17:*403-414, 1976.
137. F. Buchthal, O. Svensmark, and H. Simonsen, Relation of EEG and seizures to phenobarbital in serum. *Arch. Neurol. 19:*567-572, 1968.
138. O. Faero, K. W. Kastrup, E. Lykkegaard Nielsen, J. C. Melchior, and I. Thorn, Successful prophylaxis of febrile convulsions with phenobarbital. *Epilepsia 13:*279-285, 1972.
139. I. Thorn, A controlled study of prophylactic long-term treatment of febrile convulsions with phenobarbital. *Acta Neurol. Scand., Suppl. 60:* 67-73, 1975.
140. J. Z. Heckmatt, A. B. Houston, D. J. Clow, J. B. P. Stephenson, K. L. Dodd, G. T. Lealman, and R. W. Logan, Failure of phenobarbitone to prevent febrile convulsions. *Brit. Med. J. 1:*539-561, 1976.
141. C. E. Pippenger and T. S. Rosen, Phenobarbital plasma levels in neonates. *Clinics in Perinatology 2:*111-115, 1975.

142. J. Møller, *SerumKoncentrationsbestämningar av Karbamazepin inom baruneurologin in PlasmaKoncentrations bestämningar av Antiepileptika: Metodologiska och Kliniska Aspekter.* Lidingö, 1971, pp. 72-79.
143. F. Monaco, A. Riccio, P. Benna, A. Covacich, L. Durelli, M. Fantini, P. M. Furlan, M. Gilli, R. Mutani, W. Troni, M. Gerna, and P. L. Morselli, Further observations on carbamazepine plasma levels in epileptic patients. *Neurology 26:*936-943, 1976.
144. N. Simonsen, P. Z. Olsen, V. Kühl, M. Lund, and J. Wendelboe, A double blind study of carbamazepine and diphenylhydantoin in temporal lobe epilepsy. *Acta Neurol. Scand., Suppl. 60:*39-42, 1975.
145. R. J. Perchalski and B. J. Wilder, Rapid gas-liquid chromatographic determination of carbamazepine in plasma. *Clin. Chem. 20:*492-493, 1974.
146. H. Schneider, Carbamazepine: An attempt to correlate serum levels with anti-epileptic and side effects. In *Clinical Pharmacology of Antiepileptic Drugs* (H. Schneider, D. Janz, C. Gardner-Thorpe, H. Meinardi, and A. L. Sherwin, eds.). Berlin, Springer, 1975, pp. 151-158.
147. M. Dam, A. Jensen, and J. Christiansen, Plasma level and effect of carbamazepine in grand mal and psychomotor epilepsy. *Acta Neurol. Scand., Suppl. 60:*33-38, 1975.
148. A. Frigerio and P. L. Morselli, Carbamazepine: Biotransformation. In *Advances in Neurology,* vol. 11 (J. K. Penry, ed.). New York, Raven Press, 1975, pp. 295-307.
149. H. Meinardi, Other antiepileptic drugs: Carbamazepine. In *Antiepileptic Drugs* (D. M. Woodbury, J. K. Penry, and R. P. Schmidt, eds.). New York, Raven Press, 1972, pp. 487-496.
150. J. K. Penry, R. J. Porter, and F. E. Dreifuss, Ethosuximide: Relation of plasma levels to clinical control. In *Antiepileptic Drugs* (D. M. Woodbury, J. K. Penry, and R. P. Schmidt, eds.). New York, Raven Press, 1972, pp. 431-441.
151. T. R. Browne, F. E. Dreifuss, P. R. Dyken, D. J. Goode, J. K. Penry, R. J. Porter, B. G. White, and P. T. White, Ethosuximide in the treatment of absence (petit mal) seizures. *Neurology 25:*515-524, 1975.
152. B. N. Jensen, Trimethadione in the serum of patients with petit mal. *Dan. Med. Bull. 9:*74-79, 1962.
153. H. R. Chamberlin, W. J. Waddell, and T. C. Butler, A study of the product of demethylation of Tridione in the control of petit mal epilepsy. *Neurology 15:*449-454, 1965.
154. H. E. Booker and G. G. Celesia, Serum concentrations of diazepam in subjects with epilepsy. *Arch. Neurol. 29:*191-194, 1973.
155. M. Fink, P. Irwin, R. E. Weinfeld, M. A. Schwartz, and A. H. Conney, Blood levels and electroencephalographic effects of diazepam and bromazepam. *Clin. Pharmacol. Ther. 20:*184-191, 1975.
156. H. H. Dasberg, E. van der Kleijn, P. J. M. Guelen, and H. M. van Praag, Plasma concentrations of diazepam and of its metabolite N-desmethyldiazepam in relation to anxiolytic effect. *Clin. Pharmacol. Ther. 15:*473-483, 1974.

157. A. J. Bond, D. M. Hailey, and M. H. Lader, Plasma concentrations of benzodiazepines. *Brit. J. Clin. Pharmacol. 4:*51-56, 1977.
158. C. Y. Huang, J. G. McLeod, D. Sampson, and W. J. Hensley, Clonazepam in the treatment of epilepsy. *Proc. Aust. Assoc. Neurol. 10:*67-74, 1973.
159. C. Y. Huang, J. G. McLeod, D. Sampson, and W. J. Hensley, Clonazepam in the treatment of epilepsy. *Med. J. Aust. 2:*5-8, 1974.
160. F. E. Dreifuss, J. K. Penry, S. W. Rose, H. J. Kupferberg, P. Dyken, and S. Sato, Serum clonazepam concentrations in children with absence seizures. *Neurology 25:*255-258, 1975.
161. J. Naestoft, M. Lund, N. E. Larsen, and E. Hvidberg, Assay and pharmacokinetics of clonazepam in humans. *Acta Neurol. Scand. 49:*103-108, 1973.
162. E. F. Hvidberg and O. Sjo, Clinical pharmacokinetic experiences with clonazepam. In *Clinical Pharmacology of Antiepileptic Drugs* (H. Schneider, D. Janz, C. Gardner-Thorpe, H. Meinardi, and A. L. Sherwin, eds.). Berlin, Springer, 1975, pp. 242-246.
163. F. Vajda, P. Morris, O. Dummer, and P. Bladin, Studies on sodium valproate, a new anticonvulsant. In *Clinical and Pharmacological Aspects of Sodium Valproate (Epilim) in the Treatment of Epilepsy.* (N. J. Legg, ed.). Turnbridge Wells, MCS Consultants, 1976, pp. 92-100.
164. H. Meinardi, Discussion. In *Clinical and Pharmacological Aspects of Sodium Valproate (Epilim) in the Treatment of Epilepsy.* (N. J. Legg, ed.). Turnbridge Wells, MCS Consultants, 1976, p. 48.

16

Clinical Use of Plasma Concentrations of Psychotherapeutic Drugs
An Overview

Leo E. Hollister / *Psychopharmacology Research, Veterans Administration Hospital, and Department of Psychiatry and Pharmacology, Stanford University School of Medicine, Palo Alto, California, United States*

I. INTRODUCTION

Since the early 1970s advances in chemical technology have made it easier to measure plasma concentrations of drugs. The idea of monitoring treatment by use of plasma concentrations is not especially new. In psychiatry, it was possible to monitor plasma concentrations of bromide early in this century, but due to the peculiar distribution of this ion in the body, plasma concentrations were not the best guide. Use of plasma concentrations to monitor treatment really caught the imagination of clinicians during the 1940s, when it became clear that plasma concentrations of sulfonamides were quite pertinent both to obtaining cure of infection and for avoiding some of the unwanted effects. Since then, it has become possible to monitor plasma concentrations of an increasing array of drugs. Sometimes such monitoring has proven to be vital to effective clinical use, as in the case of anticonvulsant and antiarrhythmic drugs. At present, it is technically possible to measure plasma concentrations of almost all psychotherapeutic drugs. The major questions we must answer is when such measurements should be done and what we may expect from them.

II. TECHNICAL ASPECTS OF MEASUREMENT

The various methods for measuring plasma concentrations of psychoactive drugs have been well summarized in Chaps. 2 and 3. The problems may stem not from a dearth of methods but from their abundance. It is still difficult to know which method is preferred, either from the viewpoint of accuracy, or reproducibility, or economic feasibility. Different methods yield different results, so that reported values for thioridazine concentrations, for instance, have varied by as much as two orders of magnitude.

Most of the literature pertaining to plasma concentrations of psychotherapeutic drugs (with the exception of lithium ion) has appeared in the past few years. With each new technical advance the inadequacies of previous techniques became clearly evident. Consequently, many studies have been contradictory, although this problem is diminishing.

Gas-liquid chromatography (GLC) is the most widely used technique at the moment. Various detection systems, including flame ionization, microcoulometry, or electron capture, have their various proponents [1]. During the past few years, the development of sensitive and reliable nitrogen-phosphorus detectors has been a major advance, eliminating the requirement of derivatization for many drugs. Reports are still too few, using this detector, to determine whether the values reported previously using derivatization techniques will be changed.

Mass spectrometry combined with GLC (GLC-MS) is regarded by many as the most accurate of all existing techniques [2,3]. It is, however, both expensive and complex, so that it is not widely used. As these instruments become both cheaper and more reliable, which is highly likely, it may become the preferred technique.

Radioimmunoassay for measuring psychotherapeutic drugs is technically feasible. The problems associated with its use are in developing specific antigens to both the drug and its active metabolites. Separate testing must be done for parent drug and active metabolites, when these are present.

A new method based on radioreceptor assay has been used to measure neuroleptics [4]. This method does not measure plasma concentrations of drug per se, but rather measures the degree of competitive binding to brain dopamine receptors in the plasma. Values are expressed against a standard of binding for chlorpromazine, as "chlorpromazine equivalents." The attraction of this method is that it can measure total antipsychotic activity when a patient is on a mixture of antipsychotic drugs and that it uses a biological end point, receptor binding, rather than a chemical determination. In a sense, it might be compared with the use of prothrombin times to measure anticoagulant activity of coumarin derivatives rather than actual plasma concentrations of warfarin. Time will tell whether or not this technique will be preferred over direct chemical measurement.

Other techniques which have more or less languished have used fluorescence, spectrophotometry, thin-layer chromatography, and radioderivation. Each of these has major drawbacks which makes it likely that they will not find much future use.

Thus, we seem to be on the threshold of a technology that would allow the measurement of plasma concentrations of most psychotherapeutic drugs as a routine laboratory procedure. It will not always be easy, as anyone who has tried to establish such techniques in their own laboratory well knows. Accuracy is essential, for bad data are worse than none. Furthermore, such determinations will not come cheaply at a time when the costs of medical care are of urgent concern.

III. NONTECHNICAL ASPECTS OF MEASUREMENT

Some psychotherapeutic drugs have extremely complicated pharmacokinetic properties that make interpretation of plasma concentrations difficult. Antipsychotic drugs have a low and variable bioavailability when taken by mouth, the usual form of dosage. They also have a high and variable degree of protein binding in plasma. When such is the case, minor shifts in protein binding may have major consequences in the amount of available pharmacologically active drug, even when plasma levels are unchanged. Both protein binding and high lipid solubility lead to marked sequestration of drug in tissues, the consequences of which are not fully known. Accordingly, the volume of distribution of these drugs is large and highly variable. Plasma disappearance rates are biphasic and highly variable. The relatively short plasma $T_{1/2}$ of these drugs belies their prolonged clinical effects and is often an inadequate indicator of them [5]. One can readily appreciate that a simple plasma concentration is difficult to interpret under such circumstances.

The tricyclic antidepressants and benzodiazepines share many of the same kinetic properties as the antipsychotics, which creates equal difficulty in assessing the meaning of plasma concentrations. In addition, some of them form active metabolites, whose kinetic properties may differ from those of the parent drug and whose pharmacologic attributes may also be different.

Little wonder, then, that lithium is such a delightful exception. It is a simple ion which is virtually totally available when taken by mouth. It is neither protein bound nor lipid soluble, but is distributed mainly in the body water. It undergoes no metabolism and is excreted almost entirely through the kidney. One can easily appreciate that the value of measurement of plasma concentrations of lithium can not be automatically extrapolated to the other classes of drugs. (See Chap. 2 for a review of lithium measurements.)

IV. ANTIPSYCHOTIC DRUGS

No one has yet reported on clinical experience with routine monitoring of antipsychotic drugs for the treatment of schizophrenic patients. All of the studies have been experimental and have been limited to a few drugs. Most data are available on chlorpromazine and thioridazine, not only because they are among the older drugs but also because they are given in relatively high doses. This is unfortunate, as both of these drugs have serious limitations as compared with presently available drugs. Chapters 8 and 10 by Drs. Curry and Crammer have well reviewed the literature regarding these two drugs.

Two studies show a weak relationship between plasma concentrations of chlorpromazine and clinical effects. In one, virtually no therapeutic effects were seen with concentrations below 30 ng/ml, while toxic effects were seen with very high levels, such as 750-1,000 ng/ml [6]. A therapeutic range of 150 to 300 ng/ml was suggested. In another study, the antipsychotic effect was significantly related to plasma concentrations after 2 weeks of treatment, but not after 4 weeks. As it is highly unlikely that 2 weeks of treatment would be adequate for a schizophrenic, the failure to maintain a relationship between clinical efficacy and plasma levels is somewhat disturbing. Although a level of 40 ng/ml was deemed to be the lowest consonant with a therapeutic effect, only 6 of the 30 patients in this study reached that level (none exceeded 80 ng/ml) despite doses as high as 600 mg daily of chlorpromazine over a 4-week period [7]. In contrast to these positive studies, the majority of attempts to relate plasma concentrations to clinical therapeutic action have failed [8].

Plasma concentrations reported for thioridazine have been much higher, usually over 1,000 ng/ml and often as high as 5,000 ng/ml after treatment with usual therapeutic doses. One study which used a fluorimetric method of determination found a relationship between improvement in schizophrenics and plasma concentrations 2 days after a single dose of the drug [9]. The implications of such a finding, which is totally unrelated to what might be the normal case during treatment, are uncertain.

New data on haloperidol are accumulating at a rapid rate. Most studies, as reported in Chap. 11 by Dr. Evans, have related plasma concentrations to dose, not to therapeutic response. A number of studies still unpublished suggest that the therapeutic range of plasma concentrations may be between 10 and 30 ng/ml. However, many patients are treated with very high doses of the drug and attain much higher plasma concentrations, with no clear evidence that these high plasma concentrations impede progress. What we don't know at the moment is when the plasma concentration/clinical response curve begins to flatten.

As pointed out in Chap 9 by Drs. Sakalis and Traficante, measurement of plasma concentrations of fluphenazine has been exceedingly difficult. The levels attained after usual therapeutic doses of the drug are quite small, sometimes less than 1 ng/ml. Very large doses of the drug may provide levels of from 20 to 30 ng/ml, but the use of such large doses is still controversial. In any case, it is safe to say that at the moment no one has been able to define a range of therapeutic plasma concentrations of this drug. Perhaps more to the point, the release characteristics of the fatty acid ester preparations of the drug, such as fluphenazine decanoate and enanthate, have not been defined, nor the ratio of dose between these preparations and either oral or parenteral doses of fluphenazine hydrochloride.

Data concerning other antipsychotic drugs are only fragmentary; no range of effective plasma concentrations has been proposed yet for any. One study of butaperazine reported plasma concentrations of around 300 ng/ml following 40-mg doses [10]. Another reported plasma concentrations of 18,000 to 27,000 ng/ml following the same dose [11]. Different techniques give different answers, which vary by as much as two orders of magnitude.

In summary, with the exception of weak evidence of a possible relationship between plasma concentrations of chlorpromazine and therapeutic outcome, it has been impossible to define such a relationship with any other antipsychotic drug. Current practice is not to monitor plasma concentrations of these drugs, which seems to be reasonable in view of the uncertainties.

V. TRICYCLIC ANTIDEPRESSANTS

More work has related plasma concentrations of tricyclics to clinical effects than for any other psychotherapeutic drug, excepting lithium. Reports have been mixed, but enough have found a relationship to indicate that it may exist. Most compelling has been the idea that below certain plasma concentrations of drug clinical response may either be poor or suboptimal. Much of this work as well as the pharmacokinetics of these drugs has been thoroughly reviewed in Chap. 4 by Dr. Gram.

Largely for technical reasons, most measurement of plasma concentrations involve secondary amines, such as nortriptyline and desipramine, although these drugs are less often used than their tertiary amine precursors amitriptyline and imipramine. Patients with endogenous depression who were treated with nortriptyline responded best when steady-state plasma concentrations were in the range 50-139 ng/ml. At higher or lower doses, responses were poorer, suggesting an inverted U-shaped relationship between plasma concentrations and clinical response [12]. This range of therapeutic plasma concentrations was confirmed by a later study that also confirmed the adverse effects of high concentrations (140-260 ng/ml) or nortriptyline [13]. A number of studies have failed to find such a relationship between plasma concentrations of nortriptyline and therapeutic results, but unlike the positive studies, they have not used exclusively patients with endogenous depressions. As endogenous depression is the only type for which specific antidepressant efficacy of tricyclics is claimed, choice of patients is crucial.

When one measures the tertiary amine tricyclics in plasma, one must account both for the parent compounds as well as for the active demethylated metabolites. After 4 weeks of treatment with 150 mg/day of amitriptyline, a good correlation was found between plasma concentration and clinical response. Levels of combined amitriptyline/nortriptyline of less than 120 ng/ml were associated with poor clinical results [14]. These findings were subsequently confirmed by the observation that patients with a combined concentration of 95 ng/ml fared better than those whose levels were lower; improvement continued in a linear fashion as levels reached 250 ng/ml [15]. The inverted U-shaped curve of response does not seem to hold for amitriptyline as it does for nortriptyline; it is more linear.

A linear response was also found for imipramine over a range of 50-1050 ng/ml, with the exception of delusional patients [16]. A somewhat higher critical level of response was found for imipramine in a later study. All patients treated with imipramine with plasma levels of imipramine greater than 45 ng/ml and desipramine greater than 75 ng/ml did well; most of those who responded well had combined levels of drugs above 240 ng/ml, while all failures were below this level [17]. Steady-state levels greater than 70 ng/ml of protriptyline produced better outcomes than those patients who had lower levels. As with the other tertiary amines, the relationship was linear up to levels of 167 ng/ml [18].

From these data one might assume that determinations of plasma concentrations of tricyclics might be indicated for patients who have received what appears to be an adequate dose (at least 150 mg/day) but who have not shown the expected improvement. A level below those regarded as critical would mandate increased doses. Curiously enough, it has been suggested that plasma concentrations of nortriptyline should be monitored to avoid overtreating patients. Of 36 patients treated with an average daily dose of 100 mg of nortriptyline, 22 had values over the ceiling of 150 ng/ml (many well over 250 ng/ml) and had responded poorly. Only 2 patients showed confusional states and no other major side effects were noted, so that one may have some doubts about the accuracy of the method, which was not specified. However, it was suggested that the increased age of the patients might be the cause for the high levels [19]. This suggestion is reasonable, as elderly patients show a decreased rate of elimination of imipramine and amitriptyline from plasma [20].

Our experience with monitoring plasma concentrations of tricyclics in a free-rein clinical situation was illuminating [21]. Noncompliance in taking medication was suspected at one time or another in 19 patients, due to unusually low plasma concentrations in relation to the presumed dose. Attempts to correlate plasma concentrations with clinical response to amitriptyline and nortriptyline failed, probably because of the heterogeneity of the depressive syndromes being treated. Plasma concentrations were correlated highly with dose in the case of amitriptyline, less so with other drugs. Amitriptyline and imipramine generally produced plasma concentrations of the parent drug and secondary amine metabolite that were higher in ng/ml than the dose in mg/day; nortriptyline and desipramine did the opposite. Conversion of amitriptyline and imipramine to their secondary amine metabolites was variable between patients and within individual patients. Contrary to widely held belief, most patients were found to have plasma concentrations within the presumed therapeutic range for the various drugs being tested, even though the concentrations may not have been optimal. We concluded that monitoring plasma concentrations of tricyclics was of value only in specially selected situations but could not be justified as a routine procedure.

A World Health Organization collaborative study of the value of monitoring amitriptyline plasma levels came to the same conclusion. In this study, patients were carefully selected to represent only those with endogenous depression, the type most likely to respond specifically to this drug. This multiclinic trial in five centers studied 54 of these carefully selected patients. No important correlations were found between steady-state plasma levels and therapeutic outcome or corrected side effects [22].

In summary, evidence to date strongly suggests that in patients with endogenous depression, clinical response is correlated with plasma concentrations of drug. The difference in pattern between nortriptyline, on the one hand, and amitriptyline and imipramine, on the other, is not yet clear. Virtually no relationship can be shown between clinical response and plasma concentrations in patients with other types of depression. Determination of plasma concentration might be of value in detecting or confirming occasional patients who fail to comply or in deciding whether or not an increase in dose is warranted due to inadequate or suboptimal dosage. Another use of such determinations would be to explain unwanted effects that are not clearly those due to drug. Arguments for routine monitoring of plasma concentrations are not compelling.

VI. LITHIUM

Monitoring plasma concentrations of lithium is such established practice that it is difficult to imagine using the drug without it. Unlike most of those previously discussed, lithium has a remarkably low therapeutic margin. Symptoms and signs that may occur from therapeutic doses merge with those that herald toxicity. Clinical guides to toxicity are not adequate. The role of monitoring plasma levels of lithium has been reviewed extensively in Chap. 7 by Drs. Annitto and Gershon.

The usual plasma concentrations of lithium sought for therapeutic purposes are from 0.9 to 1.4 meq/liter, and for maintenance purposes 0.6 to 1.0 meq/liter. It should be emphasized that these concentrations are not absolute. If a patient does well at lower concentrations, rejoice. On the other hand, if an unresponsive patient has no remarkable toxic effects even though the plasma concentration is at the upper end ot this range, one might feel free to increase the dose. Finally, if a patient has clearly toxic symptoms, the dose should be reduced no matter what the plasma concentration may be. Laboratory tests are not meant to supplant good clinical judgment.

The values quoted are nadir values in the postabsorptive state, meaning the blood samples should be taken approximately 12 h after the last dose. If samples are drawn too close to the last dose, values may be factitiously high.

Measurement of erythrocyte concentrations of lithium have not been widely adopted. Initially, these concentrations were assumed to correlate better with clinical response than those from plasma, but proof of that assumption has been lacking. Past experience has shown that plasma concentrations are adequate for most purposes. Lithium concentrations in saliva can be measured, but no doubt most clinicians would prefer to use the more rapidly available blood.

In summary, monitoring lithium concentrations is well established as an integral part of clinical practice. The danger is that too much faith may be placed on their value to the neglect of good clinical observation.

VII. ANTIANXIETY-HYPNOTIC DRUGS

For practical purposes, antianxiety-hypnotic drugs as a class are subsumed by the benzodiazepines. Measurements of plasma concentrations of these drugs have been directed at elucidating their kinetics in man, never for monitoring treatment. As treatment both of anxiety and insomnia is purely symptomatic, and the complaints are largely subjective, one could scarcely tell an anxious patient that she should feel better because her plasma concentrations of diazepam were in the therapeutic range. Further, measurement of anxiety has really not been good enough to make fine correlations between plasma concentrations and clinical effects, even if they were desirable. One can measure sedation more accurately, plasma levels correlating well with this effect. One would scarcely want to measure the plasma concentrations of hypnotics during the night when the desired effects occur.

As pointed out in Chap. 14 by Dr. Wade, plasma concentrations of sedative-hypnotic drugs are usually of little help in assessing the severity of overdoses of these drugs. He correctly points out that many of these determinations are done hastily by laboratories that may not be highly experienced or not set up to do them on a regular basis. The pernicious practice of reporting results in "parts per million" still holds for many of these forensic laboratories, at least in the United States.

VIII. ANTICONVULSANTS

Monitoring of phenytoin began in the 1960s and was of such great clinical utility that techniques were rapidly developed so that now virtually all anticonvulsants can be monitored. Dr. Eadie has reviewed the present status of monitoring anticonvulsants in Chap. 15. His comment regarding the interpretation of the results of such laboratory determinations applies not only to anticonvulsants but also to all of those we have been discussing: "The patient's clinical state should always be the final criterion in management, and measurement of plasma . . . levels should be seen only as a means to an end." With better monitoring of phenytoin plasma concentrations, it became increasingly evident that some clinical failures which led to coadministration of another anticonvulsant were really due to inadequate doses of phenytoin. Thus, the tendency has been to use single-drug treatment whenever possible. It is rather remarkable that this drug, now 40 years into clinical practice, should remain so preeminent.

Monitoring plasma concentrations of anticonvulsants that either have a low therapeutic margin, such as phenytoin and carbamazepine, or which provide indefinite signs of clinical toxicity, such as ethosuximide, may be warranted. On the other hand, drugs which show objective clinical signs indicating their effects, such as drowsiness associated with phenobarbital, primidone, or clonazepam, scarcely need close monitoring.

Despite the long period in which it has been possible to measure plasma concentrations of anticonvulsants, tests of reliability between various laboratories purporting to measure concentrations of these drugs in plasma have been far from encouraging. Thus, such tests should not always be the sole basis for changing treatment unless they have been confirmed or unless there is a good clinical reason for making a change.

IX. CONCLUSIONS

The ability to monitor plasma concentrations of various psychotherapeutic drugs represents one of the great technological advances in chemical methodology. Like all technologies, the question might be raised: Just because something is possible, need it be done? There is little doubt that monitoring plasma levels of lithium and of anticonvulsants has made such treatment both safer and more effective. Monitoring plasma concentrations of tricyclic antidepressants will probably prove to be valuable, but largely for special patients or for special situations. Arguments for monitoring plasma concentrations of antipsychotic drugs are weak, but the evidence one way or another is still fragmentary. There seems to be no good reason for monitoring levels of antianxiety or hypnotic drugs, which generally have a large margin of safety and suitable clinical criteria of response.

REFERENCES

1. E. Usdin, The assay of chlorpromazine and metabolites in blood, urine, and other tissues. *CRC Crit. Rev. Clin. Lab. Sci. 2:*347-391, 1971.
2. D. C. Hobbs, W. M. Welch, M. J. Short, W. A. Moody, and C. D. Van der Velde, Pharmacokinetics of thiothixene in man. *Clin. Pharmacol. Ther. 16:*473-478, 1974.
3. J. T. Biggs, W. H. Holland, S. Chang, P. P. Hipps, and W. R. Sherman, Electron beam ionization mass fragmentographic analysis of tricyclic antidepressants in human plasma. *J. Pharmaceut. Sci. 65:*261-268, 1976.
4. I. Creese and S. H. Snyder, A simple and sensitive radioreceptor assay for antischizophrenic drugs in blood. *Nature 270:*180-182, 1977.
5. L. E. Hollister, Psychiatric disorders. In *Drug Therapy: Principles and Practice of Clinical Pharmacology and Therapeutics* (G. S. Avery, ed.). Sydney, ADIS Press, 1976, pp. 796-844.

6. L. Rivera-Calimlim, L. Castaneda, and L. Lasagna, Effects of mode of management on plasma chlorpromazine in psychiatric patients. *Clin. Pharmacol. Ther. 14:*978-986, 1973.
7. B. Wode-Helgodt, S. Borg, B. Fyrö, and G. Sedvall, Clinical effects and drug concentrations in plasma and cerebrospinal fluid in psychotic patients treated with fixed doses of chlorpromazine. *Acta Psychiatr. Scand. 58:* 149-173, 1978.
8. J. Kane, A. Rifkin, F. Quitkin, and D. F. Klein, Antipsychotic drug blood levels and clinical outcome. In *Progress in Psychiatric Drug Treatment* (D. F. Klein and R. Gittelman-Klein, eds.). New York, Brunner/Mazel, 1976, pp. 399-408.
9. L. A. Gottschalk, R. Biener, E. P. Noble, H. Birch, D. E. Wilbert, and J. F. Heiser, Thioridazine plasma levels and clinical response. *Compr. Psychiatry 16:*323-337, 1975.
10. J. M. Davis, D. S. Janowsky, H. J. Sckerke, H. Manier, and M. El-Yousef, The pharmacokinetics of butaperazine in serum. In *Advances in Biochemical Psychopharmacology,* vol. 9: *Phenothiazines and Related Drugs* (I. S. Forrest, C. J. Carr, and E. Usdin, eds.). New York, Raven Press, 1974, pp. 457-461.
11. G. M. Simpson, R. Lament, T. B. Cooper, J. H. Lee, and R. B. Bruce, The relationship between blood levels of different forms of butaperazine and clinical response. *J. Clin. Pharmacol. 13:*288-299, 1973.
12. M. Asberg, B. Cronholm, F. Sjöqvist, and D. Tuck, Relationship between plasma level and therapeutic effect on nortriptyline. *Brit. Med. J. 3:*331, 1971.
13. V. E. Ziegler, P. A. Clayton, J. R. Taylor, B. T. Co, and J. T. Biggs, Nortriptyline plasma levels and therapeutic response. *Clin. Pharmacol. Ther. 20:*458-463, 1976.
14. R. A. Braithwaite, R. Goulding, G. Theano, J. Bailey, and A. Coppen, Plasma concentration of amitriptyline and clinical response. *Lancet 1:* 1297-1300, 1972.
15. V. E. Ziegler, B. T. Co, J. R. Tayloe, P. J. Clayton, and J. T. Biggs, Amitriptyline plasma levels and therapeutic response. *Clin. Pharmacol. Ther. 19:*795-801, 1976.
16. A. H. Glassman, J. M. Perel, M. Shostak, S. J. Kantor, and J. L. Fleiss, Clinical implications of imipramine plasma levels for depressive illness. *Arch. Gen. Psychiatry 34:*197-204, 1977.
17. N. Reisby, L. F. Gram, P. Bech, A. Nagy, G. O. Petersen, J. Ortmann, I. Ibsen, S. J. Dencker, O. Jacobsen, O. Drautwald, I. Sondergaard, and J. Christiansen, Imipramine: Clinical effects and pharmacokinetic variability. *Psychopharmacology 54:*263-272, 1977.
18. J. T. Biggs and V. E. Ziegler, Protriptyline plasma levels and antidepressant response. *Clin. Pharmacol. Ther. 22:*269-273, 1977.
19. S. A. Montgomery, R. A. Braithwaite, and J. L. Crammer, Routine nortriptyline levels on treatment of depression. *Brit. Med. J. 2:*166-167, 1977.

20. A. Nies, D. S. Robinson, M. J. Friedman, R. Green, T. B. Cooper, C. L. Ravaris, and J. O. Ives, Relationship between age and tricyclic antidepressant plasma levels. *Amer. J. Psychiatry 134:*7, 1977.
21. L. E. Hollister, Monitoring of tricyclic antidepressant plasma concentrations. *JAMA 241:*2530–2533, 1979.
22. A. Coppen, K. Ghose, S. Montgomery, V. A. Rama Rao, J. Christiansen, P. L. Mikkleson, H. M. van Praag, F. van de Poel, E. J. Minsker, V. G. Kozulja, N. Matussek, G. Kungkunz, and A. Jorgensen, Amitriptyline plasma-concentration and clinical effect. (A World Health Organization Collaborative Study.) *Lancet 1:*63–66, 1978.

Author Index

Numbers in brackets are reference numbers and indicate that an author's work is referred to although his name is not cited in the text. Italic numbers give the page on which the complete reference is listed.

A

F

H

I

K

L

Q

R

S

U

V

W

X

Y

Z

Subject Index

A

D

E

V

Y

Z